Shaped Beam Radiosurgery

Antonio A.F. De Salles
(Editor-in-Chief)

Alessandra A. Gorgulho • Nzhde Agazaryan
Ben Slotman • Michael Selch
(Co-Editors)

Aaron J. Burwick • Raymond A. Schulz
(Managing Editors)

Shaped Beam Radiosurgery

State of the Art

Springer

Editor-in-Chief
Antonio A.F. De Salles
Department of Neurosurgery
David Geffen School of Medicine at UCLA
10495 Le Conte Ave., Suite 2120
Los Angeles, CA 90095
USA
adesalles@mednet.ucla.edu

Co-Editors
Alessandra A. Gorgulho
Department of Neurosurgery
UCLA Medical Center
David Geffen School of Medicine at UCLA
300 UCLA Medical Plaza, Suite B212
Los Angeles, CA 90095
USA
a_gorgulho@yahoo.com

Nzhde Agazaryan
David Geffen School of Medicine at UCLA
200 UCLA Medical Plaza, Suite B265
Los Angeles, CA 90095
USA
nagazaryan@mednet.ucla.edu

Ben Slotman
Department of Radiation Oncology
VU University medical center
De Boelelaan 1117, 1081 HV, Amsterdam
The Netherlands
bj.slotman@vumc.nl

Michael Selch
Department of Radiation Oncology
David Geffen School of Medicine at UCLA
200 UCLA Medical Plaza, Suite B265
Los Angeles, CA 90095
USA
mselch@mednet.ucla.edu

Managing Editors
Aaron J. Burwick
Novalis Circle, Brainlab Inc.
3 Westbrook Corporate Center
Suite 400, Westchester, IL 60154
USA
aaron.burwick@brainlab.com

Raymond A. Schulz
Varian Medical Systems, Inc.
Varian Surgical Sciences
3100 Hansen Way
Palo Alto, CA 94304
USA
raymond.schulz@varian.com

ISBN 978-3-642-42823-4 ISBN 978-3-642-11151-8 (eBook)
DOI 10.1007/978-3-642-11151-8
Springer Heidelberg Dordrecht London New York

Cover design: eStudioCalamar, Figueres/Berlin

Printed on acid-free paper

Springer is part of Springer Science+Business Media (www.springer.com)

Foreword

In previous decades the notion of multidisciplinary care was embraced to bring increasingly complex treatment modalities safely and expeditiously to patients. Stereotactic radiosurgery is exemplary of such a mutual effort. In this regard, the paradigm of bringing together the neurosurgeon, radiation oncologist, diagnostic radiologist, and medical physicist into collaboration served the development of the medical science and our patients well.

We now enter an era of an enhanced and more sophisticated understanding of anatomy, molecular biology, radiation biology, genetics, and imaging science as it relates to stereotactic based radiation treatments. The technology we use has continued to improve in its flexibility, accuracy and precision giving us the ability to maximize therapeutic benefit while minimizing morbidity. This progress, however, comes with concomitant increase in complexity of structure and process.

Stereotactic radiation techniques such as stereotactic radiosurgery (SRS) and stereotactic body radiation therapy (SBRT) serve as a paradigm for breaking down the silos of traditional department-based medical disciplines by setting up integrated practice units for the benefit of the patient. We come together out of necessity to address the complexity of the processes. Barriers to this integration remain, but will continue to be addressed and overcome. The techniques developed by the collaboration now allow for the lessons learned from SRS in the brain to be applied to the spine, pancreas, prostate, kidney, and with motion management, to the lung and liver. The application of SRS and SBRT now abound in curative as well as palliative settings – and with new notions of the treatment of oligometastasis, it shows promise to convert heretofore incurable cancer into a chronic disease.

Even more exciting, the frontiers of research afford the possibility of using radiation in the SRS/SBRT context to manipulate signaling pathways of cancer cell growth and immune response (Danger Theory) for the benefit of the patient. Radiation biologists are developing a new understanding of the nuances of the radiation interaction with cancerous and normal tissues to achieve genetic changes that can be translated to enhance apoptosis, expedite healing, prevent excessive repair reaction of normal tissue, and even stimulate the production of neurotransmitters in cases of neurodegenerative diseases.

The chapters ahead review the progress made and set out possibilities for the future. The future of this complex discipline, stereotactic radiation, is indeed bright.

Los Angeles, CA, USA — Michael L. Steinberg

Contents

Part I

Basic Principles

Evolution of Stereotactic Radiosurgery 1

Antonio A.F. De Salles

1.1 Introduction

Four photon-energy radiosurgery devices have been competitive in the market due to their uniqueness and specific advantages over the other systems (see Chap. 2). In the near future, these systems will compete with the evolution of non-photon delivery systems, such as proton beam systems. Inexpensive proton beam systems have been on the radar for many years. Now, one such device still five times more expensive than the photon delivery systems is making its way into the market and may be successful due to potentially better dose distributions (Kjellberg et al. 1983). However, the intrinsic advantage of the proton beam with its Bragg peak delivery has yet to match the current developments of the photon beam exploitations, such as multiple beams (200+ gamma beams), continuous beam delivery with shaping and modulation (LINACs), 150+ non-isocentric nodes of the Cyberknife® (Accuray Inc, Sunnyvale, CA), or the tomographic capabilities of Tomotherapy® (TomoTherapy, Madison, WI). Systems combining all the predicates of these four systems are also likely to gain market share. An example is the VERO™ (Brainlab AG, Feldkirchen, Germany), already in use in Europe.

Little has improved on the generation of energy; what has improved is the capability of beam manipulation. This became possible with the integration of fast computer calculation of radiation dosimetry (see Chap. 5). It made possible the introduction of three-dimensional imaging to treatment planning, relaying this information to smart robotic machines capable of delivering intricate plans, including shaping and modulation of the radiation beam. As the advances of this field continue depending on the image capabilities, we will discuss the landmarks of imaging integration and speculate the impact of the imaging development in the future of stereotactic radiation.

A.A.F. De Salles
Department of Neurosurgery and Radiation Oncology,
David Geffen School of Medicine at UCLA,
10495 Le Conte Ave., Suite 2120, Los Angeles,
CA 90095, USA
e-mail: adesalles@mednet.ucla.edu

1.2 Three- and Four-Dimensional Imaging

Stereotactic radiosurgery was initiated with anteroposterior and lateral X-rays (Leksell 1951). These two projections were able to give precision to the stereotactic technique, allowing calculation of X, Y, and Z coordinates of a point inside of the stereotactic space. It also allowed calculation of the volume of an ellipsoid projection to the two 2D planes (Bova and Friedman 1991). This depended on collimator size to obtain the functional lesion desired, as envisioned by Leksell, which was then possible with the radiofrequency technique. Therefore, at the inception of radiosurgery, Leksell was trying to mimic a radiofrequency heat lesion for functional procedures in the brain. When radiosurgery started to be applied to ablate arteriovenous malformations, the need for better definition of the volume of radiation came into demand (Friedman and Bova 1989). Rough approximation of the lesion volume was then initially tried (De Salles et al. 1987), however the integration of computed tomography to treatment planning brought the revolution capable of tumor volume definition with the possibility to integrate the radiation delivery with the true lesion volume. This brought about

A.A.F. De Salles et al. (eds.), *Shaped Beam Radiosurgery*,
DOI: 10.1007/978-3-642-11151-8_1, © Springer-Verlag Berlin Heidelberg 2011

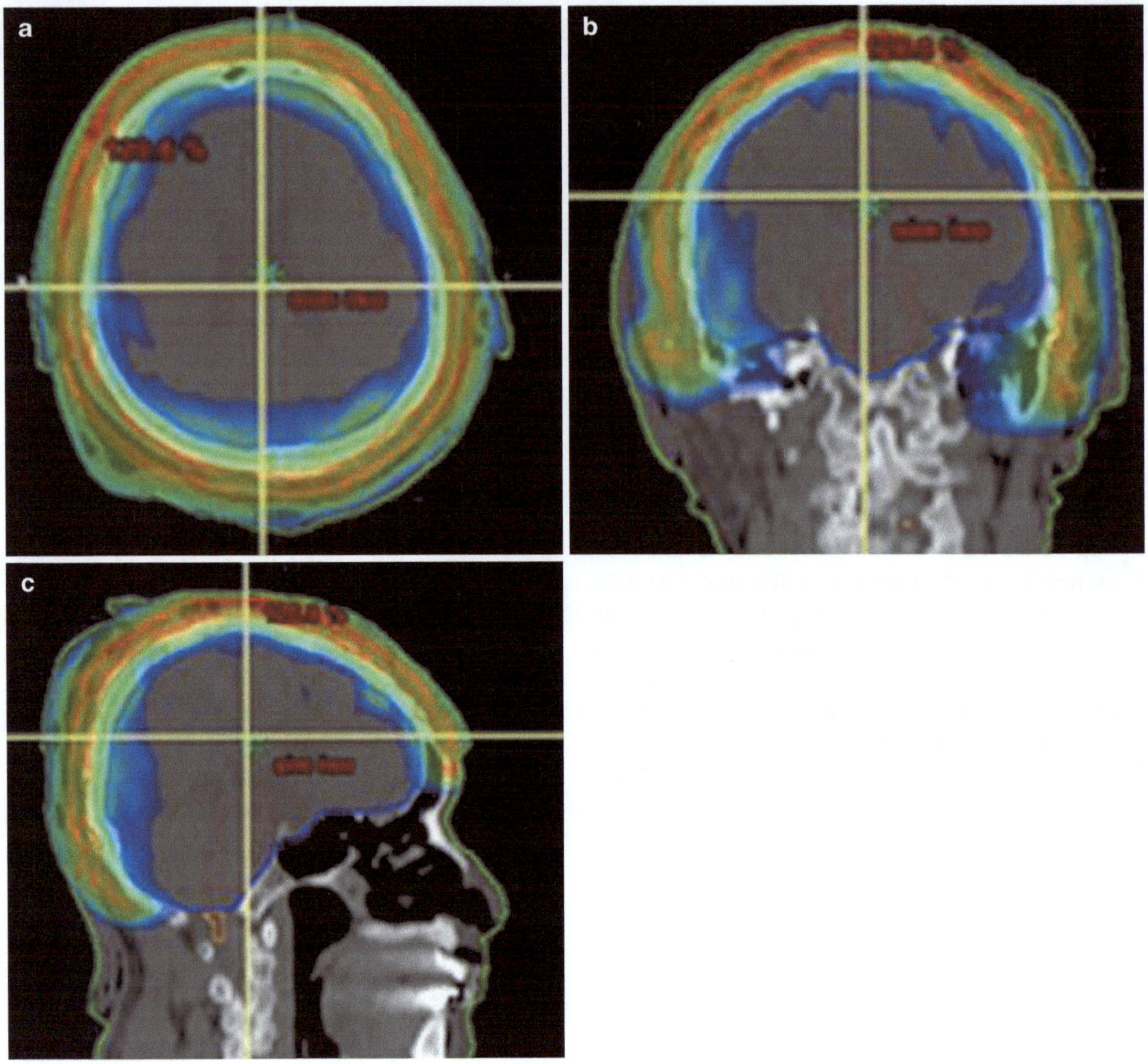

Fig. 1.1 Skull sarcoma planned with Rapid Arc. Axial (**a**), Coronal (**b**), and Sagittal (**c**)

the proposal of modulation of the radiation beam as the next step, allowing the treatment of previously difficult to treat pathologies (Fig. 1.1). Now the possibility of registering the movement of lesions for moving targets, such as those in the liver and lung, has brought into reality radiosurgery of lesions throughout the body, revolutionizing the field of radiation therapy with stereotactic body radiation therapy (SBRT) and demanding 4D treatment planning, competing with gated radiation delivery (see Chaps. 24–26).

1.3 Image Fusion

The desire to merge images of different modalities was initiated to bring the high definition of 3D visualization of lesions on magnetic resonance imaging (MRI) and computed tomography (CT) scans into the radiosurgery planning. This effort required the transport of the information obtained by MRI and CT into the stereotactic space (De Salles et al. 1987). The need to fuse images was further stimulated by the identification of distortions of the MRI, hampering the quality of the stereotactic calculations. Fusion of MRI and CT of the same patient allowed for the MRI distortions correction (Alexander et al. 1995), improving visualization of the lesions and still maintaining the stereotactic exquisite precision. This advance permitted the delivery of effective single dose of radiation to targets in the brain and now in the whole body (De Salles et al. 1997; De Salles et al. 2004).

1.4 Functional Image Integration

The integration of functional imaging into treatment planning, promises the improvement of stereotactic radiosurgery results. Advanced functional imaging such as functional MRI with fiber tracking can now be used in brain pathologies such as arteriovenous malformation (AVMs) (Hauptman et al. 2008), and implementation of molecular imaging such as metionine and fluorodopa scans, as well as with well-established fluoro-deoxy-glucose positron emission tomography (PET) are useful tools in treating tumors of the brain (Melega et al. 2010). This likely will lead to a new capability of preserving function from radiation damage and directing radiation to the functional portions of the pathology. Moreover, head and neck cancers and tumors in other locations can now be functionally localized and brought into the treatment planning by computed tomography fused to PET (CT-PET) fusion allowing for more specific delivery of radiation (Fig. 1.2).

1.5 Anatomical Integration

1.5.1 Atlas

Historical atlases have helped neurosurgeons integrate knowledge accumulated by electrophysiology and classic anatomy to advanced imaging techniques. The integration of three-dimensional imaging to historical atlases, pioneered by Talairach and Tournoux (1988), became commonplace in commercial software for neurosurgery. Now it is becoming commonplace for SBRT pioneered by Brainlab technology (see Chap. 3). These robust guidelines for planning

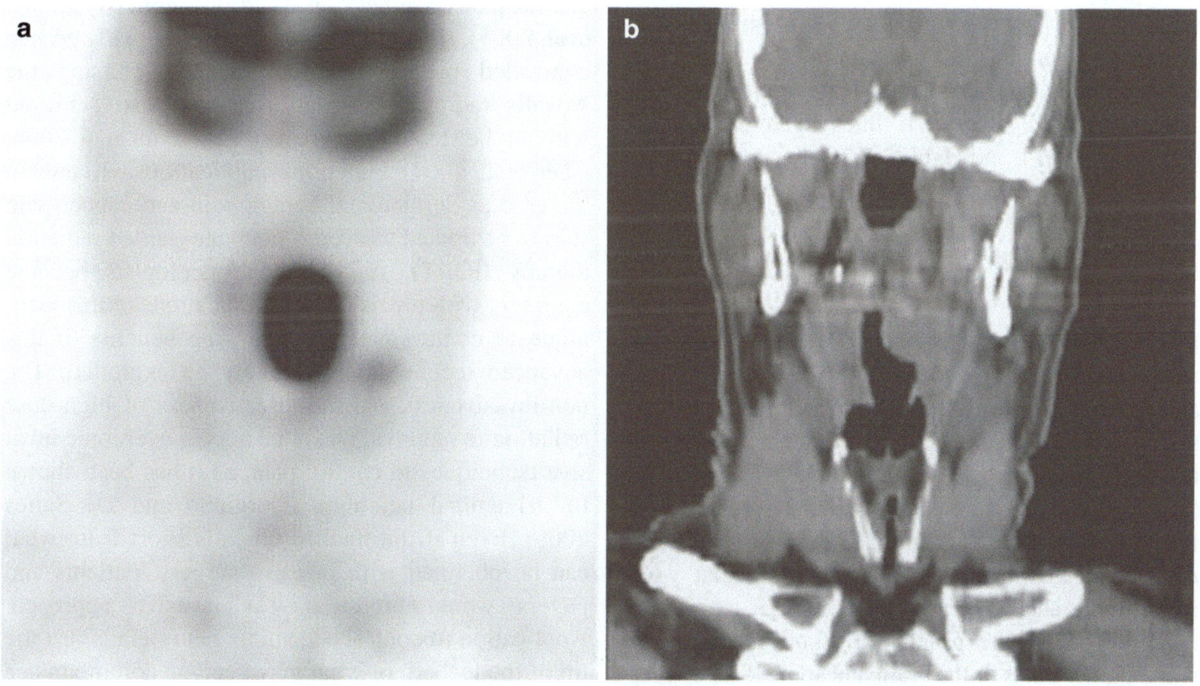

Fig. 1.2 CT fused to fluoro-deoxy-glucose PET (CT-FDG-PET) fusion for stereotactic planning of a head and neck tumor. Notice that the molecular image alone has poor anatomic definition (**a**), CT alone has poor lesion definition (**b**), merging both images it is possible to precisely localize the most active portion of the tumor to be treated (**c**)

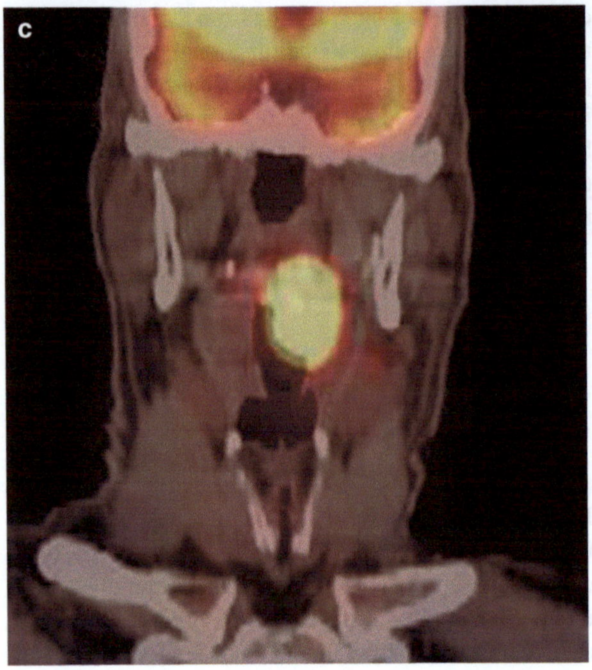

Fig. 1.2 (continued)

radiation delivery have expedited segmentation of structures to be avoided, thereby making this approach readily applicable in clinic without the need of tedious segmentation by a knowledgeable professional. This becomes important with techniques of inverse treatment planning such as intensity modulation radiation therapy (IMRT), volumetric intensity modulated arc therapy (VMAT), and Hybrid Arc delivery (Fig. 1.1).

1.5.2 Fiber Tracking

Imaging techniques have evolved beyond the ability of the practitioner to use them clinically. Fiber tracking and its integration with localization and treatment planning software is an example of such technical advance over clinical practice. While practitioners are still using almost exclusively anatomical visualization of lesions, fiber tracking could revolutionize dose distribution in neurological applications. Understanding that white matter tracts should be avoided from high exposure of radiation due to the paucity of blood supply to the white matter tracts in the brain and spine leads to preservation of important functional pathways. White matter tracts are served with one fourth of the blood supply available to the gray matter. As much of the permanent damage caused by radiation is secondary to vascular obstruction with ensuing ischemia, avoidance of large dose to these brain-sensitive portions can be achieved with integration of fiber tracking information in relation to lesion locations and functionality of the brain. This is now possible with currently available software used in Novalis® radiosurgery (Brainlab AG, Feldkirchen, Germany) treatment planning (Fig. 1.3).

1.6 Functional Applications

Accuracy and precision of linear accelerator radiosurgery has been well established by several groups (De Salles et al. 2001; Friedman and Bova 1992; Rahimian et al. 2004; Solberg et al. 2004). This application allows precise and accurate placement of high doses of radiation to specific regions of the brain and spine (Frighetto et al. 2004; De Salles and Medin 2009; Smith et al. 2003), even daring positioning of isocenters close to vital structures such as the brainstem (Gorgulho et al. 2006). Trigeminal neuralgia (De Salles et al. 1997), cluster headaches (De Salles et al. 2006), central pain (Frighetto et al. 2004), epilepsy (Selch et al. 2005), are all functional disorders already proven controlled by stereotactic radiosurgery using the Novalis radiosurgery platform, now also achieved without the stereotactic frame (Agazaryan et al. 2008; Chen et al. 2004). Functional applications will tend to increase as dermatomal benign pain and cancer pain start to be treated with current image-guided radiation therapy (IGRT). As radiation oncologists become confident with precision and applications of this technique to control patient's pain, the benefits of this advanced technology will likely be exploited. The non-invasiveness and the effectiveness of high-dose radiation to ganglia and spinal nerves overcome invasive techniques to control pain, as it has been shown for trigeminal neuralgia (Gorgulho and De Salles 2006). Even if the final result falls short from what can be obtained with invasive surgery, patients and payers would prefer a less invasive approach. Application to control trigeminal neuralgia is just the tip of the iceberg of what may become commonplace in cancer and benign pain control (See Chaps. 4, 17–20, 28). Manipulation of the radiation strength to achieve functional changes in the neural tissue is still

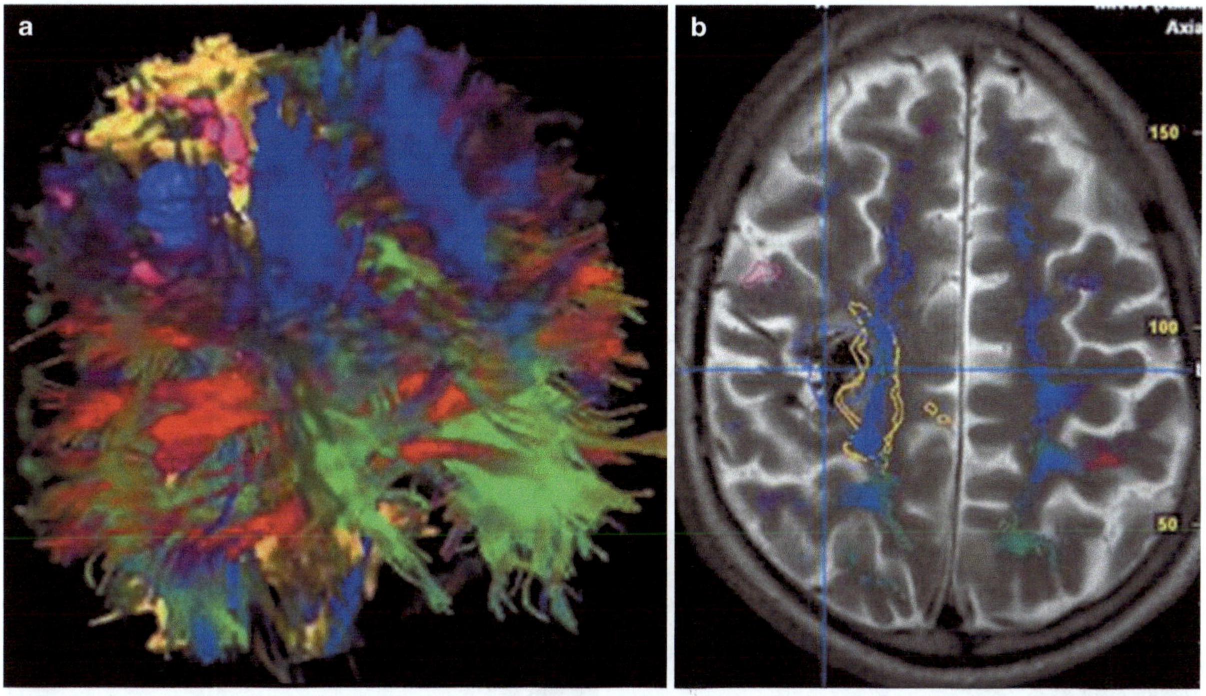

Fig. 1.3 The application of fiber tracking in radiosurgery is still at its infancy. The universe of fibers in the brain is depicted in (**a**). An AVM imbedded in the *right white* matter tracks and motor area is shown for planning centered in the *cross lines*. High dose should be avoided in the medial periphery of the AVM where the fibers are seen in *blue* (**b**)

an unexploited field. Radiation may modulate function of cells to profit the patient with functional disorders. An example is the experimental work showing that low dose of radiation, i.e., radiation in the penumbral zone of the high radiation beam, affect cells leading to over production of neurotransmitters and growth factors (De Salles et al. 2001). The latter reaction may be similar to the phenomenon of repair with cellular proliferation and overproduction of collagen type IV material, which occurs in the vasculature of the AVM nidus treated by radiosurgery (Jahan et al. 2006).

1.7 Stereotactic Brain and Spine Radiation

Radiosurgery has revolutionized the treatment of benign and metastatic brain tumors (See Chaps. 7–15). Single-dose radiation, a novelty for neurosurgeons and radiation oncologists alike, became common practice with the explosion of imaging and precision-oriented radiation technology during the last two decades of the twentieth century. Now, the knowledge of radiation biology accumulated over 100 years is being applied to stereotactic radiotherapy to decrease treatment side effects (see Chap. 6). Challenging short schemes of radiation and taking advantage of the ability to reproduce patient's positioning in relation to the radiosurgery device without invasive fixation have brought the possibility of hypofractionation to resection cavities (Soltys et al. 2008) and giant AVMs (Xiao et al. 2010). Proven safe schemes of radiation for preservation of specialized sensory structures as optic and cochlear nerves, brainstem, pituitary gland, and spinal cord are used to approach previously untouchable pathologies. For example, preservation and improvement of vision in optic sheath meningiomas, exquisite preservation of the acoustic nerve function in treatment of acoustic neuromas (Selch et al. 2004), preservation of hormonal capabilities in pituitary lesions (Selch et al. 2006), and treatment of intrinsic medullar tumors and AVMs (De Salles et al. 2004; Selch et al. 2009).

1.8 Stereotactic Body Radiation Therapy

The accuracy required for stereotactic radiosurgery and the effectiveness of single-dose treatment of metastatic disease in the brain has spearheaded the development of precision-oriented radiation therapy (De Salles et al. 2008). Stereotactic body radiation therapy (SBRT) became the new and exciting effort in radiation oncology. The ability to exchange number of fractions for precise delivery of high doses has revolutionized the management of malignances in the lung (Fig. 1.4), liver, pancreas, and prostate. This ability may represent not only new more effective treatment of focal disease (Fig. 1.5), but also more comfort for the patient with savings of health dollars. Further development of these applications is the exciting part of stereotactic radiation therapy reflected in the Part III and IV of this book.

1.9 Conclusion

A revolution in radiation therapy started with the use of single high-dose delivery using the exquisite accuracy and precision of the work of functional stereotactic surgeons. This revolution hinged on the explosion of computed imaging technology, initially with the CT

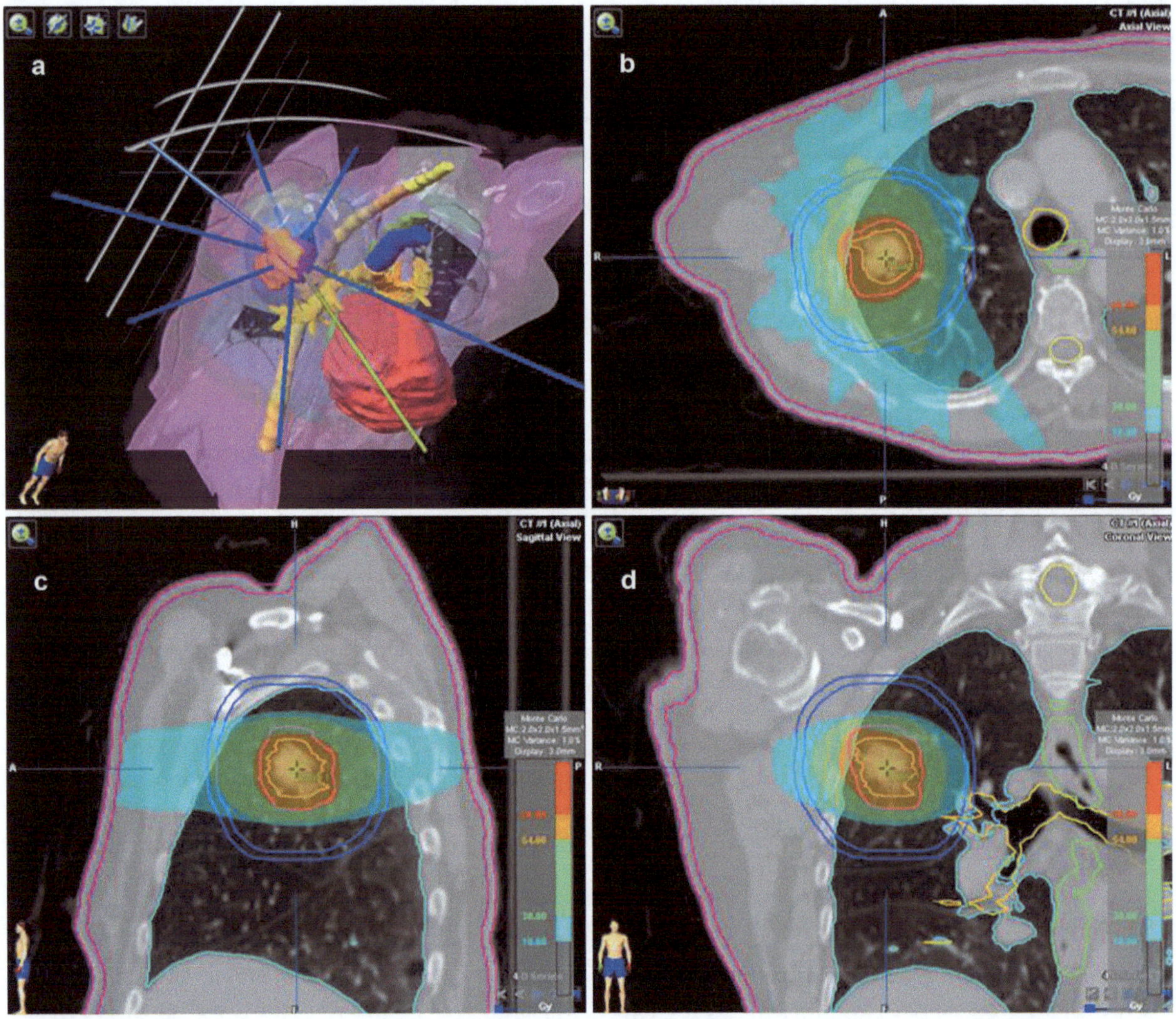

Fig. 1.4 Stereotactic radiosurgery planning for a lesion in the right lung upper lobe. Treatment for this lesion requires tracking of lung movement for gated delivery or 4D imaging capability. (**a**) Notice the 3D automatic reconstruction of organs at risk, trachea, spinal cord, heart. (**b**) Coronal, (**c**) Sagittal and (**d**) Coronal views of the radiosurgery planning

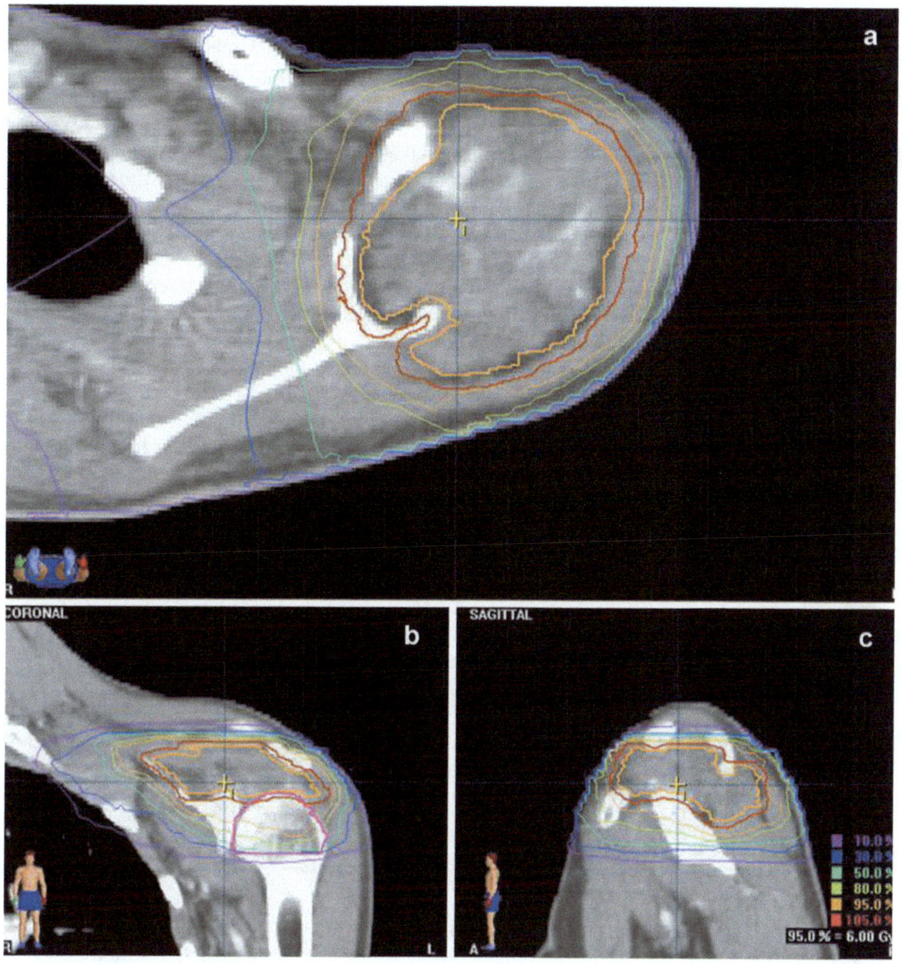

Fig. 1.5 Hypofractionated intensity modulated radiation therapy plan for a Brachial Plexus AVM presenting with left arm pain (five daily fractions of 6Gy). (**a**) Axial (**b**) Coronal and (**c**) Sagittal views of the radiosurgery plan

followed by the integration of MRI. The application of fiber tracking, functional MRI, and molecular imaging is the next step of the specificity of this revolution. The precision of the stereotactic frame gave way to image-guided technology, and challenged the dogmas established in radiation biology creating room for fewer fractions with high dose, enhanced effectiveness, decreased side effects, more comfort for the patient and likely decrease in health care dollar expenditure. The pages of this text reflect the accomplishments of this revolution.

References

Agazaryan N, Tenn SE, De Salles AAF, Selch MT (2008) Image-guided radiosurgery for spinal tumors: methods, accuracy and patient intrafraction motion. Phys Med Biol 53(6):1715–1727

Alexander E 3rd, Kooy HM, van Herk M, Schwartz M, Barnes PD, Tarbell N, Mulkern RV, Holupka EJ, Loeffler JS (1995) Magnetic resonance image-directed stereotactic neurosurgery: use of image fusion with computerized tomography to enhance spatial accuracy. J Neurosurg 83(2):271–276

Bova FJ, Friedman WA (1991) Stereotactic angiography: an inadequate database for radiosurgery? Int J Radiat Oncol Biol Phys 20(4):891–895

Chen JCT, Girvigian M, Greathaouse H, Miller M, Rahimian J (2004) Treatment of trigeminal neuralgia with linear accelerator radiosurgery: initial results. J Neurosurg 101 (Suppl 3):346–350

De Salles AAF, Medin P (2009) Functional spine radiosurgery. In: Ryu S, Gerszten PC (eds) Spine radiosurgery. Thieme, New York, pp 134–141

De Salles AAF, Asfora WT, Abe M, Kjellberg RN (1987) Transposition of target information from the magnetic resonance and CT-scan images to the conventional x-ray stereotactic space. Appl Neurophysiol 50:23–32

De Salles AAF, Solberg T, Medin P, Vassilev V, Cabatan-Awang C, Selch M (1997) Linear accelerator radiosurgery for trigeminal neuralgia. Radiosurgery 2:173–182

De Salles AAF, Melega WP, Lacan G, Steele LH, Solberg TD (2001) Radiosurgery with a 3 mm collimator in the subthalamic nucleus and substantia nigra of the vervet monkey. J Neurosurg 95:990–997

De Salles AAF, Pedroso AG, Medin P, Agazaryan N, Solberg T, Cabatan-Awang C, Espinosa DM, Ford J, Selch MT (2004) Novalis® radiosurgery shaped beam and intensity modulated radiosurgery and stereotactic radiotherapy for spine lesions. J Neurosurg 101(Suppl 3):435–440

De Salles AAF, Gorgulho A, Golish S, Medin P, Malkasian D, Solberg T, Selch M (2006) Technical and anatomical aspects of Novalis® Radiosurgery stereotactic radiosurgery sphenopalatine ganglionectomy. Int J Radiat Oncol Biol Phys 66:S53–S57

De Salles AAF, Gorgulho AA, Selch M, De Marco J, Agazaryan N (2008) Radiosurgery from the brain to the spine: 20 years experience. Acta Neurochir Suppl 101:163–168

Friedman WA, Bova FJ (1989) The University of Florida radiosurgery system. Surg Neurol 32(5):334–342

Friedman WA, Bova FJ (1992) Linear accelerator radiosurgery for arteriovenous malformations. J Neurosurg 77(6):832–841

Frighetto L, De Salles AAF, Cabatan-Awang C, Ford J, Solberg T, Selch MT (2004) Linear accelerator thalamotomy. Surg Neurol 62(2):106–113

Gorgulho AA, De Salles AAF (2006) Impact of radiosurgery on the surgical treatment of trigeminal neuralgia. Surg Neurol 66:350–356

Gorgulho A, De Salles AAF, McArthur D et al (2006) Brainstem and trigeminal nerve changes after radiosurgery for trigeminal pain. Surg Neurol 66:127–135, discussion 135

Hauptman JS, De Salles AAF, Espinoza R, Sedrak M, Ishida W (2008) Potential surgical targets for deep brain stimulation in treatment-resistant depression. Neurosurg Focus 25(1): E3

Jahan R, Solberg TD, Lee D, Medin P, Tateshima S, Sayre J, De Salles AAF, Vinters HV, Vinuela F (2006) Stereotactic radiosurgery of the rete mirabile in swine: a longitudinal study of histopathological changes. Neurosurgery 58(3): 551–558, discussion 551–558

Kjellberg RN, Hanamura T, Davis KR et al (1983) Bragg-peak proton-beam therapy for arteriovenous malformations. N Engl J Med 309:269–274

Leksell L (1951) The stereotaxic method and radiosurgery of the brain. Acta Chir Scand 102:316

Melega W, De Salles AA (2010) Molecular imaging of the brain with positron emission tomography. Youmans Neuro logical. Elsevier.

Rahimian J, Chen JC, Rao AA, Girvigian MR, Miller MJ, Greathouse HE (2004) Geometrical accuracy of the Novalis® Radiosurgery stereotactic radiosurgery system for trigeminal neuralgia. J Neurosurg 101(Suppl 3):351–355

Selch MT, Pedroso A, Lee SP, Solberg TD, Agazaryan N, Cabatan-Awang C, De Salles AA (2004) Stereotactic radiotherapy for the treatment of acoustic neuromas. J Neurosurg 101(Suppl 3):362–372

Selch MT, Gorgulho A, Mattozo C, Solberg TD, Cabatan-Awang C, De Salles AA (2005) Linear accelerator stereotactic radiosurgery for the treatment of gelastic seizures due to hypothalamic hamartoma. Minim Invasive Neurosurg 48(5): 310–314

Selch MT, Gorgulho A, Lee SP, De Salles AA et al (2006) Stereotactic radiotherapy for the treatment of pituitary adenomas. Minim Invasive Neurosurg 49:150–155

Selch MT, Lin K, Agazaryan N, Tenn S, Gorgulho A, Demarco JJ, De Salles AA (2009) Initial clinical experience with image-guided linear accelerator-based spinal radiosurgery for treatment of benign nerve sheath tumors. Surg Neurol 72(6):668–674

Smith ZA, De Salles AAF, Frighetto L, Wallace R, Cabatan-Awang C, Selch MT, Solberg T (2003) Linear accelerator radiosurgery for the treatment of trigeminal neuralgia. J Neurosurg 99:511–516

Solberg TD, Goetsch SJ, Selch MT, Melega W, Lacan G, De Salles AA (2004) Functional stereotactic radiosurgery involving a dedicated linear accelerator and gamma unit: a comparison study. J Neurosurg 101(Suppl 3): 373–380

Soltys SG, Adler JR, Lipani JD, Jackson PS, Choi CY, Puataweepong P, White S, Gibbs IC, Chang SD (2008) Stereotactic radiosurgery of the postoperative resection cavity for brain metastases. Int J Radiat Oncol Biol Phys 70(1): 187–193

Talairach J, Tournoux P (1988) Co-planar stereotaxic atlas of the human brain. 3-dimensional proportional system: an approach to cerebral imaging. Thieme Medical Publishers, New York

Xiao F, Gorgulho AA, Lin CS, Chen CH, Agazaryan N, Viñuela F, Selch MT, De Salles AAF (2010) Treatment of giant cerebral arteriovenous malformation: hypofractionated stereotactic radiation as the first stage. Neurosurgery 67(5): 1253–1259

Delivery Techniques

2

Ben Slotman

2.1 Introduction

The role of stereotactic irradiation has been established for the treatment of various benign and malignant intracranial lesions and diseases. The history of current stereotactic radiosurgery starts, after some early experiments in the 1950s and 1960s, in 1968, when Leksell and Larsson started their clinical work with the Gamma Knife. This device was developed to deliver high doses of radiation with great precision to small targets in the brain. A few decades ago, the widespread availability of linear accelerators (linacs) had lead to investigations on their use for single fraction stereotactic radiosurgery (SRS) and fractionated stereotactic radiotherapy (SRT). Special circular collimators were developed to allow for the use of narrow beams. Linac-based radiosurgical technologies were further advanced by incorporating improved stereotactic positioning devices and methods to measure the accuracy of various components. Since the 1990s, beam shaping is predominantly being achieved by the use of high-definition multileaf collimators (micro-MLCs). Just as in non-stereotactic radiotherapy, these MLCs also make it possible to deliver intensity-modulated SRS and SRT. In the last decade, dedicated linac-based devices were developed, including the Brainlab Novalis® Radiosurgery system (Fig. 2.1) and the Accuray Cyberknife (Fig. 2.2). The original version of the Novalis Radiosurgery system uses a 6 MV

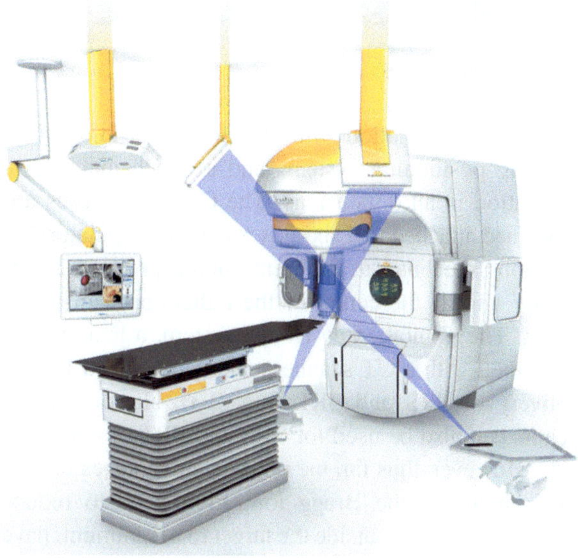

Fig. 2.1 Novalis Tx

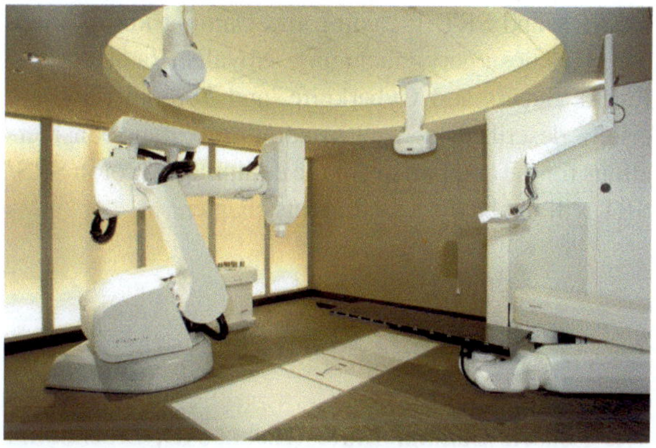

Fig. 2.2 Cyberknife

B. Slotman
Department of Radiation Oncology,
VU University medical center, De Boelelaan 1117,
1081 HV, Amsterdam, The Netherlands
e-mail: bj.slotman@vumc.nl

A.A.F. De Salles et al. (eds.), *Shaped Beam Radiosurgery*,
DOI: 10.1007/978-3-642-11151-8_2, © Springer-Verlag Berlin Heidelberg 2011

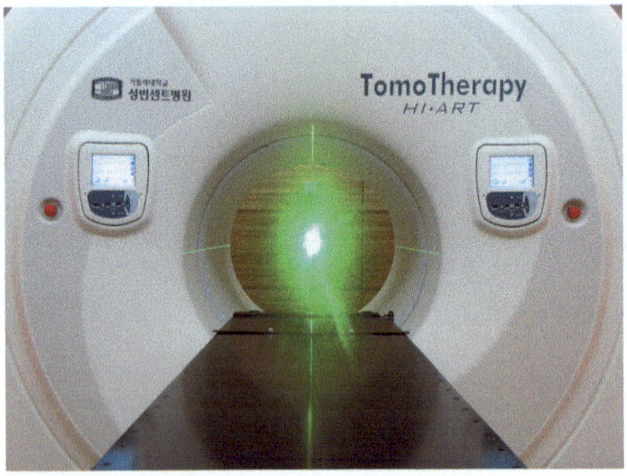

Fig. 2.3 Tomotherapy

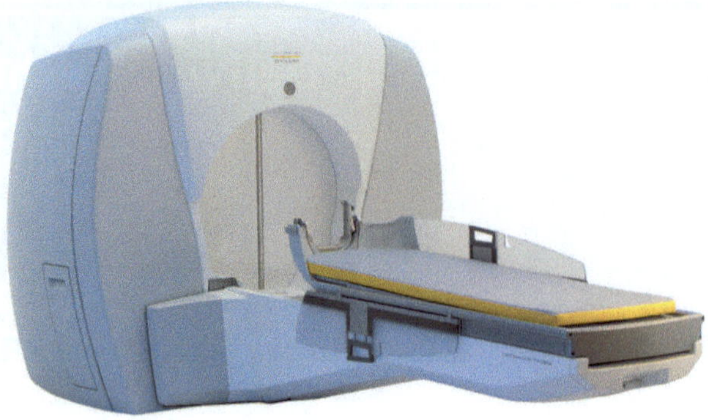

Fig. 2.4 Gamma knife

linac, in combination with infrared and kilovoltage imaging positioning systems and a couch that allows adaptation in all dimensions. The Cyberknife uses a 6 MV linac attached to a six-axis robotic manipulator that positions the linac at different source positions, constantly aiming the center of the radiation beam at the target. The Tomotherapy Hi-Art system, a linac that is combined with a CT scanner, can also be used for the delivery of SRS and SRT (Fig. 2.3). Narrow proton beams can also be used for SRS and SRT of small targets. However, thus far, the physical advantages of protons, including the Bragg ionization peak to reduce doses to the tissue outside the target to a minimum, have not yet been substantiated in clinical studies. The high cost and limited number of facilities available are important factors that preclude the more widespread use of protons in SRS. A small proportion of patients currently treated with protons receive stereotactic proton-beam radiosurgery. In this chapter, various types of equipment for SRS and SRT, including the Gamma knife, linac-based radiosurgery, including Novalis Radiosurgery, Elekta Access and Cyberknife, and Tomotherapy, are briefly described, as well as some important considerations for the comparison of the equipment. Proton SRS/SRT will not be discussed in this chapter.

2.2 Gamma Knife and RGS-System

The Leksell Gamma Knife (Elekta AB, Stockholm, Sweden) was developed for SRS about 40 years ago and is currently being used in over 200 sites throughout the world. The system consists of about 200 Cobalt-60 sources that are all directed to a single focal point. Leksell Gamma Knife Perfexion (Fig. 2.4) is the current high-end model with improved access to the intracranial structures and improvements in workflow, such as automated collimator changes. This leads to better shielding and more flexibility. A derivative of the Gamma knife, the RGS system with 30 Cobalt-60 radiation sources contained in a revolving hemispheric shell, was more recently developed. A secondary collimator is formed by a coaxial hemispheric shell with six groups of five collimator holes, which are arranged in the same pattern as the radiation sources. These systems, as a result of their design, can only be used to treat intracranial lesions in a single fraction (SRS). A head ring, attached to the head of the patients is used for immobilization and localization. For the generation of treatment plans and the delivery of treatment of irregularly shaped lesions, multiple isocenters are used.

2.3 Linac Radiosurgery

An adapted linear accelerator can also be used for very precise stereotactic treatments. Since a number of decades, linear accelerators are being used for SRS/SRT and clinical results are similar to those obtained with a Gamma Knife. Initially, a floor stand was needed for support of the treatment couch. More recent couches have sufficient stability for SRS and SRT treatment themselves. For single-fraction SRS, in general an invasive frame or head ring is being used. As this cannot easily be used for fractionated treatments over a longer period of time, noninvasive systems have been developed making use of dental and occipital impressions, or fixation using ears and nose bridge.

These fixation systems can be used as a frame of reference for imaging, treatment planning, and stereotactic treatment delivery. Some of the current noninvasive fixation systems, such as the Brainlab mask system; have similar precision as the systems using an invasive head ring for fixation (Solberg et al. 2008).

With linac-based SRS/SRT, stereotactic treatment of lesions outside the brain is also possible. Stereotactic radiotherapy has proven its benefit for various indications and this is a rapidly expanding field. For the treatment of extracranial lesions, positioning and immobilization systems have been developed, one of which is the Elekta Stereotactic Body frame. With the introduction of improved imaging devices, including cone beam CT on the linacs, such frames are no longer required. In the early years, predominantly circular collimators were used to obtain sharp beams with rapid dose fall off. A number of arcs were used with one or more isocenters. For irregular lesions, customized blocks were used with a large number of static fields. In the 1990s, the circular collimators and customized blocks were mostly replaced by high definition multileaf collimators. These micro-MLCs are similar to the standard MLCs of the linacs, with the exception of having smaller leaf sizes (2.5–3 mm versus 5 or 10 mm), smaller maximal field sizes, and improved dosimetry specifications. The micro-MLCs were initially used to create "shaped" static fields. Subsequently, they were used for dynamic conformal arc therapy, where the treatment aperture changes during irradiation according to the shape of the target and presence of critical structures. Nowadays, micro-MLCs are also used to deliver intensity-modulated SRS/SRT, by not only changing the shape of the aperture, but also changing the fluency within the field. Current linear accelerators capable of performing SRT also have imaging devices for Kilovoltage and/or Megavoltage imaging and eventually cone beam CT scanning. Two linear accelerator-based systems, which were specifically developed for SRS/SRT, the Brainlab Novalis Radiosurgery and Accuray Cyberknife, will be discussed in more detail.

2.4 Novalis Radiosurgery

Novalis Radiosurgery (Brainlab AG, Feldkirchen, Germany) is an integrated system featuring treatment planning, automated patient positioning, image-guidance, and treatment delivery for intra- and extracranial SRS and SRT. More than 150 systems have been installed. Image-guided target positioning takes place with reference of the treatment isocenter to internal or external localization markers. The original version of Novalis Radiosurgery is a single energy 6 MV dedicated linac with a built in micro-MLC, which is also capable of delivering dynamic arcs and intensity-modulated radiosurgery (IMRS). The maximum dose rate is 800 MU/min. Image-guided radiotherapy (IGRT) is provided by the ExacTrac® system that automatically aligns the target volume with the treatment beam based on infrared tracking of external body markers. It also uses automated registration of bony structures and implanted radiopaque markers using stereoscopic X-ray imaging. The Exactrac 6D Couch enables fast and precise couch correction in all directions to account for any misalignment or rotation. For the treatment of tumors that move with respiration, a respiratory gating system, which makes use of implanted markers, can be used. The most recent version, Novalis TX®, is a dual energy, dedicated linac that includes a new micro-MLC (120 leafs, of which 64 of 2.5-mm width in the center), stereo-KV imaging, and an On Board Imager including cone beam CT scan. The maximum dose rate is 1,000 MU/min. The new delivery technology RapidArc (Varian medical systems, USA), is also available on this linac. RapidArc is a volumetric intensity-modulated arc therapy, which can deliver the required dose distribution with one or a few arcs. For most treatments, this can be performed within a few minutes. During the rotation, the dose rate, micro-MLC setting, and speed of the gantry change simultaneously. Early studies using this technique indicate that it can also be used for SRS/SRT (Slotman et al. 2008). RapidArc combines high conformity with significantly shorter treatment times, which reduce the risk of patient or tumor movement, is more comfortable for the patient and allows a higher throughput of patients.

2.5 Cyberknife

The Cyberknife uses a 6 MV linac (maximum dose rate 800 MU/min), which is connected to a robotic manipulator that positions the linac at different source positions with the center of the radiation beam directed toward the target. During treatment, an image-processing system acquires X-ray images of the patient and compares the actual images with images in a database, to determine the direction and amount of motion. About 140 Cyberknife systems have been installed. In contrast to the linac-based systems, where compensation for misalignment due motion is being performed by a change in table position and/or gating of the radiation beam (i.e., turning the beam on when the target volume is in the desired position and turning the beam off when it is not), the Cyberknife system uses the robotic linac to compensate for it. Using this technique, tracking of the target volume is possible. A collimator changer is available for automatic exchange between collimators. The Cyberknife uses X-ray imaging to sense internal anatomy, while information on the motion of the patient surface is detected with an infrared imaging system. The Cyberknife uses a series of images from both sensors (infrared and X-ray), synchronizes one with the other, and calculates a motion pattern. This pattern correlates the external motion to the internal motion. Using the Cyberknife, it is possible to track tumors moving with respiration.

2.6 Tomotherapy Hi-Art

The Tomotherapy Hi-Arts system is a linac (6 MV, output 850 MU/min) combined with a CT scanner. Tomotherapy was developed in the 1990s. At present, more than 150 units are installed worldwide. For the delivery of the treatment, it uses a fan beam, which is modulated by a binary MLC. The leaves rapidly cross the width of the fan beam. The beam is subdivided into small "beamlets" which, depending on opening and closing of the leaves, will receive a high- or low dose-intensity. The leaves are pneumatically driven and can change between these open and closed states in a very rapid fashion. The treatment is delivered in a helical fashion with continuous and synchronous motion of gantry and couch, similar to a CT scanner. The Tomotherapy Hi-Art system includes integrated systems for treatment planning, patient set-up, CT-guided treatment, quality assurance, and recording and verification. Treatment planning differs from linac-based IMRT planning in that no beam angles, beam weights, and MLC patterns have to be determined. A Radionics head ring can be used for immobilization for SRS and SRT treatments, but it is not used for localization. Using the MV beam, CT images are acquired before each treatment and compared with the planning CT scan. For SRT, a single isocenter can be used for several targets.

2.7 Discussion

Apart from differences in costs for purchase, operation, and maintenance, every system has its specific advantages and disadvantages. The choice for a type of equipment should be based on wishes concerning functionality, applicability, flexibility, etc. It is important to consider at least the former points and the following discussion. In general, the specific role for SRS and SRT is disappearing. Differences between stereotactic techniques and other forms of image-guided radiotherapy and intensity-modulated radiotherapy are only gradual. Some types of equipment, such as a Gamma Knife, can only be used for the treatment of intracranial lesions. Linac-based systems, including Tomotherapy, allow for treatment of the rapidly expanding field of extracranial targets as well. There are a number of indications for intra- and extracranial treatments, where fractionated SRT has radiobiological advantages over single fraction SRS. Invasive head rings can only be used for SRS, while mask or frameless systems can be used for both SRS and SRT.

Integration of the system from image acquisition, contouring, treatment planning, setup, delivery to verification, is important for high throughput and reduces the risk of errors. Imaging is of crucial importance in high-precision radiotherapy. Cone beam CT offers the benefit of imaging the tumor (and not only the bony structures as with conventional X-ray imaging) before treatment with the patient in treatment position. Some systems are able to achieve more homogenous dose-distributions than others. In addition, it is important to choose a modern treatment planning system for a correct calculation of the delivered dose. Monte Carlo algorithms have a clear benefit over more conventional algorithms used in treatment planning software. Because of the risk of secondary tumors (Xu et al. 2008), especially in patients with benign lesions, children or patients with a good prognosis, a peripheral dose as low as possible, should also be considered as a factor in the decision-making process. The maximum dose rate influences treatment time. Because of the fraction sizes, which are generally used in SRS and SRT, this is an important factor to consider. Treatment time is related to patient and tumor motion (Purdie et al. 2007), patient comfort and the number of patients that can be treated per machine per day. The way in which the dose is delivered to the target volume is also a factor to consider. Radiobiological studies have shown differences in response when irradiation was given to a volume as a whole, or in smaller parts (Mackonis et al. 2007). The clinical consequences of this factor need to be determined. When SRS or SRT is combined with conventional radiotherapy, an integrated plan with integrated delivery using RapidArc has advantages over standard conventional SRS/SRT plans (Lagerwaard et al. 2008). The maximum field size and the possibility to use noncoplanar techniques are additional important factors when comparing different types of equipment.

References

Lagerwaard FJ, Verbakel WFAR, van der Hoorn E, Slotman BJ, Senan S (2008) Volumetric modulated arc therapy (RapidArc) for rapid, non-invasive stereotactic radiosurgery of multiple brain metastases. Int J Radiat Oncol Biol Phys 72(S1):S530

Mackonis EC, Suchowerska N, Zhang M, Ebert M, McKenzie DR, Jackson M (2007) Cellular response to modulated radiation fields. Phys Med Biol 52:5469–5482

Purdie TG, Bissonnette JP, Franks K, Bezjak A, Payne D, Sie F, Sharpe MB, Jaffray DA (2007) Cone-beam computed tomography for on-line image guidance of lung stereotactic radiotherapy: localization, verification, and intrafraction tumor position. Int J Radiat Oncol Biol Phys 68:243–252

Slotman BJ, Lagerwaard FJ, Verbakel WF, van der Hoorn E, Senan S (2008) A novel approach for highly conformal irradiation of vestibular Schwannoma using a single volumetric aperture based intensity modulated arc. Int J Radiat Oncol Biol Phys 72(S1):S4236–S4237

Solberg TD, Medin PM, Mullin J, Li S (2008) Quality assurance of immobilization and target localization systems for frameless stereotactic cranial and extracranial hypofractionated radiotherapy. Int J Radiat Oncol Biol Phys 71:S131–S135

Xu XG, Badnarz B, Paganetti H (2008) A review of dosimetry studies on external-beam radiation treatment with respect to second cancer induction. Phys Med Biol 53:R193–R241

3 Image-Guidance in Shaped Beam Radiosurgery and SBRT

Steve Tenn and Nzhde Agazaryan

3.1 Introduction

From its inception, the practice of radiation oncology has relied on its practitioner's ability to determine the location of the disease being treated. This may be accomplished through direct physical examination by the physician or through inference based on clinical knowledge of the disease process. In all cases, the best clinical outcomes are obtained when the disease location can be determined sufficiently well to completely encompass the intended target in prescribed ionizing radiation fields, as well as to protect healthy tissue from the same fields. Thus, radiation oncology has always relied on the best image guidance methods available at the time in order to obtain the maximum therapeutic ratios for successful treatment. Image guidance has two major roles to play in the practice of radiation oncology. First, it allows one to detect the location of disease within the patient for delineation of the target region. Second, it allows one to locate the specified target region at the time of treatment so that the patient can be positioned correctly with respect to the treatment field. The ability to detect both diseased and normal tissues has been greatly enhanced through advances in imaging technologies such as computed tomography (CT), magnetic resonance imaging (MRI), ultrasound (US), single-photon emission tomography (SPECT), and positron emission tomography (PET). Each technique has specific advantages that can be utilized in radiotherapy. Due to its geometric accuracy in rendering patient anatomy and ability to estimate electron density in patients, the CT scanner has become ubiquitous in radiation oncology departments for virtual treatment simulation (Aird and Conway 2002). MRI and PET images are also being utilized with increasing frequency in institutions that have access to these technologies. For example, it is relatively routine at many institutions to obtain MRI images in addition to the CT simulation scan for treatment planning of brain and spinal disorders such as metastatic disease. The exquisite soft tissue contrast obtained from MRI studies can be invaluable in determining the location and extent of some diseases that cannot be visualized in CT imaging alone. In contrast to MRI and CT imaging that are used primarily to obtain anatomical information through physical differences in tissues, PET imaging is a functional imaging modality utilizing radioisotope-labeled tracers to detect regional differences in tissue uptake and metabolism (Ford et al. 2009). The application of these imaging technologies allows clinicians to accurately delineate the active disease sites to be targeted for treatment as well as the normal tissues that are at risk of treatment complication from excess dose. Combining the improvements in target delineation with advances in external beam and stereotactic radiosurgery delivery methods such as three-dimensional conformal radiotherapy (3D-CRT) and intensity modulated radiotherapy (IMRT) have improved our ability to closely conform the prescribed dose distribution to target shapes with rapid dose decrease outside of the target area, thus restricting the dose received by normal

S. Tenn (✉) and N. Agazaryan
Department of Radiation Oncology,
David Geffen School of Medicine at UCLA,
200 UCLA Medical Plaza, Suite B265, Los Angeles,
CA 90095, USA
e-mail: stenn@mednet.ucla.edu

A.A.F. De Salles et al. (eds.), *Shaped Beam Radiosurgery*,
DOI: 10.1007/978-3-642-11151-8_3,

tissues. However, the extremely conformal dose distributions and steep dose gradients now achievable also increase the risks of unintended target underdose leading to suboptimal response or excessive normal tissue dose leading to possible complications if the fields are not delivered accurately. While the concepts of planning target volumes (PTV) and planning organ at risk volumes (PRV) that include margins for location uncertainties have been introduced by the ICRU (ICRU 1999) to help address this issue, the goal of increasing therapeutic ratio, in many cases, drives the practice of radiation oncology toward higher target doses, as well as better normal tissue sparing. This requires accurate positioning and delivery of treatment fields, an area in which imaging plays an increasingly important role. As noted above, incorporating imaging technologies into the treatment delivery process has improved our ability to detect and also accurately localize delineated targets. The current technologies used for treatment delivery image guidance include X-ray imaging (Jaffray et al. 1999), gamma-ray seed tracking (Alezra et al. 2009), ultrasound imaging (Fuss et al. 2004), infrared (IR) imaging (Meeks et al. 1998; Wang et al. 2001), video imaging (Milliken et al. 1997), electromagnetic transponder (Willoughby et al. 2006), and recently MR (Fallone et al. 2009). Application of these technologies to guide the delivery of external beam radiotherapy is colloquially referred to as image-guided radiotherapy or IGRT for short. This chapter will detail the treatment delivery image-guidance technologies available for shaped beam radiosurgery with Novalis® Radiosurgery and Novalis Tx®.

3.2 Image-Guidance Technologies Available on Novalis Tx

Several technologies and methods are currently available for accomplishing image-guided patient setup on the Novalis Tx. These include Megavoltage (MV) electronic portal imaging device (EPID), kilovoltage (kV) planar, and tomographic imaging via sources and imagers attached to the gantry, kV imaging via sources and imagers attached to the floor and ceiling of the treatment vault, IR and video optical guidance.

3.2.1 Varian Portal Imaging

Portal imaging with film or an electronic imager was one of the first X-ray image guidance techniques developed for radiotherapy (Byhardt et al. 1978; Lam et al. 1987). The portal images are acquired for a given treatment field (or portal) by delivering a small amount of radiation (usually a few monitor units) from the treatment beam through the patient with field collimating devices (blocks, MLC, etc.) in place. The patient's anatomy in the portal image can then be compared to that in simulation images acquired on analog simulators or, more currently, with digitally reconstructed radiographs (DRRs) that are generated from three-dimensional (3D) CT simulation images. Translational and rotational offsets between anatomic features in the DRRs and those in the portal images indicate the shift necessary to correct the patients' position for accurate treatment from that particular treatment portal. Following the advent of portal image guidance, studies were conducted to determine target positioning accuracy when setup is based on surface landmarks alone. Lam and coworkers (Lam et al. 1987) at Johns Hopkins noted that when using skin landmarks, "a margin of 1 cm around the tumor is barely sufficient if a 5% accuracy in dose delivery is desired." Other studies comparing portal image positioning to skin landmark setup have found the most common causes of geometric misalignment were errors in field centering, block positioning, and body positioning/orientation (Byhardt et al. 1978). The use of portal images to verify and, if necessary, correct tattoo-based setup on a weekly basis has now become a standard image guidance approach to improve patient positioning. Electronic portal imaging on the Novalis Tx is accomplished with Varian's Portal Vision™ (PV) consisting of an amorphous silicon flat panel detector (aS1000) mounted to the linac gantry via robotic arm (Exact Arm) and managed by the IAS3 image acquisition system (Fig. 3.1). The aS1000 is a high-resolution flat panel imager consisting of a $1,024 \times 768$ array of solid-state detectors covering an area of 40×30 cm^2 (linear pixel size 0.392 mm). The IAS3 acquisition system features short image acquisition times, real-time display capability, signal integration mode for use with portal dosimetry, and high-quality (14 bit

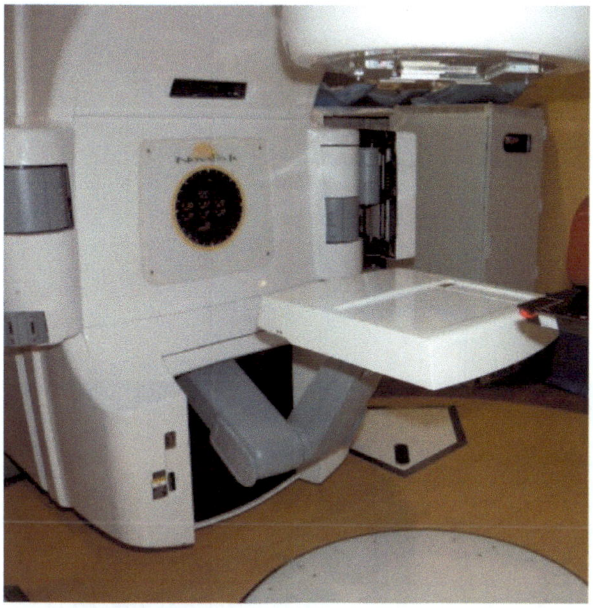

Fig. 3.1 Varian's Portal Vision™ (PV) imager is shown in extended position

digital analog conversion) image acquisition. These features allow high-resolution images to be acquired with low patient dose.

3.2.2 Varian OBI kV X-Ray Imaging

The primary limitation of MV imaging with the treatment beam is a lack of soft tissue contrast (Fig. 3.2). In order to address this shortcoming while providing an image acquisition perspective similar to that of the treatment beam, investigators began mounting kV imaging systems to the linac gantry (Biggs et al. 1985; Jaffray et al. 1999). With their lower photon energy and small focal spot size, kV systems can provide diagnostic quality planar images of the patient while in treatment position. Typically, these imaging systems are mounted to the gantry so that the image axes (vector from object to image) are perpendicular or oblique to the treatment beam axis. This mounting allows images to be acquired even while the treatment beam is active.

Gantry-mounted kV imaging is available on the Novalis Tx in the form of Varian's On-Board Imager (OBI) (Varian Medical Systems, Inc., Palo Alto, California) system (Fig. 3.3). Varian's OBI configuration places the kV X-ray source and imager so that the image axis is orthogonal to the treatment beam axis. The imager and the source are each mounted to the gantry via robotic support arms (Exact Arm). The arms can be extended to place the imaging axis through isocenter for acquiring setup images and then retracted to move the imaging system out of the way during treatment.

OBI can be used to acquire orthogonal pairs of images that are registered with corresponding DRRs for 3D translational shift detection. As with the MV Portal Vision described above, DRRs corresponding to the kV X-ray source and imager configuration must be generated from CT simulation data for comparison with the acquired radiographs. Registration of the

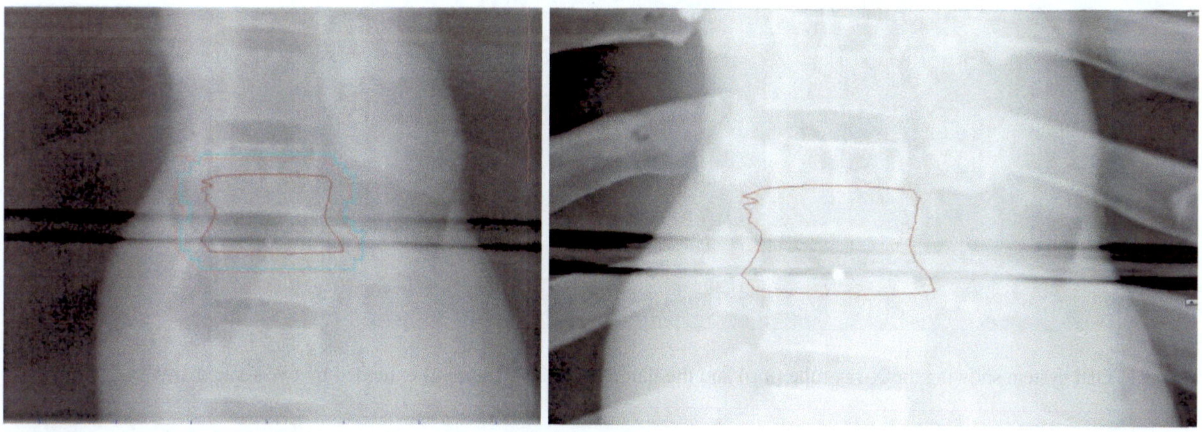

Fig. 3.2 Comparison of Megavoltage (MV) port image (*left*) versus kilovoltage (kV) Varian's On-Board Imager (OBI) (*right*)

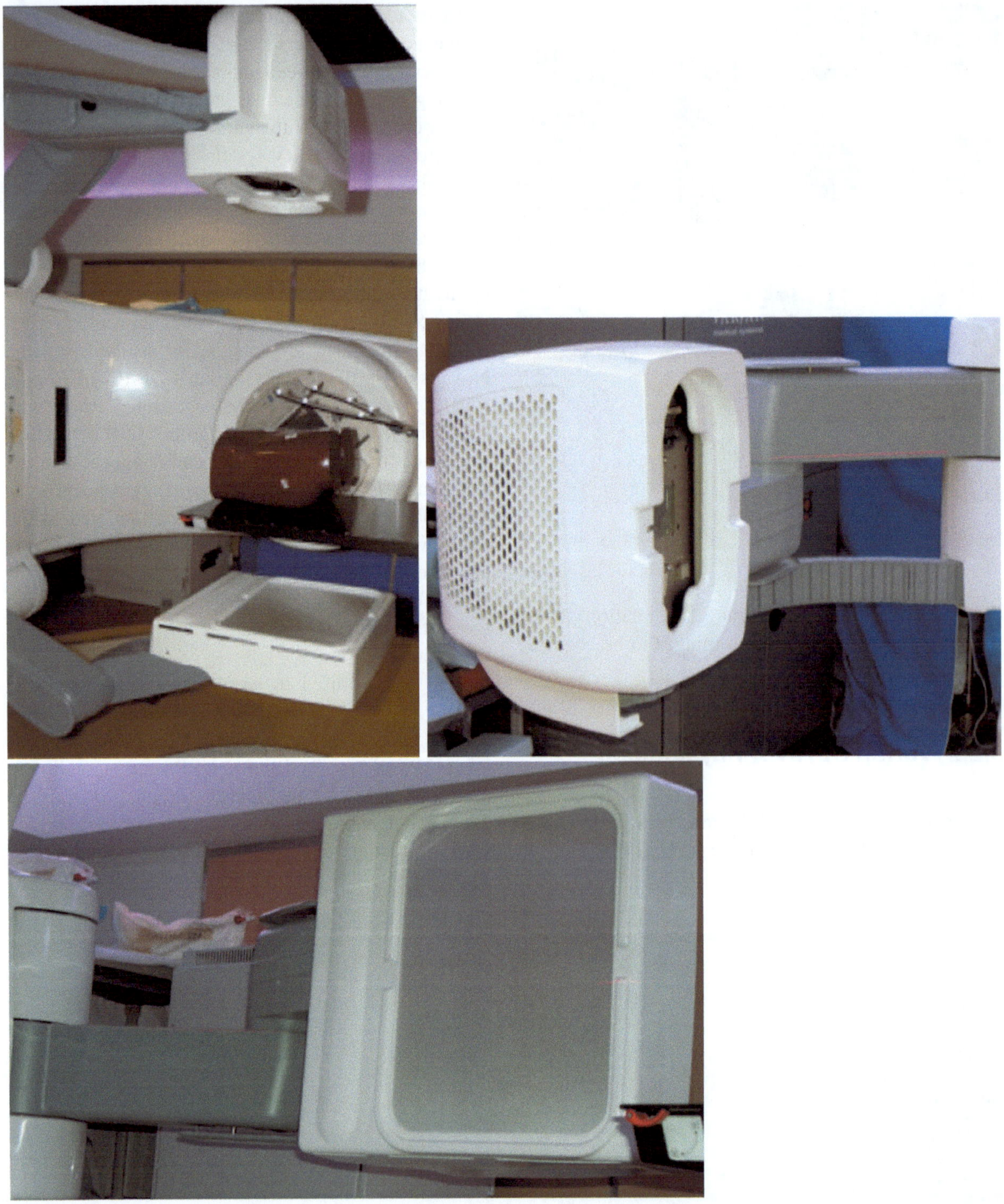

Fig. 3.3 OBI system showing the X-ray tube (*top*) and the flat panel imager (*bottom*) extended by two Exact Arms

orthogonal image pair (a process called 2D/2D match) with the corresponding DRR pair can detect 3D anatomic displacements and indicate the shifts necessary to properly place the target with respect to the linac isocenter. The registration or matching process, described more fully below, can be accomplished automatically by computer workstation or manually by the operator. The OBI system can also be used to acquire

3D CT images via cone beam CT (CBCT) reconstructions (Jaffray et al. 2002; Yin et al. 2005). CBCT images are generated by rotating the gantry while acquiring planar images (up to 700) in a cine acquisition mode. A tomographic reconstruction is made from the set of planar images. Several acquisition and reconstruction methods are available for CBCT on the Novalis Tx. In "half-scan" acquisition mode, the gantry rotates through 200° during which up to 700 individual planar kV images are acquired. "Full-scan" acquisition mode requires 360° of rotation while images are acquired. There are also full-fan or half-fan reconstruction modes. To acquire images for a full-fan reconstruction the imager must be centered over the gantry's rotational axis. Thus, the complete anatomic region to be imaged can be viewed in each image. This provides a maximum reconstruction diameter of 25 cm. If larger fields of view are required (up to 45 cm) a half-fan reconstruction is utilized. Here the imager is slightly offset perpendicularly to the gantry rotational axis so that more laterally located anatomy will be included in each planar image. The gantry must rotate through a full 360° in order to acquire all images needed for this reconstruction. The 3D image obtained with CBCT can be used to detect target misalignment in all six dimensions (translation and rotation). This is typically accomplished by computer registration of the CBCT data with the simulation CT set (a process called 3D/3D match). Manual match is also an option where the operator drags and rotates the CBCT image in three orthogonal windows until the two images visually coincide with each other. While all 6° of target orientation can be detected with 3D/3D match, only the three translations and couch rotation (yaw) can be corrected for.

3.2.3 Brainlab ExacTrac®

A stereoscopic image guidance system, Brainlab's ExacTrac X-ray 6D system, is available on the classic Novalis, Novalis Tx, and can be installed with many other linear accelerators. ExacTrac integrates infrared (IR) tracking with oblique stereoscopic kV X-ray imaging for fast and accurate patient positioning. Due to its speed and accuracy, this is the workhorse image guidance system for patient positioning on the classic Novalis and Novalis Tx at many institutions. The IR tracking component can update marker positions every 50 ms or less and is employed to track patient or table position in real time. The IR system electronic hardware consists of infrared emitters and detectors mounted to the ceiling of the linac vault. On older systems, two independent cameras were mounted separately. On the newest systems, the IR light source and cameras are integrated into a single unit, along with a video camera (Fig. 3.4). Following a calibration procedure, the camera system can accurately detect the 3D positions of IR reflecting markers relative to the linac reference frame.

IR markers can be used to track target position in two ways. In the first method, a group of markers (typically four or more) are attached to the anterior surface of the patient or patient immobilization device (Fig. 3.5). The markers are placed on the patient for the

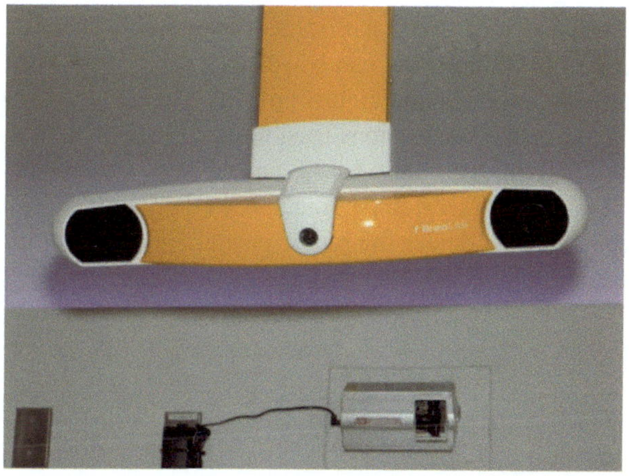

Fig. 3.4 ExacTrac's integrated video and IR camera system

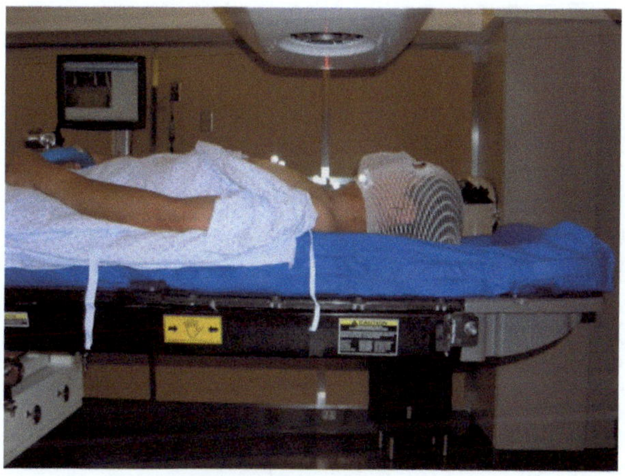

Fig. 3.5 Infrared (IR) reflective markers are shown attached to a patient's chest and mask for a C-spine treatment

acquisition of the simulation CT and are linked geometrically, during treatment planning, with the isocenter position. With an assumption that the marker positions are linked to the target position, tracking the markers consequently tracks the target. With this method the patient can be continuously monitored for movement during treatment. The second method does not require markers to be attached directly to the patient. Instead, an array of markers (Reference Star) is attached to the treatment couch (Fig. 3.6). As long as the target remains fixed relative to the treatment couch, the target position can be tracked via the reference star. The main advantage provided by tracking with the reference star is that couch movements are tracked directly and small patient movements that do not relate to target motion (e.g., respiration during spine treatment) are ignored, making automated positioning more reliable. Similar arguments can be made for the cranial array with reflective markers; hence, corrective table shifts can be reliably performed with the reference star and cranial array.

While the IR system is used for tracking a patient's position in real time based on surface- or couch-mounted markers, ExacTrac's X-ray component is employed to detect the target position intermittently and more directly through internal anatomic features. The X-ray system allows positioning based on anatomy that may be more strongly associated with the target than surface landmarks. Some useful radiographic features are skeletal anatomy, implanted fiducials, and in some cases such as solid tumors in the lung or tumors in the bone, the tumor itself may be visualized. ExacTrac's X-ray system is composed of 2 kV sources mounted to the vault floor next to the linac gantry and two flat panel image detectors mounted to the ceiling above the treatment couch (Fig. 3.7). The arrangement allows images to be acquired for a greater range of gantry positions than if the sources and imagers were positioned in the plane of gantry rotation. By mounting the sources and imagers to fixed positions in the treatment vault rather than to the mobile gantry the accuracy of the system is not affected by the mechanical precision of the linac.

The X-ray subsystem is calibrated in a procedure similar to that of the IR system. The procedure accomplishes two objectives. First, it calibrates the geometric framework of the imaging system to an accuracy on the order of a few tenths of a millimeter. Second, it registers the coordinate system of the X-ray system with that of the IR system. Following proper calibration, target displacements relative to isocenter can be accurately detected by the X-ray imaging system and are then compensated for by robotic couch translations and rotations. The IR system tracks and guides these corrective movements. The ExacTrac system uses 2D/3D image registration to detect offsets in all six

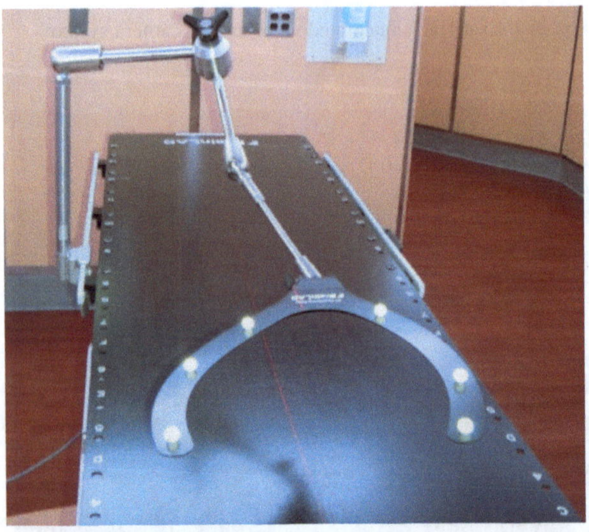

Fig. 3.6 Reference Star IR marker array attached directly to the treatment couch

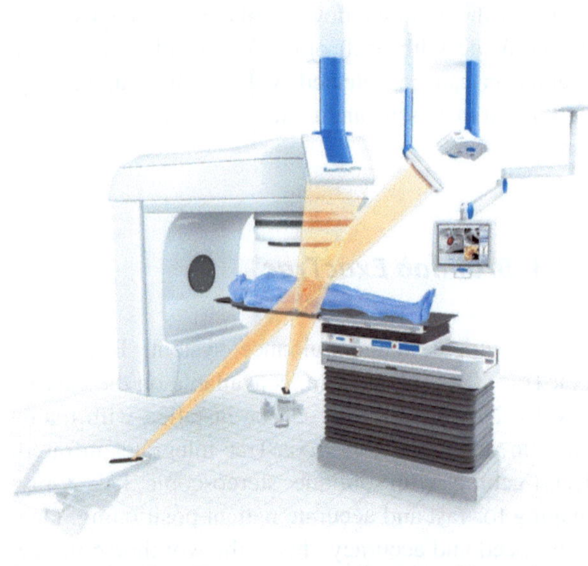

Fig. 3.7 ExacTrac X-ray system configuration. X-ray tubes are located in the floor lateral to the gantry and flat panel imagers are mounted to the ceiling

spatial degrees of freedom (three translational and three rotational). The registration process is automatic and takes only a few seconds to accomplish on a modern workstation. An option to manually register the images is also available, but this method can only correct for translational offsets. ExacTrac is also capable of performing 2D/2D registration for a single image in a process called Snap Verification (SV). Snap Verification was implemented to address the problem that for some gantry angles one of the kV X-ray imagers' field of view is partially or fully obscured by the gantry (Fig. 3.8). For these gantry angles, it may be desirable to detect whether the patient has moved without taking extra time to move the gantry out of the way and acquire full stereoscopic imaging. SV is essentially a monoscopic image guidance method that allows the operator to acquire a single kV image and predict whether the target has shifted from the proper setup location. Because SV is a monoscopic imaging method, only translations and rotations parallel to the image plane are accurately detectable. Movements normal to the image plane and rotations along axes within the image plane cannot be resolved sufficiently well to determine the full 6D target position from a single image. Therefore, SV can only be used to estimate or predict whether a given amount of motion has occurred. For example, if a translation of 1 mm were detected in the image plane by SV then the actual 3D translation may have been more due to possible out of plan motion. It is still possible however that the actual 3D motion may have been less than 1 mm because the 2D/2D fusion results may be inaccurate due to rotations that make projectional changes in bony anatomy. In an initial study of the sensitivity and specificity of Snap Verification to detect movement, it has been found that for detecting 1.5 mm 3D movement, monoscopic imaging with 1.2-mm threshold maximizes the sum of sensitivity and specificity with 95% negative predictive value. (Agazaryan et al. 2009). That is, when SV predicts that no movement has occurred greater than 1.2 mm in 2D, 95% of the time there has been no movements greater than 1.5 mm in 3D.

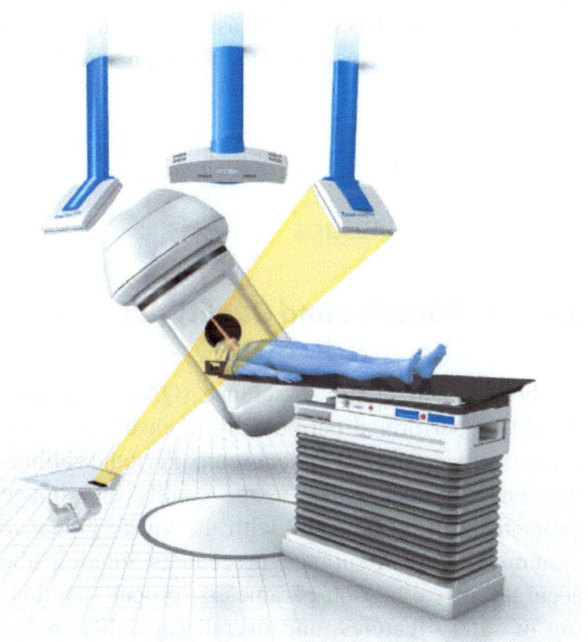

Fig. 3.8 Certain gantry rotation angles can block the X-ray camera system leaving only one imager available to image

The ExacTrac system is also capable of performing gated or event-triggered image guidance to compensate for respiratory-induced target motion. In this mode, the system tracks a patient's respiratory motion through movement of IR markers attached to the abdomen or chest. The kV X-ray system is triggered to acquire images at specific, user defined, phase point in the respiratory cycle. This allows pairs of stereoscopic images to be acquired of the target position at different points in the breathing cycle. The patient can then be positioned so that the target is located at isocenter for a given phase point in the respiratory cycle based on the corresponding image set. ExacTrac also sends a gating signal to the linac based on the respiratory cycle for beam hold and beam enable so that the beam is only turned on while the target is transiting the isocenter. The gating window and phase points for triggering localization X-rays are all user definable.

3.3 Registration Methods

There are several image registration methods utilized by the image guidance technologies on the Novalis Tx. Varian OBI implements both 2D-2D matching and 3D/3D matching depending on the image types obtained. The ExacTrac system makes use of both fiducial point-based registration and 2D-3D registration methods. Both portal image registration and Snap Verification described previously are examples of 2D-2D image registration and guidance. For 2D-2D registration, planar images taken at the time of treatment are compared with corresponding reference planar images depicting the correct anatomical orientation that should be observed if setup is correct. The test image is translated, rotated, and scaled if necessary, until a best match is obtained. The shifts needed to accomplish this match are related to the shifts needed to correct patient setup. Each 2D-2D image registration can correct for translations in the plane of the acquired image and rotations perpendicular to this plane (in plane rotations). Thus, given two orthogonal images and two DRRs the 3D translations and two of the rotations needed to correctly position the target can be estimated. Recently, 2D-3D and 3D-3D image registration techniques that are able to accurately determine the target position in all six geometric dimensions (three translational and three rotational degrees of freedom) have been developed. 2D-3D image guidance refers to the registration of pairs of 2D images acquired at the time of treatment with 3D images (typically CT studies) in order to detect target position and orientation. 3D-3D image guidance refers to the registration of in-room 3D image sets (e.g., in-room MV CT (Mackie et al. 1993), kilovoltage (kV) CT (Uematsu et al. 1996), and gantry-mounted kV cone beam CT (CBCT) (Jaffray et al. 2002)) with 3D simulation CT images in order to detect the target's 6D position.

2D-3D image registration differs from 2D-2D registration in that 3D data from the reference image set provides additional information necessary to accurately detect all translational and rotational displacements. Two types of algorithms are typically employed to accomplish 2D-3D registration on modern image guidance systems. The first method utilizes a library of DRRs that are pre-generated from the 3D reference set image set (Fu and Kuduvalli 2008). The library contains DRRs that are generated by rotating the 3D data set by various amounts and calculating the projected image for the rotations. Several minutes of computation time are needed to generate the library, which is completed before treatment begins. With the patient on the treatment couch, X-ray image pairs are acquired. The first step in the registration process is a fast 2D-2D match that provides an initial course estimate of translational and in plane rotational offsets. The corrections are refined by searching the library for DRRs that match the X-ray image pairs in order to estimate the rotations. Finally, the match converges on a final solution through small translation and rotation incremental steps once the rotational deviations have been removed. The entire process takes a few seconds to complete allowing for fast target realignment and resumption of treatment. This method is used by the CyberKnife radiosurgery system. The second method does not require pre-generated DRRs. Instead, the registration process proceeds in an online or real-time fashion with the reference 3D image set being iteratively translated and rotated by small amounts (Agazaryan et al. 2008). During each iteration, a pair of DRRs are generated and compared with the acquired images. The algorithm proceeds until the generated DRRs match the acquired images within a tolerance limit. The orientation of the CT set that generated the matching DRRs represents the current orientation of the patient and the set of translations and rotations needed to bring the patient into correct alignment are fully determined. This method is used by the ExacTrac system. A limitation of 2D image registration methods is their reliance on anatomy that can be visualized in planar images. Thus, their use is typically limited to cases where the target is closely associated with skeletal anatomy or when radiopaque fiducial markers can be introduced near the target. Because 3D imaging modalities produce better soft tissue contrast 3D-3D image guidance techniques can be used to localize soft tissue targets that are not strongly associated with radiopaque landmarks. Examples include targets in the thorax and abdomen. 3D-3D registration is accomplished by iteratively translating and rotating the reference set with respect to the test set until a best match is found. The match is typically assessed using mutual information as the objective to be optimized (Maes et al. 1997).

3.4 Technical Issues

3.4.1 Calibration and Quality Assurance

Calibration and quality assurance (QA) procedures should be performed periodically to ensure safe and accurate image-guided patient setup. Periodic calibration ensures that proper image quality and image geometry will be obtained with the image guidance system. Quality assurance procedures monitor the accuracy of calibration parameters, proper functioning of safety features, and overall capability of the systems. In this section, a brief summary of calibration and QA for the different Novalis Tx image guidance systems is provided. The calibration and QA procedures can be categorized into those dealing with geometric accuracy and those dealing with image quality.

3.4.1.1 OBI Calibration

Calibration of the OBI system begins with mechanical (geometric) alignment of the ExactArms for both the X-ray source and the imager panel. The calibration is accomplished by moving the ExactArm into predefined geometrical configurations (joint angles and arm positions). The procedure identifies correct positioning for the source and imager through their range of motion. Mechanical axis calibrations are followed by isocenter calibration. Isocenter calibration determines the distance from the X-ray source and image acquisition plane locations to the linac isocenter. These two procedures ensure that the ExactArm geometry is well defined and in agreement with parameters in the algorithms used for image reconstruction and registration. Once mechanical calibration has been accomplished image quality calibration procedures should be performed. These procedures ensure that optimal image quality will be obtained from the system. The first step in optimizing image quality is to detect and correct pixel readout variations that can lead to image artifacts. The readout variations are typically due to imager aging and temperature variations. To detect the pixel variations dark field (without radiation) and flood field (with radiation) images are acquired. From these a pixel-by-pixel correction map is generated for the imager. A drift field image is also created. This image is simply a subtraction image of two dark field images taken sequentially with a set amount of time between acquisitions. The image can detect pixel values that have changed or "drifted" over a given time interval. From this information, a map is created that contains locations of pixels that have excessive drift. These pixel values can be replaced by the average of neighboring pixel values in image generated for display.

3.4.1.2 CBCT Calibration

Calibration for CBCT has additional steps beyond those performed for planar kV imaging. Because small mechanical shifts in imaging components can occur during gantry rotation for CBCT acquisition a geometric calibration of the system at a series of gantry angles must be performed. The procedure identifies shifts in imager components with respect to the isocenter location at these different gantry angles for accurate image reconstruction. Other calibration procedures are also performed that reduce ring artifacts, correct for beam hardening, and calibrate the Hounsfield Units (HU) accuracy in reconstructed images. These procedures help to maintain high image quality that is necessary for accurate image registration.

3.4.1.3 ExacTrac Calibration

ExacTrac calibration serves to accurately define the geometry of both the IR and X-ray systems as well as to align their frames of reference with the linac coordinate system. Two phantoms are available for calibration of the latest version of the system. The first phantom is the isocenter phantom (Fig 3.9), which has four IR reflective spheres on its surface and is scored with crosshairs for alignment with the setup lasers or light field crosshairs. After aligning this phantom with the setup lasers, the locations of the IR spheres identify the linac isocenter position and linac geometric axes orientation for the IR camera component of ExacTrac. The second phantom (Fig. 3.9) registers the X-ray component to the IR system. The phantom is

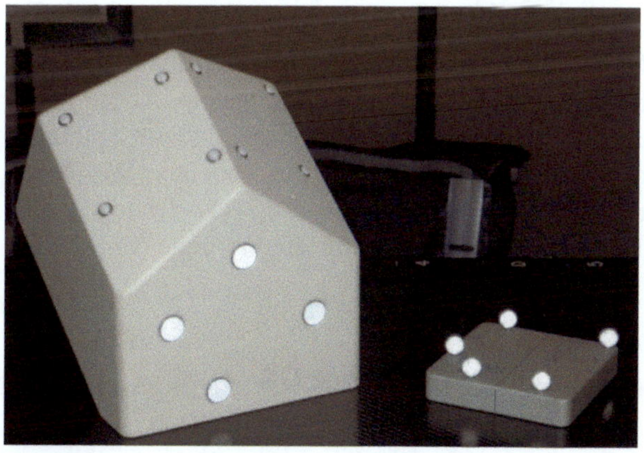

Fig. 3.9 ExacTrac calibration phantoms. X-ray phantom on *left* with eight metal fiducials on the upper facets of the phantom. IR phantom on *right* with crosshairs etched on surface for alignment with the setup lasers

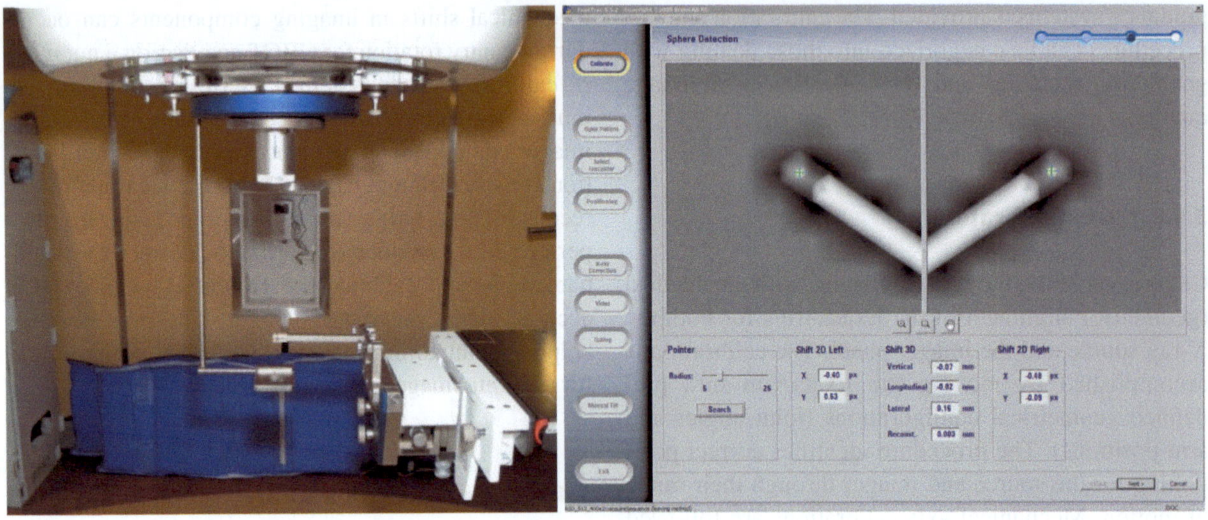

Fig. 3.10 Winston Lutz test setup and example result from ExacTrac

positioned at a preset position with respect to isocenter that is identified by the IR cameras using four IR reflective markers. Eight metallic fiducials also embedded on the surface of the phantom are imaged with the kV X-ray component once the phantom is in position at the isocenter. The geometry of the metallic fiducials in each X-ray image provides a complete geometric calibration of the X-ray component and registers its coordinate system to that of the IR tracking component providing complete system integration.

It is important to note that the entire ExacTrac system is registered with isocenter via the calibration procedure described above. Because the ExacTrac coordinate system is linked with isocenter through the setup lasers, it is imperative that these setup lasers be made to coincide with the linac isocenter before calibrating the ExacTrac system. At our institution, the lasers are made to coincide with a stereotactic cone collimated radiation isocenter. We locate this isocenter via Winston–Lutz (W–L) test (Lutz 1988) using a 7.5-mm radiosurgery cone (Fig. 3.10).

3.4.2 Image Guidance QA

Periodic quality assurance of the image guidance systems is necessary to ensure the accuracy and image quality of the systems. Yoo and coworkers have described a detailed list of quality assurance procedures for the Varian OBI system (Yoo et al. 2006). QA procedures include checking the digital graticule for isocenter coincidence using a phantom with radiopaque fiducial that can be accurately placed at isocenter, checking 2D/2D match accuracy with a similar phantom, and checking image quality and geometric accuracy of CBCT using the Catphan 504 phantom. The authors suggest that QA checks involving isocenter coincidence should be performed on a daily or weekly basis depending on the frequency with which the systems are utilized. Quality assurance for the ExacTrac system as practiced at our institution consists of daily isocenter coincidence verification by the morning linac warm-up therapists and monthly recalibration of the entire system by a physicist following a Winston–Lutz test. The daily isocenter coincidence test ensures that the ExacTrac-identified isocenter coincides with the laser-identified isocenter. The procedure consists of aligning the isocenter phantom to the setup lasers and acquiring two X-ray images of the phantom. The ExacTrac system then performs 6D registration and reports the detected offset from its stored isocenter location. On days that radiosurgery treatments are performed an abridged Winston–Lutz test (Gantry angles 0°, 90°, and 180° with no couch rotations) is carried out before treatments begin. Following the W–L test, ExacTrac X-ray images are acquired of the tungsten ball at isocenter. The system identifies the ball position in each image and calculates the ball's 3D offset from ExacTrac's saved isocenter location.

3.4.3 Fiducial Versus Anatomic Registration

As noted previously, the use of implanted radiopaque fiducials is favored for image guidance techniques utilizing planar imaging where soft tissue targets are not strongly associated with skeletal anatomy. Common sites for implanted fiducial marker use are tumors in the lung, liver, pancreas, and prostate (Figs. 3.11 and 3.12). The markers are implanted either directly into the tumor or in healthy tissue surrounding the tumor. As long as the fiducials remain fixed with respect to target anatomy, the target position can be inferred from the fiducial positions at the time of treatment.

Image registration based on discrete implanted fiducial markers is accomplished by matching, in space, one group of discrete points to another group that may be shifted and rotated with respect to the first. Essentially, the method solves for the vector and rotation matrix that bring the fiducial points in a test image into alignment with those in a reference image. The translation vector can be found simply from the displacement between the centroids of the two fiducial groups. Finding the rotation matrix then becomes a matter of solving what is known as the Orthogonal Procrustes problem (Schonemann 1968). Several algorithms are available to solve for the rotations including use of singular value decomposition (SVD), iterative methods, and quaternions (Arun et al. 1987; Horn et al. 1988). Fiducial point registration will produce correct 6D alignment given that three or more fiducials are arranged non-linearly, non-symmetrically, and that the two groups are similar and without deformation. In practice, fiducials are typically attached to tissues that can deform over both short and long intervals of time. The fiducials may become dislodged and migrate from their initial implantation site. Image acquisition will also introduce a small amount of uncertainty in the geometry of the fiducial group. For example, artifacts and slice thickness in CT studies can introduce uncertainty into the positions of metallic fiducials. These distortions and uncertainties in the fiducial group geometry lead to uncertainty in the registration result (Fitzpatrick et al. 1998). Several techniques can be used to reduce uncertainty associated with fiducial point-based image guidance. In order to detect rotations as well as translations more than one fiducial (preferably three or more) is needed. Implanting multiple fiducials

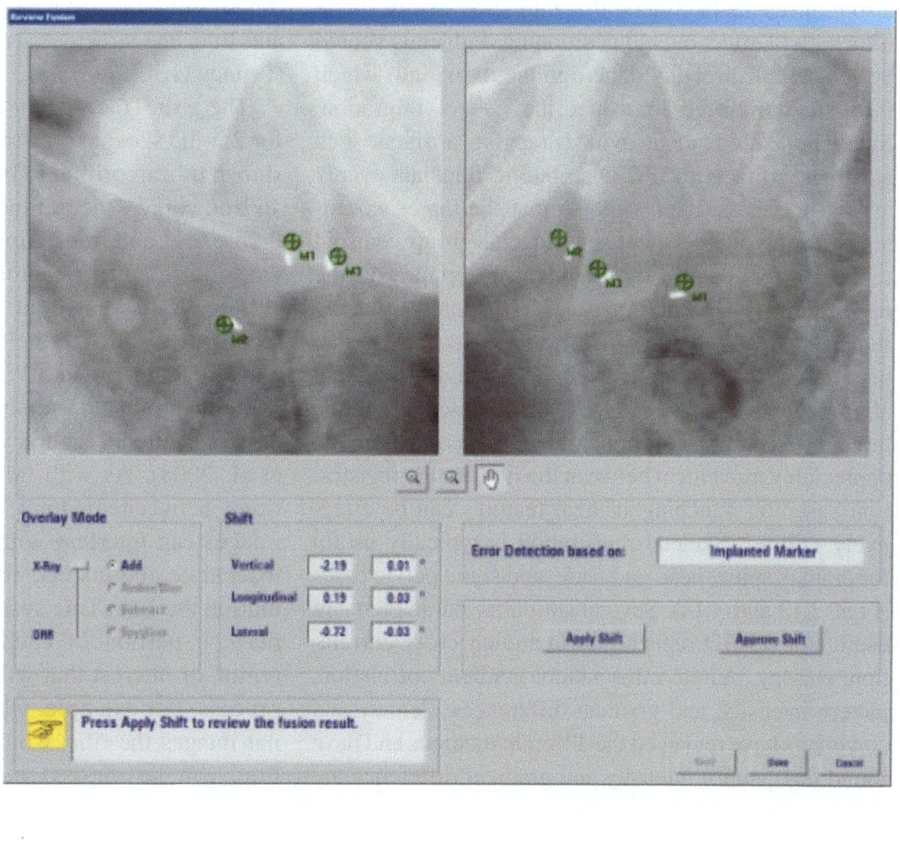

Fig. 3.11 Prostate fiducials as seen on ExacTrac kV X-ray. The crosshairs are positioned over the markers for fiducial-based registration

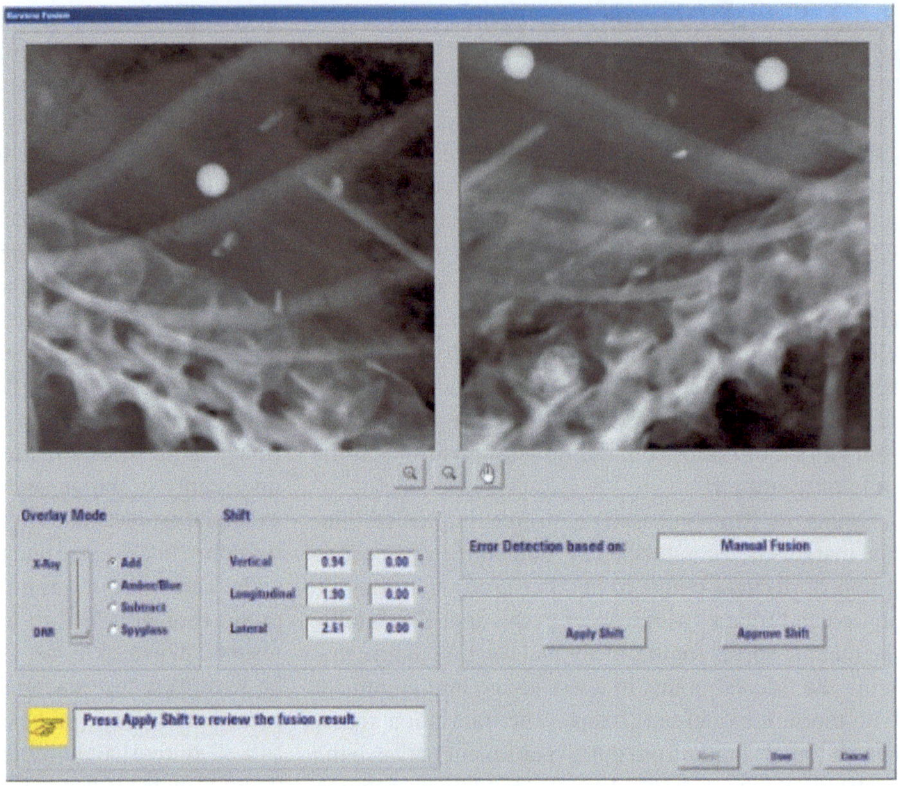

Fig. 3.12 Fiducials in lung as seen from ExacTrac kV X-rays. The white circles are ExacTrac IR markers attached to the patient's chest

also reduces the likelihood that migration of any single fiducial will affect overall positioning. Fiducials should be selected that readily adhere to the tissue into which they are introduced to reduce the risk of migration. Small fiducials tend to reduce imaging artifacts such as streak artifacts in CT. Distributing fiducials evenly around the target if possible so that the target isocenter is closely aligned with the fiducial group centroid reduces errors caused by rotational uncertainty in the registration (Fitzpatrick et al. 1998). Finally, spacing fiducials as widely as practicable reduces rotational uncertainty for targets that require accurate rotational alignment (Fitzpatrick et al. 1998). In cases where the target is fixed to or near bone such that there will not be appreciably movement between the two, image registration based on matching skeletal features can be effectively utilized. Skeletal registration is typically useful for cranial, spine, head and neck, and some pelvic cases (Figs. 3.13 and 3.14). Several similarity parameters are useful for 2D/3D registration including cross correlation, entropy, mutual information, gradient correlation, pattern intensity, and gradient differences. Penney and coworkers have reviewed the different methods and have found that pattern intensity and gradient difference are robust similarity measures when soft tissue structures and thin line structures are present within the images (Penney et al. 1998).

The ExacTrac system utilizes gradient correlation for 2D-3D skeletal registration. Phantom studies have shown this algorithm to be quite accurate. Agazaryan and coworkers determined that rotational errors of 0.2° ± 0.1° and translational errors of 0.1 mm can be detected in spine phantom setup with the ExacTrac system (Agazaryan et al. 2008). In a study of cranial localization for frameless SRS treatments with Novalis Radiosurgery, Wurm and coworkers, using a skull phantom, determined that overall ExacTrac system translational accuracy was 1.04 ± 0.47 mm (Wurm et al. 2008). As with fiducial registration, deformations between anatomy in the reference and test images can interfere with the registration producing inaccurate alignments. To reduce the effect of deformation the ExacTrac system allows users to block or mask a portion of each image leaving a reduced region of interest that will be used in the registration process. For example, when registering thoracic spinal images the ribs, which can move due to respiration, can be masked out and not included in the

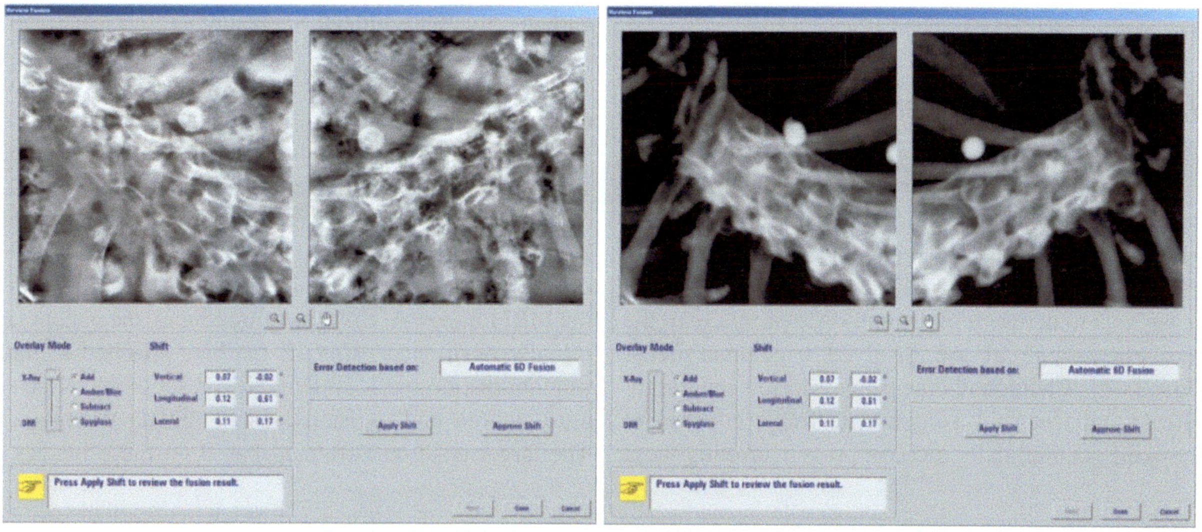

Fig. 3.13 Spine anatomy as seen on ExacTrac X-ray images and corresponding digitally reconstructed radiograph (DRR)

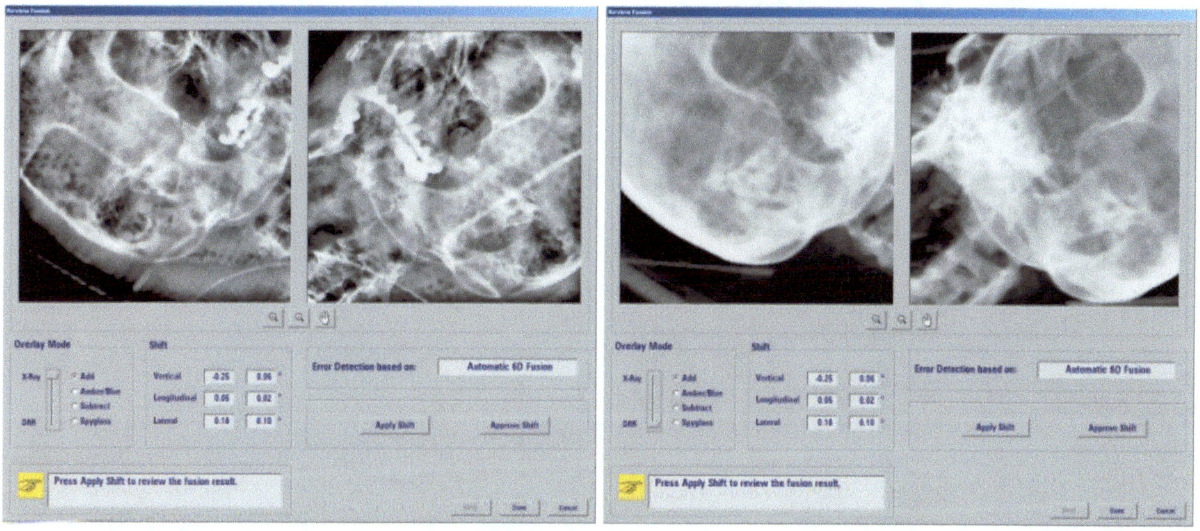

Fig. 3.14 Cranial anatomy as seen on ExacTrac kV X-rays

information for registration. Thus, changes in rib position due to respiration will not affect registration and accurate targeting of the spine. Three-dimensional imaging techniques such as CBCT that can directly image soft tissues are useful for soft tissue tumors that are not strongly associated with skeletal anatomy. In many instances, the target can be located directly in the CBCT image and registered manually with the simulation CT scan. Treatment of tumors in the thorax and abdomen are good candidates for this type of image guidance. Automatic registration can also be performed on the Varian system. The registration is accomplished via maximization of mutual information (Wells et al. 1996). In the current software version, this is a global registration in as much as it uses all anatomy in both images to accomplish the match. Therefore, the registration result must be verified visually to ensure that the region containing the target is properly aligned between the two images. In cases where a patient's anatomy has significant deformation relative to the simulation images the registration may fail to give a reasonable result.

3.5 Case Illustrations

3.5.1 Frameless Trigeminal Treatment

Single fraction radiosurgery is a treatment option offered at our institution for patients with intractable trigeminal neuralgia. The treatment is performed using a small diameter (4 mm) radiosurgery cone with six or seven arcs to deliver a maximum dose of 90 Gy to the root entry zone of the involved trigeminal nerve (Fig. 3.15). Traditionally the patients have been immobilized and localized using a rigid frame attached to the skull via minimally invasive posts. Currently these patients are immobilized using moldable masks and localized using ExacTrac.

The patient is CT scanned in the Brainlab head and neck localization system using contrast with 1.5-mm slice thickness. The simulation CT scan is registered with a constructive interference steady state (CISS) MRI image on which the trigeminal nerve can easily be identified (Chavez et al. 2005). Contrast enhancement of arteries in the CT scan aid reliable registration with the MRI images. At the time of treatment, the patient is initially positioned using IR markers attached to the immobilization mask system. Next a set of kV X-rays are acquired and registered using 2D/3D technique. The target position is refined based on these images.

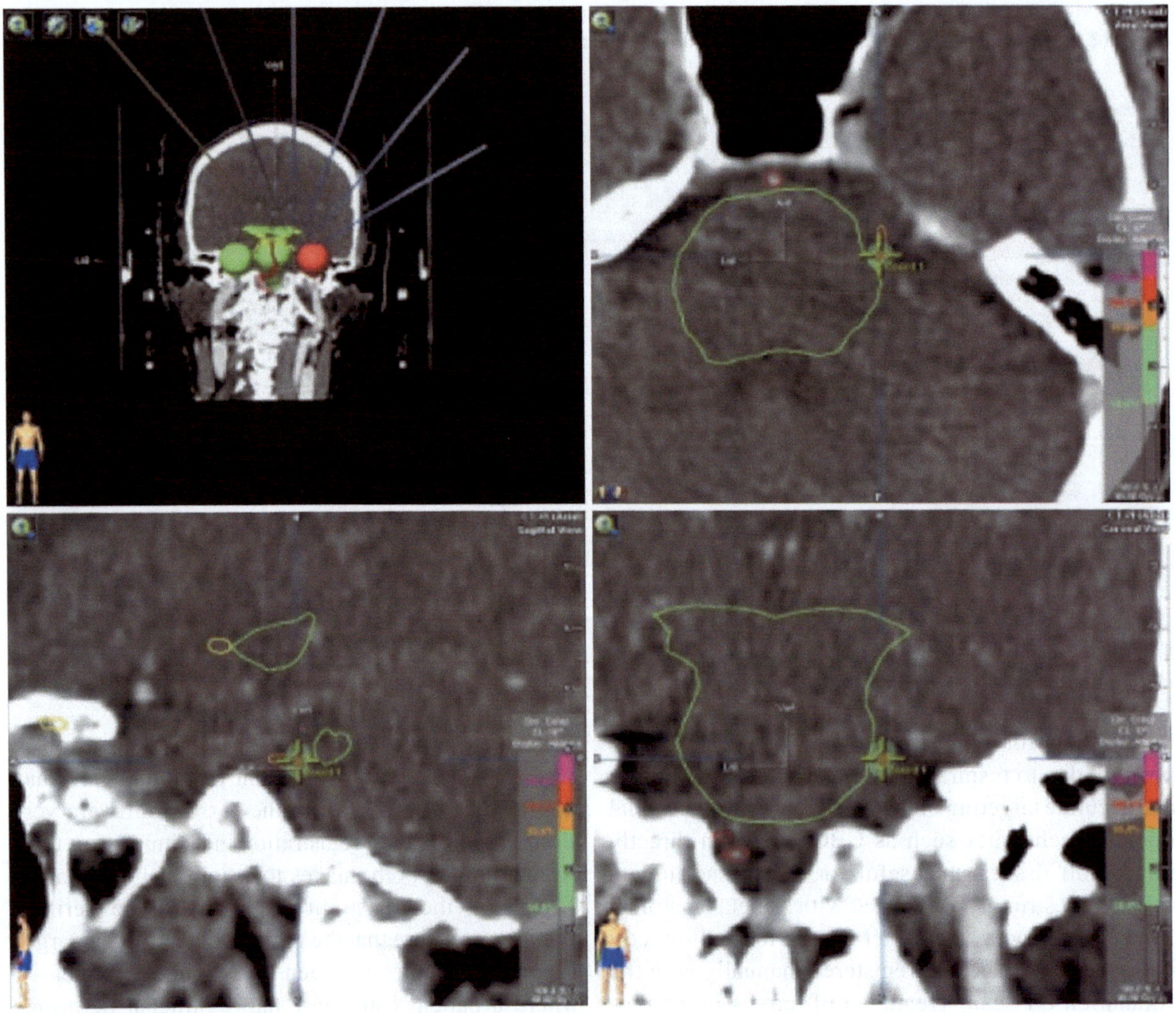

Fig. 3.15 Trigeminal plan as seen on computed tomography (CT) and constructive interference steady state (CISS) magnetic resonance imaging (MRI)

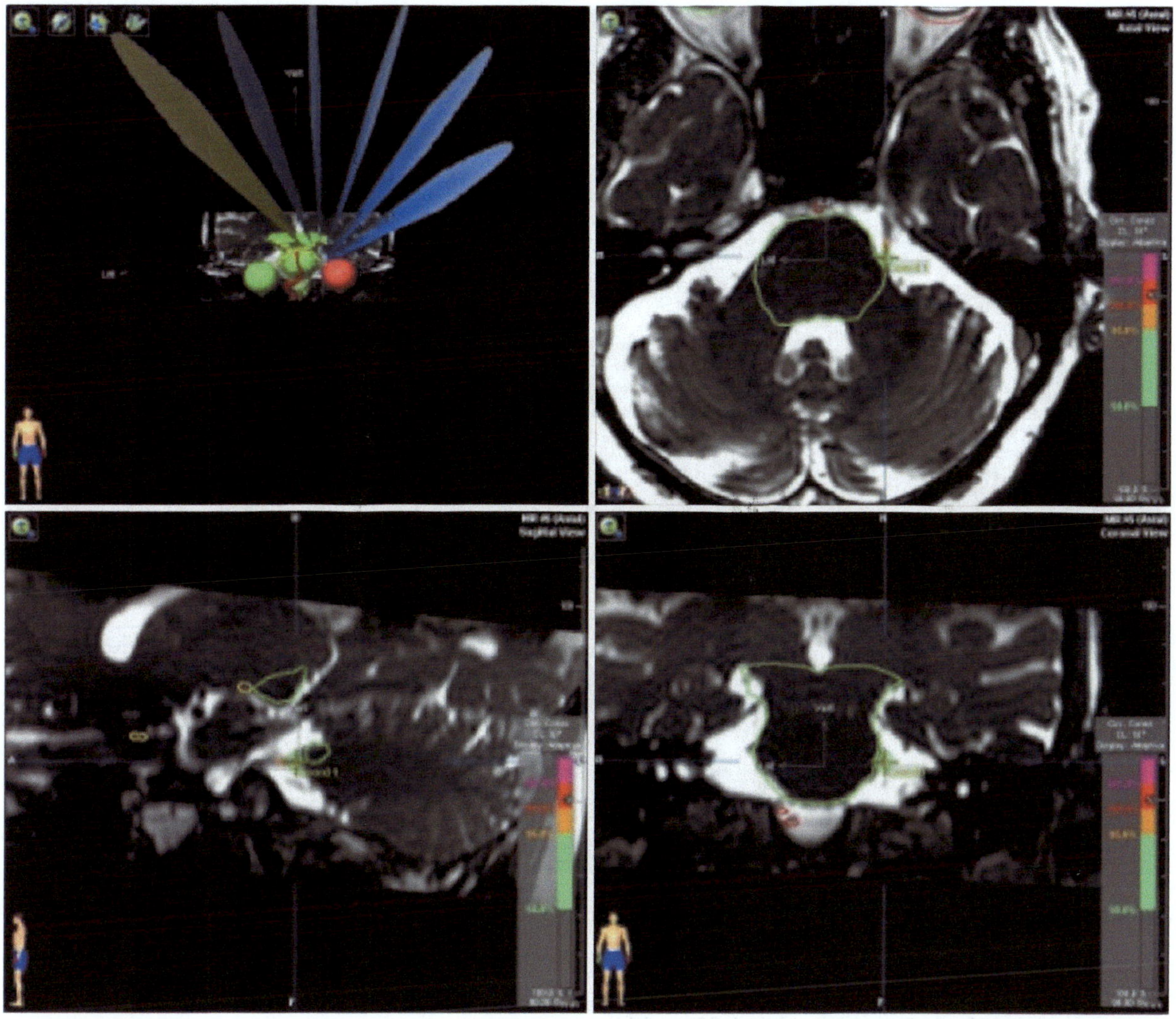

Fig. 3.15 (continued)

CBCT is then acquired as an independent verification of the setup. Finally, a verification set of images is acquired with ExacTrac before the first arc is delivered. No shifts will be necessary following verification unless the patient has moved within the mask. Preceding each subsequent arc a verification set of ExacTrac images is acquired with full 6D registration. Unlike the rigid frame system, the mask system allows some patient movement (Murphy et al. 2003). Imaging between each arc allows us to detect and correct for any patient movement that occurs during a delivery. If ExacTrac detects target movement more than 0.5 mm, the patient is repositioned and another set of verification images is acquired before treatment continues. Each arc takes approximately 3 min to deliver. The total treatment delivery time using this technique is approximately 45 min including time for setup, imaging, and corrections.

3.5.2 Spinal Radiosurgery

Single fraction spinal radiosurgery is performed at our institution for a number of indications including spinal mets, schwannomas, and AVMs. Dose is delivered either by arcs (dynamic conformal arcs or Rapid Arc) or by static intensity modulated fields (Fig. 3.16). Spine metastases are typically treated 12–16 Gy in a single fraction while limiting the cord dose. Following the practice at

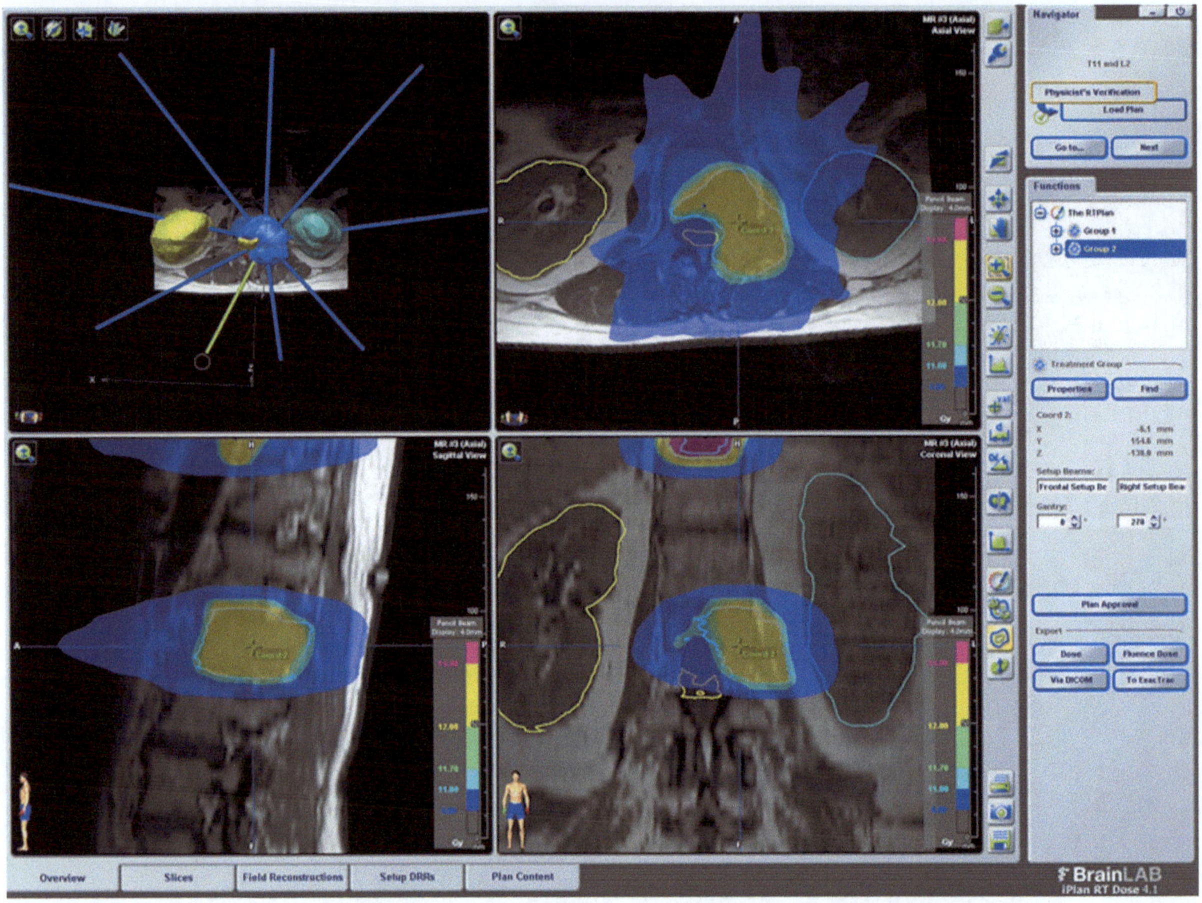

Fig. 3.16 Example spine plan with 12 Gy dose (Spine Plan.JPG)

Henry Ford Hospital, we contour the cord 6 mm superior and 6 mm inferior to the tumor and limit 90% of this volume to receive less than 10 Gy (Ryu et al. 2007).

Spine radiosurgery patients are immobilized in Body Fix Blue Bags (Elekta) and imaged with 1.5-mm thick CT images. MRI scans are also acquired and fused to the simulation CT scan for target identification and contouring. At the time of treatment, the patients are repositioned on the treatment couch using IR reflective markers for initial positioning. An initial pair of kV X-ray images are acquired and fused to the simulation images to refine the setup.

Couch shifts necessary to bring the target into proper alignment are performed and a set of verification images are acquired to confirm proper alignment has been performed. Similar to trigeminal treatments, a full set of verification images are acquired before each arc or field to detect and correct for small shifts that the patient may make during treatment.

3.5.3 Lung SBRT

For limited stage NSCLC or small peripheral mets to the lung hypofractionated SBRT treatment may be indicated. A typical lung SBRT treatment at our institution consists of three fractions of 18 Gy to a total of 54 Gy. The treatment plan consists of coplanar dynamic conformal arcs or in cases where normal tissue sparing is paramount we will treat with coplanar intensity modulated fields (Fig. 3.17).

Before simulation, two to three radiopaque fiducial markers may be implanted near the tumor. These markers can be visualized on both CT and planar kV imaging studies. A 4D CT scan is acquired for target contouring purposes along with a standard "free breathing" scan that is used as the reference simulation scan for treatment planning. The 4D CT acquisition is reconstructed at 0%, 50%, and 100% phases of the respiratory cycle (full exhale, mid inhale, and full

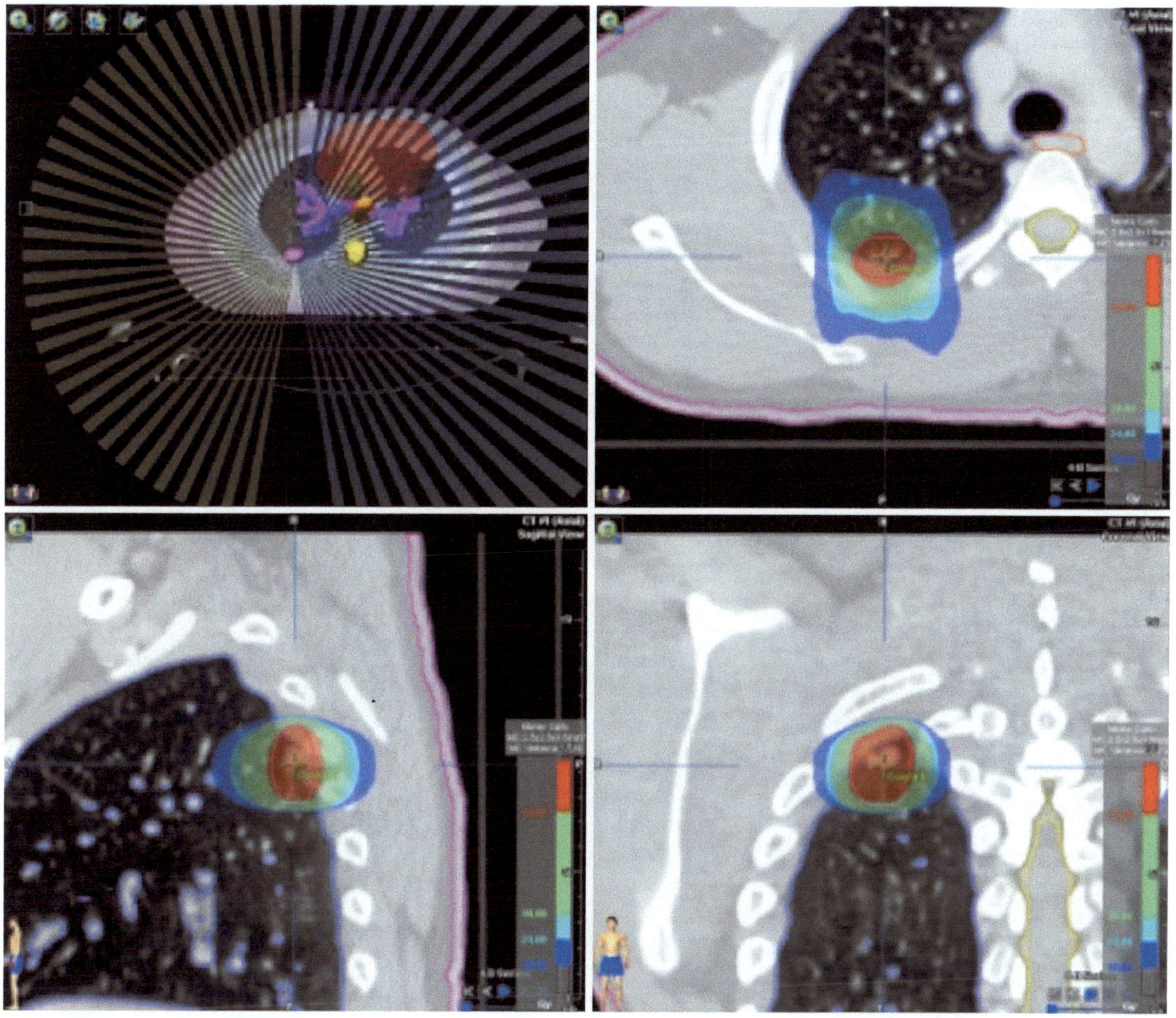

Fig. 3.17 Example Lung SBRT plan

inhale, respectively) and exported to the treatment planning system (iPlan Dose) in order to define the target ITV. The treatment plan is created with heterogeneity correction turned off for the purpose of calculating monitor units. Heterogeneity correction is turned on and Monte Carlo dose calculation available in the iPlan Dose TPS is used to evaluate the dose distribution to the target and organs at risk. At the time of treatment, the patient is repositioned on the treatment couch in the Blue Bag. ExacTrac kV X-ray images are acquired at the exhale pause for patient positioning. Fiducial match is then employed for target registration. CBCT is also acquired for lung SBRT patients as an independent verification (Fig. 3.18). The tumor is usually visible in the CBCT images and in some cases the physician will chose to modify patient positioning based on the CBCT images. In some instances, the physician has chosen not to implant radiopaque fiducial markers in the patient and for these cases CBCT is the primary image guidance method for patient setup. However, tumor motion can lead to artifacts on CBCT reconstructions that increase setup uncertainty.

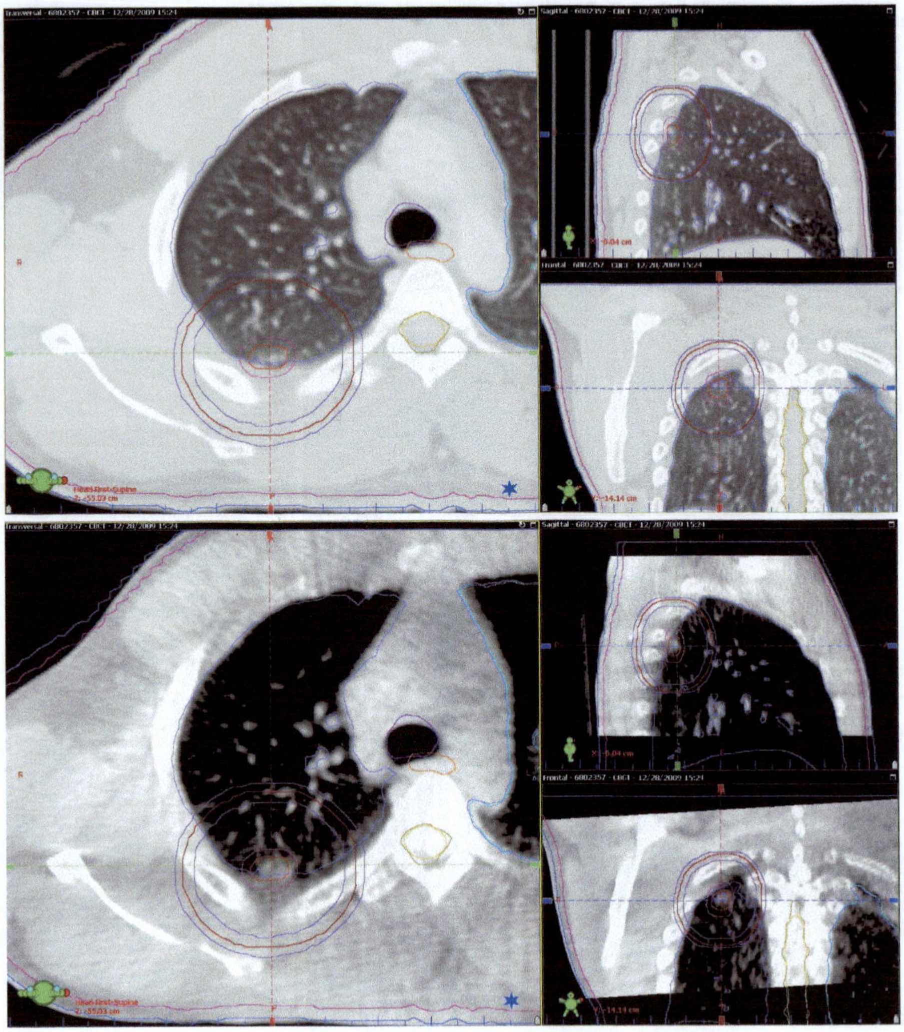

Fig. 3.18 Lung SBRT CT sim scan (*top*) and cone beam CT (CBCT) (*bottom*) showing alignment for treatment

3.5.4 Future Development

Current image guidance techniques rely almost exclusively on rigid registration methods. That is, the registration methods do not account for deformations between the reference and test images. As noted, nonskeletal human anatomy is easily deformed and methods to register images that account for these deformations can improve the accuracy of dose localization. These methods, collectively known as deformable image registration, are in development and are being tested for use in the clinic (Hill et al. 2001). Already deformable image registration is being used in some IGRS systems such as the CyberKnife (Accuray) for spine registration (Muacevic et al. 2006). Deformable image registration is also an enabling technology for another treatment advancement under active development known as adaptive radiation therapy or ART (Yan et al. 1997). Adaptive radiotherapy is a feedback-driven method of changing or adapting radiotherapy treatment plans in response to anatomic changes. ART utilizes 3D images of the patient acquired while the patient is on treatment. Dose from the current treatment plan can be calculated on the new images and evaluated. If anatomy changes during treatment due to tumor progression/regression, weight loss, and other causes the current treatment plan may no longer be optimal. A new treatment plan can be created and optimized for the patient's current anatomy. Ultimately, as technology improves and dose calculations can be carried out much faster, this process may be accomplished in real time, while the patient is being treated to account for intra-fraction patient motion (Men et al. 2009; Gu et al. 2009). In order to keep track of dose to different tissues over the course of treatment these tissues must, ideally, be registered between the original planning images and the current planning images; a task requiring rapid image segmentation and deformable registration (Gu et al. 2010).

References

Agazaryan N, Tenn SE, Desalles AA, Selch MT (2008) Image-guided radiosurgery for spinal tumors: methods, accuracy and patient intrafraction motion. Phys Med Biol 53:1715–1727

Agazaryan N, Tenn S, Selch MT, Rehs J, Erbel S, Remmert G (2009) Monoscopic imaging for intra-fraction motion management. In: 11th international congress of the IUPESM. Munich

Aird EG, Conway J (2002) CT simulation for radiotherapy treatment planning. Br J Radiol 75:937–949

Alezra D, Shchory T, Lifshitz I, Pfeffer R (2009) SU-FF-J-48: Localization accuracy of a gantry-mounted radioactive tracking system in the clinical radiation therapy environment. Med Phys 36(6):2486

Arun KS, Huang TS, Blostein SD (1987) Least-squares fitting of two 3-D point sets pattern analysis and machine intelligence. IEEE Trans PAMI 9:698–700

Biggs PJ, Goitein M, Russell MD (1985) A diagnostic X ray field verification device for a 10 MV linear accelerator. Int J Radiat Oncol Biol Phys 11:635–643

Byhardt RW, Cox JD, Hornburg A, Liermann G (1978) Weekly localization films and detection of field placement errors. Int J Radiat Oncol Biol Phys 4:881–887

Chavez GD, De Salles AAF, Solberg TD, Pedroso A, Espinoza D, Villablanca P (2005) Three-dimensional fast imaging employing steady-state acquisition magnetic resonance imaging for stereotactic radiosurgery of trigeminal neuralgia. Neurosurgery 56:E628, Discussion E

Fallone BG, Murray B, Rathee S, Stanescu T, Steciw S, Vidakovic S, Blosser E, Tymofichuk D (2009) First MR images obtained during megavoltage photon irradiation from a prototype integrated linac-MR system. Med Phys 36: 2084–2088

Fitzpatrick JM, West JB, Maurer CR Jr (1998) Predicting error in rigid-body point-based registration. IEEE Trans Med Imaging 17:694–702

Ford EC, Herman J, Yorke E, Wahl RL (2009) 18F-FDG PET/CT for image-guided and intensity-modulated radiotherapy. J Nucl Med 50:1655–1665

Fu D, Kuduvalli G (2008) A fast, accurate, and automatic 2D-3D image registration for image-guided cranial radiosurgery. Med Phys 35:2180–2194

Fuss M, Salter BJ, Cavanaugh SX, Fuss C, Sadeghi A, Fuller CD, Ameduri A, Hevezi JM, Herman TS, Thomas CR Jr (2004) Daily ultrasound-based image-guided targeting for radiotherapy of upper abdominal malignancies. Int J Radiat Oncol Biol Phys 59:1245–1256

Gu X, Choi D, Men C, Pan H, Majumdar A, Jiang SB (2009) GPU-based ultra-fast dose calculation using a finite size pencil beam model. Phys Med Biol 54:6287–6297

Gu X, Pan H, Liang Y, Castillo R, Yang D, Choi D, Castillo E, Majumdar A, Guerrero T, Jiang SB (2010) Implementation and evaluation of various demons deformable image registration algorithms on a GPU. Phys Med Biol 55:207–219

Hill DL, Batchelor PG, Holden M, Hawkes DJ (2001) Medical image registration. Phys Med Biol 46:R1–R45

Horn BKP, Hilden HM, Negahdaripour S (1988) Closed-form solution of absolute orientation using orthonormal matrices. J Opt Soc Am A 5:1127–1135

ICRU (1999) Prescribing, recording and reporting photon beam therapy (supplement to ICRU Report 50). ICRU, Bethesda

Jaffray DA, Drake DG, Moreau M, Martinez AA, Wong JW (1999) A radiographic and tomographic imaging system integrated into a medical linear accelerator for localization of bone and soft-tissue targets. Int J Radiat Oncol Biol Phys 45:773–789

Jaffray DA, Siewerdsen JH, Wong JW, Martinez AA (2002) Flat-panel cone-beam computed tomography for image-guided radiation therapy. Int J Radiat Oncol Biol Phys 53:1337–1349

Lam WC, Partowmah M, Lee DJ, Wharam MD, Lam KS (1987) On-line measurement of field placement errors in external beam radiotherapy. Br J Radiol 60:361–365

Lutz W., Winston KR, Linear accelerator as a neurosurgical tool for stereotactic radiosurgery. Neurosurgery. 1988 Mar;22(3): 454–64.

Mackie TR, Holmes T, Swerdloff S, Reckwerdt P, Deasy JO, Yang J, Paliwal B, Kinsella T (1993) Tomotherapy: a new concept for the delivery of dynamic conformal radiotherapy. Med Phys 20:1709–1719

Maes F, Collignon A, Vandermeulen D, Marchal G, Suetens P (1997) Multimodality image registration by maximization of mutual information. IEEE Trans Med Imaging 16: 187–198

Meeks SL, Bova FJ, Friedman WA, Buatti JM, Moore RD, Mendenhall WM (1998) IRLED-based patient localization for linac radiosurgery. Int J Radiat Oncol Biol Phys 41:433–439

Men C, Gu X, Choi D, Majumdar A, Zheng Z, Mueller K, Jiang SB (2009) GPU-based ultrafast IMRT plan optimization. Phys Med Biol 54:6565–6573

Milliken BD, Rubin SJ, Hamilton RJ, Johnson LS, Chen GT (1997) Performance of a video-image-subtraction-based patient positioning system. Int J Radiat Oncol Biol Phys 38:855–866

Muacevic A, Staehler M, Drexler C, Wowra B, Reiser M, Tonn JC (2006) Technical description, phantom accuracy, and clinical feasibility for fiducial-free frameless real-time image-guided spinal radiosurgery. J Neurosurg Spine 5: 303–312

Murphy MJ, Chang SD, Gibbs IC, Le QT, Hai J, Kim D, Martin DP, Adler JR Jr (2003) Patterns of patient movement during frameless image-guided radiosurgery. Int J Radiat Oncol Biol Phys 55:1400–1408

Penney GP, Weese J, Little JA, Desmedt P, Hill DL, Hawkes DJ (1998) A comparison of similarity measures for use in 2-D-3-D medical image registration. IEEE Trans Med Imaging 17:586–595

Ryu S, Jin JY, Jin R, Rock J, Ajlouni M, Movsas B, Rosenblum M, Kim JH (2007) Partial volume tolerance of the spinal cord and complications of single-dose radiosurgery. Cancer 109:628–636

Schonemann PH (1968) On two-sided orthogonal Procrustes problems. Psychometrika 33:19–33

Uematsu M, Fukui T, Shioda A, Tokumitsu H, Takai K, Kojima T, Asai Y, Kusano S (1996) A dual computed tomography linear accelerator unit for stereotactic radiation therapy: a new approach without cranially fixated stereotactic frames. Int J Radiat Oncol Biol Phys 35:587–592

Wang LT, Solberg TD, Medin PM, Boone R (2001) Infrared patient positioning for stereotactic radiosurgery of extracranial tumors. Comput Biol Med 31:101–111

Wells WM 3rd, Viola P, Atsumi H, Nakajima S, Kikinis R (1996) Multi-modal volume registration by maximization of mutual information. Med Image Anal 1:35–51

Willoughby TR, Kupelian PA, Pouliot J, Shinohara K, Aubin M, Roach M III, Skrumeda LL, Balter JM, Litzenberg DW, Hadley SW, Wei JT, Sandler HM (2006) Target localization and real-time tracking using the Calypso 4D localization system in patients with localized prostate cancer. Int J Radiat Oncol Biol Phys 65:528–534

Wurm RE, Erbel S, Schwenkert I, Gum F, Agaoglu D, Schild R, Schlenger L, Scheffler D, Brock M, Budach V (2008) Novalis frameless image-guided noninvasive radiosurgery: initial experience. Neurosurgery 62:A11–A17, Discussion A7–8

Yan D, Vicini F, Wong J, Martinez A (1997) Adaptive radiation therapy. Phys Med Biol 42:123–132

Yin FF, Guan H, Lu W (2005) A technique for on-board CT reconstruction using both kilovoltage and megavoltage beam projections for 3D treatment verification. Med Phys 32:2819–2826

Yoo S, Kim GY, Hammoud R, Elder E, Pawlicki T, Guan H, Fox T, Luxton G, Yin FF, Munro P (2006) A quality assurance program for the on-board imagers. Med Phys 33: 4431–4447

4 Frame-Based and Frameless Accuracy of Novalis® Radiosurgery

Javad Rahimian, Joseph C.T. Chen, Michael R. Girvigian, Michael J. Miller, and Rombod Rahimian

4.1 Introduction

Stereotactic Radiosurgery (SRS) is a method of precisely delivering high doses of radiation to destroy targeted areas of abnormal tissue. Stereotactic Radiosurgery (SRS) and Stereotactic Radiotherapy (SRT) are effectively being used in the treatment of arteriovenous malformations (AVM), trigeminal neuralgia (TN), and malignant or benign brain tumors, while minimizing the amount of radiation delivered to surrounding normal tissue (Khan 2003). Over 50 years ago the first trigeminal neuralgia case was treated radiosurgically by Lars Leksell (Leksell 1951). Leksell developed the SRS procedure to destroy dysfunctional loci using Orthovoltage X-rays, and particle accelerators. He subsequently introduced the Gamma Knife™ (Elekta, Stockholm, Sweden) device using 60Co sources (Leksell 1968). Linear Accelerator (LINAC) based SRS technique was first proposed by Borje Larsson in 1974 (Larsson et al. 1974). This technique is based on methods of geometric superposition, using at least 300° of multiple non-coplanar arcs converged at the target to give a spherical dose distribution with rapid dose fall-off. LINAC-based SRS systems, such as the X-knife™ (Radionics, Burlington, MA, USA) system, are more common than Gamma Knife systems, and can be less expensive. The clinical differences between Gamma Knife systems and LINAC-based systems are insignificant. Both systems use stereotactic frames for immobilization and localization. The frame-based procedure involves placement of a stereotactic frame on the patient's skull, localization of the target coordinates using an imaging technique, treatment planning, and finally the treatment delivery. There are two advantages to the frame-based SRS technique, i.e., sub-millimeter geometric accuracy of treatment delivery system, and high conformity with steep dose gradients. Various SRS techniques have been developed and clinically used. These include Gamma Knife, LINAC-based SRS, frameless SRS[3] (Cyberknife®, Novalis® Radiosurgery), and charged particle accelerators such as proton beam SRS (Khan 2003).

Recent advances in frameless stereotaxy and image-guidance enable us to perform most if not all SRS procedures without the placement of a stereotactic head frame on the patient's skull. Rather, a proprietary aquaplast head mask and a frameless image-guided radiosurgery system (IGRS) are used.

J. Rahimian (✉)
Department of Radiation Oncology, Southern California Permanente Medical Group, 4950 Sunset Blvd, 90047 Los Angeles, CA, USA and
Department of Radiation Oncology, University of California, Los Angeles, CA, USA
e-mail: javad.x.rahimian@kp.org

J.C.T. Chen
Department of Neurological Surgery, Southern California Permanente Medical Group, Los Angeles, CA, USA and
Department of Neurological Surgery, University of Southern California, Los Angeles, CA, USA

M.R. Girvigian
Department of Radiation Oncology, Southern California Permanente Medical Group, 4950 Sunset Blvd, 90047 Los Angeles, CA, USA and
Department of Radiation Oncology, University of Southern California, Los Angeles, CA, USA

M.J. Miller
Department of Radiation Oncology, Southern California Permanente Medical Group, 4950 Sunset Blvd, 90047 Los Angeles, CA, USA

R. Rahimian
Department of Biological Sciences, University of California, Irvine, CA, USA

A.A.F. De Salles et al. (eds.), *Shaped Beam Radiosurgery*,
DOI: 10.1007/978-3-642-11151-8_4,

This method requires the full integration of advanced imaging, noninvasive immobilization, infrared cameras, patient positional tracking, a 6-Dimensional (6-D) Robotic couch, and organ motion-management methods. The proper integration of these methods has resulted in fundamental changes in implementation, therapeutic strategies, and approaches of stereotactic radiosurgery. With the introduction of IGRS systems, such as ExacTrac® X-Ray (Brainlab AG, Feldkirchen, Germany), we are able routinely to identify and treat very small lesions throughout the body. Furthermore, utilizing various medical imaging techniques such as PET/CT imaging, MRI and/or angiography, we may be able to detect these lesions and treat them with an IGRS technique. Thus, the aim to dispense with the invasiveness of the stereotactic head-frame fixation, without losing the inherent accuracy of the frame-based stereotactic approach. This allows patients to lie comfortably on the procedure table without anesthesia. Furthermore, the ExacTrac frameless IGRS system monitors and compensates for patient's intra-fraction movements.

New techniques have been developed for image-guided radiosurgery based on either stereoscopic or cone beam CT imaging systems, and utilization of 6-D robotic movement of the patient couch system. Other techniques based on surgical implantation of fiducial markers into the target lesions or nearby anatomy, have also been clinically introduced and utilized.

Precise deliveries of prescribed dose, regardless of frame based SRS or frameless IGRS technique, requires a comprehensive quality assurance program. There are numerous publications investigating the spatial accuracy and quality assurance of frame based Gamma Knife (Khan 2003), and LINAC-based SRS systems (Drzymala et al. 1994; Ramaseshan and Heydarian 2003; Verellen et al. 1999; Yeung et al. 1994). We have outlined comprehensive quality assurance in our previous publication for the frame-based SRS system, Novalis® Radiosurgery (Brainlab AG, Feldkirchen, Germany) (Rahimian et al. 2004).

The purpose of this study is to evaluate in a phantom the accuracy of the Novalis Radiosurgery image-guided frameless system, and compare it with the previously reported (Rahimian et al. 2004) frame-based results. We will outline a quality assurance program based on our experimental findings.

4.2 Materials and Methods

We have evaluated the accuracy of the Novalis Radiosurgery system, which is a dedicated LINAC-based radiosurgery system with stereoscopic imaging capabilities, infrared camera monitoring, and the capability of tracking patient intra-fraction movements. The system consists of two floor-mounted kilovolt X-ray tubes, two ceiling-mounted amorphous silicon flat panel detectors, and two ceiling-mounted infrared (IR) cameras for IR–based positioning and tracking of the patients. The patient couch top movement is controlled by a robotic mechanism, and is capable of moving the patient in position in 6-D. The ExacTrac Version 5.0.2 6-D image-guided frameless system enables us to image the patient at any couch position using the Frameless Radiosurgery Positioning Array (FRPA) (Fig. 4.1), which corrects for possible patient intra-fraction movements or couch isocentricity errors. FRPA consists of six infrared markers with fixed geometry, without the infrared imaging ambiguities occasionally encountered with manual placement of the markers directly on the mask system. This system helps to eliminate the micro-adjustments required between couch positions for the frame-based system that were necessary previously.

The Novalis Radiosurgery Linear Accelerator system has a stringent isocentricity standard with maximum field size of $10 \times 10\ cm^2$, equipped with 26 pairs of leaves in the micromultileaf collimator (mMLC). The leaf width of the mMLC is 3.0, 4.5, and 5.5 mm, respectively. In addition, cones of various sizes ranging from 4 mm to 20 mm can be attached to the gantry. The planned radiation dose is delivered using multiple arcs converged at the isocenter using either cones or mMLC. Furthermore, conformal static beams, Intensity Modulated Radiosurgery (IMRS) planning, and dynamic

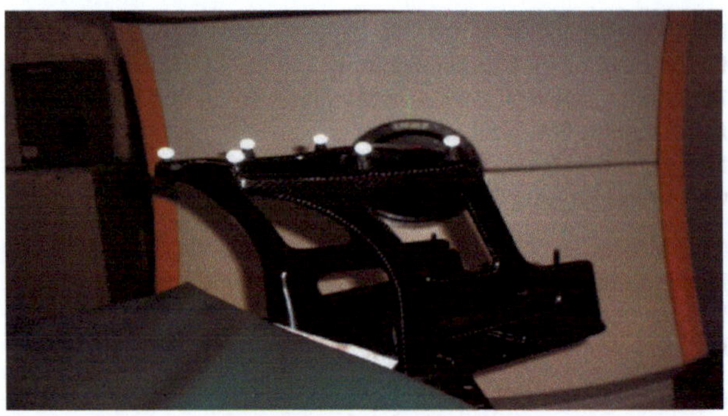

Fig. 4.1 The Brainlab frameless radiosurgery positioning array

conformal arc dose delivery are available (Chen et al. 2007). The total spatial error in the Novalis Radiosurgery technique is accumulated by target localization using a combination of the following methods (Rahimian et al. 2004): MR imaging, CT imaging, MR-CT fusion, CT-Angiography image fusion, dose planning, mechanical errors, gantry isocentricity, patient positioning, patient intra-fraction movements, target positioning overlays, and the radiation dose delivery system.

4.2.1 Phantom Measurements

The isocentric accuracy of the gantry (Fig. 4.2), as well as the patient support system (Fig. 4.3) was measured with the Winston-Lutz test. The details of the test are described elsewhere (Khan 2003; Lutz et al. 1988). Given an acceptable mechanical isocentricity, the lasers are set to converge at the isocenter. For this test, the Brainlab Isocenter Phantom (I.P., Fig. 4.4) is placed on the couch at the isocenter using the room lasers. The Brainlab I.P. consists of three horizontal and vertical crosshairs to align it with the room ceiling and wall lasers. In addition, the I.P. has five infrared markers that are used to calibrate the IR–based positioning and tracking of the 6-D robotic couch system. We use the I.P. to measure the overall accuracy of the IR-based 6-D Robotic couch-infrared camera system, as well as the ExacTrac stereoscopic X-ray-DRR auto fusion software. The Brainlab I.P. is positioned randomly on the couch. The pendant controlling the robotic system is pressed to take the phantom to the isocenter. The deviation of the position of the cross-hairs of the phantom from the lasers' cross-hairs are measured four times, and averaged to determine the spatial deviations introduced by the IR-actuated 6-D positioning and tracking system.

As part of daily calibration, we use the Brainlab X-ray phantom (Fig. 4.5) to calibrate the ExacTrac

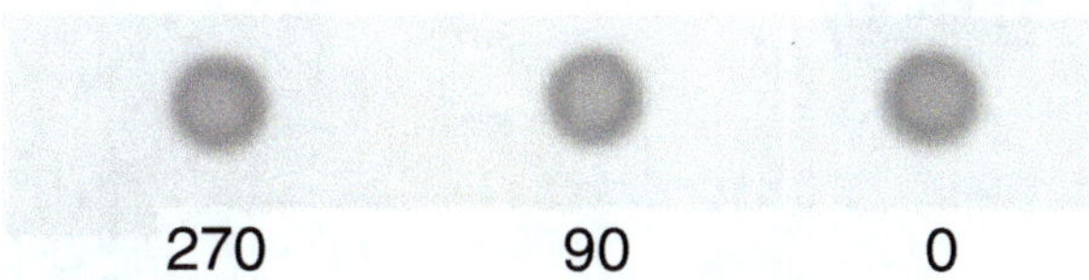

Fig. 4.2 Winston-Lutz test of the Gantry rotation at 270°, 0°, and 90° positions

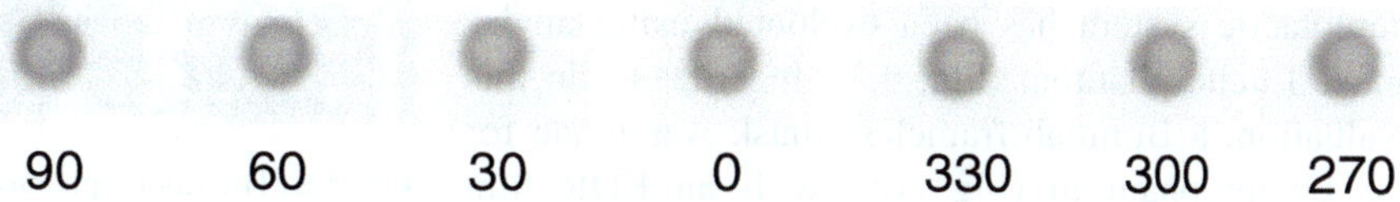

Fig. 4.3 Winston-Lutz test of the couch rotation at 0°, 90°, 63°, 36°, and 10° couch positions

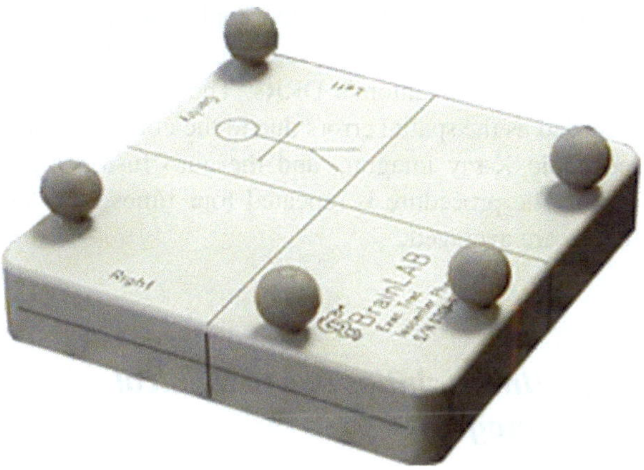

Fig. 4.4 Brainlab isocenter phantom

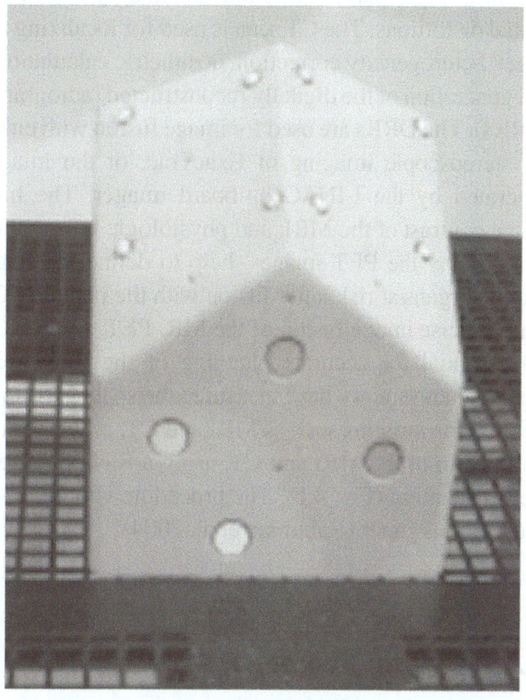

Fig. 4.5 Brainlab's X-ray–detectors calibration phantom

X-ray and the amorphous silicon detector system. The ExacTrac imaging system and its auto-fusion software must be evaluated after satisfactory daily calibration of the X-ray-detector system. This calibration is performed by positioning the I.P. carefully at the isocenter, and then taking two stereoscopic images of the phantom. These stereoscopic images are then auto fused with the phantom's DRRs. The shifts are then recorded as the spatial errors due to the composite stereoscopic X-ray imaging, and the auto fusion algorithm. The procedure is repeated four times, and the results are averaged.

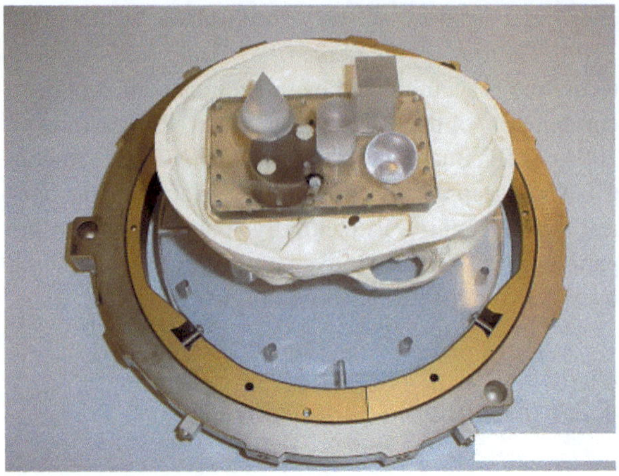

Fig. 4.6 Radionics' geometric phantom

4.2.2 Uncertainties due to Medical Imaging

Precise definition of a target for treatment by stereotactic radiosurgery requires medical images with thin slice thickness, high spatial resolution, and images free of any spatial distortions. The CT scan is used for localizing the target, heterogeneity correction, dosimetric calculations, and generation of the digitally reconstructed radiographs (DRRs). The DRRs are used for image fusion with either the stereoscopic imaging of ExacTrac, or the images generated by the LINAC on-board imager. The high image contrast of the MRI, and physiologic information provided by the PET images, help to define the target and the organs at risk, after fusion with the planning CT scan. Precise image fusion of the MR, PET, and the CT are essential for accurate planning of the SRS treatments. Therefore, we have measured the spatial errors of the imaging systems such as MRI and CT, as well as the auto fusion of the MRI and CT, using a Radionics geometric phantom (Fig. 4.6). The procedure is outlined in our previous paper (Rahimian et al. 2004).

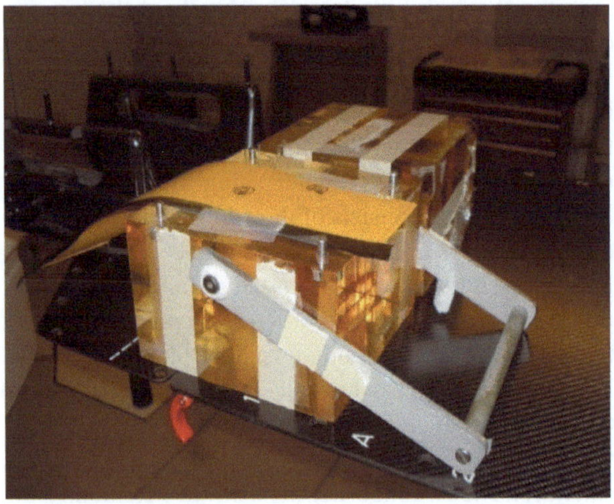

Fig. 4.7 The Lucite phantom with an EDR film

4.2.3 Overall Geometric Accuracy Test

The overall geometric accuracy of our Novalis Radiosurgery version 5.02 image guided frameless stereotactic system has been evaluated using an inhouse Lucite phantom (Fig. 4.7). In order to do this evaluation, a Brainlab frameless mask was made for the Lucite phantom (Fig. 4.8) with an EDR film

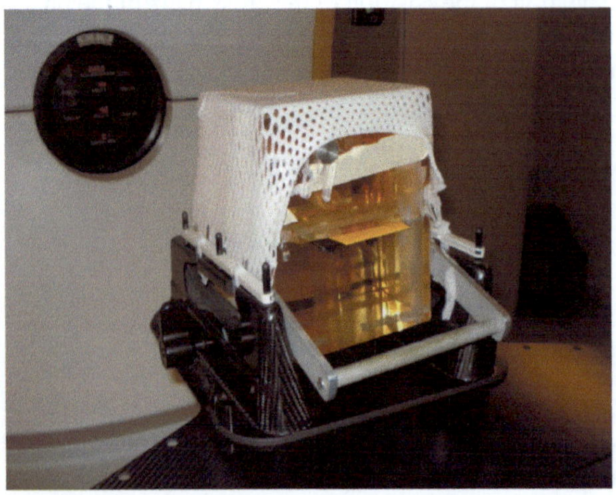

Fig. 4.8 The Lucite phantom with a Brainlab mask

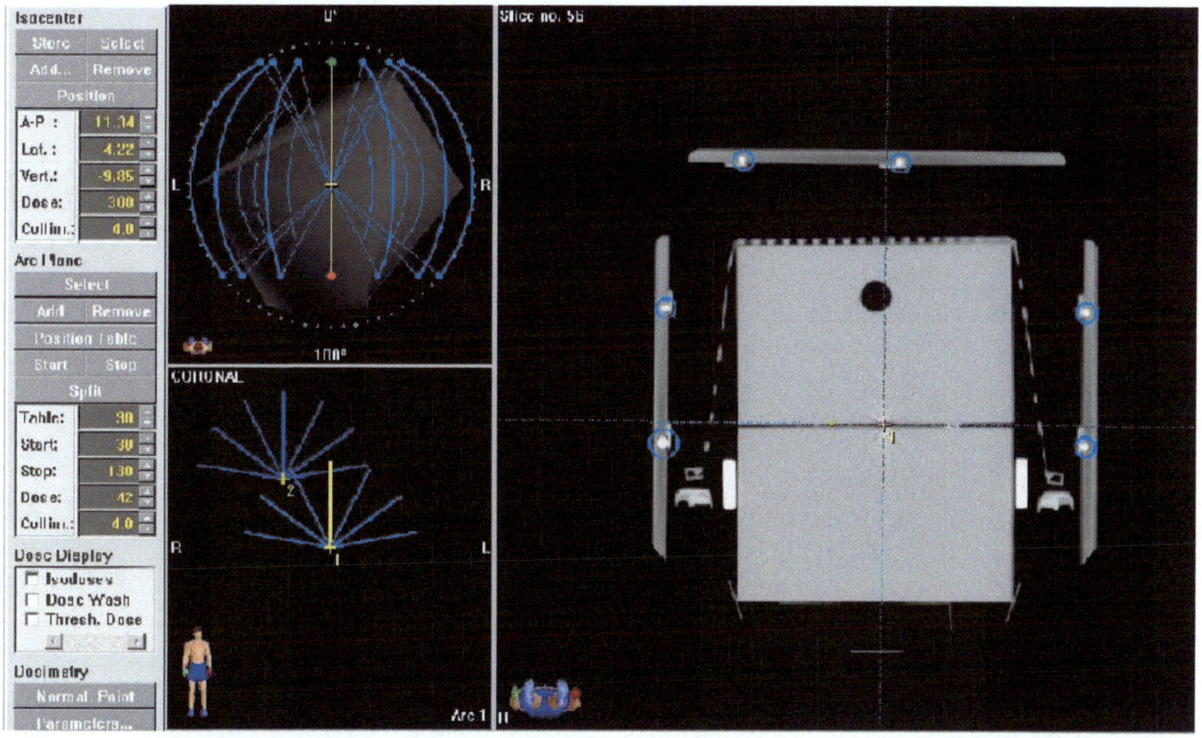

Fig. 4.9 Seven circular arcs with 4 mm cone, and 300 cGy at the isocenter was planned for each of the two BB markers

sandwiched between the two parts of the phantom. A target defined by a 1.5 mm diameter spherical BB marker was taped on the film parallel to the X-Y plane of the stereotactic coordinate system inside the phantom. CT images of the phantom were acquired by a GE 16-slice CT system (GE Medical Systems, Waukesha, Wisconsin) using a 512×512 matrix and a 1.25 mm slice thickness, with the Brainlab head and neck localizer. The BB marker was defined as the target on the CT images (Fig. 4.9). The same protocol used in our institution for the treatment of trigeminal neuralgia (Chen et al. 2004) was used (7 non-coplanar circular arcs with a 4 mm cone) to plan and treat the marker using the stereoscopic image guidance. Localization of the targets in the phantom is done with the Brainlab treatment planning system (BrainSCAN® version 5.31). The treatment was given using the IGRS system of the Brainlab treatment planning system. The phantom was imaged at each couch angle, and the images were fused with the DRR's using the auto fusion option of the ExacTrac software. The ExacTrac X-ray correction was applied until the phantom was within an acceptance criterion of 0.5 mm, and 0.5°. A second set of stereoscopic images were taken for verification before each arc exposure of the EDR film. The EDR film was developed, and scanned in high resolution using Vidar Dosimetry-Pro scanner, and RIT Technology software. The same technique was repeated for a second target. The displacement of the centroid of the optical density on the film, and the position of the marker was calculated using the RIT Technology software, and averaged for the two targets.

4.3 Results

Table 4.1 summarizes the average, and the standard deviations of all the components contributing to inaccuracies of the frameless IGRS system. The cumulative root mean square (RMS) value of the inaccuracies involving the frameless IGRS procedure was calculated to be 0.64±0.39 mm. This includes inaccuracies involving gantry isocentricity, CT and MR imaging, MR-CT fusion, stereoscopic imaging, DRR auto fusion, and IR–based positioning and tracking of the 6-D robotic couch system. The overall

Table 4.1 Mean errors for frameless IGRS

Descriptions	Mean error (mm)	S.D.
MR	0.22	0.10
CT	0.12	0.14
MR-CT fusion	0.41	0.30
Gantry isocentricity	0.30	0.10
Couch isocentricity	–	–
Lasers	–	–
Target positioner box	–	–
Exactrac X-ray system and auto-fusion	0.22	0.10
Infrared actuated 6-D robotics	0.20	0.10
Total rms frameless IGRS	0.64	0.39
Average geometric error in this study	0.48	0.55

accuracy of the frameless system was verified with the two targets defined in our Lucite phantom, using a treatment plan with seven non-coplanar circular arcs, and a 4 mm cone as described above. A geometric accuracy of 0.48 ± 0.55 mm was achieved on two different targets treated in the phantom (Fig. 4.10). The geometric accuracy of the Novalis Radiosurgery frameless system depends significantly on the landmarks used for auto fusion in the ExacTrac TM software. Table 4.2 summarizes our previously published (Rahimian et al. 2004) average, and standard deviations of all the components contributing to inaccuracies of the Novalis Radiosurgery frame-based system. Table 4.3 compares the overall precision of the Novalis frame-based, and frameless image guided stereotactic radiosurgery systems. There are no statistically significant differences between the overall precision of the Novalis frame-based, and the frameless IGRS systems.

4.4 Discussion

For over five decades, frame based stereotactic radiosurgery has been successfully used to treat patients with intracranial lesions and neurological disorders. There are two advantages to the frame based SRS

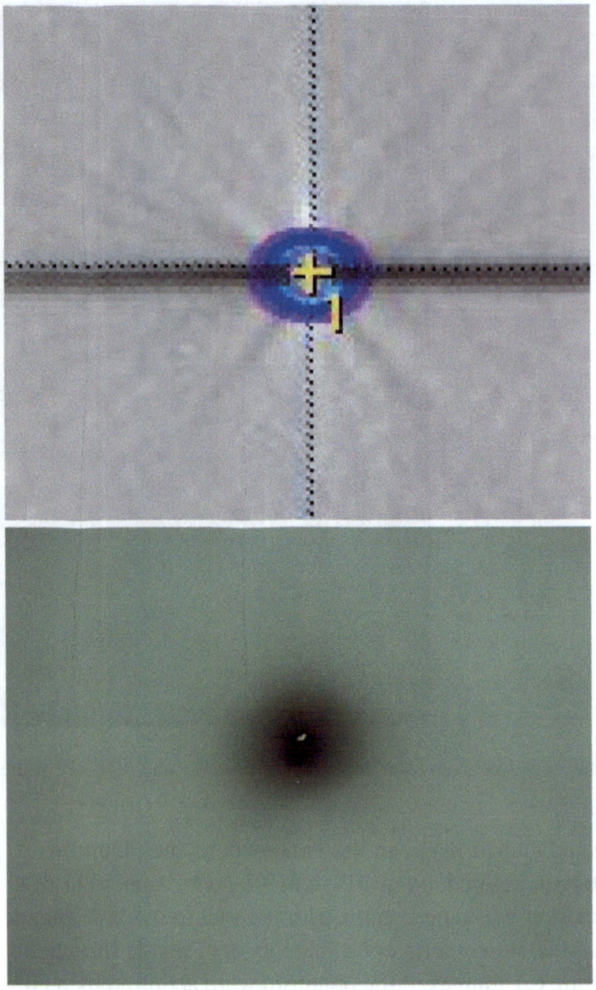

Fig. 4.10 The isodose plan (*top*) and the film developed after exposure to 300 cGy. The PinPrick is where the BB was positioned (*bottom*)

Table 4.2 Frame-based mean errors

Descriptions	Mean (Rahimian et al. 2004) error (mm)	S.D.
MR	0.22	0.10
CT	0.12	0.14
MR-CT fusion	0.41	0.30
Gantry isocentricity	0.30	0.10
Couch isocentricity	–	–
Lasers	0.20	0.10
Target positioner box	0.20	0.10
Total frame based rms with couch microadjustments	0.63	0.39

Table 4.3 Frame-based and frameless error comparison

Descriptions	Mean error (mm)	S.D.
MR	0.22	0.10
CT	0.12	0.14
Fusion	0.41	0.30
Gantry isocentricity	0.30	0.10
Couch isocentricity	0.60	0.15
Lasers	0.20	0.10
Target positioner box	0.20	0.10
Exactrac X-ray system and auto-fusion	0.22	0.10
Infrared actuated 6-D robotics	0.20	0.10
Total errors, frame based	*0.87*	*0.41*
Total frame based error with couch microadjust ments	0.63	0.39
Total error frameless IGRS	0.64	0.39
Average geometric error in this study	0.48	0.55

technique, i.e., sub millimeter geometric accuracy of treatment delivery system, and high conformity with steep dose gradients. However, there are many disadvantages. Frame placements require application by a neurosurgeon under local anesthesia, and nursing staff time. The frame is placed on a long lever couch mount. Heavy breathing during treatment can move the couch mount relative to the gantry isocenter, introducing possible inaccuracies due to patient motion. Frame-based head fixation can be painful, and the limitation of head movement can be intolerable to many patients. In general, one cannot treat lesions with a fractionated treatment schedule when using stereotactic frame placement. Furthermore, there is a risk of epidural hematoma, cranial fracture, and cerebrospinal fluid (CSF) leak following the application of head pins. Finally, laceration of the scalp with patient movement is possible, especially in young children. The advantages of a frameless image guided radiosurgery system include the following:

- Non-invasive treatment
- Minimal to no pain
- No need for anesthetics or sterilization of equipment
- Improved patient workflow
- Flexibility in treatment planning and treatment delivery
- Fractionated treatment is possible
- Collision of the mask system with the gantry is not a limiting factor with the Novalis Radiosurgery frameless system, thus utilization of the full gantry range of motion around the patient is possible for treatment delivery.
- The frameless mount and array is placed on the table top or table extension, limiting possible inaccuracies due to patient motion related to heavy breathing during treatment.

Each step in the chain of SRS treatment planning, from start to finish, may introduce an error. The overall precision of the SRS technique cannot be better than the least accurate single step in the chain of an optimal treatment plan (Mack et al. 2002). Thus, stringent geometric accuracy and precision is required for treating stereotactic radiosurgery patients. The spatial errors are best estimated using a systematic approach to isolate independent contributing factors (Yeung et al. 1994). Therefore, in this study we have determined the inaccuracies in each step of the procedure for the Novalis Radiosurgery frameless system. These inaccuracies include medical imaging, MR-CT image fusion, treatment planning, gantry isocentricity, stereoscopic imaging, ExacTrac auto fusion algorithm, infrared camera system, and finally the IR–based positioning and tracking of the patient 6-D robotic couch system. We then compared these results with our data for the frame-based treatment published previously. Table 4.3 summarizes various parameter accuracies of the Brainlab frame-based and frameless SRS systems. The geometric accuracy of the frameless image guided system showed comparable results with the frame based SRS system. The greatest overall error is due to MRI-CT fusion and lower resolution MRI images. We have improved the spatial errors introduced by the MRI imaging and MRI-CT fusion by acquiring our MRI images using 512×512 matrices with a slice thickness of 1.0–1.2 mm, using a smaller field of view, and 3-D volumetric acquisition utilizing General Electric's MRI 3-D Spoiled Gradient-Echo Pulse Sequence (SPGR) or 3-D Fast Imaging Employing Steady-State Acquisition (FIESTA) pulse sequences (Chen et al. 2007).

Our treatment results of the 2 BB targets placed on the EDR film, based on our IGRS trigeminal neuralgia protocol, revealed an accuracy of 0.48 ± 0.55 mm. This is in line with total system RMS value of 0.64 ± 0.39 mm calculated for the Novalis Radiosurgery frameless radiosurgery system. Figure 4.11 shows the isocenter on the pre, and post MR images of a patient treated for left trigeminal neuralgia using 4 mm cone, and 90 Gy to the isocenter. The figure shows the enhancement of the left trigeminal nerve. The geometric deviation between the isocenter, and the maximum MR contrast enhancement after the treatment measured to be 0.83 mm confirming the geometric accuracy of the frameless technique (Rahimian et al. 2009). Further, Fig. 4.12 shows the before, and 2 month after-images of a 0.17 mL (4 × 7.3 mm) lesion treated with a dose of 25 Gy to the isocenter, confirming the accuracy of the hit using the Novalis Radiosurgery frameless radiosurgery system (Chen et al. 2007, 2009).

Wurm et al. (2008) performed routine phantom studies and reported an overall system accuracy of 1.04 ± 0.47 mm; the average in plane deviations for the *x* and *y* axis of 0.02 ± 0.96 mm and 0.02 ± 0.70, respectively. In this study, they have excluded the errors introduced by the MRI image distortions and the MRI-CT fusion from the chain of events for treatment planning.

Vinci et al. (2008) evaluated the accuracy of coplanar conformal therapy using ExacTrac image guidance by measuring the two-dimensional (2D) dose distributions in cranial orthogonal anatomical planes. Dose distributions were measured in the axial, sagittal, and coronal planes using a CIRS (Computerized Imaging Reference Systems, Inc.) anthropomorphic head phantom with a custom internal film cassette. These isodose distributions were compared with the isodose planned using BrainSCAN planning software. Their study showed systematic errors in the measurement technique were 0.2 mm or less along all three anatomical axes. Random error averaged 0.29 ± 0.06 mm for the ExacTrac acceptance criteria of 1 mm/1°,

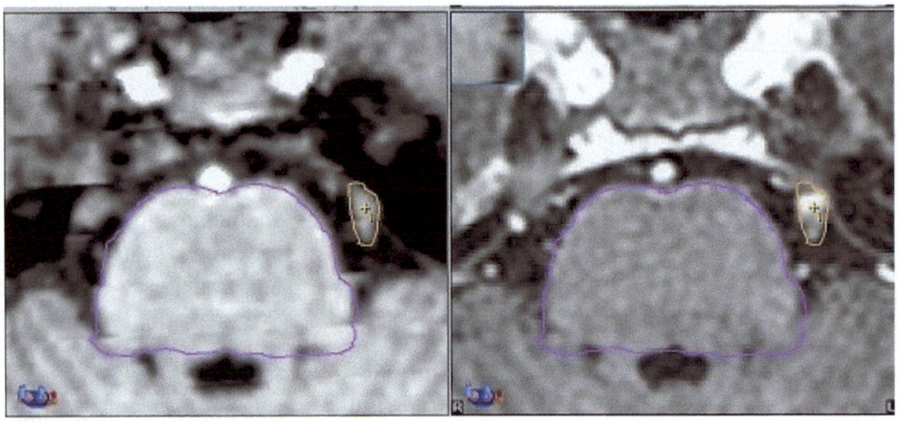

Fig. 4.11 The pre and post treatment images of the left trigeminal neuralgia. Note the enhancement of the nerve after the treatment with 90 Gy to the isocenter

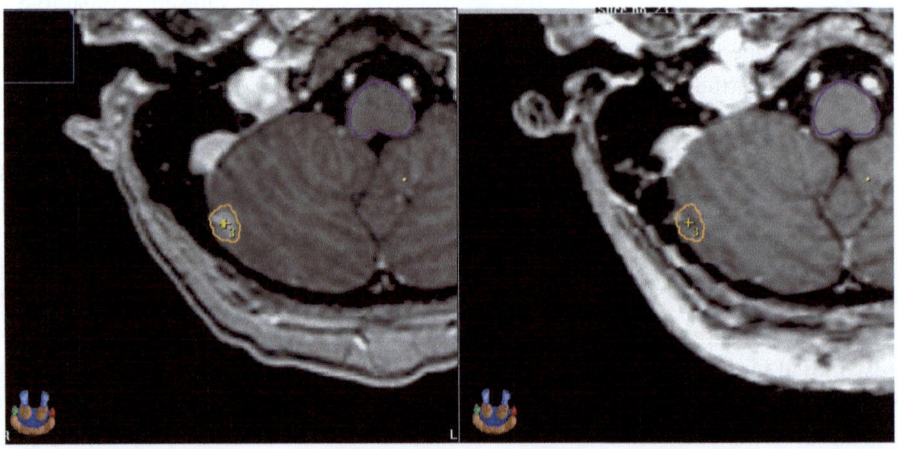

Fig. 4.12 The pre and post frameless IGRS treatment images of a 0.17 mL (4.0 mm × 7.3 mm) lesion with 25 Gy to the isocenter. The post treatment images are taken 2 month after the treatment

and 0.15±0.02 mm for the acceptance criteria of 0.4 mm/0.4°. Alignment error (displacement between midpoints of planned and measured 70% isodose contours) exhibited measured values as great as 0.9, 0.3, and 1.0 mm along the P–A, R–L, and I–S axes, respectively. The authors concluded that their goal of achieving accuracy of delivery of 1 mm or better in each of the three major anatomical axes was almost, but not quite achieved. This was not because of the accuracy of the image guidance system, but likely due to inaccuracy of laser isocenter and other systematic errors.

The literature supports our own results, that the greatest inaccuracies in the entire SRS technique are fusion inaccuracies, gantry isocentricity, and MRI distortions (Guideline 2002; Brommeland and Hennig 2000; Wood and Henkelman 1999). MRI scans are prone to image artifacts and image distortions due to an inhomogeneous magnetic field, ferromagnetic materials, spatial variations in magnetic susceptibility, and nonlinear magnetic field gradients (Wood and Henkelman 1999). It has been previously shown that the T1 MRI image sequence is more prone to distortion than the T1 3D Spoiled Gradient-Echo Pulse Sequence (SPGR) and the 3D Fast Imaging Employing Steady-State Acquisition (FIESTA) sequences, or their equivalent (Mack et al. 2002). We have a quality assurance program in place for our MRI system that includes imaging a MRI phantom to show the resolution, and distortion. Comprehensive tests of the magnetic field uniformity, as well as gradient field measurements are performed by a GE service man bimonthly or as needed. Image fusion programs in the planning system, and at the ExacTrac computer, can potentially introduce errors in the target positioning due to misregistration. In this study we have evaluated the effects of medical imaging, and image fusion on the overall spatial accuracy of stereotactic radiosurgery.

The LINAC is tested daily for accurate isocentricity as part of the quality assurance program using the Winston-Lutz test (Khan 2003; Lutz et al. 1988). The gantry isocentricity can drift over time (we experienced it ranging from 0.10 mm to 0.60 mm), over our 0.30 mm tolerance. In addition, Table 4.4 outlines our quality assurance frequencies as well as the tolerance limits. The overall RMS values of all the tolerances, excluding the couch, are calculated to be 0.68 mm. The recommended tests, and their frequencies, as well as the tolerances in Table 4.4 may be used as a quality assurance guide. Adherence will ensure higher quality treatments.

Table 4.4 Quality assurance frequency and tolerance

Descriptions	Frequency	Max. error tolerance
MRI image resolution and distortion phantom	Monthly	≤0.30 mm
MRI external magnetic field homogeneity	Bimonthly	–
MRI gradient *X*, *Y*, *Z* plane calibration checks	Bimonthly	≤0.30 mm
CT image resolution phantom	Annually	≤0.30 mm
Gantry isocentricity Winston-Lutz test	Daily	≤0.30 mm
Infra-red camera calibration	Daily	≤0.20 mm
6-D robotic couch and ExacTrac auto-fusion	Daily	≤0.25 mm
Novalis couch isocentricity (IGRS corrects for Couch)	Monthly	≤0.75 mm
Cumulative RMS of tolerances for frameless IGRS system		≤0.68 mm

In our experience the bi-valve style mask (Fig. 4.13) with a mouth piece, is a better mask to immobilize the patients for frameless radiosurgery. Other mask systems have shown patient motion inside the mask. Figure 4.14 shows the daily treatment isocenter marked on the mask due to the patient movement inside the mask. The patient was treated by image guidance however, correcting for his intra-fraction movements.

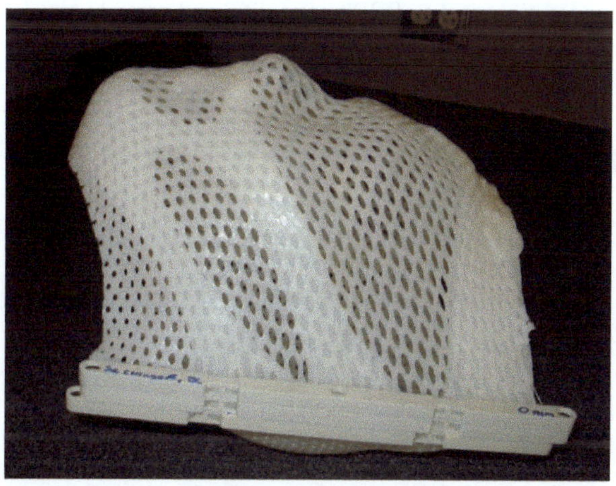

Fig. 4.13 The Brainlab bi-valve IGRS mask with mouthpiece

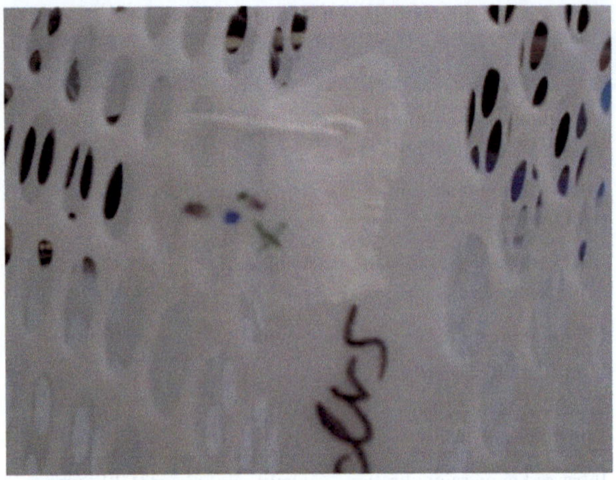

Fig. 4.14 Patient fractional day to day isocenter movement marked on the mask. Patient intra-fraction movements were corrected by image guidance

4.5 Conclusion

The accuracy of target localization achieved with the Brainlab frameless technique approaches that attainable with invasive stereotactic frames. However, since the ExacTrac™ auto fusion software relies heavily on the bony landmarks, special care must be taken with the frameless system by taking at least one image for positioning and one image for verification per bed position, to ensure accurate treatment of the patients. Our highest spatial errors were due to inaccuracies with image fusion, gantry isocentricity, and image distortions. This is in line with the published data (Ryken et al. 2001; Vinci et al. 2008; Wurm et al. 2008). A comprehensive quality assurance program is outlined in this paper to ensure high quality SRS treatments, and provide possibly better clinical outcomes.

References

ACR practice Guideline (2002) ACR practice guideline for the performance of Stereotactic radiosurgery. ACR practice Guideline. pp 567–572

Brommeland T, Hennig R (2000) Mechanical accuracy of a new stereotactic guide. Acta Neurochir (Wien) 142(4):449–454

Chen JCT, Girvigian M, Greathouse H, Miller M, Rahimian J (2004) Treatment of trigeminal neuralgia with linear accelerator radiosurgery: initial results. J Neurosurg 101(Suppl 3):346–350

Chen JCT, Rahimian J, Girvigian MR, Miller MJ (2007) Contemporary methods of radiosurgery treatment with the Novalis linear accelerator system. Neurosurg Focus 23(6):E4

Chen JCT, Bugoci DM, Girvigian MR, Miller MJ, Arellano A, Rahimian J (2009) Control of brain metastases using Novalis ExacTrac frameless image-guided radiosurgery. Neurosurg Focus 27(6):E6

Drzymala RE, Klein EE, Simpson JR, Rich KM, Wasserman TH, Purdy JA (1994) Assurance of high quality linac-based stereotactic radiosurgery. Int J Radiat Oncol Biol Phys 30(2):459–472, Sep 30

Khan FM (2003) Physics of radiation therapy, 3rd edn. Lippincott Williams & Wilkins, Philadelphia, pp 507–520, Chapter 21

Larsson B, Lidén K, Sarby B (1974) Irradiation of small structures through the intact skull. Acta Oncol 13(6):512–534

Leksell L (1951) The stereotactic method and radiosurgery of the brain. Acta Chir Scand 102:316–319

Leksell L (1968) Cerebral radiosurgery. I. Gammathalamotomy in two cases of intractable pain. Acta Chir Scand 134: 585–595

Lutz WA, Winston KR, Maleki N (1988) A system for stereotactic radiosurgery with a linear accelerator. Int J Radiat Oncol Biol Phys 14:373

Mack A, Czempiel H, Kreiner HJ, Durr G, Wowra B (2002) Quality assurance in Stereotactic space. A system test for verifying the accuracy of aim in radiosurgery. Med Phys 29(4):561–568

Rahimian J, Chen JCT, RAO AA, Girvigian MR, Miller MJ, Greathouse HE (2004) Geometrical accuracy of the Novalis stereotactic radiosurgery system for trigeminal neuralgia. J Neurosurg 101(Suppl 3):351–355

Rahimian J, Girvigian MR, Chen JCT, Rahimian R, Miller MJ (2009) Geometric accuracy of frameless based image guided stereotactic radiosurgery of trigeminal neuralgia using Brainlab's ExacTrac 6-D robotic system. Int J Radiat Oncol Biol Phys 75(Suppl 3):S676

Ramaseshan R, Heydarian M (2003) Comprehensive quality assurance for stereotactic radiosurgery treatments. Phys Med Biol 48:199–205

Ryken T, Meeks S, Pennington E, Hitchon P, Traynelis V, Mayr N, Bova F, Friedman W, Buatti J (2001) Initial clinical experience with frameless stereotactic radiosurgery: analysis of accuracy and feasibility. Int J Radiat Oncol Biol Phys 51(4):1152–1158

Verellen D, Linthout N et al (1999) Assessment of the uncertainties in dose delivery of a commercial system for LINAC-based stereotactic radiosurgery. Int J Radiat Oncol Biol Phys 44(2):421–433

Vinci JP, Hogstrom KR, Neck DW (2008) Accuracy of cranial coplanar beam therapy using an oblique, stereoscopic x-ray image guidance system. Med Phys 35(8):3809–3819

Wood ML, Henkelman RM (1999) Artifacts. In: Stark DD, Bradley WG (eds) Magnetic resonance imaging, vol 1, 3rd edn. Mosby, St. Louis, pp 215–230

Wurm RE, Erbel S, Schwenkert I, Gum F, Agaoglu D et al (2008) Novalis frameless image-guided noninvasive radiosurgery: initial experience. Neurosurgery 62(Supp 5):A11–18

Yeung D, Palta J, Fontanesi J, Kun L (1994) Systematic analysis of errors in target localization and treatment delivery in Stereotactic radiosurgery (SRS). Int J Radiat Oncol Biol Phys 28(2):493–498

Monte Carlo Treatment Planning

5

Matthias Fippel

5.1 Introduction

Conventional dose calculation algorithms, such as Pencil Beam (PB) are proven effective for tumors located in homogeneous regions with similar tissue consistency such as the brain. However, these algorithms tend to overestimate the dose distribution in tumors diagnosed in extracranial regions such as in the lung and head and neck regions where large inhomogeneities exist. Due to the inconsistencies seen in current calculation methods for extracranial treatments and the need for more precise radiation delivery, research has led to the creation and integration of improved calculation methods into treatment planning software. Most advanced are Monte Carlo (MC) algorithms to compensate for this under dosage in extracranial calculations and to improve radiation treatment planning accuracy for clinical practice.

MC is a stochastic method for solving complex equations numerically. MC techniques are based on pseudo random numbers generated by computer algorithms called random number generators. They are used to simulate a huge number of tracks (also called histories) of individual photons and electrons including all daughter particles. MC dose calculation requires a virtual model of the medical linear accelerator (LINAC) head including the beam collimating system. This model is based on technical information from the LINAC vendor and basic data measured on-site. MC also requires a three-dimensional CT scan of the patient's tissue to create an internal model of the patient and to calculate the dose distribution of the radiation emitted by the LINAC.

This chapter introduces the physical background to MC dose calculation developed for Radiosurgery and its integration into the treatment planning software iPlan® RT Dose from Brainlab. It allows the reader to understand the behavior of the MC algorithm and how it will be integrated into the clinical environment.

5.1.1 Background

Current cancer treatment techniques allow precise dose deposition in the target volume and an improved protection of the normal tissue. Accurate dose calculation is essential to assure the efficacy of these techniques. Conventional dose calculation methods, like the PB algorithm, are of high quality in regions with homogeneous tissue, e.g., within the brain. However, for treatments in the head and neck or in the thorax regions, i.e., in regions consisting of bone, soft tissue, and air cavities, an improved accuracy is required. For example, the PB algorithm is known to overestimate the dose in the target volume for the treatment of small lung tumors. The reason is, the PB algorithm calculates dose by scaling PB dose distribution kernels in water to take the tissue heterogeneities into account, but this method has accuracy limitations in these regions. MC dose calculation algorithms, on the other hand, provide more accurate results especially in heterogeneous regions.

M. Fippel
Brainlab AG, Kapellenstrasse 12,
85622 Feldkirchen, Germany
e-mail: matthias.fippel@brainlab.com

A.A.F. De Salles et al. (eds.), *Shaped Beam Radiosurgery*,
DOI: 10.1007/978-3-642-11151-8_5, © Springer-Verlag Berlin Heidelberg 2011

5.1.2 Monte Carlo Particle Transport Simulation

In radiotherapy, stochastic MC techniques are applied to numerically solve the transport problem of ionizing radiation within the human body. Here the radiation is decomposed into single quantum particles (photons, electrons, positrons). The motion of these particles through the irradiation device and the human tissue is simulated by taking into account the material properties of the different components of the LINAC head and the tissue properties in each volume element (voxel). The photons, electrons, and positrons interact with the electrons of the atomic shells and the electromagnetic field of the atomic nuclei. This interaction can cause ionization events. The corresponding interaction properties are based on quantum physics. For the LINAC head, these properties can be calculated using the known atomic composition of the different components; for the patient, they can be calculated based on the CT images and the Hounsfield Unit (HU) in each voxel. The interaction properties are given as total and differential cross sections. Total cross sections characterize the interaction probabilities of a particle with a given energy in a medium with a definite atomic composition. Differential cross sections characterize the probability distribution functions for the generation of secondary particles with definite secondary particle parameters like energy and scattering angle. The random numbers in a MC simulation are required to sample the specific parameters from these probability distribution functions. For example, the path length of a photon with given energy is sampled from an exponential distribution function based on the linear attenuation coefficients along the straight line from the starting position to the interaction point. The type of the photon interaction (photoelectric absorption, Compton scatter, or pair production) is sampled from the total cross sections of these processes. After sampling the secondary particle parameters from the differential cross sections, the secondary particles are simulated in a similar manner. This procedure causes a particle history beginning with an initial particle and many daughter particles in multiple generations. The process stops if the remaining energy falls below some minimum energy (also called cut-off energy) or all particles have left the region of interest. Figure 5.1 shows two examples of possible particle histories.

The MC simulation of charged particles (electrons and positrons) is more complicated and more time consuming than the simulation of photons because the number of interactions per length unit is much higher.

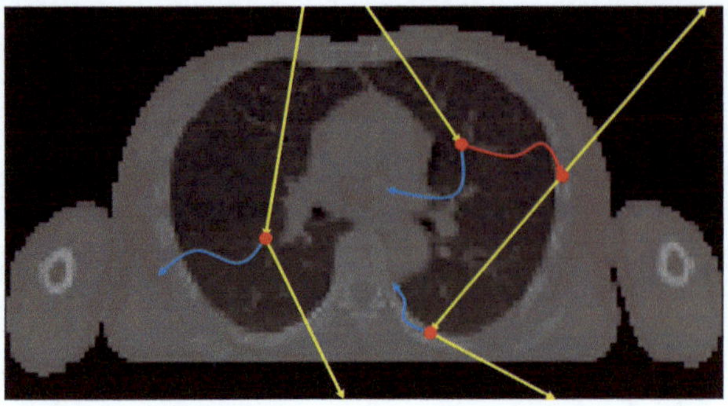

Fig. 5.1 Schematic representation of two particle history examples within the patient model. Illustrated are photons (*yellow*), electrons (*blue*), and positrons (*red*). The red dots represent interactions of the particles with atoms of the tissue

However, the so-called condensed history technique allows the simulation of charged particles in a reasonable time. Using this technique, a large number of elastic and semielastic interactions are grouped together into one particle step and is modeled as multiple-interaction with continuous energy loss of the electrons and positrons along their paths.

At each charged particle step, the amount of absorbed energy is calculated and accumulated in a three-dimensional matrix. Later this matrix is transformed into dose by dividing the energy in each voxel by the mass of the voxel. Generally, a huge number of particle histories must be simulated in a MC calculation. Otherwise, the number of energy deposition events per voxel is small. This leads to a large variance of the dose value in each voxel and the dose distribution becomes noisy. The effect of noisy dose distributions can be observed at the isodose lines if they appear too jagged. Sometimes it is difficult to distinguish between physical and statistical fluctuations. Therefore, it is important to calculate a smooth dose distribution with small statistical variance. This statistical variance per voxel decreases with increasing number of histories N_{hist} as $1/\sqrt{N_{hist}}$, i.e., the statistical variance can be decreased by a factor of 2 if the number of histories is increased by a factor of 4. This behavior contributes to the long calculation times of MC algorithms.

In general, MC dose algorithms consist of at least two components. One component is a virtual model of the treatment device. It is used as particle source and provides particle parameter (position, angle, energy, charge) distributions close to reality. The second component takes the particles generated by the first component as input. It models the particle transport through the patient and calculates the dose distribution. It is useful to subdivide the first component, the model of the LINAC head, into further subcomponents.

For more general information about all issues associated with clinical implementation of Monte Carlo-based external beam treatment planning we refer to the review by Reynaert et al. (2007) or the AAPM Task Group Report No 105 (2007). The following description illustrates MC treatment planning for Shaped-Beam Radiosurgery as implemented in the Brainlab iPlan RT Dose system.

5.2 iPlan® Monte Carlo Algorithm

5.2.1 Background

The iPlan RT Dose Monte Carlo algorithm is based on the X-ray Voxel Monte Carlo (XVMC) algorithm developed by Iwan Kawrakow and Matthias Fippel (Kawrakow et al. 1996; Fippel et al. 1997; Fippel 1999; Fippel et al. 1999; Kawrakow and Fippel 2000; Fippel et al. 2003; Fippel 2004).

This MC algorithm consists of three main components (see Fig. 5.2). The first component is used as particle source. It models the upper part of the LINAC head (target, primary collimator, flattening filter) and generates photons as well as contaminant electrons from the corresponding distribution. The particles are then transferred to the second component, the model of the collimating system. Depending on the field configuration, the particles are absorbed, scattered, or passed through. The surviving particles are transferred to the patient dose computation engine. In this third component, the radiation transport through the patient geometry is simulated and the dose distribution is computed. In the following sections, the three components of iPlan MC are characterized in more detail.

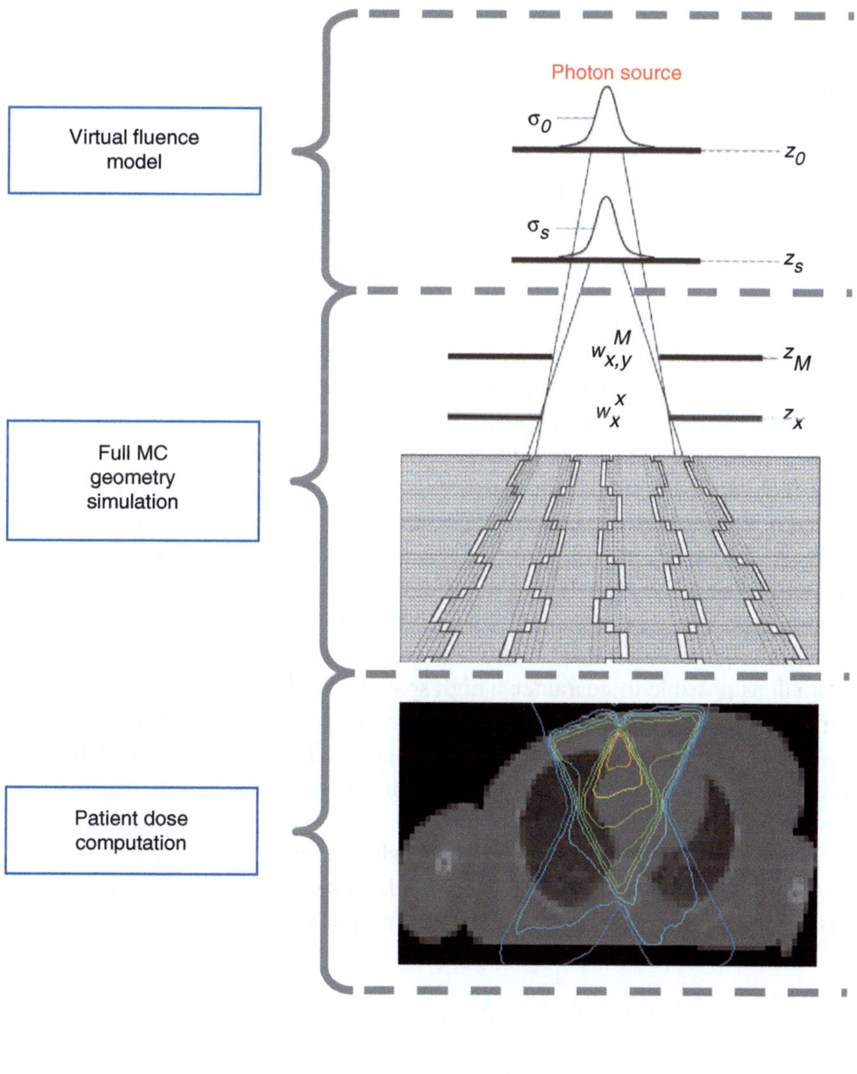

Fig. 5.2 Components of the iPlan Monte Carlo dose engine

5.2.2 Virtual Energy Fluence Model (VEFM)

The geometries of the target, the flattening filter, and the primary collimator do not change when the field shape is changed. Therefore, it can be assumed that the phase space of photons and charged particles above the jaws and the multileaf collimators (MLCs) is independent on the field configuration. To model this phase space, a Virtual Energy Fluence Model (VEFM) is employed. With some extensions this model is based on the work by Fippel et al. (2003).

It consists of two or three photon sources with two-dimensional Gaussian shape and one charged particle (electron) contamination source. The photon sources model bremsstrahlung photons created in the target and Compton photons scattered by the primary collimator and flattening filter materials. For the photon sources various parameters are required. For example, the distances of the sources to the nominal beam focus is either estimated or taken from the technical information provided by the LINAC vendor. The Gaussian widths (standard deviations) as well as the relative weights of the photon sources are fitted using measured dose distributions in air. Additional horn correction parameters are also fitted from these measurements. They model deviations of the beam profile from an ideal flat profile.

The measurements in air have to be performed by a qualified medical physicist in the clinic using an empty water phantom. It is necessary to measure profiles and in-air output factors (head scatter factors) for a variety of field sizes representing the range of treatment field sizes. The profiles must be measured in different directions and with different distances to the beam focus. It is recommended to use an ionization chamber with built-up cap for the measurements. The cap increases the number of electrons in the chamber with the aim of an improved measurement signal. It also removes electrons coming from the LINAC head. The cap should be as small as possible to guarantee a high spatial resolution. Therefore, it should consist of a material with high density, e.g., brass or some similar material. The thickness of the cap is estimated such that the depth of dose maximum is reached.

The measured profiles are normalized using the in-air output factors. In this way, they provide absolute dose profiles per monitor unit (MU). Then the data can be used as representation of a photon fluence distribution in air versus field size. On the other hand, based on the model assumptions a theoretical fluence distribution in air is calculated analytically. By minimizing the deviations between both distributions, the free model parameters are adjusted.

The VEFM also requires information about the photon energy spectrum as well as the fluence of charged particle contamination at the patient's surface. This information is derived from a measured depth dose curve $D_{meas}(z)$ in water for the reference field size (field size used for the dose – monitor unit calibration). The curve $D_{meas}(z)$ is used to minimize the squared difference to a calculated depth dose curve $D_{calc}(z)$. Based on the model assumptions, $D_{calc}(z)$ is given by

$$D_{calc}(z) = w_\gamma \int_{E_{\min}}^{E_{\max}} dE \; p(E)\, D_{mono}(E,z) + w_e D_e(z).$$

The set of monoenergetic depth dose curves $D_{mono}(E,z)$ in water is calculated using the MC dose engine and the geometric beam model parameters derived after fitting the measured profiles in air. The set is calculated for a table of energies reaching from the minimum energy of the spectrum $E_{\min}$ up to an energy that is somewhat larger than the maximum energy $E_{\max}$. This allows usage of $E_{\max}$ as a further fitting parameter. In contrast to the original paper (Fippel et al. 2003), the energy spectrum $p(E)$ is modeled by

$$p(E) = N\left(1 - \exp(-l\,E)\right)\exp(-b\,E), \;\; E_{\min} \le E \le E_{\max}.$$

The free parameters l, b and the normalization factor N are fitted. For $E_{\min}$ and $E_{\max}$ usually fixed values are taken, but it is possible to adjust them also, because sometimes the maximum energy of the spectrum can be different from the nominal photon energy setting in MV. The parameter w_γ is the total weight of all photon sources. It is calculated by $w_\gamma = 1 - w_e$ with w_e being the weight of the electron contamination source. The parameter w_e is also fitted using the measured depth dose in water and the formula on $D_{calc}(z)$. It requires the depth dose MC computation of a pure electron contamination source in water $D_e(z)$. Because most of the electrons originate in the flattening filter, the location of the electron source is assumed to be the foot plane of the filter. The energy spectrum of the electrons is estimated by an exponential distribution as described by Fippel et al. (2003).

5.2.3 Modeling of the Collimating System

The components of the collimating system (jaws and MLC) are modeled in different ways. The rectangle given by the positions of both jaw pairs are used to define the sampling space of the initial particles. That means only photons and electrons are generated going through the jaw opening.

The MLC is simulated with two different precision levels selected by the user of iPlan RT Dose. In the Monte Carlo Options dialog, it is possible to choose between the MLC models "Accuracy optimized" (default setting) and "Speed optimized." Depending on this selection and depending on the type of the MLC, one of the MLC models represented in Fig. 5.3 is used for the Monte Carlo simulation. The model of an ideal MLC (*upper left* MLC in Fig. 5.3) will be used, if the MLC model "Speed optimized" is selected. This model neglects both, the air gaps between neighbor leaves as well as the corresponding tongue and groove design. On the other hand, the thickness of the MLC, the widths of the leaves, the material of the leaves, and the rounded leaf tips (if available) are correctly taken into account with the "Speed optimized" selection. The influence of the "Speed optimized" MLC model on the dose accuracy depends on the beam set up. It is expected to be small for conformal beams, but it can be larger for Intensity Modulated Radiotherapy (IMRT) beams. Therefore, it is recommended to use the "Speed optimized" option only for the intermediate planning process. The final dose calculation should be performed with an "Accuracy optimized" model. The "Accuracy optimized" model always takes the correct tongue and groove design depending on the MLC type into account (see Fig. 5.3 for a representation of the different leaf designs).

The algorithm behind these models is entirely based on the work published by Fippel (2004). It is a full MC geometry simulation of the photon transport. It takes into account Compton interactions, pair production events, and photoelectric absorptions. Primary and secondary electrons are simulated using the continuous slowing down approximation. In this approach, the geometries are defined by virtually placing planes and cylinder surfaces in the 3D space. The planes (and surfaces) define the boundaries between regions of different materials. In general, MLC regions consist of a tungsten alloy and air. For these materials photon cross section tables pre-calculated using the computer code XCOM (Berger and Hubbell 1987) as well as electron stopping power and range tables pre-calculated using

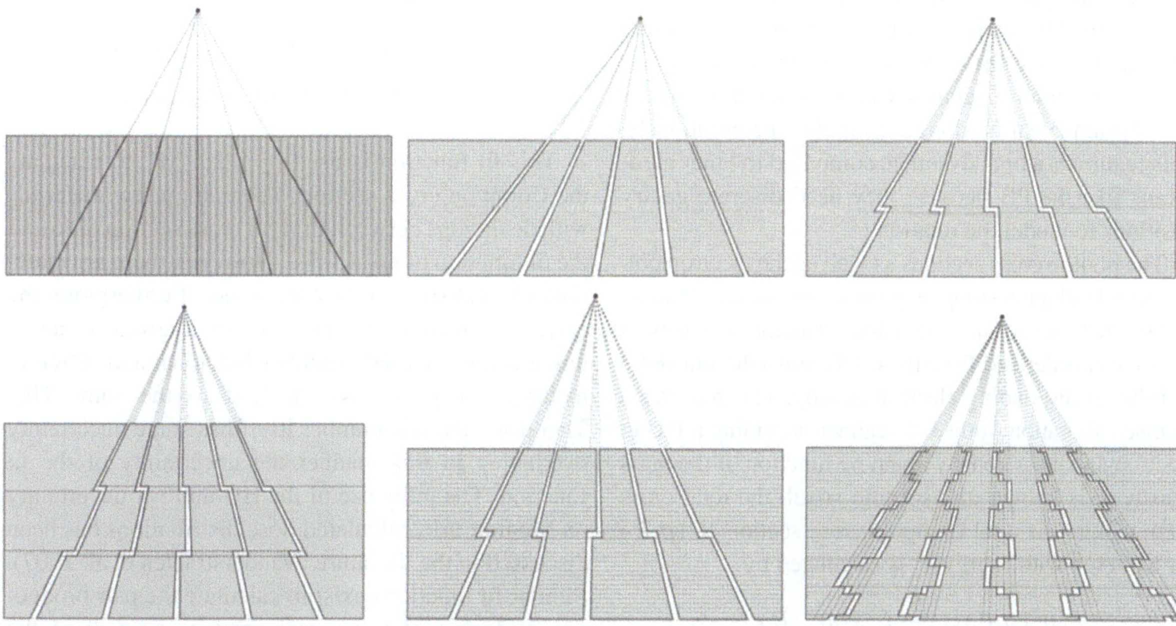

Fig. 5.3 Different multileaf collimator (MLC) leaf designs (from *upper left* to *lower right*): ideal MLC (no leakage radiation), tilted leaves (Siemens), step design (Elekta), tongue and groove design (Varian), Varian Millennium, Brainlab m3. Represented are only four leaf pairs per MLC

the ESTAR software (Berger 1993) are used. The particle ray-tracing algorithm is based on bit masks and bit patterns to identify the region indices. In extension to the original paper, further MLC models have been implemented.

5.2.4 MC Patient Dose Computation Engine

The MC algorithm to simulate the transport of photons and electrons through human tissue is based on the publications by Kawrakow et al. (1996), Fippel (1999), Kawrakow and Fippel (2000). It is a condensed history algorithm with continuous boundary crossing to simulate the transport of secondary and contaminant electrons. It takes into account and simulates delta electrons (free secondary electrons created during electron–electron interactions) as well as bremsstrahlung photons. For the MC photon transport simulations, Compton interactions, pair production events, and photoelectric absorptions are considered. Several variance reduction techniques like electron history repetition, multiple photon transport, or Russian roulette speed up the dose computation significantly compared to general-purpose MC codes, e.g., EGSnrc (Kawrakow 2000). The MC particle histories can run in parallel threads, therefore the code fully benefits from the use of multiprocessor machines. Gantry rotations (static or with dynamic leaf motion) are simulated continuously. This feature is a big advantage compared to other algorithms like the PB because they need discrete gantry positions to model the rotation.

The photon cross sections as well as the electron collision and radiation stopping powers are calculated using a 3D distribution of mass densities. The mass density in each voxel is derived from the CT Hounsfield unit (HU) and the corresponding electron density. This requires a precise calibration of the CT scanner providing a HU to electron and mass density mapping function. If the mass density ρ is known in a specific voxel, the total cross section, e.g., the total Compton cross section $\mu_C(\rho,E)$ for a photon with energy E is calculated by

$$\mu_C(\rho,E)=\frac{\rho}{\rho^W}f_C(\rho)\mu_C^W(E).$$

The function $\mu_C^W(E)$ is the tabulated Compton cross section in water, ρ^W is the mass density of water, and

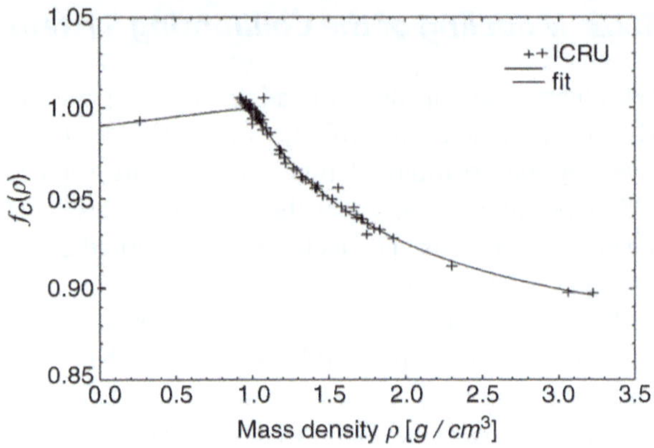

Fig. 5.4 Compton cross section ratio *versus* mass density for all materials of ICRU report 46 (crosses). The line represents a fit to these data. This function is used by iPlan MC to calculate the Compton cross section

the function $f_C(\rho)$ is a fit function based on analyzing ICRU cross section data for body tissues (ICRU 1992). The factorization into a function depending only on ρ and a second function depending only on E is an approximation. However, the data of ICRU Report 46 (1992) imply that this approximation is possible for human tissue. Figure 5.4 shows the Compton cross section ratio $f_C(\rho)$ as function of mass density ρ for all materials from ICRU Report 46. The line in Fig. 5.4 represents a fit to these data. It is given by

$$f_C(\rho)\approx\begin{cases}0.99+0.01\rho/\rho^W, & \rho\le\rho^W\\ 0.85+0.15\rho^W/\rho, & \rho\ge\rho^W\end{cases}$$

This fit function is used by iPlan MC to calculate the Compton cross section. There are a few materials with deviations between the real cross section ratio and the fit function of up to 1.5%. However, these are materials like gallstone or urinary stones. Furthermore, the correct elemental composition in a given voxel is unknown. Only a HU number is known and different material compositions can lead to the same HU. Therefore, the HU number itself has some uncertainty overlaying in this manner the uncertainty of the fit function. The influence of the HU number uncertainty on Monte Carlo calculated dose distributions has been discussed in the literature (Vanderstraeten et al. 2007). Similar fit functions exist to calculate the pair production and photoelectric cross sections as well as the electron collision and radiation stopping powers. Their dependencies on the mass density of course differ from $f_C(\rho)$.

The function $f_C(\rho)$ is also used to convert mass densities ρ into electron densities n_e or *vice versa.* The relation is given by

$$n_e = n_e^W \frac{\rho}{\rho^W} f_C(\rho)$$

with n_e^W being the electron density of water.

5.2.5 Monte Carlo and Pencil Beam

The MC dose calculation algorithm cannot be used without the PB algorithm. This is a restriction, but it has been implemented into the treatment planning software because of three main advantages:

- It allows the user to cross check the results by two almost independent dose calculations.
- It provides a smooth transition from clinical experience based on PB dose calculations to a more accurate experience based on Monte Carlo dose calculation.
- The faster PB algorithm can be used for the intermediate planning process. Later, the user can switch to Monte Carlo to fine-tune the treatment plan.

Therefore, commissioning of the MC dose calculation algorithm requires commissioning of the PB algorithm.

5.3 iPlan Monte Carlo Parameters

5.3.1 Background

The user of the software has some influence on the MC dose calculation accuracy, the dose calculation time, and the dose result type. This can be done using the Monte Carlo Options dialog. Four parameters can be influenced:

- Spatial resolution (in mm)
- Mean variance (in %)
- Dose result type ("Dose to medium" or "Dose to water")
- MLC model ("Accuracy optimized" or "Speed optimized")

5.3.2 Spatial Resolution

The spatial resolution defines the size of the internal MC dose computation grid. It does not mean however that the final MC grid size is exactly equal to the value of the parameter. The MC voxels are constructed by combining an integer number of pixels from the original CT cube. Therefore, the final sizes of the voxels are only approximately equal to the value of the spatial resolution parameter. They can also be different for the three spatial directions. Furthermore, they cannot be smaller than the initial pixel sizes. The selection of this parameter has a strong influence on the calculation time. Decreasing this parameter by a factor of 2 can increase the calculation time by a factor of about 6. A spatial resolution of 4–5 mm might be a good choice for the intermediate planning process or for large tumors and large field sizes. Final dose calculations for small tumors should be performed with a spatial resolution of 2–3 mm.

5.3.3 Mean Variance

The mean variance parameter is used to estimate the number of particle histories needed to achieve this variance per beam in percent of the maximum dose of that beam. Because everything here is normalized per beam, the final variance in the Planning Target Volume (PTV) can be smaller. For example, if we have five overlapping beams in the PTV and each beam is calculated with 2% variance, then the variance in the PTV is about 1%. In the nonoverlapping regions it remains 2%. Because of the $1/\sqrt{N_{hist}}$ law mentioned above, the calculation time increases by a factor of 4 if the mean variance is decreased by a factor of 2. The default setting is 2%; the final calculation should be 1% or smaller.

5.3.4 Dose Result Type

The iPlan RT Dose application allows the calculation of two different dose types. The default setting "Dose to medium" means real energy dose, i.e., the energy absorbed in a tissue voxel divided by the mass of the

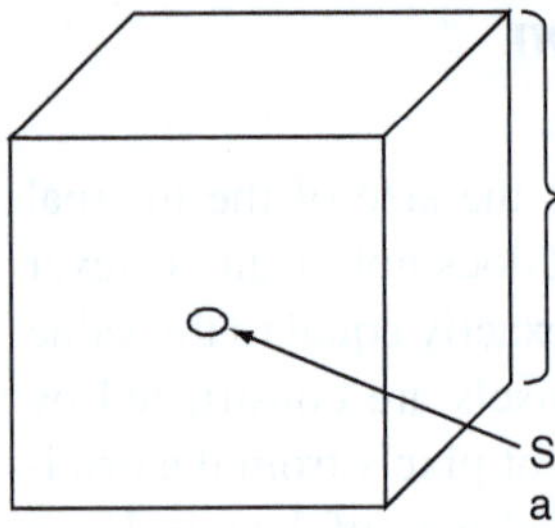

Fig. 5.5 The difference between "Dose to medium" and "Dose to water." "Dose to medium" should be calculated if the user is interested in the average dose within the whole voxel. "Dose to water" should be calculated if the user has more interest in the dose within small soft tissue cells surrounded by bone material, e.g., in bone marrow

voxel. "Dose to water," on the other hand, means energy absorbed in a small cavity of water divided by the mass of the water cavity, whereas some tissue, e.g., bone, surrounds the small cavity in the corresponding voxel (see Fig. 5.5). There is no visible difference between "Dose to medium" and "Dose to water" for most of the human soft tissue types. However, "Dose to water" can be up to 15% larger compared to "Dose to medium" for bony tissues (AAPM 2007). This is because of the high-density bone causing a higher fluence of secondary electrons in the water cavity and accordingly causing a higher dose compared to the case of the cavity filled also with bone. Therefore "Dose to water" should be selected if the user wants to know the dose in soft tissue cells within a bony structure, e.g., in bone marrow (see Fig. 5.5). The relation between "Dose to water" D_W and "Dose to medium" D_M is calculated by

$$D_W = D_M (S/\rho)^W_M,$$

with $(S/\rho)^W_M$ being the unrestricted electron mass collision stopping power ratio for water to that for the medium averaged over the spectrum of the photon beam. This ratio is approximately 1.0 for soft tissues with a mass density of about 1.0 g/cm^3. It increases up to ~1.15 for bony tissues of mass density up to 2.0 g/cm^3.

5.3.5 MLC Model Precision

The MLC model precision can be either "Accuracy optimized" or "Speed optimized." "Accuracy optimized" means, the MLC is modeled with full tongue-and-groove design. It takes into account the air gaps between neighbor leaves. The "Speed optimized" option neglects this effect. It employs a model of an ideal MLC (see Sect. 5.2.3 and Fig. 5.3). Therefore, this option shortens the calculation time. Section 5.2.3 contains more detailed information.

5.4 MC Treatment Planning in Extracranial Radiosurgery

Especially for small- and medium-sized lung tumors, conventional PB dose calculation increases the uncertainty on the calculated dose. Because of the approximated modeling of secondary electron transport, the accuracy of PB dose calculation depends strongly on the location and the size of the tumor. This is represented in Figs. 5.6–5.9. Figure 5.6 shows PB and MC dose distributions for a treatment plan with eight conformal beams of the Novalis® Radiosurgery system. The field diameters of the m3 micro-MLC range from about 40–80 mm. The monitor unit (MU) prescription is calculated based on the PB dose distribution. The dose distribution is recalculated using the MC algorithm and the same number of MU. The magnified PB isodose line representation in the left lower screen shot of Fig. 5.6 differs significantly from the MC isodose lines in the right lower screen shot. Especially at the interface between lung tissue and tumor tissue, the influence of secondary electrons on the calculated dose distribution is visible. As shown by MC, in reality there is some under-dosage at the edge of the tumor. This effect is not reproduced correctly by PB calculation. On the other hand, there is good agreement between PB and MC at the interface between soft tissue and tumor tissue. Therefore, smaller inaccuracies of the PB might be clinically insignificant. The Dose Volume Histograms (DVHs) for the Planning Target Volume (PTV) of both dose distributions is shown in Fig. 5.7. The average dose of MC compared to PB is in the order of 5% lower. That means the PB error is about 5%. Figure 5.8 shows a second treatment plan calculated for 11 beams of the Novalis Radiosurgery system. In contrast to Fig. 5.6, here the size of the tumor is smaller leading to average field diameters of about 30 mm. Furthermore, this time the tumor is located almost in the center of one

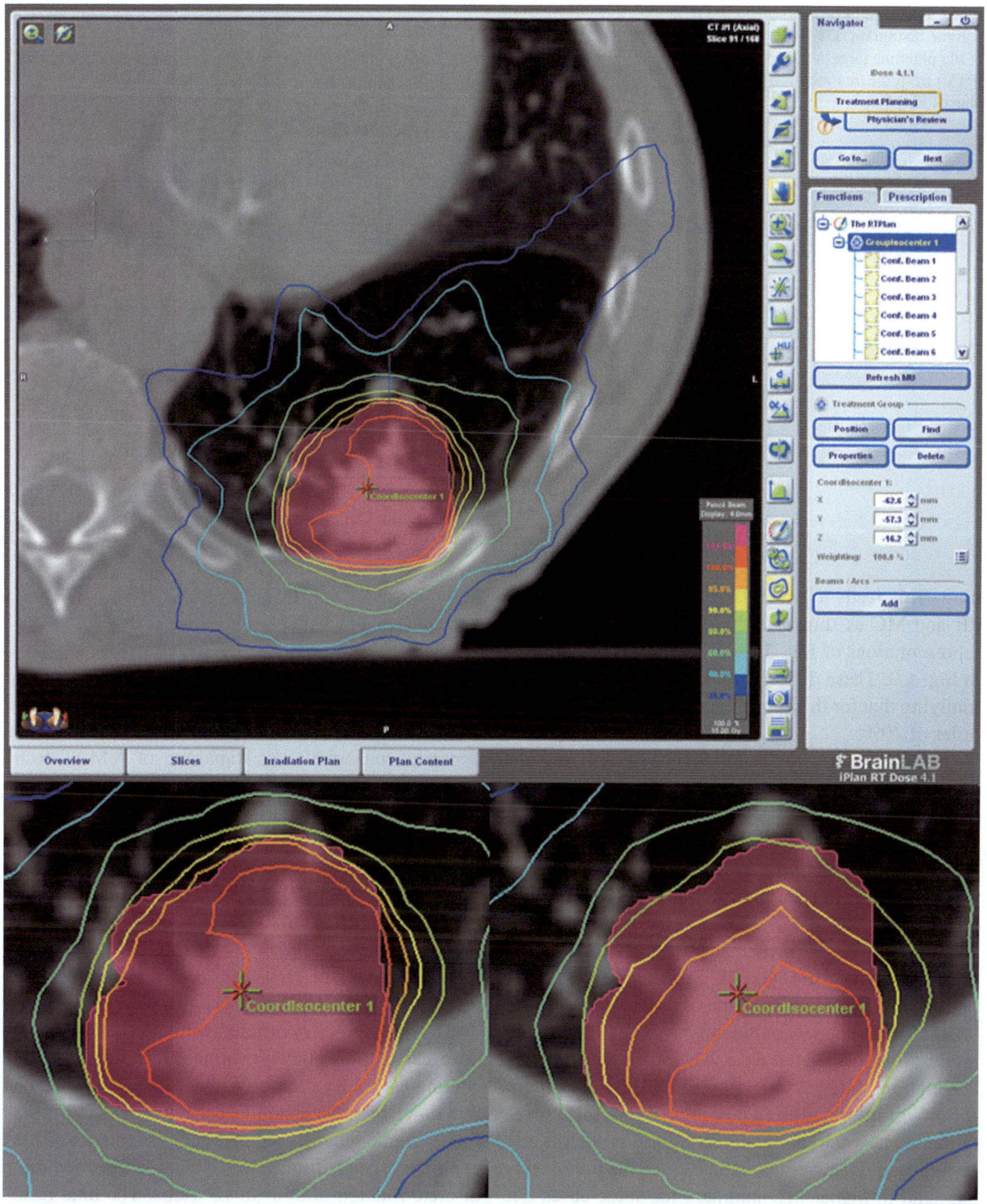

Fig. 5.6 Screen shots of a patient with medium sized lung tumor. The isodose prescription is based on the pencil beam algorithm (*upper picture*). The lower magnified screen shots compare the two algorithms, PB (*left*) and Monte Carlo (MC) (*right*)

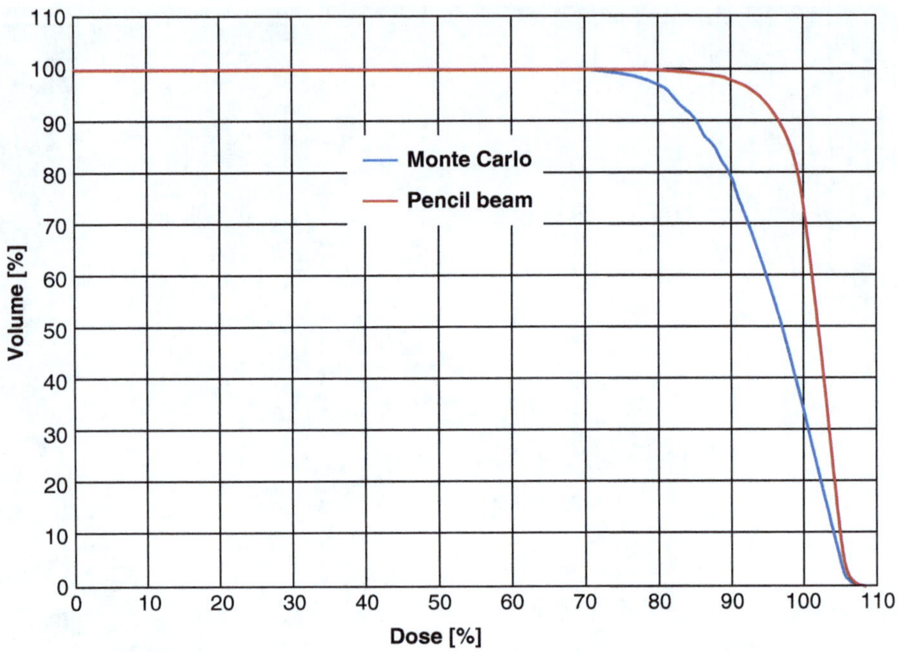

Fig. 5.7 MC and PB dose volume histogram (DVH) of the planning target volume (PTV) from the treatment plan of Fig. 5.6

lung. This leads to much larger differences between PB and MC as shown in the magnified isodose line representations of Fig. 5.8 and the DVHs of the PTV in Fig. 5.9. These differences are in the order of 20% implying that for this tumor type the PB error is in the order of 20%.

The following conclusion should be drawn from these observations. For small-and medium-sized lung tumors, PB dose calculations are highly inaccurate. It is furthermore difficult to estimate the error of the PB dose calculation. It can be 20% or more if the tumor is small and entirely surrounded by lung tissue, but it can be 5% or lower if the tumor is larger and at least partly interfacing to soft tissue. This makes it difficult to relate PB calculated dose distributions to the clinical outcome of the treatments. MC on the other hand, significantly reduces the uncertainty of the calculated dose. Therefore, much better correlation analysis between dose and treatment follow-up information is possible. When this correlation is known, treatment prescription protocols can be adjusted. Depending on the type of the tumor, this can lead to higher MU numbers for some cases but also to lower MU numbers for other cases. Lower MU numbers are always beneficial for the patient, because normal tissue and organs at risk are better protected in this case.

5.5 Dynamic Treatments and Moving Patients (4D)

Many treatment techniques involve dynamic delivery devices. For example, in dynamic IMRT, leaves move continuously from control point to control point. With dynamic conformal arc, RapidArc or VMAT techniques, also the gantry moves continuously during rotation. Semi-analytical algorithms (Pencil Beam, Collapsed Cone, AAA, etc.) have to discretize these motions to calculate dose distributions. This causes calculation artifacts. For example, a continuous gantry rotation performed in 10° steps produces toes in the lower dose region. They can be minimized by decreasing the step size. However, dose calculation time increases linearly with increasing number of steps.

This is completely different with Monte Carlo. MC dose calculation allows continuous leaf motion and continuous gantry rotation without increasing calculation time. To understand this behavior, the gantry rotation example will be used here. Let us assume the MC algorithm spends time T to simulate N histories for a discrete rotation of 360° in 10° steps. The final result will have a statistical variance s. The number of histories per step is $N/36$ and the calculation time per step is $T/36$. To perform the simulation in 2° steps and with the same variance s of the final dose distribution, then

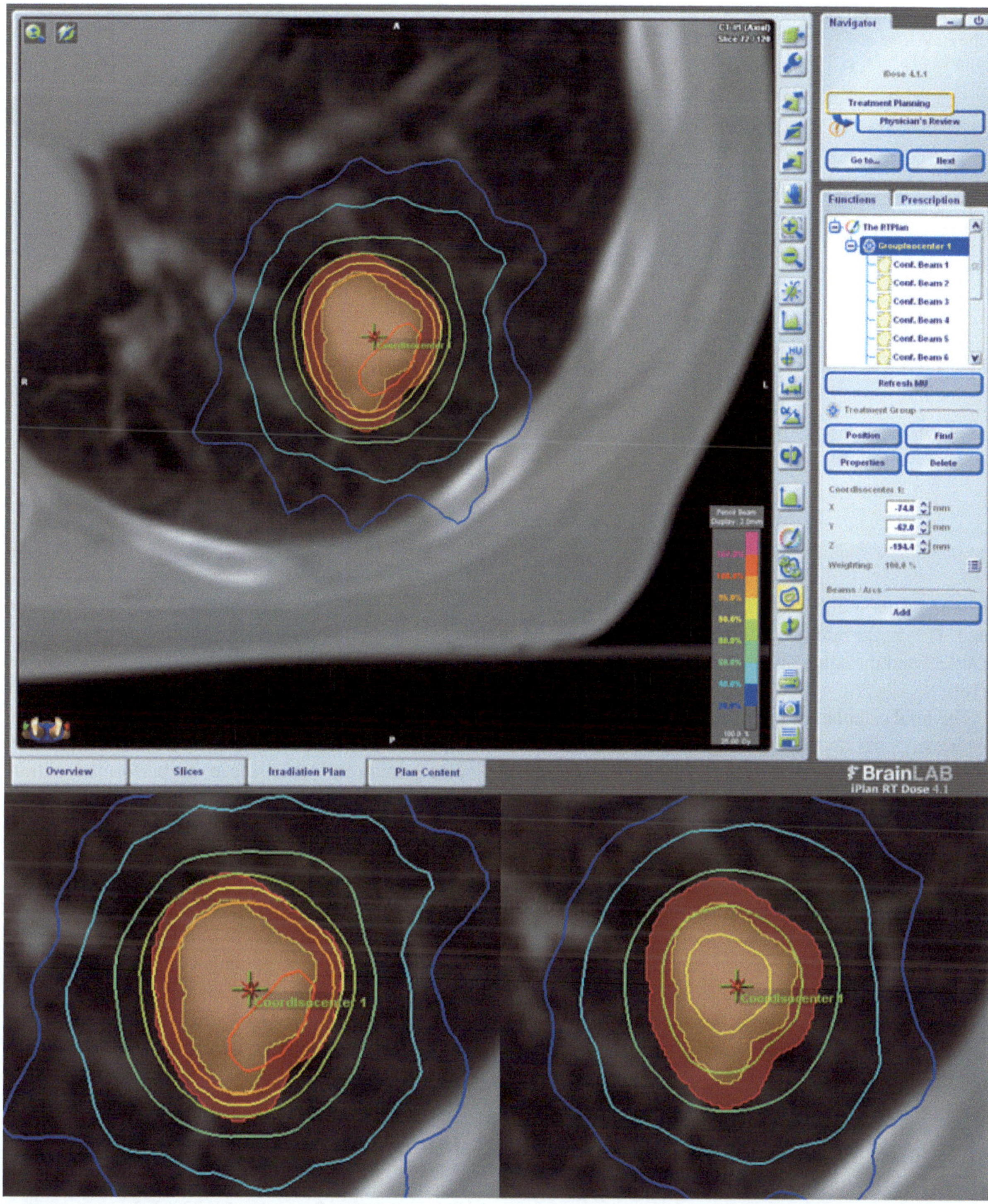

Fig. 5.8 Screen shots of a patient with small sized lung tumor. The isodose prescription is based on the pencil beam algorithm (*upper picture*). The lower magnified screen shots compare the two algorithms, PB (*left*) and Monte Carlo (MC) (*right*)

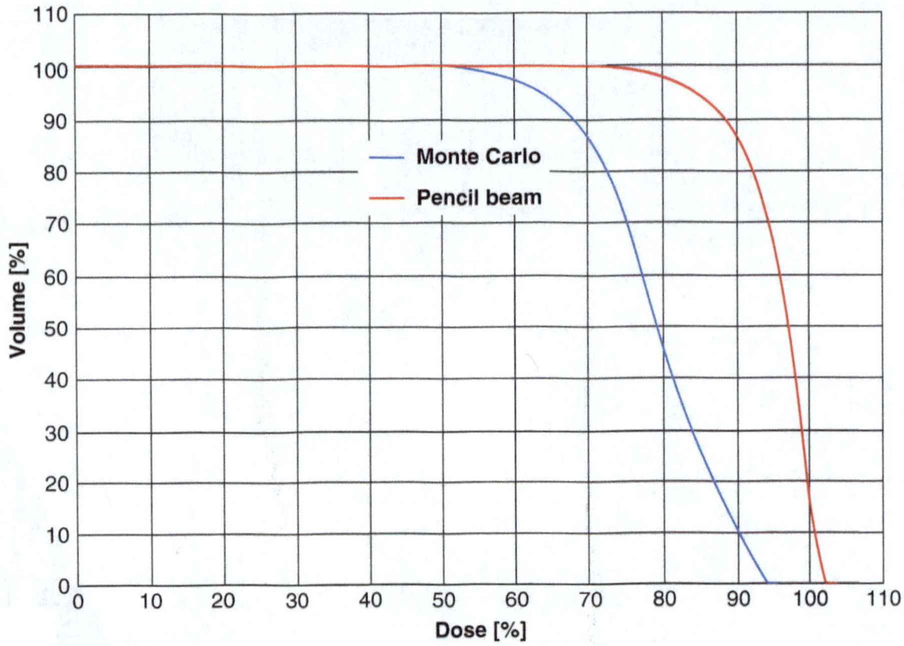

Fig. 5.9 MC and PB DVH of the PTV from the treatment plan of Fig. 5.8

the same total number of N histories must be calculated. That is, the number of histories per step decreases to *N*/180 and the calculation time per step decreases to *T*/180.

The total calculation time *T* and the total number of histories *N* only depend on the variance *s* of the final result but not on the number of steps. Therefore, in a MC simulation it is possible to make the steps arbitrarily small and finally all motions and rotations can be performed continuously.

The discussion above can be extended to 4D treatment planning, e.g., to calculate the dose for a dynamic CT movie showing respiratory motion of the patient. The dose distribution for each of the respiratory phases can be calculated with lower statistical accuracy, a lower number of histories, and less calculation time. The total calculation time will depend only on the statistical variance of the sum dose distribution in the reference CT.

Although PB dose calculation is still much faster than MC for single beams and single dose points, MC dose distributions can be calculated for small tumors within seconds on present-day workstations during the intermediate planning process and with relaxed accuracy parameters. The final dose calculation with more precise parameter settings can be performed within minutes. The calculation time is independent on the delivery technique, i.e., it is almost the same for arcs and static beams. It only depends on the size of the tumor and the accuracy parameters outlined in Sect. 5.3

MC is ideally suited for all kinds of dynamic delivery devices and moving patient anatomies. Because of the increasing relevance of dynamics in treatment planning and delivery, Monte Carlo will become the standard dose calculation engine in future.

5.6 Conclusion

For cranial treatments in radiosurgery, conventional dose calculation using the Pencil Beam algorithm has been proven to be accurate. In extracranial regions, especially for the treatment of small lung tumors it is shown that MC dose calculation should be the method of choice.

References

AAPM Task Group Report No 105 (2007) Issues associated with clinical implementation of Monte Carlo-based external beam treatment planning. Med Phys 34:4818–4853

Berger MJ (1993) ESTAR, PSTAR, and ASTAR: computer programs for calculating stopping-power and range tables for electrons, protons, and helium ions. Technical Report NBSIR 4999 National Institute of Standards and Technology, Gaithersburg

Berger MJ, Hubbell JH (1987) XCOM: photon cross sections on a personal computer. Technical Report NBSIR National Institute of Standards and Technology, Gaithersburg, 87–3597

Fippel M (1999) Fast Monte Carlo dose calculation for photon beams based on the VMC electron algorithm. Med Phys 26:1466–1475

Fippel M (2004) Efficient particle transport simulation through beam modulating devices for Monte Carlo treatment planning. Med Phys 31:1235–1242

Fippel M, Kawrakow I, Friedrich K (1997) Electron beam dose calculations with the VMC algorithm and the verification data of the NCI working group. Phys Med Biol 42:501–520

Fippel M, Laub W, Huber B, Nüsslin F (1999) Experimental investigation of a fast Monte Carlo photon beam dose calculation algorithm. Phys Med Biol 44:3039–3054

Fippel M, Haryanto F, Dohm O, Nüsslin F, Kriesen S (2003) A virtual photon energy fluence model for Monte Carlo dose calculation. Med Phys 30:301–311

ICRU Report No 46 (1992) Photon, electron, proton and neutron interaction data for body tissues. International Commission on Radiation Units and Measurements, Bethesda

Kawrakow I (2000) Accurate condensed history Monte Carlo simulation of electron transport. I. EGSnrc, the new EGS4 version. Med Phys 27:485–498

Kawrakow I, Fippel M (2000) Investigation of variance reduction techniques for Monte Carlo photon dose calculation using XVMC. Phys Med Biol 45:2163–2183

Kawrakow I, Fippel M, Friedrich K (1996) 3D electron dose calculation using a voxel based Monte Carlo algorithm (VMC). Med Phys 23:445–457

Reynaert N, van der Marck SC, Schaart DR, van der Zee W, van Vliet-Vroegindeweij C, Tomsej M, Jansen J, Heijmen B, Coghe M, De Wagter C (2007) Monte Carlo treatment planning for photon and electron beams. Radiat Phys Chem 76:643–686

Vanderstraeten B, Chin PW, Fix M, Leal M, Mora G, Reynaert N, Seco J, Soukup M, Spezi E, De Neve W, Thierens H (2007) Conversion of CT numbers into tissue parameters for Monte Carlo dose calculations: a multi-centre study. Phys Med Biol 52:539–562

Fractionation in Radiobiology: Classical Concepts and Recent Developments

6

Steve P. Lee

6.1 Introduction

Well-focused radiation treatments such as the one utilizing stereotactic guidance for both benign and malignant tumors have gained significant popularity over the recent decades. Historically, executing the treatment course over several weeks with daily fraction of relatively low dose (termed conventional or standard fractionation) has been established as the norm for major portion of the past century. This has largely been guided by the established quantitative doctrines of clinical or classical radiation biology. However, a new trend has apparently emerged to deliver significantly fewer fractions of treatment (called hypofractionation) or even single-dose irradiation. That one can now seemingly violate the long-held tenet of fractionation radiobiology results largely from the physical advantage of ultra-precision-oriented technology, made possible by more sophisticated computerized treatment planning. Nevertheless, some new biological insights have been offered by recent investigators with renewed quantitative theories, in order to account for the observed clinical efficacy of hypofractionation. The synopsis below aims to present the shifting development in fractionation practice from the classical radiobiology viewpoints, with the emphasis on the evolution of mathematical modeling so pervasive in the clinical application of the biological principles. Readers interested in a more in-depth coverage of the background information are urged to first browse through the author's earlier review on the subject, which followed a thread of synthesis of central ideas behind quantitative radiobiology (Lee et al. 2006). In order to maintain a self-sufficient amount of information, however, much of the previously presented exposition is summarized and at times included verbatim here for the reader's convenience. The main addition to the antecedent discussion is the presentation of recent development of theoretical models designed to quantify more accurately the observed efficacy of hypofractionation and thus justify its clinical practice.

For the purpose of adhering to the conventionally accepted yet simultaneously logical terminology, the author shall first define the following terms:

Stereotactic: any treatment technology employing fixation device for any part of the patient's body with target localization based on a 3-D frame of reference, with the purpose of achieving millimeter range accuracy, whether intracranially (intra-CNS if spine is included) or extracranially (extra-CNS).
Radiosurgery: single-dose irradiation.
Radiotherapy: multi-fractionated irradiation.

In particular, *stereotactic body radiotherapy* (SBRT) pertains to stereotactic treatment using hypofractionated regimen for extra-CNS disease (nowadays usually refers to five or fewer fractions – for reasons beyond what science might dictate but chosen rather arbitrarily for healthcare reimbursement purpose), while *stereotactic radiosurgery* (SRS) and *stereotactic radiotherapy* (SRT) refer to treatment using single-dose and conventional fractionation scheme, respectively. The phrase "conventional" or "standard" fractionation is meant for a treatment scheme in which typically 1.8–2 Gy per fraction is used, while "hypofractionation" often involves fractional dose significantly higher than such range.

S.P. Lee
Department of Radiation Oncology, David Geffen School of Medicine at UCLA, 200 UCLA Medical Plaza, Suite B265, Los Angeles, CA, USA 90095
e-mail: splee@mednet.ucla.edu

A.A.F. De Salles et al. (eds.), *Shaped Beam Radiosurgery*,
DOI: 10.1007/978-3-642-11151-8_6, © Springer-Verlag Berlin Heidelberg 2011

The ubiquitous term of *intensity-modulated radiation therapy* (IMRT) actually describes the intervening process of a computerized technique, with the ultimate aim of obtaining an optimal dosimetric outcome through *inverse* planning (as opposed to *forward* planning which depends on the traditional trial-and-error efforts by physicists and dosimetrists). The by-product of the technique, that the intensity is being modulated (necessitated by the dependence on the agile movements of multi-leaf collimators, MLC), is a rather undesirable consequence since it precipitates in unpredictable heterogeneous dose distribution that carries much biological uncertainty. When coupled with stereotactic approach, the terms IMRS or IMSRS, IMSRT, and IMSBRT are all self-explanatory based on the definitions given above.

Another popular technique, *image-guided radiotherapy* (IGRT), pertains to a separate effort by clinicians to mitigate against motion or set-up uncertainty whether during or in-between radiation fractions. The more comprehensive extension of IGRT, *adaptive radiotherapy* (ART), aims to accommodate the ever-changing spatial extents of the intended target volumes as well as the dose-constraining normal tissues throughout the entire time course of the patient's treatment.

Physical techniques to ensure tight conformation of radiation dose deposition over the irregularly shaped target volumes by means of stereotaxis can encompass a wide variety of approaches such as MLC-mediated shaped-beam technology (e.g., Novalis® Radiosurgery) or superimposing spherical point dose distributions of different diameters (e.g., Cyberknife®, Gamma Knife®). Optimization of dosimetric outcome can be achieved by modifying several physical parameters such as the direction of individual radiation beam trajectory, its intensity (or dose rate), the number of fields, the couch position or motion, and so on. All these attempts to achieve ultra-precision-oriented radiotherapy have precipitated in many biological and clinical consequences that warrant continuous investigations and perhaps scrutiny. In general, one can say that biological analysis lags behind the advancement in physics technology. The readers are encouraged to adhere to the author's suggestion of visualizing the interplay between biology and physics as "four-dimensional" problems as outlined in the previous work (Lee et al. 2006). Radiobiologic issues brought about by the advances in treatment technology such as volume effect, dose coverage, conformality and heterogeneity, normal tissue organization, partial tumor dose escalation or underdosage, etc., have been presented, but by no means does such superficial survey imply their lack of importance. The discussion below pertains to only a partial portion of what needs to be understood as the foundation of our knowledge in clinically relevant radiobiology. A serious omission is the new insights gained from modern genetic and molecular biology, which might in the near future impose a paradigm shift in our clinical practice of radiation oncology.

6.2 Fractionation in Classical Radiobiology

Radiation therapy with the aim of controlling cellular proliferation such as in malignant or even benign tumors is fundamentally a *biologic* therapy, with its ultimate goal being the termination of the tumor's reproductive or clonogenic growth. Nevertheless, it may also injure the surrounding normal tissues due to its inability to distinguish subcellular targets of different types of cells. To strive for the maximization of the therapeutic ratio – defined as an abstract ratio of tumor cell killing over normal tissue damage – has thus become the decisive goal for generations of radiotherapists since ionizing radiation was first used for therapeutic purpose more than a century ago.

6.2.1 The 4 R's of Fractionation Radiobiology

Initially, it took several decades of trials and errors before clinicians realized that the best way to yield the highest therapeutic ratio would be by *fractionation* rather than single-dose treatment (Coutard 1932). In other words, when a course of treatment is split into multiple fractions of small doses each given separately in time, the resulting clinical or biological effect is different from when the sum of the total dose is given all at once and quite often yields better therapeutic outcome. Clearly, some biological processes seem to occur during the time interval in-between the fractions. As more data had been gradually collected via laboratory investigations, these biological processes were identified and summarized conveniently as the "4 R's of fractionation radiobiology" (Withers 1975): *reoxygenation*, *repopulation*, *repair*, and *redistribution*. Rather than reiterating here their individual definitions as described previously (Lee et al. 2006), it is informative to present those pertinent concepts abided by generations of radiation therapists. Namely, fractionation allows the usually hypoxic center of an expanding tumor to *reoxygenate* during the interval between fractions, thus enhancing more tumor cell killing mediated by oxygen radical formation. During the time of a radiation treatment course, both normal tissue progenitor cells and malignant cells may *repopulate*, and the outcome of such competing processes may influence the therapeutic efficacy. In comparison with single-dose irradiation, fractionation can spare normal cells which seem to *repair* radiation-induced "sublethal damages" (SLDs) relatively better than malignant ones. Finally, due to cell cycle phase *redistribution*, fast-cycling cells such as in cancer are more prone to radiation killing than slow or dormant ones characterizing many normal tissues.

6.2.2 The Need for Quantification: Empirical Power Laws

As the biological effects of fractionation were identified, a subsequent question naturally arose: how much dose per fraction over how long of a time course should be given-thus rendering clinical radiobiology into effectively a quantitative discipline. The first such quantitative guideline was published by Strandqvist (1944) who borrowed empirically from a certain "Law of Photochemistry" (Schwarzschild 1900): Given the intensity (i.e., dose per time) of light, *I*, and the time of exposure, *T*, for a certain degree of photochemical effect, Ψ, one could express the following relationship:

$$D \equiv I \cdot T = \psi \cdot T^{k}. \qquad (6.1)$$

where the dose, *D*, is equivalent to $I \cdot T$, and the exponent *k* is a parameter characterizing such "power-law" relationship. This equation predicts a linear curve on a log*D* vs. log*T* display for the same effect Ψ, with the slope of the line dictated by *k*.

Various quantitative schemes were invented over several decades to interpret more complex clinical observations, yet the approaches largely followed the original framework of utilizing phenomenologically oriented entities with empirical assumption of the power laws (Ellis 1967; Kirk et al. 1971; Orton and Ellis 1973; Sheline et al. 1980). However, as more was learned about the underlying mechanisms of radiation effect on cells and tissues, the phenomenological guidelines based on power-laws were replaced by more mechanistically sound biophysical models.

6.2.3 Mechanistic Models and Cell Survival Curves

Equipped with precise ways of measuring a given amount of radiation dosage as well as the clonogenic potential of the surviving cells, one can quantify the radiation cytotoxic effect as a function of radiation dose with the intervening mechanism interpreted using biophysical models. The most elementary assumption is the "target-cell hypothesis" or "hit theory" (Alpen 1998) that within each cell there exist critical targets which, when hit with ionizing radiation particles in a random fashion, may lead to consequential loss of cellular reproductive integrity.

Laboratory techniques of quantifying the ability of cells to maintain clonogenesity were created, and many experimentally obtained "survival curves" were published. The first mammalian cell study was reported by Puck and Marcus (1956) in 1956. When plotted as a semi-logarithmetical graph of log *SF* (surviving fraction) vs. radiation dose *D*, most revealed a very similar shape with a "curvy shoulder" at the low-dose region in contiguity with a relatively linear tail toward the high-dose region (Fig. 6.1a). Various biophysical models have been proposed since, and up until recent times a clear champion has been the *linear-quadratic* (LQ) model (Fowler 1989). Based on this model, a versatile theoretical framework has been developed to correlate biological effects of radiation treatments using a variable range of dose rates or fractionation schemes (Brenner and Hall 1991; Brenner et al. 1991). Before we embark on its detailed description, it is however crucial to review another less popular but perhaps more mechanistically robust model: the *single-hit, multitarget* (SH-MT) model.

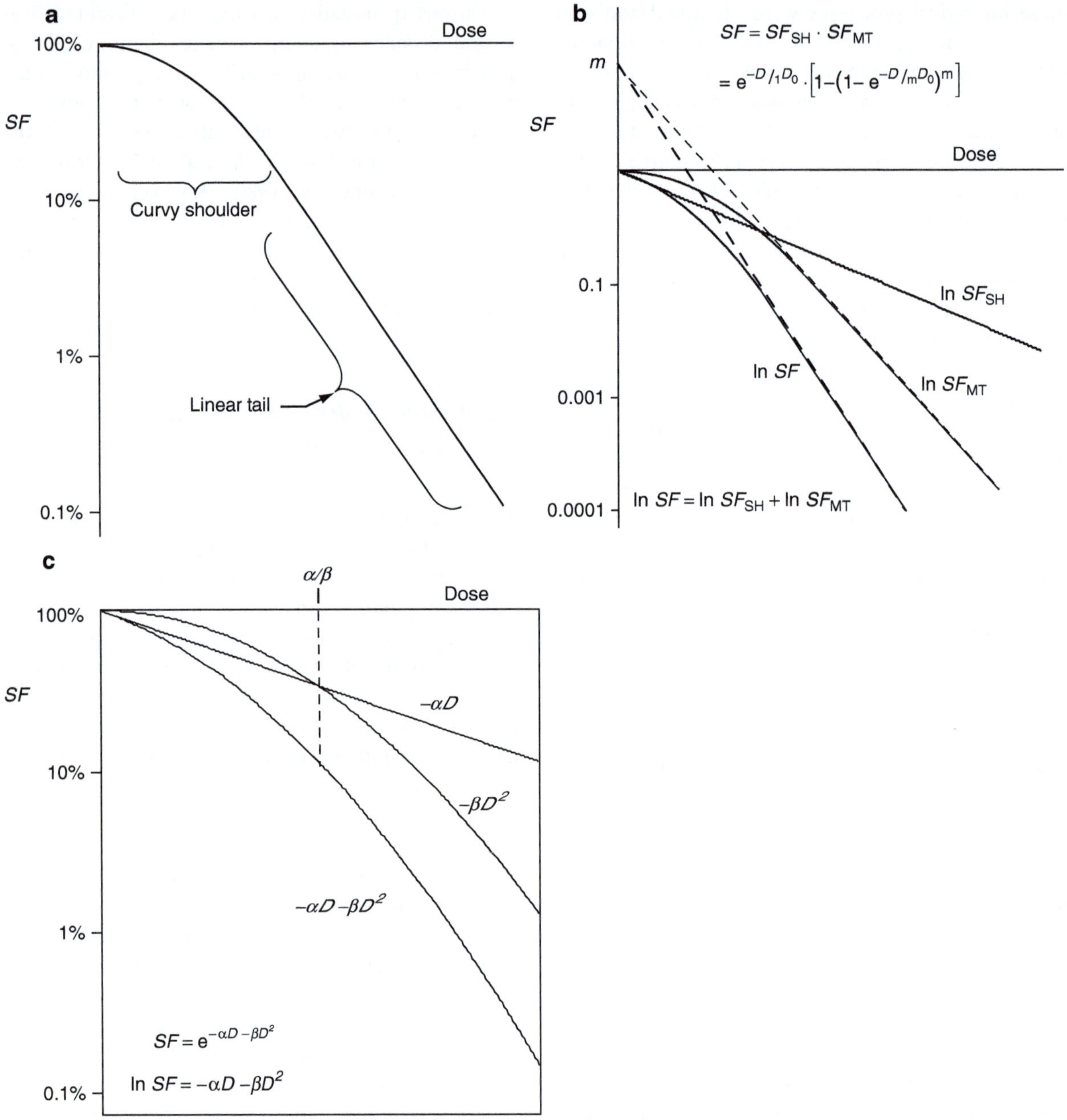

Fig. 6.1 (**a**) Typical radiation cell survival curve as logarithm of *surviving fraction* (*SF*) vs. *dose* in linear scale. It appears to have a *curvy shoulder* and a *linear tail*, thus reflecting probably two independent biophysical processes. (**b**) Single-hit, multitarget (SH-MT) model. The "extrapolation number," *m*, corresponds to the intercept on the vertical axis of a straight line back-extrapolated from the linear tail portion of the survival curve. (**c**) Linear-quadratic (LQ) model. In contrast to (b), the tail portion is not linear, but continuously bending as governed by the quadratic term

6.2.4 Single-Hit, Multitarget Killing (SH-MT) Mode

This model follows the assumption of two independent mechanisms of cell killing and adequately describes the shape of a typical radiation survival curve (Alpen 1998; Withers and Peters 1980). The first, or *single-hit* component comes from a straightforward theorization based on a Poisson process of radiation action on a critical target within each cell, which after being "hit" by the ionizing particle alone will cause irreversible cell death. The expression for the surviving fraction due to this process (SF_{SH}) can be expressed as

$$SF_{\mathrm{SH}} = e^{-D/_1D_0},$$

where D is the radiation dose, and $_1D_0$ is the dose at which the survival fraction becomes e^{-1} (~37%) of its original value (i.e., a parameter defining the intrinsic radiation sensitivity), that translates, *on the average*, to one lethal hit per target. On a survival curve presented as a semi-log plot of lnSF vs. D, the negative reciprocal of $_1D_0$ yields the slope of the expected straight line (Fig. 6.1b).

The second independent mode of cell killing by radiation is thought to result from cell death due to cumulative (though not necessarily synchronous) injuries elicited at *all* of several, say, m, multiple intracellular targets. By repeated interpretations using Poisson process for each of the m target-inactivations, one can derive the following expression for the surviving fraction (SF_{MT}):

$$SF_{\mathrm{MT}} = 1-\left(1-e^{-D/_mD_0}\right)^m,$$

where $_mD_0$ is another biological parameter characterizing the effectiveness of the radiation particle to inactivate these targets. Thus, the combined effect of radiation in this two-component model becomes:

$$SF = e^{-D/_1D_0}\left[1-\left(1-e^{-D/_mD_0}\right)^m\right]. \tag{6.2}$$

The semi-log plot based on the above equation shows a survival curve with an initially convex "shoulder" at low-dose range, but eventually tends into a straight line as D increases (Fig. 6.1b).

6.2.5 Linear-Quadratic (LQ) Model

According to this model, the surviving fraction after a single treatment of radiation dose D can be characterized by the following equation (Alpen 1998; Fowler 1989; Thames et al. 1982):

$$SF = e^{-\alpha D-\beta D^2}, \tag{6.3}$$

where α and β are tissue-specific parameters governing intrinsic radiation sensitivity. However, the survival curve *takes on a continuously bending downward trend* rather than becoming nearly a straight line at high-dose range (Fig. 6.1c). The linear component might be seen as the result of the single-hit mechanism described above. The mechanistic origin of the quadratic component, however, has been somewhat controversial (Brenner and Hall 1992; Yaes et al. 1992). Furthermore, because of its alleged inadequacy in explaining the observed clinical success of hypofractionation practice nowadays and thus attracting heavy scrutiny (Kirpatrick et al. 2008; Timmerman et al. 2007), the LQ model deserves some close inspection here. Its mechanistic explanation can be traced back to 1940s when Lea and Catcheside (1942) published their study of chromosome aberrations in *Tradescantia* microspores: Let $n(t)$ denote the number of radiation-induced lesions (such as SLDs) at time t. First, assume the formation of these lesions to be proportional to I, the intensity (or dose per time) of the radiation, with a constant ξ. Second, assume the repair of lesions is exponential (i.e., follows first-order kinetics) with a rate constant μ. Then one can express a pair of differential equations as

$$\frac{dn(t)}{dt} = \xi I - \mu n(t) \qquad \text{for } 0 \le t \le T$$

$$\frac{dn(t)}{dt} = -\mu n(t) \qquad \text{for } T \le t \le \infty$$

Finally, assume that permanent cell lethality results from *the interaction between one sublethal lesion and another one* such that an irreversible chromosomal aberration is formed, then the incidence rate of such interactions will be proportional to $n(t)\cdot n(t) = [n(t)]^2$. One can then readily derive a mathematical expression for the number of permanent lethal lesions and find it to be directly proportional to $(IT)^2 \equiv D^2$ (thus the *quadratic* component). Moreover, such expression is seen to be dictated by a *repair factor*, G, as a function of T and μ:

$$G(\mu,T) = \frac{2}{\mu T}\left[1-\frac{1}{\mu T}(1-e^{-\mu T})\right]. \tag{6.4}$$

Equation 6.4 has been derived in other more generalized approaches, e.g., by Kellerer and Rossi (1972) using microdosimetric analysis for their *theory of dual radiation action*, or by Thames 1985)with an *incomplete repair* (IR) model. It plays an important role in establishing the theoretical framework of determining equivalent biological effects of various brachytherapy techniques, fractionated teletherapy, and indeed any variable range of dose rates or fractionation schemes (Lee et al. 2006; Brenner and Hall 1991).

One might note that the LQ theory has never been created empirically by using a mathematical "trick" of keeping only the first two orders of a polynomial "power-series expansion" as suggested by some investigators (Timmerman et al. 2007). In fact, were one to adhere to such hypothetical notion with the addition of "higher order" terms in a polynomial function, it would result in bending the semi-log survival curve further downward at high-dose range, in contrast to the assertion that it should swing upward to fit the observed survival data better (Fig. 6.2). Therefore, the argument of a truncated power-series expansion as the motive behind the LQ formulation should be avoided.

Regardless of its true mechanistic origin, the LQ model is useful because of its simplicity and the fact that it does describe the shape of the survival curves adequately. From fitting in vitro and in vivo data, Brenner has argued that it is valid at least for single-dose range of about 2–15 Gy (Brenner 2008). One of the most attractive roles of the LQ model stems from its ability to explain the differential sensitivities of the so-called *acutely responding* vs. *late-responding* tissues to fractionated radiotherapy (Fig. 6.3a), thus establishing the theoretical advantage of fractionation – even *hyperfractionation* (with relatively smaller dose per fraction given more than once per day) – when treating malignant tumors (mostly acutely responding) embedded within late-responding normal tissues (Withers et al. 1982). Indeed, for a fractionated radiotherapy course with n fractions of dose per fraction, d, the overall effect is given by:

$$SF = e^{-n(\alpha d + \beta d^2)}. \tag{6.5}$$

On the survival curve plot, this amounts to repeating by n times the initial fractional amount of cell survival resulting from dose d, each picking up successively where it ends from the previous treatment after complete repair of SLD during the interfractional interval (Fig. 6.3b). The net result is the sparing of the irradiated tissues, with an "effective slope" of an essentially linear overall survival curve becoming less steep the more fractionated the treatment is. Furthermore, it is seen that by fractionation the late-responding tissue is spared relatively more than the acutely responding tissue due to its "curvier" shape (signifying higher capacity for SLD repair) of its single-dose survival curve in the small-dose range of clinical interest (Fig. 6.3c). The late-responding tissues are hence much more sensitive to the variation in fractionation size than the acutely responding tissues (Thames et al. 1982; Withers et al. 1982).

The validity of Eq. 6.5 depends on the assumption that cellular damage events are repaired sufficiently in between fractions. With a typical half-life of such repair measured in hours, the condition is usually satisfied for daily (24-h) inter-fractional interval. A useful corollary can be derived from the consideration of "incompletely repaired" events (i.e., the IR model, (Thames 1985)) when the inter-fractional interval is shortened to a significant degree or during continuous low-dose rate (LDR) irradiation via brachytherapy. We can see from Fig. 6.3b that, as the dose per fraction (or dose rate) approaches zero, the progressively more "spared" survival curve becomes less steep and ultimately has a limiting effective slope characterized by the single-hit component only (α, or ${}_1D_0$), since this is the component of damage that is not repairable in time (Withers and Peters 1980).

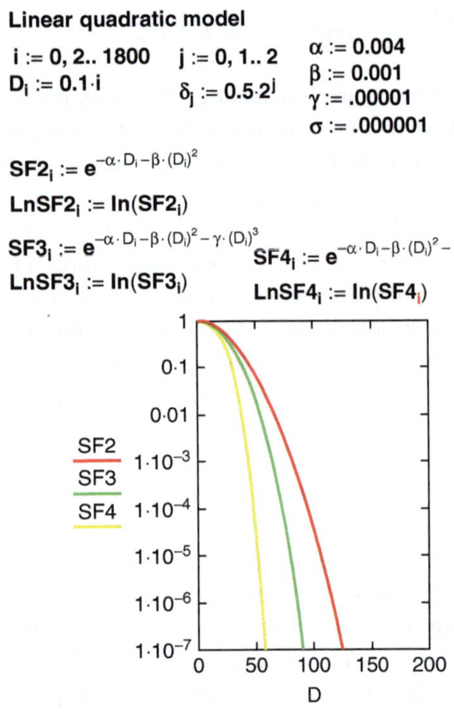

Fig. 6.2 Mathcad™ worksheet showing the incorporation of higher order terms (up to fourth power) in a hypothetical power series expansion of a cell survival curve. In keeping with the notion that any additional contribution of radiation dose, even in higher power terms, should effect cell death, all terms must thus have negative sign. It can be seen that the higher the number of terms, the more the terminal portion of the curve bends downward rather than upward

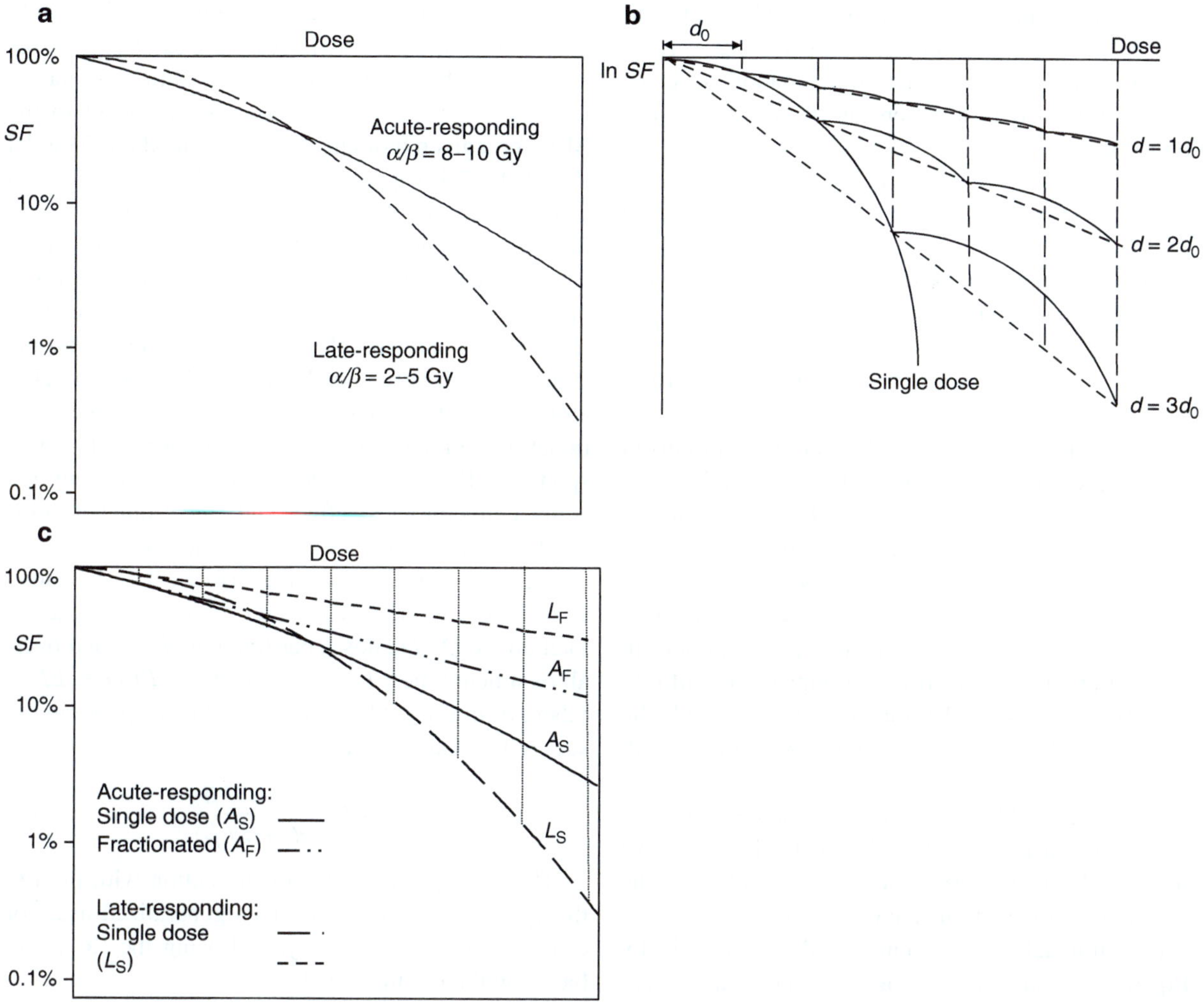

Fig. 6.3 (**a**) Distinct shapes of survival curves between *acute-responding* and *late-responding* tissues. The former is characterized by larger α/β ratio and dominated by the linear component, the latter by a smaller α/β and dominated by the quadratic component. (**b**) Fractionation effect and survival curve. Here the effects of three fractionation schemes are shown, with respective dose per fraction of d_0, $2d_0$, and $3d_0$. Upon fractionation, the initial portion of the single-dose curve is repeated successively, so long as near-complete repair of sublethal damages takes place in-between the fractions. Clearly, the smaller the dose per fraction, the more sparing of the tissue at a certain dose, or the higher the total dose is required to achieve certain biological effect. (**c**) Differential sparing effects of fractionation upon *acute-* vs. *late-responding* tissues. Fractionation spares the late-responding tissue more because of the "curvier" shape of its survival curve (L_S cf. L_F), while the acute-responding tissue is spared relatively less (A_S cf. A_F)

To account for repopulation of cells which is especially relevant when the tissue under consideration is an acutely responding (i.e., rapidly proliferating) type, a *treatment time* factor is introduced (Fowler 1989):

$$SF = e^{-n(\alpha d + \beta d^2) + \frac{\ln 2 (T - T_k)}{T_p}}, \tag{6.6}$$

where T is the overall treatment time, T_k is the "kick-off" time point when "accelerated repopulation" (Withers et al. 1988) begins after the treatment starts, and T_p is the effective doubling time of the clonogenic cells.

6.2.6 Biologically Effective Dose (BED)

Based on the LQ model, Barendsen (1982) and Fowler (1989) have suggested a quantity termed *biologically effective dose* (BED), which proved to be very convenient in quantifying radiobiological effects and even enabled sensible comparisons among various clinical trials using different fractionation schemes (Fowler 1992). With a dimension of dose (Gy), it is defined as:

$$BED \equiv nd\left(1+\frac{d}{\alpha/\beta}\right)-\frac{\ln 2(T-T_k)}{\alpha \cdot T_p}. \quad (6.7)$$

For late-responding tissues only, the treatment time factor (i.e., repopulation) can be neglected, and

$$BED \equiv nd\left(1+\frac{d}{\alpha/\beta}\right). \quad (6.8)$$

This abstract quantity can best be conceptualized by its representation on the multi-fractionation survival curves (Fig. 6.4; Lee et al. 1995). One can see that the numerical value of BED for any fractionation scheme is equivalent to the total physical dose needed to cause the same degree of biological effect (cell survival) using an "ultrafractionated" regimen in which d approaches zero and n approaches infinity ($d \to 0$, $n \to \infty$) such that the product, nd, equals the given total dose, D (Barendsen 1982; Yaes et al. 1991).

Using the SH-MT model, Withers and Peters (1980) have analyzed in detail the change in the "effective slope" of the multifraction survival curve, $D_{0(\mathrm{eff})}$, as the size of dose per fraction changes. Such a cell survival plot – although more complicated mathematically (Eq. 6.2) – shows a limiting maximal (least steep) slope characterized by the single-hit mechanism only (${}_1D_0$) as the dose per fraction (or dose rate) approaches zero. It is thus analogous to the ultrafractionation scheme of which the total dose is equivalent to the BED for a given biological effect, using the LQ model (Fig. 6.4). This supports the notion that BED is indeed a mechanistically sound quantity measuring the "isoeffect" dose for any fractionation scheme with respect to a particular process of radiation killing (i.e., single-hit, or the linear component in the LQ theory), which represents the nonrepairable damage to the chromosome that results directly in cell lethality (Brenner and Hall 1992; Lea and Catcheside 1942). Thus, given any fractionation regimen delivering a total dose D, its corresponding BED is a unique entity quantifying the equivalent biological effect and free from any arbitrarily chosen "reference" fractionation scheme.

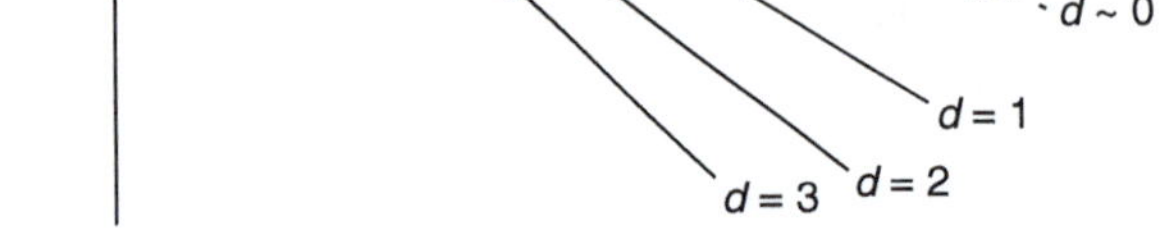

Fig. 6.4 Concept of biologically effective dose (BED) as depicted on survival curves. Only late effects are considered. Each line from the origin represents the "effective" survival curve for a multifraction regimen using dose per fraction, *d*. For a given total physical dose, *D*, a BED as a function of *d*, BED(*d*), can be visualized as the isoeffective total dose of a regimen in which *d* approaches zero asymptotically (Redrawn from Lee et al. 1995)

We can derive readily the "isoeffect conversion" relation for two fractionation regimens with respective total doses, D_1, D_2, doses per fraction, d_1, d_2, and overall treatment times, T_1, T_2: For isoeffect, $BED_1 \equiv BED_2$; then, from Eq. 6.8 by considering late-responding tissues only (Withers et al. 1983):

$$D_1 = D_2\frac{(d_2+\alpha/\beta)}{(d_1+\alpha/\beta)}. \quad (6.9)$$

The concept of BED (in conjunction with the LQ theory) can be applied for much generalized use. For example, for brachytherapy, and using the IR model based on the LQ theory:

$$BED = D\left(1+\frac{G(\mu,T)\cdot D}{\alpha/\beta}\right), \quad (6.10)$$

where μ is the rate constant for SLD repair, T is the time of continuous irradiation, and $G(\mu, T)$ is given as in Eq. 6.4 (Lea and Catcheside 1942; Thames 1985; Oliver 1964).

6.2.7 TCP and NTCP

Clinically, the terms *tumor control probability* (TCP) and *normal tissue complication probability* (NTCP) are more useful than BED in providing patients a quantitative sense of radiobiological consequence. They are defined, according to Poisson statistics, as:

$$TCP = e^{-M \cdot SF_M}, \quad (6.11)$$

$$NTCP = e^{-N \cdot SF_N}, \quad (6.12)$$

where M is the number of clonogenic cells in the tumor (or "tumorlets"), N is the *functional subunits* (FSUs, at times called *tissue rescue units*, TRUs) for normal tissue, and SF_M and SF_N are the respective surviving fractions as functions of radiation dose and intrinsic radiation sensitivity (per Eq. 6.5 or 6.6) (Withers and Peters 1980). When plotted against dose (thus termed dose–response curves), both TCP and NTCP present as sigmoid curves.

It is not an exaggeration to say that almost all clinical efforts in the entire history of radiation therapy have been designed to separate the TCP and NTCP curves in order to maximize the therapeutic ratio. For example, using ultra-precision-oriented treatment techniques such as stereotactic irradiation, the NTCP curve is effectively pushed to the right in relation to the TCP curve. Hence, tumor dose escalation is feasible at a minimal expense of normal tissue damage. This has recently transpired into promising outcomes for SRS and SBRT by escalating tumor dose far beyond the usual level attained in conventional fractionation. However, it might have also prompted some practitioners to question the validity of the LQ model since the theory has allegedly failed to predict such clinical success. One might further perceive an apparent disadvantage of using conventional level of dose per fraction and conclude that higher fractional dose is actually more beneficial *in principle* – in contrast to standard fractionation or even hyperfractionation that was once championed by classical radiobiology teaching (Fowler 1989; Withers and Peters 1980). This may not necessarily be the case, since the reality might lie in the fact that the traditional level of dose has simply not been sufficiently high to reach beyond the steep portion of the sigmoid TCP curve. This is especially true for most malignancies which are notorious for having low local control rates with conventional dosage, such as high-grade gliomas, liver or lung cancers (and perhaps even prostate cancer - a special case for which much radiobiological discussion has been centered upon what the true α/β value should be). One should keep in mind that the biological effect of radiation as depicted in the BED expression (Eq. 6.7 or 6.8) depends not only on *dose per fraction*, but also on the *total dose*. Classical radiobiology has advocated hyperfractionation mainly due to its theoretical advantage of sparing late-responding tissues (Withers et al. 1982) (which might be independently achieved via stereotactic positioning in SRS/SBRT), but has never discounted the likely benefit of tumor dose escalation regardless of fractionation patterns.

Nevertheless, is there really "new" biology, unforeseen by classical theories, being revealed in view of the recently established clinical efficacy of SRS/SBRT? The answer is certainly positive. From the discussion about the mechanistic origin of the survival curve models so far, there is no doubt that all hypothesized mechanisms are at best still elementary, with other possible concomitant biological processes summarily ignored. For example, the LQ formulation in Eq. 6.5 considers only one R of the "4 Rs" – repair, while Eq. 6.6 adds another R: repopulation. This kind of methodical approach is generic in any mechanistically constructed quantitative model, since the aim is to start with basic assumptions then adding complexity in a well-controlled stepwise fashion. It remains to be seen what other relevant biological or clinical processes should be included to further improve the therapeutic efficacy of fractionated radiation treatment.

Flickinger et al. (2003) have attempted to fit the clinically observed SRS dose–response data with the LQ model by logistic regression. However, without constraining the biological parameters such as α and β to be nonnegative as specified in the model's original hypothesis, the α/β values obtained for various clinical endpoints including cranial neuropathy and angiographic obliteration of vascular malformations turned out to be negative. Rather than attributing such unrealistic results as due to the disregard of the LQ model's mechanistic origin, the authors called for other explanations such as vasculature as the alternative biological target for SRS instead of the traditionally believed mitotic arrest of proliferative cells. Similar arguments have also been discussed by others, all pointing out the apparent inconsistency of the LQ model in quantifying the observed clinical data for SRS/SBRT. For example, Kirkpatrick et al. called for the consideration of vascular and stromal damages by high-dose radiation, as well as radioresistant tumor subpopulations such as cancer stem cells (Kirpatrick et al. 2008; Bao et al. 2006).

6.3 Alternative Models to Explain Efficacy of Single-Dose or Hypofractionation Treatment

6.3.1 SH-MT vs. LQ Models

The two-component models such as SH-MT and LQ models are useful in describing the shape of the single-dose survival curve. At the low-dose range often utilized by the conventional fractionation scheme, the two models may predict pretty much identical survival results. However, at higher-dose range the two curves seem to deviate from each other, since the SH-MT model predicts an eventual straight line while the LQ curve continues to bend downward (Fig. 6.5). This divergent behavior turns out to be of crucial importance when one wishes to apply these models to single-dose irradiation (SRS) as well as hypofractionation schemes such as used in SBRT. Since the LQ model involves simpler mathematic formulation, it has gained wider popularity. Advocates of SBRT, however, soon observed that the LQ theory would "break down" at these larger fractional dose levels (often 5–20 Gy or even higher) as it tends to overestimate radiation toxicity. It was pointed out that most single-dose survival curves do often tend to straight line at higher-dose range, thus explaining why LQ theory might have lost its appeal for SBRT supporters. Not surprisingly, interest in the SH-MT model was revived for the quantification of SBRT hypofractionation results. Yet the notorious mathematic complexity of SH-MT model

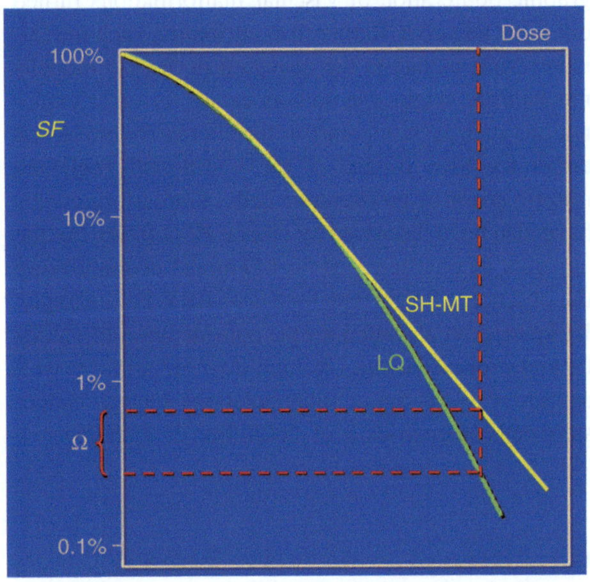

Fig. 6.5 Difference in biological effect at high-dose range between the predictions of the SH-MT (*yellow*) and the LQ (*green*) models. The amount of difference in surviving fraction, Ω (albeit depicted in logarithmic scale) for certain dosage can be measured by the different intersections the *vertical dashed line* makes with either survival curve. Clearly, the LQ model overestimates cell lethality at high-dose range in comparison with the SH-MT model

Table 6.1 Main differences between the LQ and the SH-MT models

LQ	SH-MT
"Shoulder" due to predominantly two hits	"Shoulder" due to sum of two or more hits (targets)
Math is easier to handle	Math is harder to handle
Linear-additivity of BED is a versatile tool	Linearly additive form of BED not found easily
Terminal slope of semi-log survival curve is "continuously bending"	Terminal slope of semi-log survival curve is straight
Could overestimate cell killing at higher dose	Could underestimate cell killing at higher dose

(Eq. 6.2) has limited its acceptance, until more recently newer models begin to appear to circumvent such problem. Before the presentation of these newer models, it is useful to summarize the major differences between the SH-MT and the LQ models (Table 6.1).

6.3.2 Hybrid Models for Hypofractionation Schemes: Universal Survival Curve Model

To mitigate the difficulty posed by the mathematic expression of the SH-MT model and simultaneously exploit the applicability of LQ model at low-dose range, some newer "hybrid" models have been proposed. A versatile formulation named *universal survival curve* (USC) model has been published by Park et al. (2008). The essence of this model is to capitalize on a simple mathematical trick well known for the SH-MT model: by back extrapolation of the terminal straight-line portion of the SH-MT survival curve toward the abscissa, one encounters the familiar entities of the so-called *extrapolation number* (m in Eq. 6.2) and the quasi-threshold dose (D_q) (Fig. 6.6). By simple geometric argument, it is found that the surviving fraction as a function of the dose d is given as

$$\ln SF = \frac{-d + D_q}{D_0}, \tag{6.13}$$

where the parameter D_0 in the denominator is an abbreviated expression of $_mD_0$ in the SH-MT model (Eq. 6.2) that characterizes the terminal slope of the survival curve at high-dose range, and d is the dose variable.

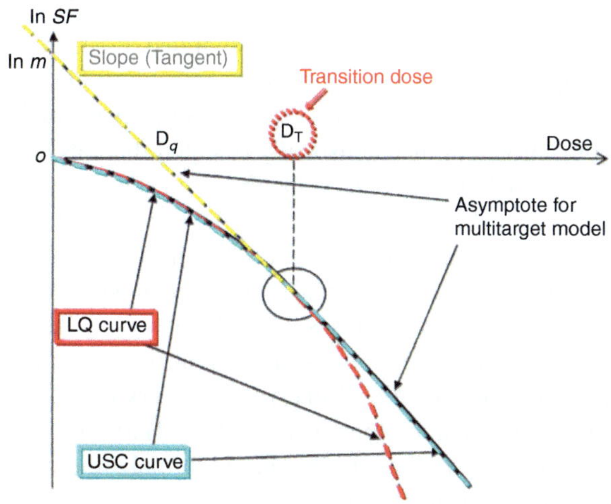

Fig. 6.6 The USC model (*cyan dashed line*) is a hybrid between the LQ model (*red dashed line*) at low-dose range and the SH-MT model at high-dose range, the latter with a terminal straight line that can be back extrapolated toward the vertical axis (*yellow dashed line*) (From Park et al. 2008)

Thus, the portion of the survival curve at a relatively large-dose range – say $d \geq D_T$ where D_T is known as the *transition dose* – can be specified entirely by the two parameters D_q and D_0. For $d \leq D_T$, one only needs to adhere to the LQ model with its well-appreciated mathematic simplicity (which is also determined by two biologic parameters α and β). To summarize:

$$\ln SF = -\alpha d - \beta d^2 \qquad \text{for } d \leq D_T \quad (6.14a)$$

$$\ln SF = \frac{-d + D_q}{D_0} \qquad \text{for } d \geq D_T \quad (6.14b)$$

The proponents of this model then impose on certain mathematic constraints at D_T: namely, the two curves must meet in a manner such that they are "smoothly continuous" (such that the whole curve becomes "differentiable" at D_T). In so doing, the two separate functions expressing the survival fraction as well as their first derivatives must be equal at D_T, and one can then obtain the interrelations among the various biologic parameters as

$$\beta = \frac{(1 - \alpha D_0)^2}{4 D_0 D_q} \quad (6.15)$$

$$D_T = \frac{2 D_q}{1 - \alpha D_0} \quad (6.16)$$

When repeating with n fractions in a multi-fractionated treatment regimen,

$$\ln SF = -n(\alpha d + \beta d^2) \qquad \text{for } d \leq D_T \quad (6.17a)$$

$$\ln SF = -n\left(\frac{d - D_q}{D_0}\right) \qquad \text{for } d \geq D_T \quad (6.17b)$$

Analogous to the formulation of BED in Eq. 6.8, the expressions for BED in this hybrid model become

$$BED = D\left(1 + \frac{d}{\alpha / \beta}\right) \qquad \text{for } d \leq D_T \quad (6.18a)$$

$$BED = \frac{D - nD_q}{\alpha D_0} \qquad \text{for } d \geq D_T \quad (6.18b)$$

The authors of the USC model further seek out the appropriate expressions for *single fraction equivalent dose* (SFED, for the convenience of intercomparisons among SRS or SBRT results) as well as *standard effective dose* (SED, based on a 2-Gy per fraction regimen). The USC model was used to fit experimental data from a clonogenic assay of a H460 non-small cell lung cancer (NSCLC) cell line and resulted in seemingly better fit than the LQ model over the high-dose (10–16 Gy) range. To illustrate its clinical application, an extensive list of published SBRT experiences in the treatment of early-stage NSCLC has been analyzed and presented by tabulating SFED, BED, and SED values, assuming α/β of 10 Gy (Park et al. 2008).

6.3.3 Hybrid Models for Hypofractionation Schemes: Other Proposals

Over time, the LQ model has been modified and extended to alleviate the apparent inconsistency at high-dose range (Guerrero and Li 2004; Wang et al. 2007; Carlone et al. 2005), but most of the proposed mathematic formulations have been rather complicated beyond the reach of routine clinical application. For example, Guerrero and Li (2004) proposed a *modified LQ* (MLQ) model by imposing a "shifting" factor δ for the expression of $G(\mu, T)$ in Eq. 6.4, such that

$$G(\mu T) \rightarrow G(\mu T + \delta D).$$

They further imposed that, at relatively extreme (small and large) ranges of dose, the MLQ model should agree with the previously published *lethal-potentially lethal* (LPL) model by Curtis (1986) because of the notion that it works better than LQ model. The value of δ could thus be determined accordingly. The resulting MLQ model is seen to reproduce the LQ prediction at low fractional dose, but at high fractional dose it agrees with LPL-predicted behavior.

A close resemblance to the USC model is the linear-quadratic-linear (LQ-L) model proposed by Astrahan (2008). It relinquishes the mechanistic argument of the SH-MT model as used in the USC formulation, and directly imposes a straight line beyond a *transition dose*, again denoted as D_T:

$$\ln SF = -\alpha d - \beta d^2 \qquad \text{for } d \le D_T \quad (6.19a)$$

$$\ln SF = -\alpha D_T - \beta D_T^2 - \gamma(d - D_T) \text{ for } d \ge D_T \quad (6.19b)$$

where γ characterizes the slope of the terminal linear portion of the semi-log survival curve beginning at D_T. Both γ and D_T are empirical parameters that can only be inferred from experimental observations (although the author claims that D_T in many occasions seems to approximately equal to twice the value of α/β). Various historic publications, including the original survival curve by Puck and Marcus (1956) as well as animal experiment data by Thames and Withers (1980), were fitted using the LQ-L model with reasonable agreements. The celebrated isoeffect plots of Withers et al. (1982) were also fitted with the author's formulation of BED based on the LQ-L model, and a better fit than what LQ would predict was seen in particular for the lungs.

The publication of the USC model has stimulated several letters to the editor, each with its proposed alternative version of survival curve model (Kavanagh and Newman 2008; McKenna and Ahmad 2009; Tomé 2008). Specifically, Kavanagh and Newman 2008 proposed a model that introduced a concept of "dose-dependent increase in exponential rate of cell kill for the shoulder," as well as one of "low-dose hypersensitivity" with a decaying exponent. McKenna and Ahmad 2009) likewise introduced a modifier for the quadratic term in the LQ model Tomé (2008) introduced a modifier for the quadratic term as well by decreasing β (or increasing α/β) with increasing dose. As one can see, all these proposals suffer from either a lack of true mechanistic reasoning or an elaborated mathematic complexity that is too cumbersome to be useful in routine clinical practice. The present author possesses a conviction that mechanistically oriented theories such as the SH-MT and the LQ models are most useful since they often allow for systematic addition of complexity one layer at a time on top of the most elementary hypothesis. Such theoretical construct can better serve to generate new hypothesis when the observed data do not agree with the model's prediction. It is also more pedagogically sound, in tune with a remark by the distinguished radiobiology teacher Eric Hall that "the function of a radiation biologist is to make the clinician think" (Hall 1994).

6.4 Conclusion

In this brief update of the author's prior exposition (Lee et al. 2006), the fundamental concepts behind the standard practice of multi-fractionated radiation therapy have been reviewed. With the increasingly popular use of single-fraction or hypofractionated regimens as done in SRS or SBRT, the apparent violation of the conventional wisdom in classical radiobiology now begs for new insights. Modifications of the old quantitative models in order to explain the clinical efficacy of hypofractionation have been proposed and reviewed here. In general, most of these new models aim to mitigate the lack of applicability of the popular LQ model at high fractional dose range. Most are unfortunately more complicated mathematically, and some are frankly created without keeping the original mechanistic spirit in the biophysically derived theories. Meanwhile, new biological processes were hypothesized as alternatives to what have been preached in classical radiobiology. Most of the findings based on molecular or subcellular investigations remain qualitative gestures, or if quantitative at all might be embedded within the current mathematic frameworks without creating significant practical difference. Perhaps, in the eyes of clinicians and patients eager to exploit the logistic and technical advantages of SRS or SBRT, it may be legitimate to describe the clinical efficacy of ultra-precision-oriented yet hypofractionated radiotherapy as the ultimate product of "bad biology (in the sense of lacking true understanding) compensated by good physics."

References

Alpen EL (1998) Theories and models for cell survival. In: Alpen EL (ed) Radiation biophysics, 2nd edn. Academic Press, San Diego, pp 132–287

Astrahan M (2008) Some implications of linear-quadratic-linear radiation dose-response with regard to hypofractionation. Med Phys 35:4161–4172

Bao S, Wu Q, McLendon RE, Hao Y, Shi Q, Hjelmeland AB, Dewhirst MW, Bigner DD, Rich JN (2006) Glioma stem cells promote radioresistance by preferential activation of the DNA damage response. Nature 444:756–760

Barendsen GW (1982) Dose fractionation, dose rate and isoeffect relationships for normal tissue response. Int J Radiat Oncol Biol Phys 8:1981–1997

Brenner DJ (2008) The linear-quadratic model is an appropriate methodology for determining isoeffective doses at large dose per fraction. Semin Radiat Oncol 18:234–239

Brenner DJ, Hall EJ (1991) Conditions for the equivalence of continuous to pulsed low dose rate brachytherapy. Int J Radiat Oncol Biol Phys 20:181–190

Brenner DJ, Hall EJ (1992) The origins and basis of the linear-quadratic model (Letter). Int J Radiat Oncol Biol Phys 23:252

Brenner DJ, Huang Y, Hall EJ (1991) Fractionated high dose-rate versus low dose-rate regimens for intracavitary brachytherapy of the cervix: equivalent regimens for combined brachytherapy and external irradiation. Int J Radiat Oncol Biol Phys 21:1415–1423

Carlone M, Wilkins D, Raaphorst G (2005) The modified linear quadratic model of Guerrero and Li can be derived from mechanistic basis and exhibits linear-quadratic-linear behavior. Phys Med Biol 50:L9–L15

Coutard H (1932) Roentgen therapy of epitheliomas of the tonsillar region, hypopharynx, and larynx from 1920 to 1926. Am J Roentgenol 28:313–331, and 343–348

Curtis SB (1986) Lethal and potentially lethal lesions induced by radiation – a unified repair model. Radiat Res 106: 252–270

Ellis F (1967) Fractionation in radiotherapy. In: Deeley TJ, Woods CAP (eds) Modern trends in radiotherapy, vol 1. Butterworths, London, pp 34–51

Flickinger JC, Kondziolka D, Lunsford LD (2003) Radiobiological analysis of tissue responses following radiosurgery. Technol Cancer Res Treat 2(2):1–6

Fowler JF (1989) The linear-quadratic formula and progress in fractionated radiotherapy. Br J Radiol 62:679–694

Fowler JF (1992) Intercomparisons of new and old schedules in fractionated radiotherapy. Semin Radiat Oncol 2:67–72

Guerrero M, Li X (2004) Extending the linear-quadratic model for large fraction doses pertinent to stereotactic radiotherapy. Phys Med Biol 49:4825–4835

Hall EJ (1994) ASTRO Gold Medal: the function of a radiobiologist is to make the clinician think. Int J Radiat Oncol Biol Phys 29:891–892

Kavanagh BD, Newman F (2008) Toward a unified survival curve: in regard to Park et al. (Int J Radiat Oncol Biol Phys 2008;70:847–852) and Krueger et al. (Int J Radiat Oncol Biol Phys 2007;69:1262–1271). Int J Radiat Oncol Biol Phys 71:958–959

Kellerer AM, Rossi HH (1972) The theory of dual radiation action. Curr Top Radiat Res 8:85–158

Kirk J, Gray WM, Watson ER (1971) Cumulative radiation effect. Part I. Fractionated treatment regimens. Clin Radiol 22:145–155

Kirpatrick JP, Meyer JJ, Marks LB (2008) The linear-quadratic model is inappropriate to model high dose per fraction effects in radiotherapy. Semin Radiat Oncol 18:240–243

Lea DE, Catcheside DG (1942) The mechanism of the induction by radiation of chromosome aberrations in *Tradescantia*. J Genet 44:216–245

Lee SP, Leu MY, Smathers JB, McBride WH, Parker RG, Withers HR (1995) Biologically effective dose distribution based on the linear quadratic model and its clinical relevance. Int J Radiat Oncol Biol Phys 33:375–389

Lee SP, Withers HR, Fowler JF (2006) Radiobiological considerations. In: Slotman BJ, Solberg T, Wurm R (eds) Extracranial stereotactic radiotherapy and radiosurgery. Taylor & Francis, New York, pp 131–176

McKenna F, Ahmad S (2009) Toward a unified survival curve: in regard to Kavanagh and Newman (Int J Radiat Oncol Biol Phys 2008;71:958–959) and Park et al. (Int J Radiat Oncol Biol Phys 2008;70:847–852). Int J Radiat Oncol Biol Phys 73:640

Oliver R (1964) A comparison of the effects of acute and protracted gamma-radiation on the growth of seedlings of *Vicia faba*. II. Theoretical calculations. Int J Radiat Biol 8:475–488

Orton CG, Ellis F (1973) A simplification in the use of the NSD concept in practical radiotherapy. Br J Radiol 46:529–537

Park C, Papiez L, Zhang S, Story M, Timmerman R (2008) Universal survival curve and single fraction equivalent dose: useful tools in understanding potency of ablative radiotherapy. Int J Radiat Oncol Biol Phys 70:847–852

Puck TT, Marcus PI (1956) Action of X-rays on mammalian cells. J Exp Med 103:653–666

Schwarzschild K (1900) On the law of reciprocity for bromide of silver gelatin. Astrophys J 11:89

Sheline GE, Wara WM, Smith V (1980) Therapeutic irradiation and brain injury. Int J Radiat Oncol Biol Phys 6:1215–1228

Strandqvist M (1944) Studieren über die kumulative Wirkung der Röntgen-strahlen bei Fraktionierung. Acta Radiol 55(Suppl):1–300

Thames HD (1985) An 'incomplete-repair' model for survival after fractionated and continuous irradiations. Int J Radiat Biol 47:319–339

Thames H, Withers H (1980) Test of equal effect per fraction and estimation of initial clonogen number in micro-colony assays of survival after fractionated irradiation. Br J Radiol 53:1071–1077

Thames HD, Withers HR, Peters LJ, Fletcher GH (1982) Changes in early and late radiation responses with altered dose fractionation: implications for dose-survival relationships. Int J Radiat Oncol Biol Phys 8:219–226

Timmerman R, Bastasch M, Saha D, Abdulrahman R, Hittson W, Story M (2007) Optimizing dose and fractionation for stereotactic body radiation therapy. In: Meyer JL (ed) IMRT, IGRT, SBRT – Advances in the treatment planning and delivery of radiotherapy, vol 40, Front Radiat Ther Oncol. Karger, Basel, pp 352–365

Tomé WA (2008) Universal survival curve and single fraction equivalent dose: useful tools in understanding potency of ablative radiotherapy: in regard to Park et al. (Int J Radiat

Oncol Biol Phys 2008;70:847–852). Int J Radiat Oncol Biol Phys 72:1620

Wang JZ, Mayr NA, Yu WTC (2007) A generalized linear-quadratic formula for high-dose-rate brachytherapy and radiosurgery. Int J Radiat Oncol Biol Phys 69:S619–S620

Withers HR (1975) The 4R's of radiotherapy. In: Lett JT, Alder H (eds) Advances in radiation biology, vol 5. Academic Press, New York, p 241

Withers HR, Peters LJ (1980) Biological aspects of radiation therapy. In: Fletcher GH (ed) Textbook of radiotherapy, 3rd edn. Lea & Febiger, Philadelphia, pp 103–180

Withers HR, Thames HD, Peters LJ (1982) Differences in the fractionation response of acute and late responding tissues. In: Karcher KH, Kogelnik HD, Reinartz G (eds) Progress in radio-oncology II. Raven Press, New York, pp 257–296

Withers HR, Thames HD, Peters LJ (1983) A new isoeffect curve for change in dose per fraction. Radiother Oncol 1: 187–191

Withers HR, Taylor JMG, Maciejewski B (1988) The hazard of accelerated tumor clonogen repopulation during radiotherapy. Acta Oncol 27:131–146

Yaes RJ, Patel P, Maruyama Y (1991) On using the linear-quadratic model in daily clinical practice. Int J Radiat Oncol Biol Phys 20:1353–1362

Yaes RJ, Patel P, Maruyama Y (1992) Response to Brenner and Hall (Letter). Int J Radiat Oncol Biol Phys 23:252–253

Part II

Cranial Radiosurgery

Radiosurgery for Arteriovenous Malformations

7

Antonio A.F. De Salles and Alessandra A. Gorgulho

7.1 Introduction

Radiosurgery became widely used and accepted due to its remarkable results on the treatment of previously unresectable arteriovenous malformations (Hosobuchi 1987; Kjellberg et al. 1983; Steiner 1972). The work of the pioneers was repeated, confirmed, and expanded bringing better understanding of dose (Karlsson et al. 1997; Pedroso et al. 2004), volume (Ellis et al. 1998), brain eloquence (Pollock et al. 2004), angioarchitecture (Yuki et al. 2010), fractions of radiation (Lindvall et al. 2003; Veznedaroglu et al. 2004; Xiao et al. 2010), and staged treatment (Sirin et al. 2006). Diverse techniques have been used; allowing the challenge of previously established dogmas generated by technical limitations such as radiation field size, imaging resolution and modality, and finally the possibility of effectively, logistically, and precisely taking advantage of established radiobiology knowledge. This chapter objectively summarizes important developments in arteriovenous malformation (AVM) radiosurgery using the established dose/volume knowledge and pushing the envelope to take advantage of novel technologies that improved conformality and homogeneity of radiation volumes to tackle previously untreatable arteriovenous malformations.

7.1.1 Radiosurgical Indications

The concept of a general risk of bleeding for AVMs of the brain initially established in the literature as approximately 3% per year, confirmed by the work of the group from Helsinki in the 1990s (Ondra et al. 1990) and recently reinforced by the same institution (Hernesniemi et al. 2008), has been changing with the identification of risk factors for bleeding. The Columbia group has established several risk factors that must be taken into account when deciding on the treatment of cerebral AVMs. When analyzing risk factors for bleeding such as deep venous drainage, deep location, and hemorrhage at presentation, these investigators found that if no bleeding risk factor is present, the annual risk of bleeding is 0.9%, while if deep venous drainage is present the risk rises to 2.4%. When the AVM is in a deep location, the risk is already 3.1% and increases to 4% annually if intracranial hemorrhage was the form of presentation. If a patient presents with all these risk factors accumulated, the risk of hemorrhage reaches 34.4% per year (Al-Shahi and Stapf 2005). This important description of risk factors is of utmost importance on the decision making for treatment of an individual patient harboring an AVM in the brain. Moreover, recent evidence shows that the excess in mortality is highest in conservatively treated patients, intermediate in patients with partially occluded AVMs, and lowest in those with totally occluded AVMs (Laakso et al. 2008). The treatment of an AVM must therefore be decided minding the four options for initial management, i.e., surgery, embolization, radiosurgery, and watchful observation (Fig. 7.1).

7.1.2 Surgery

The most used classification of AVMs, the Spetzler and Martin grading system, was designed to evaluate the risks of surgery (Spetzler and Martin 1986). For

A.A.F. De Salles (✉) and A.A. Gorgulho
Department of Neurosurgery and Radiation Oncology, David Geffen School of Medicine at UCLA, 10495 Le Conte Avenue, Suite 2120, Los Angeles, CA 90095, USA
e-mail: adesalles@mednet.ucla.edu

A.A.F. De Salles et al. (eds.), *Shaped Beam Radiosurgery*, DOI: 10.1007/978-3-642-11151-8_7, © Springer-Verlag Berlin Heidelberg 2011

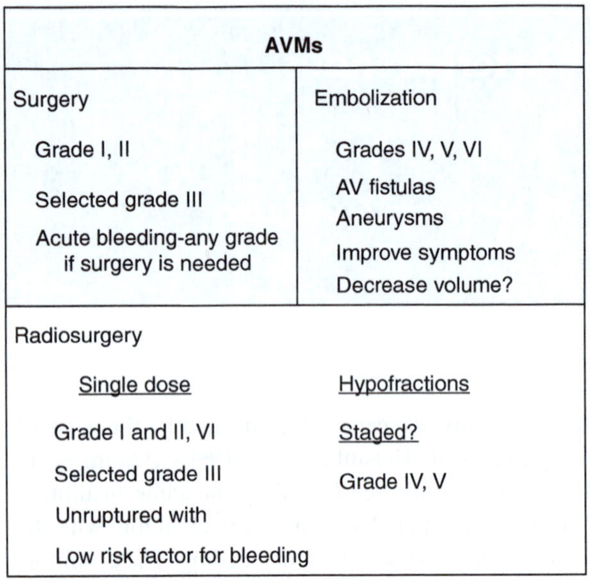

Fig. 7.1 Selection of treatment for arteriovenous malformations based on Spetzler–Martin Grade. Combination of two or even the three modalities of treatment may be necessary. Watchful observation is the option in rare situations

Table 7.1 Factors leading to AVM Grade[a] and surgical risk

	Points	Risk of new neurological deficit	
AVM size			
Small (<3 cm)	1	Grade I	0%
Medium (3-6 cm)	2	Grade II	5%
Large (>6 cm)	3	Grade III	16%
AVM location		Grade IV	27%
Non-eloquent	0	Grade V	31%
Eloquent	1	Grade VI	Surgery would lead to 100% mortality or unacceptable deficits
Venous drainage			
Superficial only	0		
Deep	1		

Modified from Spetzler and Martin (1986)
[a]Grade is addition of points from each factors, size, location, venous drainage

example, Grade I lesion has a surgical risk of causing a new neurological deficit of 0%, Grade II of 5%, Grade III of 16%, Grade IV of 27%, Grade V 31%, and Grade VI is truly inoperable because it involves diencephalon and vital areas of the brainstem (Table 7.1). These Grade VI lesions are not linked to the features of the grading system such as deep venous drainage or size; it relies only on location for grading (Fig. 7.2). The advantage of surgery over all treatment options is well accepted, as it is the only technique that immediately resolves the risk of intracranial bleeding from the AVM. It is the technique of choice when possible with acceptable neurological consequences. Therefore, only Grade I, II, and selected Grade III AVMs have surgery as the upfront treatment of choice. The other AVMs will go to surgery when there is an acute bleeding, already causing neurological deficit and an emergency surgery for decompression is necessary. In this situation, if possible, the AVM must be completely removed. It is generally accepted that Grade IV, V, and VI lesions are not operable. These lesions today are either left to follow their natural history, have adjuvant embolization followed by radiosurgery or radiosurgery alone. Treatment of these high-grade lesions is controversial, as discussed below. A randomized trial (ARUBA) is recruiting to answer this question.

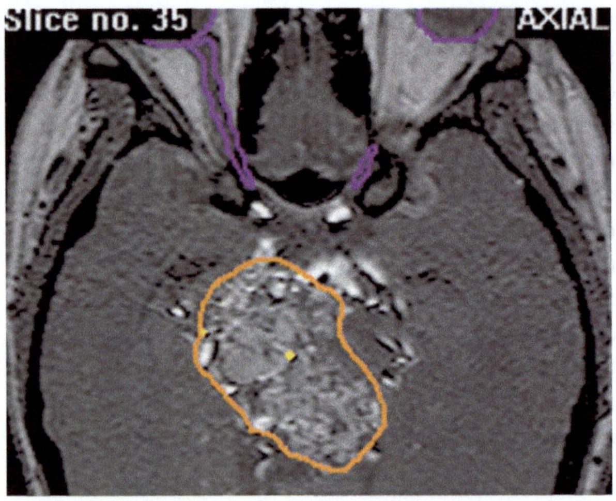

Fig. 7.2 Grade VI AVM treated with stereotactic radiotherapy, 5 fractions of 6 Gy. Notice the tight contour of the nidus

7.1.3 Embolization

Endovascular procedures revolutionized the management of vascular malformations in the brain. As AVMs are associated with flow-related aneurysms (Westphal and Grzyska 2000) and presence of large arteriovenous fistulas through the nidus low-pressure system, embolization takes an important role in the management of AVMs (Yuki et al. 2010). Embolization may provide control of large fistulas, obliteration of aneurysms in relation to the feeding vessel or circle of Willis region, decreasing the risk of intracranial bleeding. It may also improve symptoms related to high flow through the AVM nidus, such as severe headaches, seizures, and progressive neurologic deficit due to steal phenomenon. Nidus volume reduction has also been a goal of AVM embolization; however, its impact on the treatment of these lesions has been controversial (Andrade-Souza et al. 2007). This has been even more controversial when one adds the risks posed by the embolization procedure alone, which varies in the literature from 5% to 13% (Gobin et al. 1996; Yuki et al. 2010) and should be added to the risks of other procedures such as radiosurgery or surgery, since embolization is usually adjunctive to these therapies. Embolizations resulted in a mortality rate of 1.6% in published series (Gobin et al. 1996). Embolization alone will obliterate completely an AVM in approximately 11.2% of the cases. This happens usually in unique lesions with one or very few feeders.

7.1.4 Embolization and Radiosurgery

The combination of embolization and radiosurgery has been the study focus of various groups. Since volume is an important limiting factor for radiosurgery dose, its success in obliterating large AVMs, i.e., Grade IV and V AVMs, the trial of decreasing the nidus volume with various techniques of embolization was met with enthusiasm by many investigators (Dawson et al. 1990; Gobin et al. 1996; Guo et al. 1993; Mathis et al. 1995; Plasencia et al. 1999; Richling 2000; Spagnuolo et al. 2009). Recently, however it is becoming clear that embolization adds to the risk of radiosurgery and may not help the obliteration rate of AVMs (De Salles et al. 1999). As the Toronto group has reported, embolization before radiosurgery decreases the obliteration rate, even in AVMs with the same volume, location, and marginal dose (Andrade-Souza et al. 2007). Table 7.2 shows the results obtained with the association of embolization and radiosurgery over the years.

Embolization must however be associated with radiosurgery when the angioarchitecture requires, i.e., large fistulas or threatening aneurysms are associated to the AVM (Yuki et al. 2010; Westphal and Grzyska 2000) (Fig. 7.3). Its role in helping radiosurgery by

Table 7.2 Complete obliteration of AVMs treated with embolization and radiosurgery

Author		Obliteration (%)
Dawson et al.	1990	28.5
Guo et al.	1993	33.3
Mathis et al.	1995	50
Gobin et al.	1996	65
Plasensia et al.	1999	42
Richling	2000	51.7
Andrade-Souza et al.	2007	47
Spagnuolo et al.	2009	25

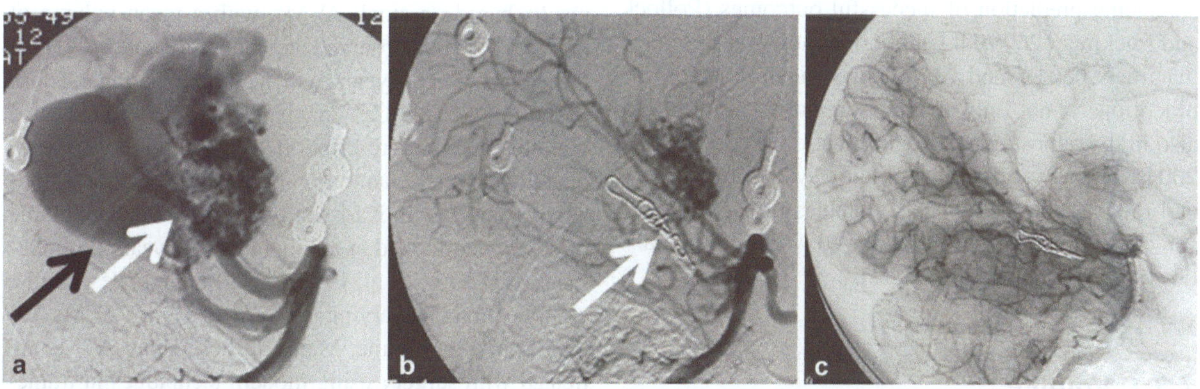

Fig. 7.3 (**a** and **d**) Spetzler–Martin Grade IV AVM with a large venous aneurysm (*black arrow*) and large flow fistula (*white arrow*) treated with coil embolization (*white arrow*) followed by radiosurgery (**b** and **e**). The prescription was 16 Gy at 90% isodose encompassing the residual AVM. Complete obliteration of the lesion 2 years after radiosurgery (**c** and **f**). This 5-year-old girl presented with intracranial bleeding

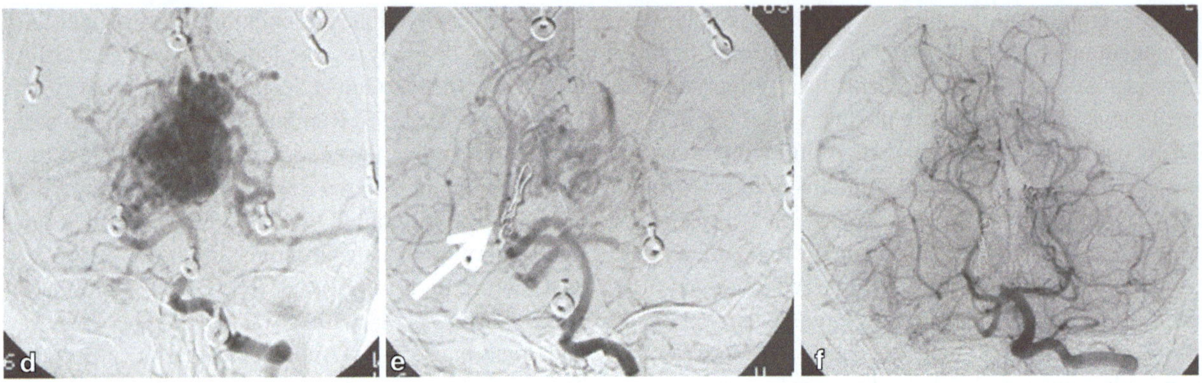

Fig. 7.3 (continued)

decreasing AVM flow or volume has not been confirmed. Precise indication of embolization associated with radiosurgery is presented in Fig. 7.1.

7.2 Defining the Complexity of an AVM: Volume and Location

AVM volume and brain function in the area harboring the AVM are the two most limiting factors when managing arteriovenous malformations. Spetzler and Martin developed the classification of AVMs thinking of surgical risks, these two factors; especially size of the lesion, reflecting its volume, took great weight in their classification (1986). Volume and brain functional eloquence are also primordial factors to evaluate risks of radiosurgery. Recent classifications directed to radiosurgery try to take advantage of other factors such as age to include in the prognostication of AVMs treated by radiosurgery, enhancing prediction of successful outcomes (Pollock and Flickinger 2008). It is important however to realize that the Spetzler and Martin classification helps the practitioners, not only for the surgical indication, but also in the radiosurgical prognostication (Pedroso et al. 2004). The use of the same grading system for surgery and radiosurgery patients also enables direct comparison of the treatment results achieved with both modalities (Andrade-Souza et al. 2005).

7.2.1 Volume

Initial work in radiosurgery was limited by size of radiation fields and techniques of radiation delivery available. Cobalt-based units limited the treatment of lesions to a maximum diameter of 3 cm for many years (Lunsford et al. 1991; Steiner et al. 1972). This limitation has been challenged by investigators using diverse approaches (Colombo et al. 1994; De Salles 1997; Friedman et al. 1995). Giant AVMs were treated by the pioneers of radiosurgery using heavy particle irradiation, i.e., proton beam or alpha particles. Here substantial and effective doses were delivered, leading to high complication rate (Hosobuchi et al. 1987; Kjellberg et al. 1983). Meticulous work by Kjellberg and collaborators to avoid complications of radiosurgery showed that as volume increased, dose should be decreased, to a point that the treatment became ineffective (Barker et al. 2003; Seifert et al. 1994). For example, to keep the risk of complication to a 5% level, the dose delivered to an AVM of 5 cm in longest diameter would be 11 Gy (Table 7.3). This dose is unlikely to obliterate an AVM based on the logarithmic predictive curve described by Karlsson et al. (1996).

The Swedish series (Karlsson et al. 1996) published results based on small AVMs, with a mean volume of only 3.6 cc. They observed an obliteration rate of 80% of the lesions within 2 years, with a minimal peripheral dose to the nidus of 23 Gy. Larger lesions cannot be treated with this minimal prescription dose without severe complications. Other Gamma-unit series reported on lesions slightly larger than Karlsson et al., with a mean volume of 4.1 cc and looked at angiograms at 3 years posttreatment (Flickinger et al. 1996). These authors described a complication rate varying from 3% to 5% for AVMs less than 8.0 cc in volume. Many of these small AVMs are treated with surgery using modern techniques in frameless stereotactic surgery. AVMs of 2.5 cm in diameter are small, considering the majority of the AVMs treated nowadays with radiosurgery in centers using particle beams or linear accelerator techniques (Table 7.3).

Table 7.3 Dose based on Kjellberg's 3% risk of radiation necrosis for AVMs

Maximum diameter (cm)[a]	Maximum radius (R) (cm)[a]	AVM vol. CC sphere assumption	Kellberg 3% non-Eloq[b]	Kellberg 3% Eloq[b]
0.70	0.35	0.18	50 Gy	38 Gy
1.00	0.50	0.53	38 Gy	28 Gy
1.50	0.75	1.78	30 Gy	20 Gy
2.00	1.00	4.22	22 Gy	16 Gy
2.50	*1.25*	*8.24*	*18 Gy*	*14 Gy*
3.00	1.50	14.24	16 Gy	13 Gy
4.00	2.00	33.76	14 Gy	12 Gy
5.00	2.50	65.94	11 Gy	8 Gy
6.00	3.00	113.94	9 Gy	6 Gy

[a]Assumption of Spheric AVM, formula: $V=(4/3)\ \pi R^3$ volume in cubic centimeters
[b]Eloq, Eloquent brain tissue

Authors using techniques with field size limitation have resorted to staged radiosurgery to treat large volume AVMs (Sirin et al. 2006). Partial irradiation of AVMs has been hampered by a higher incidence of bleeding during the obliteration waiting period (Sirin et al. 2006; Colombo et al. 1994). Complete irradiation of the nidus, including portions already embolized, may be necessary to achieve complete obliteration with the same risk of bleeding expected in the natural history of AVMs. There are, however, authors who believe that an AVM completely irradiated has a reduced risk of bleeding as the vasculature thickens toward complete obstruction of the lumen (Fig. 7.4) (Massoud et al. 2000; Karlsson et al. 1996).

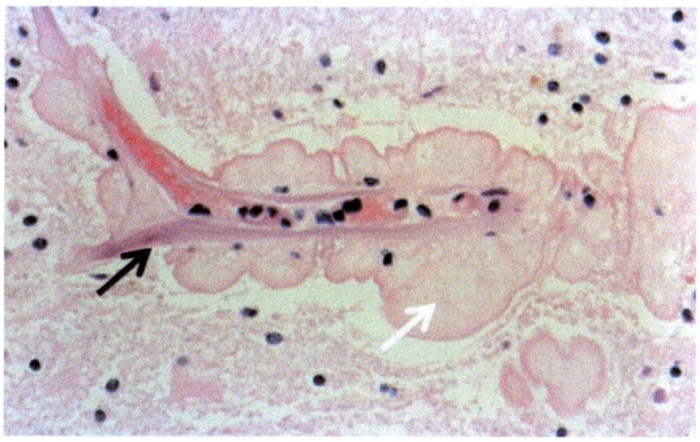

Fig. 7.4 Histology of an AVM vessel irradiated in process of obliteration (H&E). Notice the accumulation of collagen type IV in surrounding the vascular wall (*white arrow*), thickening of the muscle layer (*black arrow*), and accumulation of cells in the vascular lumen to evolve into thrombosis

7.2.2 Location

A series of 56 AVMs located in the thalamus, basal ganglia, and brainstem, with a mean volume of 3.8 cc and treated with a mean peripheral dose of 18 Gy, resulted in 43% obliteration after one radiosurgery and 57% after repeated radiosurgery. Complications after single and multiple treatments were 12–18%, respectively (Pollock et al. 2004). The Karlsson et al. series (Karlsson et al. 1997), describing AVMs with similar volumes, showed different results. The radiation dose prescribed by Pollock et al. was significantly lower due to the AVM location, therefore leading to less impressive obliteration rates. Even though the dose was decreased, the complication rate was higher in comparison to the Karlsson's group study (Karlsson et al. 1997). One should always have in mind, when deciding on the prescription dose, that AVMs in eloquent brain will most likely become symptomatic due to bleeding or radiation-induced edema. For example, Table 7.3 shows that an 8 cc AVM in non-eloquent brain is treated with 18 Gy, while one of the same volume located in eloquent brain is treated with 14 Gy (Table 7.3).

7.2.3 Dose

Development of a repair reaction in the wall of the microvasculature of the AVM nidus is sine qua non for the final obliteration of the AVM (De Salles et al. 1996; Jahan et al. 2006) (Fig. 7.4). This desirable reaction for

AVM obliteration is undesirable when the goal of the radiation delivery includes preservation of normal tissue vasculature while killing tumor cells intermingled with this normal tissue. This opposite goal explains why protracted radiation schemes, designed to preserve non-neoplastic tissues fail to obliterate AVMs (Lindqvist et al. 1986). Single dose is therefore the best approach to achieve complete obliteration of arteriovenous malformation within the shortest waiting period. Obliteration is directly proportional to the dose delivered (De Salles et al. 1996; Karlsson et al. 1997).

The highest dose delivered safely will lead to the highest rate of obliteration in the shortest period of time, therefore achieving the goal of AVM treatment, i.e., fastest decrease of symptoms and risk of hemorrhage with the lowest risk of complication. This difficult balance is the challenge of the AVM radiosurgical treatment. In the author's experience, small lesions (Table 7.3), i.e., smaller than 8.24 cc (2.5 mm largest diameter), can be treated safely with dose between 16 and 20 Gy for the goal of an approximate 90% obliteration rate in 3 years with a transient complication rate of approximately 2% (Pedroso et al. 2004). This is achieved with highly conformal and homogeneous treatments, prescription at the 90% isodose line (IDL); this is a possible prescription when using shaped beam and intensity modulation modalities in addition to minding the functional eloquence of the AVM location, see last column in Table 7.3.

The volume of functional brain tissue surrounding the AVM receiving 12 Gy, including the nidus, has been implicated as a risk factor for development of permanent symptomatic sequela from radiosurgery (Flickinger et al. 2000). It is possible to take advantage of this important information when using dose-volume histogram analysis to fine-tune the dose prescription (Fig. 7.5). It is suggested that the volume

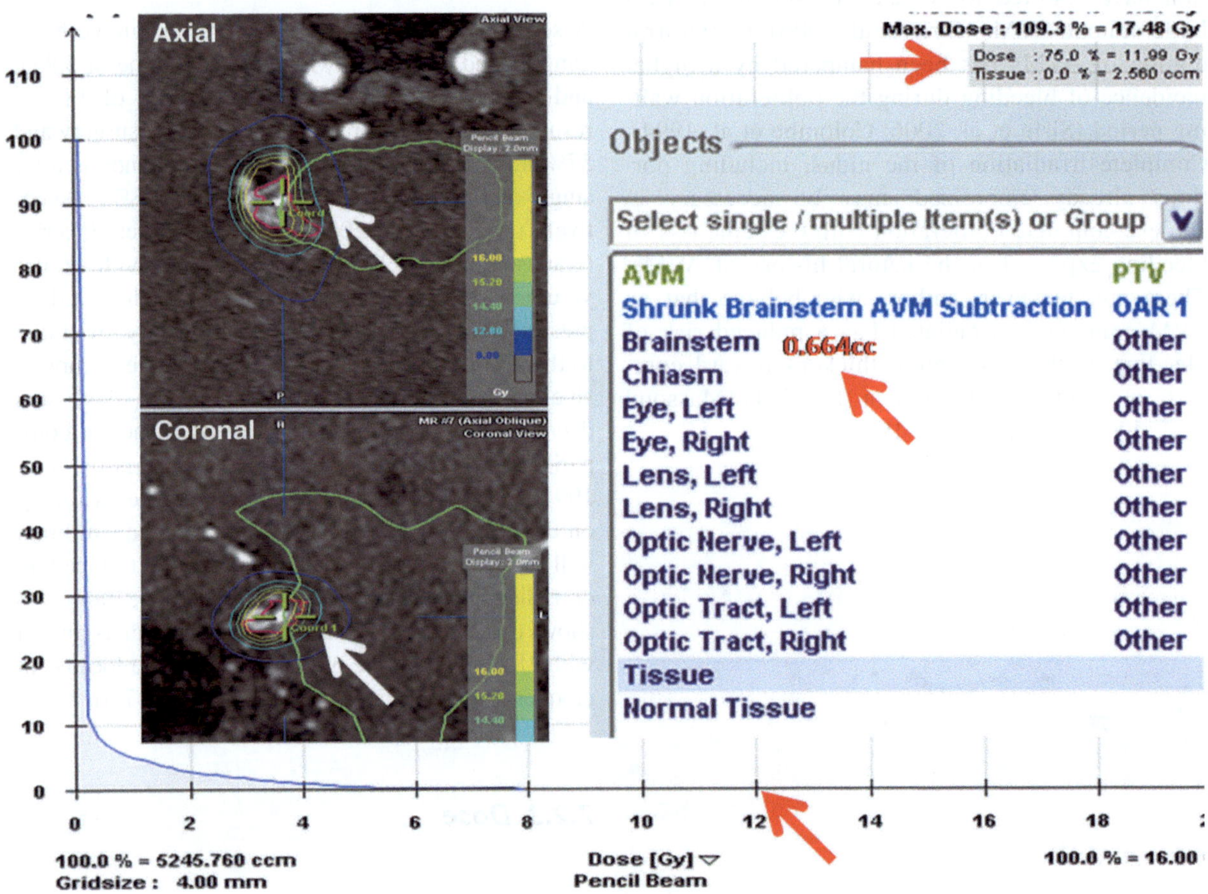

Fig. 7.5 AVM abutting and invading the right surface of the brainstem seen on axial and coronal MRIs (*white arrows*). The AVM received 16 Gy to the periphery and a maximal dose to the lesion of 17.48 Gy (*horizontal red arrow*). The dose-volume histogram demonstrates the volume of normal tissue surrounding the AVM receiving 12 Gy (*horizontal red arrow*), including the AVM volume and the volume of brainstem receiving 12 Gy (*oblique red arrows*). Notice that the software can give an estimate of the dose received by each structure listed and automatically segmented, as exemplified with the contour of the brainstem (*green brainstem outline*). Notice the dose shift away from the brainstem in this IMRT plan (*Axial*)

encompassed by the 12 Gy be smaller than 10 cc, including the AVM volume. When this is not possible with an effective dose, it may be necessary to resort to hypofractionation or staged treatment (Xiao et al. 2010; Sirin et al. 2006).

When lesions increase in size and their location is vital, like in brainstem (AVMs Grade VI); the dose has to be decreased. However, many brainstem AVMs have a small volume and although it is fair to expect lower obliteration rates, excellent results can still be obtained. Moreover, retreatment will achieve good results when repeated 3 years after the initial radiosurgery (Karlsson et al. 2007; Maesawa et al. 2000). As reflected in Table 7.3, AVMs of large volumes require decrease of the dose to a point that the treatment becomes unlikely to lead to complete response (Pedroso et al. 2004). At this point, hypofractions of radiation can be offered to decrease the volume of the AVM in preparation for a single dose within 3–4 years, when volume has been substantially reduced. Hypofractionation was not observed to increase the risk of hemorrhage during the obliteration waiting period (Xiao et al. 2010).

The hypofractionated scheme triggers obliteration to a slower path when compared to single fraction radiosurgery (Lindvall et al. 2003). However, when irradiating large and complex AVMs, the modifications into the angioarchitecture must be slow, so the safety goal is also achieved. The staged radiosurgery procedure has shown an increased bleeding rate with significant permanent sequela during the obliteration waiting period. The increased bleeding rate is probably a consequence of an unequal proportion of obliteration between the outflow portions of the AVM in comparison to the inflow portions. Neurosurgeons have met difficulty with sudden and unequal obliteration of AVMs in the past, not only with resection of giant AVMs causing the breakthrough phenomenon, but also with partial resection of the lesion causing increased risk of bleeding when residual AVM is left after surgery (Spetzler et al. 1987).

7.2.4 Hypofractional Dose

The successful management of giant cerebral arteriovenous malformations (AVMs) remains a challenge. Giant AVMs classified as high Grade, i.e., Grade IV and V in Spetzler–Martin grading presented an unacceptable surgical risk (Spetzler and Martin 1986). As discussed above, as the volume increases the ability of the current radiosurgery techniques to provide an effective dose of radiation in a single session decreases. The strategy of partially embolizing the AVM to achieve a smaller volume was met with disappointment by several investigators (Andrade-Souza et al. 2007). Therefore, strategies of maximizing the dose of radiation, using radiobiology principles of multiple fractions to preserve normal tissue and still cause a repair reaction in the vasculature of a giant AVM becomes necessary. Hypofractionation (HSRT), i.e., the maximal dose per fraction acceptable in terms of risk and yet producing a repair reaction in the AVM nidus became a testable strategy. This became more compelling when multimodality treatment gave less than desirable results for these lesions. Chang et al. reviewed their results of multimodality treatment for giant AVMs at Stanford University and reported complete cure in only 36% of patients. That was at the cost of 15% mortality plus 15% long-term morbidity (Chang et al. 2003).

Lindvall et al. pioneered the HSRT approach reporting significant occlusion rates between 2 and 8 years after HSRT using a scheme of 5 fractions of 6 Gy (Lindvall et al. 2003). Veznedaroglu et al. reviewed their results of HSRT at Jefferson University and reported a 7.2-fold greater occlusion rate of 7 Gy in 6 fractions over 5 Gy in 6 fractions cohorts (Veznedaroglu et al. 2004). However, they actually abandoned the 7 Gy scheme due to the high overall treatment related morbidity rate of 43%, a sustained complication rate of 14% and one posttreatment death from radiation reaction. We used 5 and 6 Gy fractions, to a total dose of 30 Gy, and showed that our dose scheme was safe, but obliteration was only partial. The 6 Gy fractions applied to achieve 30 Gy was statistically significantly more effective than the 5 Gy fractions to achieve 25 or 30 Gy. Prescriptions were always highly homogeneous and conformal, isodose line of prescription of 90% using shaped beam fields or intensity modulation radiation therapy (IMRT). At UCLA, HSRT is used as a preparatory procedure to decrease the AVM volume for further definite treatment with radiosurgery or surgery. Its ability to substantially diminish the AVMs volume with acceptable complication rate, meaning only transient effects, becomes very useful in the multimodality approach of these difficult giant AVMs. Currently, we recommend 6 Gy in 5 fractions in consecutive days, 1 week treatment for AVMs Grade IV, V, and VI with a large volume of the AVM extending to areas nearby the brainstem.

7.3 Planning Imaging and Prescription

Shaped beam, either with dynamic arcs or static beams, IMRT as needed and tight dose distribution without margin at the periphery of the AVM is the policy for planning all vascular lesions to be treated with radiosurgery or HSRT. Angiography is always indicated if the patient has not had an angiography at diagnosis to rule out presence of aneurysms and high flow embolizable fistulas, as the association of these entities with AVMs of the brain is frequent and they do not respond to radiation. They may also pose more risk of bleeding and cause more symptoms than the AVM nidus per se. magnetic resonance image (MRI), magnetic resonance angiography (MRA), and compute tomography (CT) angiogram are usually appropriate to develop a radiosurgery plan but may be inadequate to evaluate fistulas and some aneurysms in distal feeding arteries. These lesions may not be readily visualized using these techniques. Stereotactic angiography may be required in cases of very diffuse nidus or post-embolization when differentiation of neo-vascularization from nidus is difficult on MRA or computed tomography angiography (CTA). Figure 7.5 shows an example of a difficult AVM plan. The "hot spot" is not higher than 10–20% of the prescription dose when using shaped beam and intensity modulation technology. Also, the hot spot can be selectively placed in a strategic less eloquent region of the brain where the AVM is located. This is easily accomplished by weighting arcs, fields, or restrictions to eloquent structures when this technology is used (Fig. 7.5).

7.4 Analysis of Results and Retreatment

Our data suggest that using shaped-beam radiosurgery and prescribing with a very homogeneous dose throughout the AVM nidus leads to safe dose delivery with only transient side effects of the treatment in 2.3% of the patients. The obliteration rate is highly related to the peripheral dose, being the 18 Gy prescription at the periphery statistically significant as a predictor of complete nidus obliteration, when using single dose. Spetzler–Martin Grade of the AVM is a fair predictor of the complete obliteration of the lesion (Fig. 7.6), as it is expected that low-grade AVMs receive high dose of radiation due to their size and location in less eloquent brain regions (Pedroso et al. 2004). When using hypofractionation to treat giant AVMs (defined as AVMs with more than 5 cm in largest diameter in our reported series), we have shown that 6 Gy in 5 fractions is statistically more effective than 5 Gy in 5 fractions with only transient side effects in 5% of the patients treated. It is expected to see a decrease of approximately 50% of the volume of the AVM per year (Fig. 7.7). At 3 years, the response of the AVM nidus to the treatment reduces to minimum, therefore, at that time we repeat either hypofractionation or single dose depending on the volume of the lesion, i.e., residual lesions less than 10 cc in volume are treated with single dose and lesions of more than 10 cc are treated with repeat fractionation (Xiao et al. 2010). During the waiting period, the bleeding rate was 2.2% per year. This bleeding rate compares favorably with the natural history of AVM hemorrhage.

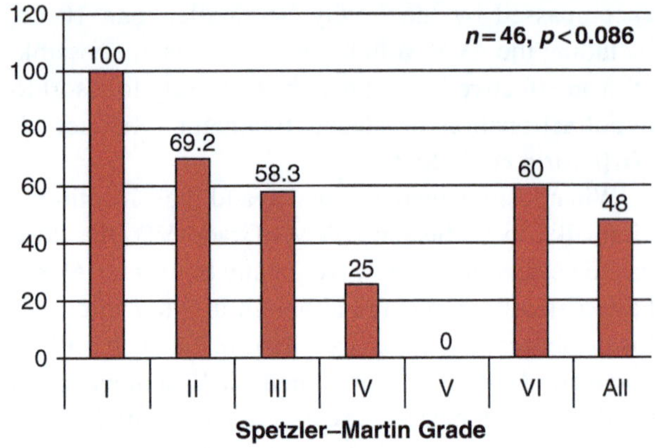

Fig. 7.6 AVMs obliteration rate based on Spetzler and Martin Grade. Less obliteration for high-grade AVMs reflects the importance of volume and eloquence on radiosurgery results. Notice that for AVMs Grade VI, where volume is not a factor in the classification with only eloquence playing a role, obliteration rate is superior to for Grade IV and V. AVMs where volume of the lesion plays important role in the classification

7.5 Spinal AVMs

Spinal radiosurgery is a relatively new application of the technique. Reliable techniques of localization of AVMs in the spine are still in development. Angiography is important for definition of the nidus in the spinal cord, however good angiographic integration with the planning software for spinal AVMs is still lacking. Exquisite MRA of the spine using 3.0 T

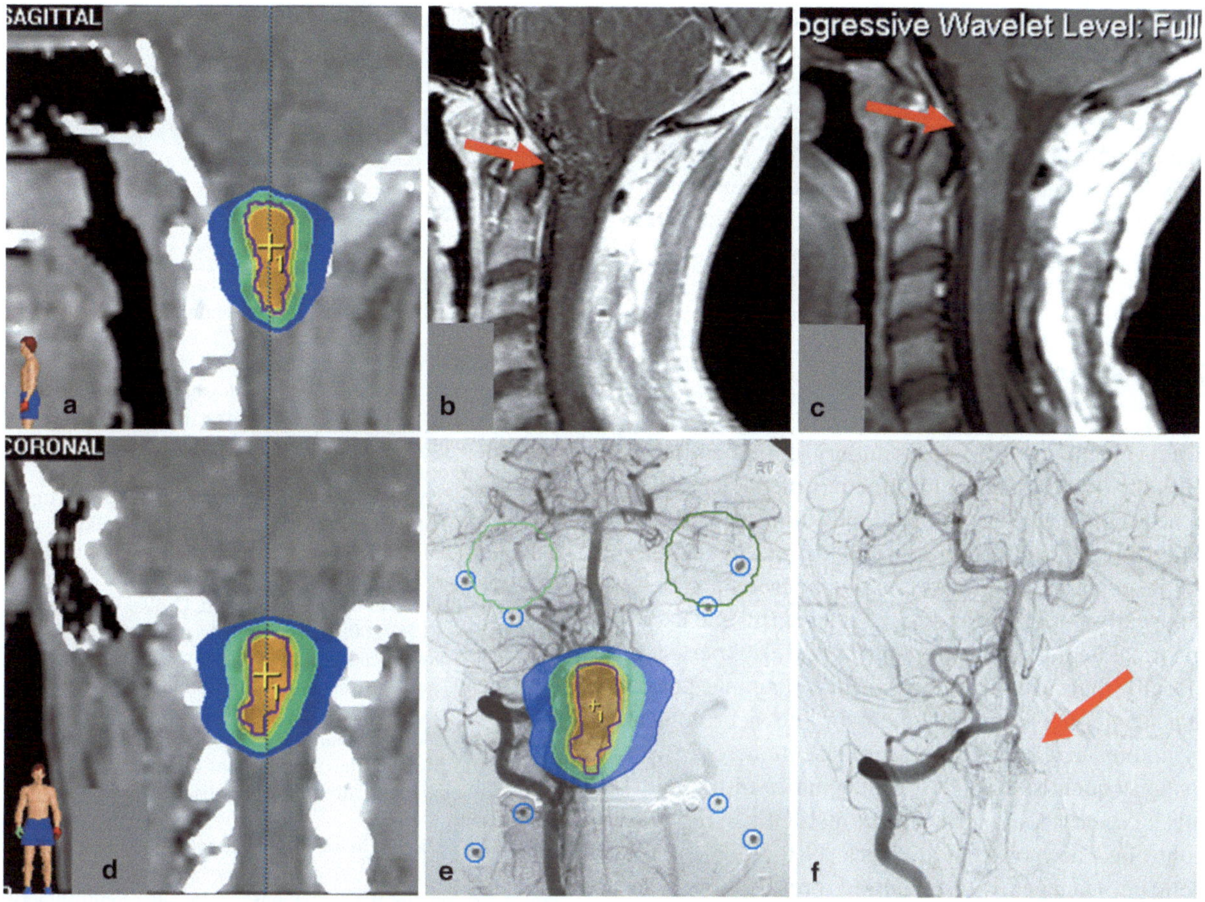

Fig. 7.7 A 22-year-old woman who bled from an AVM at the C1–C2 cord level and became quadriplegic. After emergency decompressive laminectomy, she regained her ability to walk. While still in a wheelchair, she received 12 Gy prescribed to the 90% isodose line (IL) encompassing the lesion. The volume of the lesion was 1.60 cc. (**a**) and (**d**) show the sagittal and coronal views or the radiosurgery plan exposed on CT reconstructions. *Orange* is the volume encompassed by the 90% isodose line, also seen on the angiogram in (**e**). (**b**) Shows the AVM on T1-MRI before treatment and (**c**) shows the response of the AVM to the 12 Gy radiosurgery 2 years later, notice the bright signal in the nidus, denoting obliteration process (Mobin et al. 1999). (**f**) Demonstrates almost complete obliteration of the AVM on angiogram

MRI and CT angiography have been helpful for targeting. Association of these images to standard T2- and T1-weighted MRI through the AVM location allows for definition of the nidus with a certain degree of accuracy. This shortcoming on imaging the spinal AVM nidus obviously limits the dose that one dares to deliver, compromising obliteration rate in the name of safety. As a routine, we deliver 12–14 Gy to the nidus. The plan is repeat treatment at least 3 years later if nidus is still present. Figure 7.7 shows a medullary AVM treated with this approach with remarkable response. The data existent in the literature using the CyberKnife supports hypofractionation (Sinclair et al. 2006), reflecting the difficulty to localize these lesions with certainty, the authors opted for hypofractionation to increase safety.

7.6 Management of Complications

7.6.1 Acute

Patients who have a history of seizures and are in use of anticonvulsants require special management to prevent seizure episodes in the ensuing 72 h after radiosurgery. The radiation delivery in high dose to the already low seizure threshold tissue may lead to induction of multiple seizure episodes, and even status epilepticus. This can be avoided by increasing the dose of the anticonvulsant in use, or adding a second anticonvulsant only during the post-radiosurgery 72 h. There are services that routinely use prophylactic anticonvulsants when treating AVMs; this is not the police in our service.

7.6.2 Delayed

Management of AVM radiosurgery complication is difficult on the patient and treating physician alike. When the patient has not had a bleeding episode and has not developed progressive neurological deficits, the onset of a new and progressive neurological deficit usually 6–18 months after an uneventful and exciting treatment is an extremely stressful experience. Usually the uncertainly of the final outcome generates anxiety. The management of the neurological symptoms may require long-term use of steroids with its consequent side effects. Maintenance of the minimal dose necessary to keep the patient's symptoms controlled and avoid side effects is the goal of the delicate management of steroid prescription. One should start with a high pulse of steroid, 6 mg of dexamethasone every 4 h for 1 week and decrease it rapidly at the rate of 1 mg per day to the minimal possible. Addition of a rheological agent, such as pentoxiphyline may help decrease final neurological deficit by improving flow in the penumbra of the radiation reaction. This has not been substantiated with Class I data, however it may allow early discontinuation of steroids and help the patient cope with the period of radiation reaction without the sense of hopeless and no treatment.

7.7 Conclusions

Improvement of image-guided stereotactic radiation has allowed the treatment of AVMs previously not amenable to radiosurgery. Neurosurgeons and interventional radiologists have resorted to embolization to decrease lesion size; however, this can well be accomplished with hypofractionated treatments. The success observed on the treatment of lesions in the brain is expected to be repeated in the spine and other areas of the body, see Chap. 1.

References

Al-Shahi R, Stapf C (2005) The prognosis and treatment of arteriovenous malformations of the brain. Pract Neurol 5: 194–205

Andrade-Souza YM, Zadeh G, Ramani M, Scora D, Tsao MN, Schwartz ML (2005) Testing the radiosurgery-based arteriovenous malformation score and the modified Spetzler-Martin grading system to predict radiosurgical outcome. J Neurosurgery 103:642–648

Andrade-Souza YM, Ramani M, Scora D, Tsao MN, terBrugge K, Schwartz ML (2007) Embolization before radiosurgery reduces the obliteration rate of arteriovenous malformations. Neurosurgery 60(3):443–451

Barker FG II, Butler WE, Lyons S, Cascio E, Ogilvy CS, Loeffler JS, Chapman PH (2003) Dose-volume prediction of radiation-related complications after proton beam radiosurgery for cerebral arteriovenous malformations. J Neurosurg 99(2):254–263

Chang SD, Marcellus ML, Marks MP, Levy RP, Do HM, Steinberg GK (2003) Multimodality treatment of giant intracranial arteriovenous malformations. Neurosurgery 53(1):1–11, Discussion 11–13

Colombo F, Pozza F, Chierego G, Casentini L, De Luca G, Francescon P (1994) Linear accelerator radiosurgery of cerebral arteriovenous malformations: an update. Neurosurgery 34(1):14–20

Dawson RC 3rd, Tarr RW, Hecht ST, Jungreis CA, Lunsford LD, Coffey R, Horton JA (1990) Treatment of arteriovenous malformations of the brain with combined embolization and stereotactic radiosurgery: results after 1 and 2 years. Am J Neuroradiol 11(5):857–864

De Salles AAF (1997) Radiosurgery for arteriovenous malformations of the brain. J Stroke Cerebrovasc Dis 6: 277–281

De Salles AAF, Solberg T, Mischel P, Massoud TF, Plasencia A, Goetsch S, De Souza E, Vinuela F (1996) Arteriovenous malformation animal model for radiosurgery: the rete mirabile. AJNR Am J Neuroradiol 17:1451–1458

De Salles AAF, Sun B, Solberg T, Cabatan-Awang C, Ford J, Selch M (1999) Factors relating to radiation injury after radiosurgery of arteriovenous malformations of the brain. Radiosurgery 3:168–172

Ellis TL, Friedman WA, Bova FJ, Kubilis PS, Buatti JM (1998) Analysis of treatment failure after radiosurgery for arteriovenous malformations. J Neurosurg 89(1):104–110

Flickinger J, Pollock B, Kondziolka D, Lunsford D (1996) A dose-response analysis of arteriovenous malformation obliteration after radiosurgery. Int J Radiat Oncol Biol Phys 36(4):873–879

Flickinger JC, Kondziolka D, Lunsford LD, Kassam A, Phuong LK, Liscak R, Pollock B (2000) Development of a model to predict permanent symptomatic postradiosurgery injury for arteriovenous malformation patients. Arteriovenous malformation study group. Int J Radiat Oncol Biol Phys 46(5):1143–1148

Friedman WA, Bova FJ, Mendenhall WM (1995) Linear accelerator radiosurgery for arteriovenous malformations: the relationship of size to outcome. J Neurosurg 82(2):180–189

Gobin YP, Laurent A, Merienne L, Schlienger M, Aymard A, Houdart E, Casasco A, Lefkopoulos D, George B, Merland JJ (1996) Treatment of brain arteriovenous malformations by embolization and radiosurgery. J Neurosurg 85(1): 19–28

Guo WY, Wikholm G, Karlsson B, Lindquist C, Svendsen P, Ericson K (1993) Combined embolization and gamma knife radiosurgery for cerebral arteriovenous malformations. Acta Radiol 34(6):600–606

Hernesniemi JA, Dashti R, Juvela S, Väärt K, Niemelä M, Laakso A (2008) Natural history of brain arteriovenous malformations: a long-term follow-up study of risk of hemorrhage in 238 patients. Neurosurgery 63(5):823 829

Hosobuchi Y, Fabricant J, Lyman J (1987) Stereotactic heavy-particle irradiation of intracranial arteriovenous malformations. Appl Neurophysiol 50(1–6):248–252

Jahan R, Solberg TD, Lee D, Medin P, Tateshima S, Sayre J, De Salles A, Vinters HV, Vinuela F (2006) Stereotactic radiosurgery of the rete mirabile in swine: a longitudinal study of histopathological changes. Neurosurgery 58(3): 551–558

Karlsson B, Lindquist C, Steiner L (1996) Effect of Gamma Knife surgery on the risk of rupture prior to AVM obliteration. Minim Invasive Neurosurg 39(1):21–27

Karlsson B, Lindquist C, Steiner L (1997) Prediction of obliteration after gamma knife surgery for cerebral arteriovenous malformations. Neurosurgery 40(3):425–430

Karlsson B, Jokura H, Yamamoto M, Söderman M, Lax I (2007) Is repeated radiosurgery an alternative to staged radiosurgery for very large brain arteriovenous malformations? J Neurosurg 107(4):740–744

Kjellberg RN, Hanamura T, Davis KR, Lyons SL, Adams RD (1983) Bragg-peak proton-beam therapy for arteriovenous malformations of the brain. N Engl J Med 309(5):269–274

Laakso A, Dashti R, Seppänen J, Juvela S, Väärt K, Niemelä M, Sankila R, Hernesniemi JA (2008) Long-term excess mortality in 623 patients with brain arteriovenous malformations. Neurosurgery 63(2):244–253

Lindqvist M, Steiner L, Blomgren H, Arndt J, Berggren BM (1986) Stereotactic radiation therapy of intracranial arteriovenous malformations. Acta Radiol Suppl 369:610–613

Lindvall P, Bergström P, Löfroth PO, Hariz M, Henriksson R, Jonasson P, Bergenheim AT (2003) Hypofractionated conformal stereotactic radiotherapy for arteriovenous malformations. Neurosurgery 53:1036–1043

Lunsford LD, Kondziolka D, Flickinger JC, Bissonette DJ, Jungreis CA, Maitz AH, Horton JA, Coffey RJ (1991) Stereotactic radiosurgery for arteriovenous malformations of the brain. J Neurosurg 75(4):512–524

Maesawa S, Flickinger JC, Kondziolka D, Lunsford LD (2000) Repeated radiosurgery for incompletely obliterated arteriovenous malformations. J Neurosurg 92(6):961–970

Massoud TF, Hademenos GJ, De Salles AA, Solberg TD (2000) Experimental radiosurgery simulations using a theoretical model of cerebral arteriovenous malformations. Stroke 31(10):2466–2477

Mathis JA, Barr JD, Horton JA, Jungreis CA, Lunsford LD, Kondziolka DS, Vincent D, Pentheny S (1995) The efficacy of particulate embolization combined with stereotactic radiosurgery for treatment of large arteriovenous malformations of the brain. Am J Neuroradiol 16(2): 299–306

Mobin F, De Salles AA, Abdelaziz O, Cabatan-Awang C, Solberg T, Selch M (1999) Stereotactic radiosurgery of cerebral arteriovenous malformations: appearance of perinidal T(2) hyperintensity signal as a predictor of favorable treatment response. Stereotact Funct Neurosurg 73(1–4): 50–59

Ondra SL, Troupp H, George ED, Schwab K (1990) The natural history of symptomatic arteriovenous malformations of the brain: a 24-year follow-up assessment. J Neurosurg 73(3): 387–391

Pedroso AG, De Salles AA, Tajik K, Golish R, Smith Z, Frighetto L, Solberg T, Cabatan-Awang C, Selch MT (2004) Novalis shaped beam radiosurgery of arteriovenous malformations. J Neurosurg 101(Suppl 3):425–434

Plasencia AR, De Salles AAF, Do T, Cabatan-Awang C, Solberg T, Vinuela F, Selch M (1999) Combined embolization and stereotactic radiosurgery for the treatment of large volume. High Risk Arteriovenous Malformations. Radiosurgery 3:161–167

Pollock BE, Flickinger JC (2008) Modification of the radiosurgery-based arteriovenous malformation grading system. Neurosurgery 63(2):239–243, Discussion 243

Pollock BE, Gorman DA, Brown PD (2004) Radiosurgery for arteriovenous malformations of the basal ganglia, thalamus, and brainstem. J Neurosurg 100(2):210–214

Richling B, Killer M (2000) Endovascular management of patients with cerebral arteriovenous malformations. Neurosurg Clin N Am 11(1):123–145

Seifert V, Stolke D, Mehdorn HM, Hoffmann B (1994) Clinical and radiological evaluation of long-term results of stereotactic proton beam radiosurgery in patients with cerebral arteriovenous malformations. J Neurosurg 81(5):683–689

Sinclair J, Chang SD, Gibbs IC, Adler JR (2006) Multisession CyberKnife radiosurgery for intramedullary spinal cord arteriovenous malformations. Neurosurgery 58(6): 1081–1089

Sirin S, Kondziolka D, Niranjan A, Flickinger JC, Maitz AH, Lunsford LD (2006) Prospective staged volume radiosurgery for large arteriovenous malformations: indications and outcomes in otherwise untreatable patients. Neurosurgery 58(1):17–27

Spagnuolo E, Lemme-Plaghos L, Revilla F, Quintana L, Antico J (2009) Recommendation for the management of the brain arteriovenous malformations. Neurocirugia (Astur) 20(1):5–14

Spetzler RF, Martin NA (1986) A proposed grading system for arteriovenous malformations. J Neurosurg 65(4):476–483

Spetzler RF, Martin NA, Carter LP, Flom RA, Raudzens PA, Wilkinson E (1987) Surgical management of large AVM's by staged embolization and operative excision. J Neurosurg 67(1):17–28

Steiner L, Leksell L, Greitz T, Forster DM, Backlund EO (1972) Stereotaxic radiosurgery for cerebral arteriovenous malformations. Report of a case. Acta Chir Scand 138(5):459–464

Veznedaroglu E, Andrews DW, Benitez RP, Downes MB, Werner-Wasik M, Rosenstock J, Curran WJ Jr, Rosenwasser RH (2004) Fractionated stereotactic radiotherapy for the

treatment of large arteriovenous malformations with or without previous partial embolization. Neurosurgery 55:519
Westphal M, Grzyska U (2000) Clinical significance of pedicle aneurysms on feeding vessels, especially those located in infratentorial arteriovenous malformations. J Neurosurg 92(6):995–1001
Xiao F, Gorgulho AA, Lin CS, Chen CH, Agazaryan N, Viñuela F, Selch MT, De Salles AA (2010) Treatment of giant cerebral arteriovenous malformation: hypofractionated stereotactic radiation as the first stage. Neurosurgery 67(5):1253–1259
Yuki I, Kim RH, Duckwiler G, Jahan R, Tateshima S, Gonzalez N, Gorgulho A, Diaz JL, De Salles AAF, Viñuela F (2010) Treatment of brain arteriovenous malformations with high-flow arteriovenous fistulas: risk and complications associated with endovascular embolization in multimodality treatment. J Neurosurg 113(4):715–722

Radiosurgical Management of Meningiomas

8

Alessandra A. Gorgulho, Jason S. Hauptman, and Antonio A.F. De Salles

8.1 Introduction

Meningiomas are the most common benign intracranial tumors and approximately 90% are histologically benign. Meningiomas are often classified according to their topography since location is predictive of treatment challenges. As a consequence of the limitation imposed by location, each topography has well-known rates of recurrence and complications triggered by the treatment. As a rule of thumb, small and asymptomatic meningiomas should be followed up with routine MRI scans. Usually, small meningiomas in the convexity of the skull can be safely resected. The surgical resection should aim to be complete whenever possible considering the risks of causing neurological sequela. The grade of resection correlates to the rate of recurrences. The indication of radiosurgery or stereotactic radiotherapy for these lesions is recommended in cases of partial resection or biopsy. Residual WHO I tumors are followed with serial scans, while WHO II and III are irradiated immediately after surgery. Radiation is offered to WHO I tumors when growth is confirmed. The majority of skull-base meningiomas pose surgical challenges. Surgical series show a significantly higher morbidity and mortality rates in comparison to convexity lesions. Less frequently, these lesions can be completely resected. Therefore, radiosurgery (SRS) or stereotactic radiotherapy (SRT) is the preferential treatment modality for small and asymptomatic skull-base lesions proven to be growing. Surgery should be performed if neurological symptoms require tumor decompression or if a histological confirmation is necessary. The UCLA Meningioma classification of tumors is directed to orient SRS or SRT for meningiomas with safety. Lesions distant from eloquent structures are Grade I and II and can be treated with single dose. Large meningiomas or lesions attached to the optic apparatus or causing brainstem radiological compression are treated with SRT and are classified as Grade III, Grade IV, Grade V, and Grade VI.

Radiation therapy, once reserved as adjuvant therapy for high-grade meningeal tumors, now plays a central role in the management of all meningiomas. This is a relative paradigm shift in the treatment of these generally benign lesions accounting for 15–20% of all primary intracranial tumors, affecting predominantly middle-aged patients, particularly females (Bondy and Ligon 1996; Rohringer et al. 1989). Atypical and malignant meningiomas, characterized by successive recurrences and aggressive behavior, vary in incidence from 4.7% to 7.1% and 1.0% to 3.7%, respectively (Jaaskelainen et al. 1986; Palma et al. 1997; Perry et al. 1999). There is absence of female predominance in malignant meningiomas, suggesting that the neuroendocrine anomalies apparently correlated with the etiology of benign meningiomas are not as relevant for atypical and malignant variants (Mahmood et al. 1993). Interestingly, a majority of intracranial meningiomas show alterations of chromosome 22 at the NF2 gene locus (Burger et al. 2002).

The World Health Organization (WHO) 2000 classification of histological criteria of meningiomas have useful prognostic value (Kleihues et al. 2002). WHO

A.A. Gorgulho (✉), J.S. Hauptman, and A.A.F. De Salles
Department of Neurosurgery,
David Geffen School of Medicine at UCLA, UCLA Medical Center, 300 UCLA Medical Plaza, Suite B212,
Los Angeles, CA 90095, USA
e-mail: a_gorgulho@yahoo.com; afdesalles@yahoo.com

A.A.F. De Salles et al. (eds.), *Shaped Beam Radiosurgery*,
DOI: 10.1007/978-3-642-11151-8_8, © Springer-Verlag Berlin Heidelberg 2011

Grade I meningiomas, termed well differentiated, are characterized by low mitotic activity, lack of necrosis, and absence of underlying brain invasion (Burger et al. 2002). Atypical meningiomas, designated as WHO Grade II, either have higher mitotic activity, evidence of brain invasion, or changes in histological architecture (i.e., sheath-like growth, prominent nucleoli, and increased cellularity). This classification delineates the mitotic index as the main differentiator between atypical and malignant lesions, with the latter having at least five times greater mitotic activity. Meningiomas are not necessarily stable lesions over time, as they may increase in histological grade as the successive recurrences occur. This aspect is not often discussed in the literature, and the existing series report an incidence of 4.4–18% (Hug et al. 2000; Mattozo et al. 2007; Pourel et al. 2001). Recently, Al-Mefty et al. published a series of 11 (6%) meningiomas with malignant progression out of 175 recurrent lesions. Interestingly, they found a complex karyotype present in the histologically lower-grade tumor, contradicting the stepwise clonal evolution model (Al-Mefty et al. 2004).

In addition to the impact of histological grade on frequency of recurrence, extent of surgical removal is correlated to prognosis. The Simpson classification grades the extent of tumor removal correlating it to recurrences. Grade 1 resection, associated with a 9% chance of local recurrence, requires gross total removal of all visible tumor including dural attachments. Grade 2 resection, on the other hand, constitutes gross total removal with dural cautery. Grade 2 resection is associated with a 19% recurrence rate. Partial tumor resection is termed Grade 3, and is associated with recurrence rates up to 40%. Recurrence rates significantly worsen with Grade 4 (decompression) or 5 (biopsy) procedures (Simpson 1957). Gross total resection, when possible, can lead to 85% 5-year and 75% 10-year survival rates (Johnson et al. 2008). Although the mortality rate has decreased in recent reports, a significant number of patients continue to experience adverse effects related to surgical procedures with rates ranging from 15% to 26%, particularly in the case of meningiomas of the skull base (Al-Mefty et al. 1991; Couldwell et al. 1996; DeMonte et al. 1994; O'Sullivan et al. 1997; Sekhar et al. 1994). The emergence of stereotactic radiation as an adjuvant to microsurgical resection in these cases significantly lowers posttreatment complications while maximizing chances for tumor stability and/or reduction in size (Eustacchio et al. 2002; Maruyama et al. 2004). While radiation plays less of a role in Simpson Grade 1 and 2 resections, it becomes an important adjuvant in Simpson Grades 3, 4, and 5. That being said, recent data suggests that the progression-free survival following primary stereotactic radiation for small-to-moderate sized meningiomas is equivalent to that of Simpson Grade 1 resection (Pollock et al. 2003). Therefore, this therapy is emerging as the primary treatment for smaller meningiomas without mass effect.

8.2 Stereotactic Radiation

8.2.1 *Grading of Skull-Base Meningiomas for Stereotactic Radiation*

Because of the challenges facing surgical therapy for meningiomas of the skull base, these tumors are frequently referred for radiotherapy, regardless of histological grade. Due to their tenuous location usually adjacent to a variety of radiosensitive structures, these tumors present unique challenges to the radiosurgeon as well. For that reason, they serve as a model of factors affecting the choice of radiation delivery. In 2001, a grading system was proposed to assist clinicians in deciding radiation modality and predict outcomes following stereotactic radiation (De Salles et al. 2001). This grading system was borne out of a single-center experience treating skull-base meningiomas with stereotactic radiation over an 8-year period. Stereotactic radiation, delivered either as single or fractionated stereotactic radiation, was designed to maximize tumor dose and not to violate the maximal tolerance of the optic apparatus. Grade I meningiomas are contained within the cavernous sinus or are smaller than 3 cm in non-eloquent locations (Fig. 8.1). Stereotactic radiation can be expected to achieve upward of 90% tumor control rates. In Grade II meningiomas (Fig. 8.2), tumor extends out of the cavernous sinus and involves the petrous temporal bone and/or clivus without

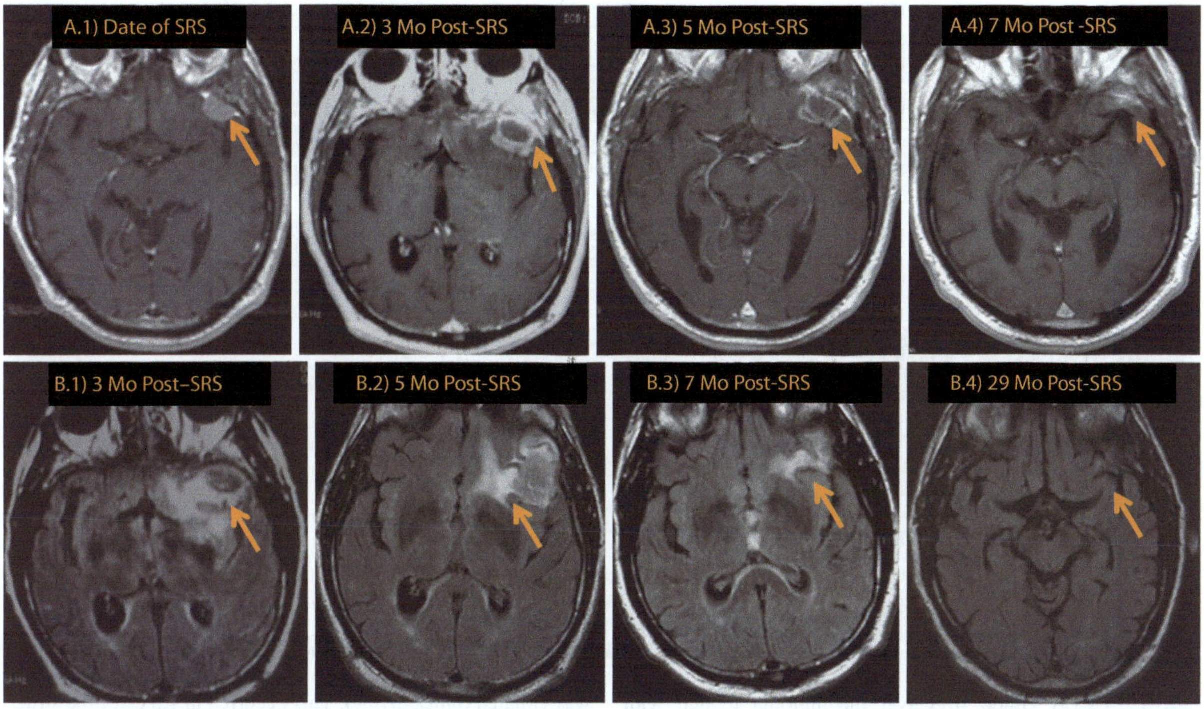

Fig. 8.1 UCLA Grade I, Meningioma in a 68-year-old man who underwent stereotactic radiosurgery (SRS) in July/2007 for a 2-cm asymptomatic left sphenoid wing tumor. The tumor was in relationship to sphenoid venous drainage. It was discovered on follow-up MRI scan performed to monitor a prior meningioma encased in left cavernous sinus, treated by SRS in 1998 (UCLA Grade I – not shown). At that time, the tumor received 16 Gy prescribed to the 90% isodose line. The maximum dose was 17.77 Gy. The dose to the optic apparatus was less than 5 Gy. It was a one isocenter plan using multileaf collimator. The 50% isodose line touched the surface of the brainstem, therefore less than 9 Gy. No signs of the cavernous sinus tumor remained, now with 12-year follow-up. In July/2007 the sphenoid wing meningioma volume was of 4.2 cc (*arrow*, **A.1**). It was treated with 4 dynamic arcs with 90% isodose covering the tumor with 17 Gy. Images show the evolution of the complication with radiation induced edema in the temporal and frontal lobes (*lower row figures*). This reaction led to seizures and mental confusion. Steroid and anticonvulsants controlled the edema and seizures within 2 months of initiation of symptoms. Notice the complete resolution of the tumor on MRI-T1-gadolinium at 7 months post-radiosurgery (*arrow*, **A.4**). Radiation-induced edema could be noticed shortly after treatment (*arrow*, **B.1**) on the MRI-Flair. It resolved overtime as can be noticed in the MRI-Flair scan obtained 29 months after radiosurgery (*arrow*, **B.4**)

evidence of brainstem compression. These patients can be expected to have more than 86% tumor control rates following radiation. Grade III meningiomas demonstrate anterior or superior extension with optic apparatus involvement. Despite their proximity to the optic nerve and tract, appropriately chosen stereotactic radiotherapy can achieve tumor control rates as high as 86% as well (Fig. 8.3). Grade IV meningiomas compress the brainstem (Fig. 8.4) and Grade V meningiomas are bilateral involving brainstem and optic apparatus (Fig. 8.5). Tumor control rates are significantly poorer for these high-grade skull-base lesions, if single fraction is used. Importantly, in this series, no patient presented with a new cranial deficit following treatment with SRT. Two patients (5%, one had Grade I tumor and the second had Grade III tumor) experienced worsening of their preoperative cranial neuropathies, though in one of these patients the worsening was transient. The optic sheath meningiomas are considered to be Grade VI and are treated with stereotactic radiotherapy only (Fig. 8.6). At UCLA, this grading system has been found to be useful when advising patients on post-radiosurgical outcome for their skull-base meningiomas. Recently it has been

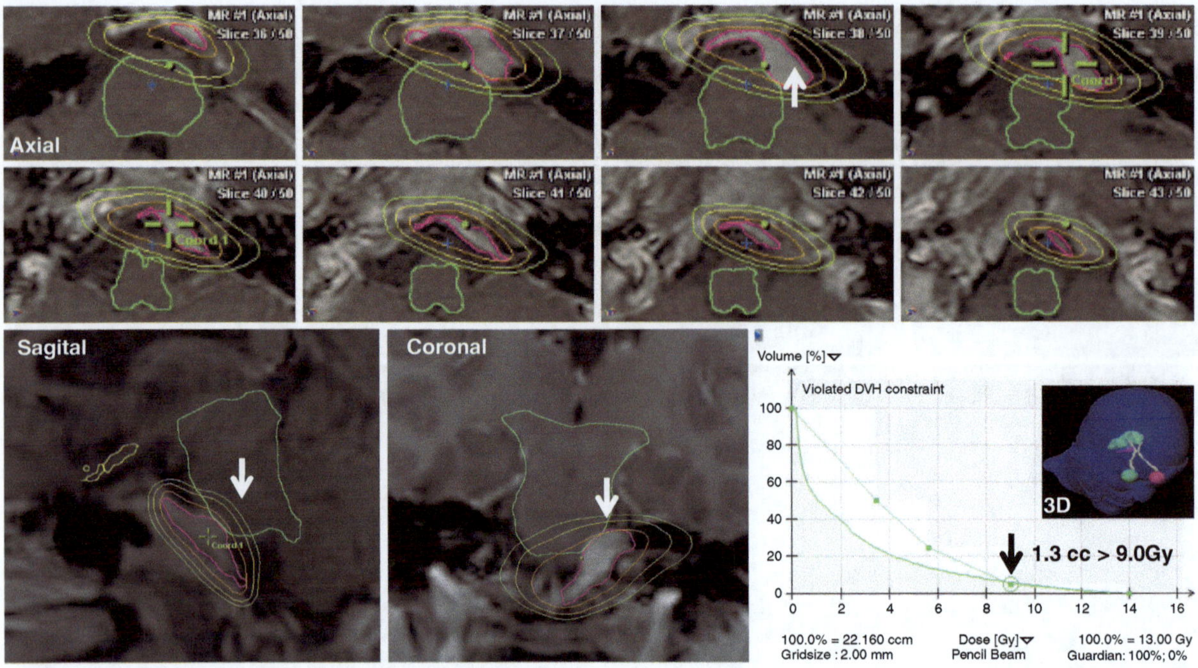

Fig. 8.2 UCLA Grade II, Clival meningioma treated with stereotactic radiosurgery (SRS). The axial pictures show the complete dose distribution of this eight IMRT-fields plan. The prescription line in orange completely encompasses the tumor and touches the brainstem where the tumor is in contact with the brainstem (*white arrows*). The dose-volume histogram shows the volume of brainstem where constrain of 9 Gy to the brainstem was violated (*black arrow*). This occurred in 1.3 cc of the structure. The tumor had a volume 2.5 cc, it was covered by 13 Gy, receiving a maximal dose of 14.3 Gy. Notice the 3D insert showing the tumor relationship with the segmented structures. The tail of the tumor was completely followed in this modern plan (See Fig. 8.4)

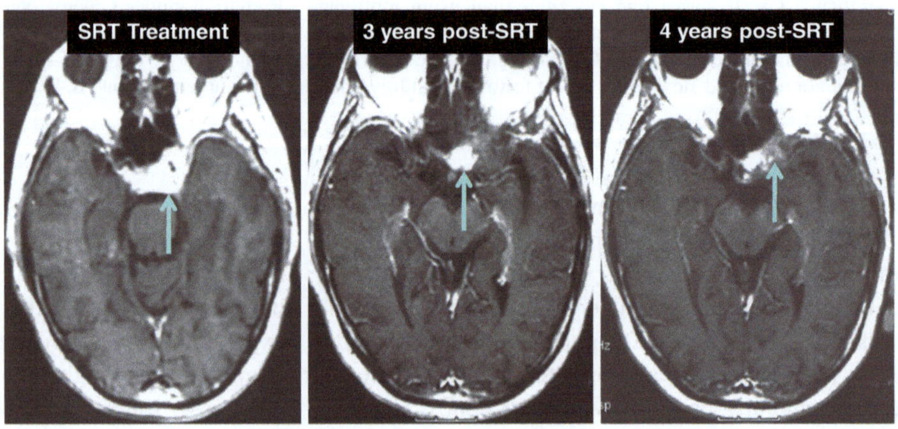

Fig. 8.3 UCLA Grade III, Meningioma involving the optic apparatus in a 58-year-old woman blind on the left eye. She was treated with stereotactic radiotherapy in attempt to preserve vision on the right eye, as tumor was involving the optic chiasm. Twenty-eight fractions of 1.8 Gy for a total of 50.40 Gy led to decrease of the tumor volume and preservation of vision (*arrow*)

modified to accommodate the increased applications of stereotactic radiosurgery for tumors away from the parasellar region and stereotactic radiotherapy for large lesions involving the skull-base and optic sheath meningiomas. This modification defines tumors smaller than 3 cm in largest diameter as Grade I when not involving structures described in the skull base, while tumors larger than 3 cm in largest diameter are already Grade III, independently of the location (Table 8.1).

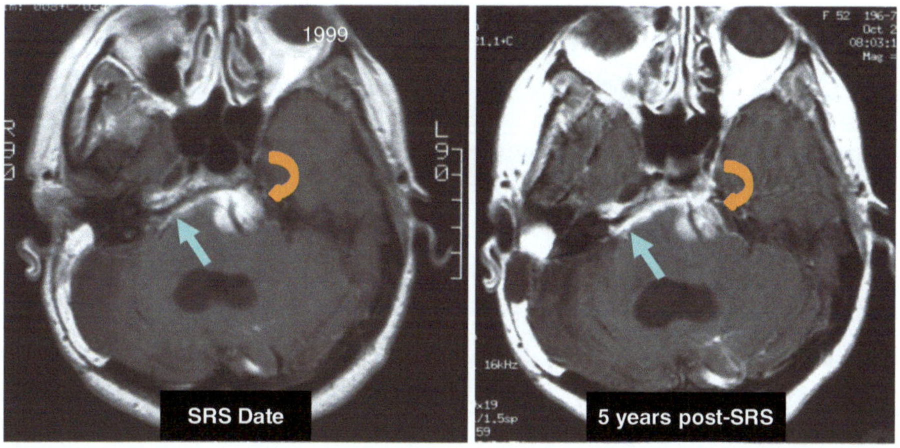

Fig. 8.4 UCLA Grade IV, WHO I meningioma in a 45-year-old woman, status posttrial of resection and radiosurgery in 1994. Radiosurgery at that time was performed with multiple isocenters at UCLA; therefore, the tail of the meningioma could not be effectively followed with the field of radiation then. Five-year follow-up MRI shows decrease of the tumor at the SRS target treated with 12 Gy, prescribed to the 50% IDL, maximal dose of 24 Gy, four isocenters. Notice also the increased diameter of the basilar artery 5 years after the treatment (*curved orange arrows*), denoting response of the tumor to the 12 Gy. The treatment failed where the tail of the tumor was not irradiated (*straight blue arrows*)

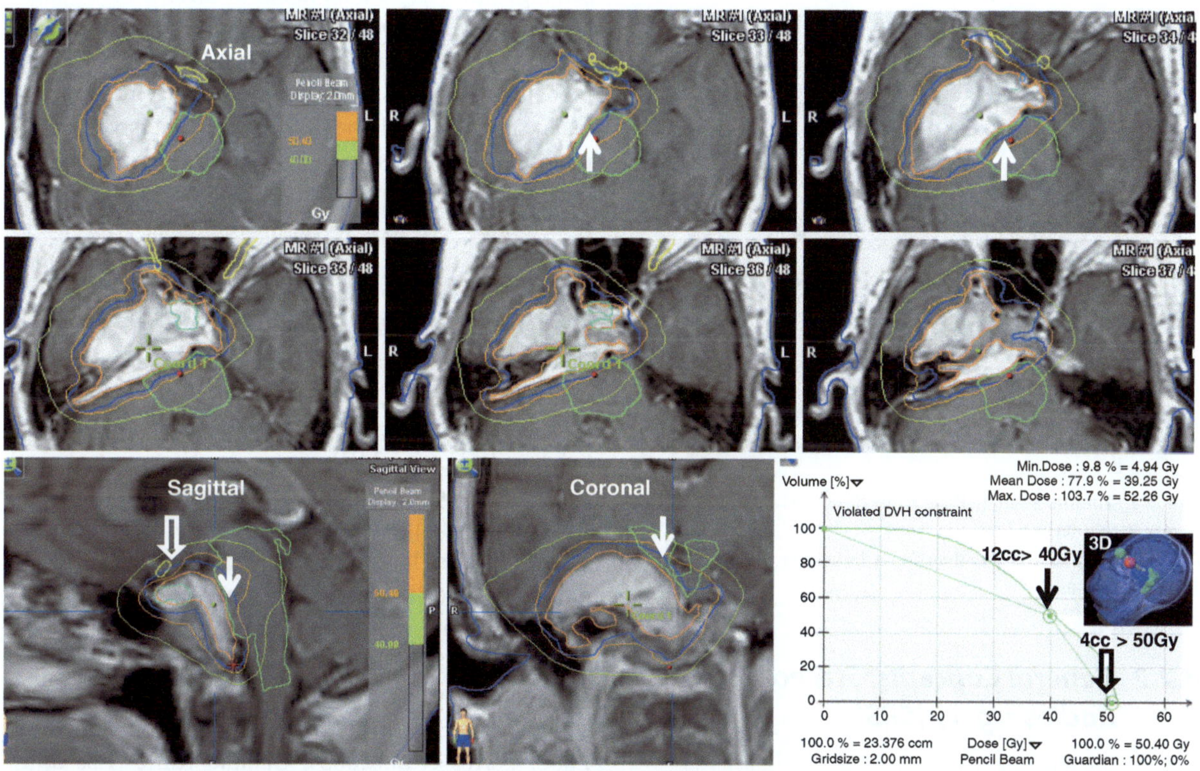

Fig. 8.5 UCLA Grade V, Clival meningioma treated with stereotactic radiotherapy (SRT) in a 47-year-old woman. The axial pictures show the dose distribution of this six IMRT-fields plan. The prescription line in orange completely encompasses the tumor and invades the brainstem where the tumor compresses it (*white arrows*). The blue line represents the 2-mm margin given in this SRT plan. Notice were the constrain placed on the optic apparatus avoids the prescribed dose to reach the optic nerve (*open white arrow,* sagittal view).The dose-volume histogram shows the volume of brainstem where constrains of 40 Gy (*black arrow*) and 50 Gy (*open arrow*) were violated. This occurred in 12 cc of the brainstem receiving more than 40 Gy and 4 cc receiving more than 50 Gy. The tumor had a volume 28.9 cc, it was covered by 50.40 Gy, receiving a maximal dose of 52.26 Gy. Notice the 3D insert showing the tumor relationship with the automatically segmented structures, compressing brainstem, optic pathways, and crossing the midline. The tail of the tumor was completely followed in this modern plan (See Fig. 8.4)

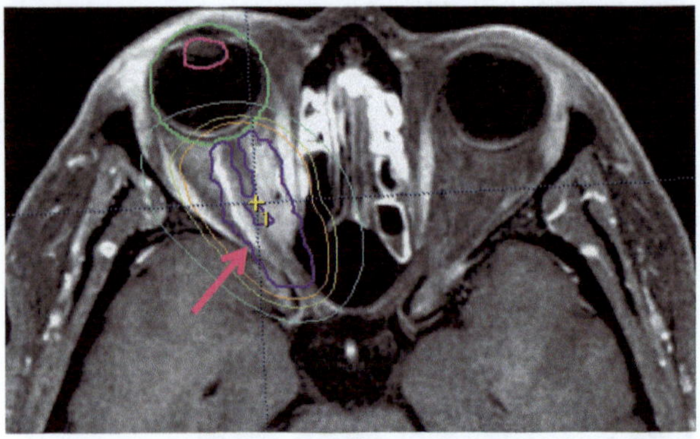

Fig. 8.6 UCLA Grade VI, Optic sheath meningioma diagnosed in a 59-year-old woman who experienced progressive proptosis (*pink arrow*) since 1998, without visual impairment. Not until 2009, she started with double vision but still 20/20 vision on the right eye. In May 2009, she underwent stereotactic radiotherapy with four dynamic arcs, 4-mm margin, 90% isodose line prescription delivering 1.8 Gy in 28 fractions, total dose of 50.40 Gy. The tumor volume was 4.49 cc. The vision has been stable since treatment. As a routine, these complex meningiomas are contoured based on fat suppression with and without contrast injection MRI sequences, with thin cuts through the region of interest

Table 8.1 UCLA Grading System for Parasellar and other locations Meningiomas

Grade I: Restricted to the cavernous sinus/parasellar region (<3 cm)
Grade II: Expansion to the clivus/petrous region
Grade III: Compression of the optic structures (>3 cm)
Grade IV: Compression of the brainstem
Grade V: Bilateral involvement of the cavernous sinus
Grade VI: Optic Sheath

Modified from De Salles et al. 2001, see Figs. 8.1–8.6 for examples

Grade I: Tumors smaller than 3 cm in largest diameter (14 cc) in any locations

Grade III: Tumors larger than 3 cm in largest diameter (14 cc) in any locations

8.2.2 General Concepts: Stereotactic Radiosurgery (SRS)

The notion of stereotactic radiosurgery (SRS) as a complement to subtotal resection of meningiomas was initially supported by the proven benefits of conventional radiation therapy, with known tumor control rates of 72–98% (Barbaro et al. 1987; Glaholm et al. 1990; Goldsmith et al. 1994; Soyuer et al. 2004; Wilson 1996). The long-term complication rate of conventional radiation therapy, however, has been reported to be from 17% to 38% in patients with more than 5 years of follow-up (Al-Mefty et al. 1990; Al-Mefty et al. 2004; Nutting et al. 1999). In a study of 748 adults who underwent radiation therapy and had long-term survival, 29% presented with some degree of neuropsychologic deficit and 12% were classified as having postradiation dementia (Crossen et al. 1994). Furthermore, in the case of higher-grade meningiomas, concerns arose as to the limitations on dosage possible with conventional radiotherapy techniques (Kokubo et al. 2000). As patients with meningiomas are expected to have long-term survival, conventional radiation therapy was replaced with stereotactic radiation, avoiding the undesired side effects of conventional radiation therapy and allowing for higher dosage delivery by achieving a focal and precise dose distribution (De Salles et al. 1993; Torres et al. 2004). Benign lesions, typically presenting with well-defined tumor borders, must be managed with focal radiation. Stereotactic radiosurgery (SRS) or stereotactic radiotherapy (SRT) may be the modality of choice, depending on involvement of eloquent structures, volume of the lesion, and proximity of radiosensitive structures. It must also be noted that malignant meningiomas treated with partial surgical resection as well as atypical meningiomas with risk of dural spread require more extensive radiation fields than their lower-grade counterparts (Mattozo et al. 2007).

Meningiomas have several characteristics making them amenable to stereotactic radiation (Kondziolka and Lunsford 1992). Meningiomas tend to be characterized by slow growth, easily imaged with contrast-enhanced CT and MRI protocols. From a technical standpoint, high dose with rapid fall off can be directed to the well-defined tumor margin with confidence. Because of the low tumor growth rates, the precisely delivered dose has time to take effect without symptoms worsening due rapid tumor growth (Fig. 8.4). The experience of stereotactic radiation using all available techniques, including linear accelerator (Hakim et al. 1998; Shafron et al. 1999; Spiegelmann et al. 2002; Torres et al. 2003), Gamma Knife (Lee et al. 2007; Iwai et al. 2003; Kobayashi et al. 2001; Kondziolka et al. 1999; Kondziolka et al. 2003; Leksell 1983; Stafford et al. 2001), and proton-beam (Vernimmen et al. 2001) has been reported, all with equitable 5-year and 10-year actuarial tumor control rates greater than 90% for WHO Grade I tumors.

Recently our institution reported a series of 161 patients who underwent SRS or SRT for treatment of 194 meningiomas arising in various locations (Torres et al. 2004). Clinical and radiographic follow-up were obtained in 128 patients harboring 156 lesions, with a mean follow-up period of 32.5 months. In this group, stereotactic radiosurgery was used to treat 79 lesions, with mean prescribed dose of 15.6 Gy. Local tumor control rates approached 92%, with clinical improvement occurred in 33.5% of the patients. Worsening of clinical symptoms was observed in 7.9% of patients who underwent SRS, with clinical complications occurring in 5% of patients.

Tumor location is an important factor to consider when deciding on radiotherapy modality. For instance, despite the dosimetric advantages of SRS, permanent cranial nerve deficit following SRS is more common in the treatment of cavernous sinus meningiomas. Tishler et al. studied 62 patients (42 with meningiomas) inside or near the cavernous sinus treated by SRS. New cranial neuropathies were found in 19% of patients. Additionally, all patients who developed optic system neuropathy (6.4%) received radiation doses higher than 8 Gy to optic apparatus (Tishler et al. 1993). Leber et al. correlated the doses delivered in the treatment of cavernous sinus lesions by SRS with incidence of optic neuropathy (Leber et al. 1998). The actuarial rate was zero for patients who received a dose of less than 10 Gy, 26.7% for patients receiving 10 to less than 15 Gy, and 77.8% for those who received doses of 15 Gy or more ($p<0.0001$). Similar findings were observed in the analysis of other series (Stafford et al. 2003), suggesting that the 8Gy dose constrain for the optic nerve when irradiating with radiosurgery is likely a safe criteria. In a recent series examining outcomes after Gamma Knife treatment of cavernous sinus meningiomas, 12% had symptom progression following margin dosages of 12 Gy (Hasegawa et al. 2007). The overall incidence of radiation neuropathy is 1.9% for patients receiving 8 Gy to a small segment of the optic nerve (Stafford et al. 2001). Morbidity after radiosurgery for meningiomas is strongly associated with tumor location and volume (Chen et al. 2001; Marks and Spencer 1991). Therefore, SRS to cavernous sinus meningiomas has generally been restricted to tumors <3 cm in greatest dimension and located several millimeters from the optic apparatus, corresponding to UCLA Grade I and II tumors (De Salles et al. 2001; De Salles et al. 1993; Lee et al. 2002; Nicolato et al. 2002) (Figs. 8.1 and 8.2). Tumors Grade III, IV, V, and VI are better candidates for stereotactic radiotherapy.

8.2.3 General Concepts: Stereotactic Radiotherapy (SRT)

Stereotactic radiotherapy (SRT), also referred to as fractionated stereotactic radiotherapy (FSRT), is a treatment option that may be undertaken when the risk of single-dose SRS is unacceptably high. SRT can be delivered using a variety of approaches, including conformal fields, dynamic arcs, and intensity-modulation. SRT is typically considered when tumors involve the optic pathways, or brainstem, or with larger lesions adjacent to eloquent structures. For example, Selch et al. reported the UCLA experience in 45 patients with cavernous sinus meningiomas treated with SRT. In this series, the median prescribed dose was 50.4 Gy and was delivered to a median tumor volume of 14.5 cc. The 3-year progression-free survival rate was 97.4% and the preexisting neurologic complaints improved in 20% of patients (Selch et al. 2004).

SRT results were recently reviewed in 317 patients with benign and atypical meningiomas in all intracranial sites. The median total dose was 57.6 Gy delivered to a median volume of 33.6 cc. The overall local control rate was 93.1%. As expected, the local tumor failure was significantly greater in patients with WHO Grade II meningiomas than in patients with WHO Grade I or unconfirmed histology. Moreover, patients with a tumor volume larger than 60 cc had a higher recurrence rate (15.5%) when compared to patients with tumor volumes smaller than 60 cc ($p<0.001$). They observed worsening of preexisting symptoms and new clinical symptoms in 8.2% and 2.5% of patients, respectively (Milker-Zabel et al. 2005).

Diffuse skull-base meningiomas not amenable to microsurgery or radiosurgery due to medical infirmity or size may also be treated by SRT. These tumors would fall in Grades III, IV and V of the UCLA grading system. Debus et al. reported on 189 patients treated by SRT for skull-base meningiomas with a mean radiation dose of 56.8 Gy and median target volume of 52.5 cc. The tumor control rates for WHO grade I and WHO grade II tumors were 98.3% and 77.7%, respectively. Preexisting cranial nerve symptoms resolved completely in 28% of the patients. Only 7% of patients showed an impairment of preexisting neurologic symptoms and 1.6% experienced new clinically significant deficits (Debus et al. 2001). These excellent results corroborate the UCLA experience with skull-base meningiomas treated with SRT (Selch et al. 2004).

Stereotactic intensity-modulated radiotherapy (IMRT) has recently emerged as an alternative to conformal field and dynamic arc plans using SRT with multileaf collimator (MLC). While in theory, IMRT may improve dosage distribution and allow for safer dose escalation (Estall et al. 2010a), the efficacy of this modality in treating complex skull-base meningiomas seems to be equivalent to SRT based on results published in the literature (Milker-Zabel et al. 2007). There may be some practical advantages in using IMRT planning, however, including increased efficiency independently by the method used to deliver IMRT (micromultileaf collimator vs. helical tomotherapy) (Estall et al. 2010a, b). In the case of larger or complex-shaped skull-base lesions, IMRT may result in lower dosages delivered to the brainstem and adjacent temporal lobe (Clark et al. 2008). Because of the highly conformal nature of IMRT targeting, there may be advantages to this modality in the treatment of histologically aggressive meningiomas, since safer dose escalation is more feasible (Pirzkall et al. 2003; Estall et al. 2010a)

8.2.4 Particular Challenges: Meningiomas of the Optic Sheath

Optic nerve sheath meningiomas, representing approximately 2% of all tumors within the orbit, typically arise from the intraorbital sheath but may also originate from the intracanalicular nerve sheath (Eddleman and Liu 2007). Patients with optic nerve sheath meningiomas were, until recently, sentenced to vision loss due to these slow-growing and difficult-to-treat tumors (Fig. 8.6). Historically, microsurgical treatment was limited to patients whose vision had already been significantly impaired. Otherwise, the incidence of visual loss with microsurgical resection was unacceptably high due to inadvertent injury to the pial vascular supply of the optic nerve (Gabibov et al. 1988). Therefore, the majority of patients with optic nerve sheath meningiomas were initially observed, even though over 85% would experience future decline in vision (Kennerdell et al. 1988; Turbin et al. 2002). The emergence of radiation therapy for the treatment of optic sheath meningiomas represented an important step forward in the management of these patients, though radiation optic neuropathy continued to be a challenge (Kupersmith et al. 1987; Wara et al. 1975). The development of SRT as a treatment alternative for these tumors became the primary therapeutic approach for optic nerve sheath meningiomas in the opinion of many authors, since SRT offers the most impressive results in terms of vision preservation (Romanelli et al. 2007). Andrews et al. reported on 30 patients with 33 optic nerve sheath meningiomas treated with SRT. Local tumor control was observed in all patients and they observed 92% of preserved vision among the optic nerves with vision before treatment. Improvement in visual acuity and/or visual field occurred in 42% of nerves. Visual loss was observed in 2 (6.6%) patients and 1 (3.3%) developed optic neuritis responsive to steroids (Andrews et al. 2002).

Baumert et al. studied the role of SRT in 39 patients with either primary or secondary optic nerve sheath meningiomas using a median dose of 54 Gy. The tumor local control was 100% after a median follow-up of 35 months. The rates of visual field stabilization, improvement, and worsening were 70%, 25%, and 4%, respectively. Additionally, new endocrinologic deficits after treatment were found in 14% of patients with primary tumors and 8% of patients with secondary tumors. The visual improvement observed in patients treated by SRT for optic sheath meningiomas was recently reported to occur within 1–3 months after treatment in 81% of patients who experienced visual improvement (Baumert et al. 2004). Homogeneity of the dose distribution becomes important when planning SRT for these tumors, since the optic nerve is frequently surrounded by tumor.

8.2.5 Particular Challenges: Petroclival Meningiomas

While many authors advocate treatment of large petroclival meningiomas including both surgical debulking and postoperative radiotherapy, the optimal treatment of small petroclival meningiomas remains controversial (Natarajan et al. 2007). Some have reported that Simpson Grade 1 and 2 resections are achievable with minimal morbidity and favorable short- and long-term outcomes (Ramina et al. 2008). Others have suggested

Table 8.2 Stereotactic Radiosurgery (SRS) and Stereotactic Radiotherapy (SRT) for Non-benign Meningiomas

Author	Year	SRS/SRT	Classification	Histology	Tumor control	Survival
Lee et al.	2007	GK	WHO	Malignant	5-year: 72%	–
				Atypical	5-year: 83%	
Ojemann et al.	2000	GK	WHO	Malignant	5-year: 26%	5-year: 40%
Stafford et al.	2001	GK	WHO	Malignant	5-year: 0%	5-year: 0%
				Atypical	5-year: 68%	5-year: 76%
Harris et al.	2003	GK	Perry et al.	Malignant	5-year: 72%	5-year: 59%
				Atypical	5-year: 83%	5-year: 59%
Huffmann et al.	2005	GK	WHO	Atypical	3-year: 95%	3-year: 93%
Hakim et al.	1998	SRS-LINAC	WHO	Malignant	67%	4-year: 22%
				Atypical	81%	4-year: 83%
Debus et al.	2001	SRT-LINAC	WHO	Atypical	3-year: 78%	–
Milker-Zabel et al.	2005	SRT-LINAC	WHO	Atypical	5-year: 89%	–
Mattozo et al.	2007	SRT-LINAC	WHO	Malignant	3-year: 0%	–
				Atypical	3-year: 83%	

Modified from Mattozo et al. 2007

that even though these lesions can be resected with rates as high as 80%, the risk of neurological morbidity approaches 40% and far exceeds the risk posed by SRS or SRT (Reinert et al. 2006). In a series presented by Roche et al., 32 patients with petroclival meningiomas treated with multi-isocentric SRS (dose 10–15 Gy) resulted in 100% progression-free survival over a mean follow-up of 52 months. Approximately 68% of patients with cranial neuropathy at presentation improved and the complication rate approached 6% (Roche et al. 2003). A second series looking at SRS also showed 92% progression-free survival and 13% neurological complication rate following SRS for petroclival meningiomas (Subach et al. 1998). This finding has led many to suggest that primary radiotherapy may be the treatment modality of choice for small asymptomatic petroclival meningiomas (Park et al. 2006).

8.2.6 *Particular Challenges: Atypical and Malignant Meningiomas*

Radiation is indicated as adjunctive therapy in all cases of atypical and malignant meningiomas (Dziuk et al. 1998; Hug et al. 2000; Milosevic et al. 1996; Ware et al. 2004). In our institution, SRS and SRT are used as rescue of recurrences after surgery and regional radiation (Torres et al. 2003; Mattozo et al. 2007). A summary of studies reporting stereotactic radiation for atypical and malignant meningiomas is presented in Table 8.2.

8.3 Combination of Surgery and Radiosurgery

Recently more conservative approaches for meningiomas have been adopted. As neurosurgeons embraced radiosurgery during the last 2 decades, it became part of the treatment planning of complex meningiomas to leave risky-to-remove residuals to be treated by SRS, improving outcomes. For instance, after reviewing 38 patients who underwent surgical resection for large sphenoid wing meningiomas that invaded the cavernous sinus, Abdel-Aziz et al. proposed that tumor portions involving the medial compartment of cavernous sinus as well as portions that infiltrate the superior orbital fissure should be left for observation or stereotactic radiation (Abdel-Aziz et al. 2004).

Maruyama et al. also proposed combining nonradical surgery and radiosurgery for the management of cavernous sinus meningiomas. Twenty-three patients had partial or subtotal surgical resection with the main aim to remove the tumor components extending outside the cavernous sinus. This was performed when the tumor was attached to or displacing the optic apparatus, brainstem, and tumors larger than 3 cm in mean diameter. The same approach was proposed when malignancy was suspected to obtain histological verification. The residual tumors underwent radiosurgery or fractionated radiotherapy depending on whether they were larger or smaller than 3 cm. Another group of 17 patients underwent SRS-only, given the presence of tumors smaller than 3 cm that were distant from optic apparatus. The 5-year actuarial local control rate was 94% (Maruyama et al. 2004). Recently, cytology of tumors located in the cavernous sinus has been obtained using frameless stereotaxis through foramen ovale biopsy. Biopsy of these tumors became part of the management of tumors in the cavernous sinus requiring a differential diagnosis (Frighetto et al. 2003).

8.4 General Management of Meningiomas

Surgical resection is still the best form of treatment for meningiomas when complete resection is possible (Simpson Grade 1 and 2), and when mass effect due to tumor size or surrounding edema warrant decompression. The state of imaging technology allows for diagnosis of benign meningioma in the great majority of the cases (Pollock et al. 2003). Therefore to obtain histological diagnosis, surgery is performed in special situations. When there is history of possible malignancy such as lymphoma invading the cavernous sinus, squamous cell carcinoma, or other malignances one may entertain a biopsy, either open or through the foramen ovale (Frighetto et al. 2003). Patients with meningiomatosis may need to have biopsy. Tumors should be followed to prove growth before radiation is offered when proven to be WHO Grade I. Single dose is the approach of choice when possible due to patient's convenience and higher odds to tumor size reduction at follow-up. As outlined previously, stereotactic radiotherapy is chosen when the risk of single-dose delivery is high, as occurs in meningiomas Grade III, IV, and V of the UCLA classification. Either single or fractionated stereotactic radiation is now performed without the application of the stereotactic frame, therefore as outpatient and without need for anesthesia.

Tumors involving the sagittal or sphenoid sinus result in more edema after single-dose radiation (Fig. 8.1). In these situations, patients may be treated with stereotactic radiotherapy instead of radiosurgery. In general, patients with parasagittal meningiomas are also at up to four times greater risk for posttreatment cerebral edema (Patil et al. 2008). Steroids are not routinely prescribed in preparation for treatment, though close follow-up may be necessary.

8.4.1 Dose Prescription

Dose distributions are made conformal using the "beam's-eye-view" technique, with radiation arcs or beams avoiding eyes and eloquent structures. Intensity modulation is used with constrains based on structure eloquence and avoidance of "hot spots" in important structures. The dose is chosen based on tumor volume using an isoeffect line generated from an integrated logistic formula. On a log-log plot of dose versus volume, this line is straight with a negative slope and has proven to be a reliable predictor of SRS complications, as previously described by Kjelberg et al. and Flickinger et al. (Kjellberg et al. 1983; Flickinger 1989). Dose is also tailored to the surrounding anatomy and typically reduced for lesions near the brainstem or cranial nerves; the optic chiasm is restricted to 8 Gy in our institution. Typically, a single dose of 12–16 Gy, and full course of fractions of 45–50.40 Gy (Figs 8.3–8.6) suffice to control meningiomas.

8.5 Conclusion

Cure, rapid recovery, and good quality of life are the aims in meningioma management. Cure is not always possible, but rapid recovery and excellent quality of life without neurological deficits caused by the treatment are reachable with the modern management of meningiomas. Currently, patients with severe neurological deficits secondary to the therapy are those who underwent aggressive surgical resection. Properly planned surgery for decompression and preservation of function using modern imaging such as fiber tracking (Kamada et al. 2005) and modern surgical techniques (Rohde et al. 2005), followed by stereotactic radiosurgery or stereotactic radiotherapy (Selch et al. 2004), can provide outstanding quality of life for patients with benign meningiomas in any location, including optic sheath meningiomas (Andrews et al. 2002). Unfortunately the same cannot be said about atypical and malignant meningiomas (Mattozo et al. 2007), where complete resection is difficult and radiation is not able to control these tumors for long term. The use of dynamic contrast-enhanced perfusion MR imaging with T2-weighted sequences measuring the endothelial permeability is useful in distinguishing these patients, allowing for planned treatment before aggressive surgery, which may compromise quality of life (Yang et al. 2003). Presently, recurrence is the rule for the malignant meningiomas, without opportunity of rescue with chemotherapy; only surgery and re-irradiation are available in the recurrence setting.

References

Abdel-Aziz KM, Froelich SC, Dagnew E et al (2004) Large sphenoid wing meningiomas involving the cavernous sinus: conservative surgical strategies for better functional outcomes. Neurosurgery 54:1375–1383, Discussion 1383–1374

Al-Mefty O, Kersh JE, Routh A et al (1990) The long-term side effects of radiation therapy for benign brain tumors in adults. J Neurosurg 73:502–512

Al-Mefty O, Ayoubi S, Smith RR (1991) The petrosal approach: indications, technique, and results. Acta Neurochir Suppl (Wien) 53:166–170

Al-Mefty O, Kadri PA, Pravdenkova S et al (2004) Malignant progression in meningioma: documentation of a series and analysis of cytogenetic findings. J Neurosurg 101:210–218

Andrews DW, Faroozan R, Yang BP et al (2002) Fractionated stereotactic radiotherapy for the treatment of optic nerve sheath meningiomas: preliminary observations of 33 optic nerves in 30 patients with historical comparison to observation with or without prior surgery. Neurosurgery 51:890–902, discussion 903–894

Barbaro NM, Gutin PH, Wilson CB et al (1987) Radiation therapy in the treatment of partially resected meningiomas. Neurosurgery 20:525–528

Baumert BG, Villa S, Studer G et al (2004) Early improvements in vision after fractionated stereotactic radiotherapy for primary optic nerve sheath meningioma. Radiother Oncol 72:169–174

Bondy M, Ligon BL (1996) Epidemiology and etiology of intracranial meningiomas: a review. J Neurooncol 29: 197–205

Burger PC, Scheithauer BW, Vogel FS (2002) Surgical pathology of the nervous system and its coverings. Elsevier, Philadelphia

Chen JC, Giannotta SL, Yu C et al (2001) Radiosurgical management of benign cavernous sinus tumors: dose profiles and acute complications. Neurosurgery 48:1022–1030, Discussion 1030–1022

Clark BG, Candish C, Vollans E et al (2008) Optimization of stereotactic radiotherapy treatment delivery technique for base-of-skull meningiomas. Med Dosim 33:239–247

Couldwell WT, Fukushima T, Giannotta SL et al (1996) Petroclival meningiomas: surgical experience in 109 cases. J Neurosurg 84:20–28

Crossen JR, Garwood D, Glatstein E et al (1994) Neurobehavioral sequelae of cranial irradiation in adults: a review of radiation-induced encephalopathy. J Clin Oncol 12:627–642

De Salles AA, Bajada CL, Goetsch S et al (1993) Radiosurgery of cavernous sinus tumors. Acta Neurochir Suppl (Wien) 58:101–103

De Salles AA, Frighetto L, Grande CV et al (2001) Radiosurgery and stereotactic radiation therapy of skull base meningiomas: proposal of a grading system. Stereotact Funct Neurosurg 76:218–229

Debus J, Wuendrich M, Pirzkall A et al (2001) High efficacy of fractionated stereotactic radiotherapy of large base-of-skull meningiomas: long-term results. J Clin Oncol 19: 3547–3553

DeMonte F, Smith HK, al-Mefty O (1994) Outcome of aggressive removal of cavernous sinus meningiomas. J Neurosurg 81:245–251

Dziuk TW, Woo S, Butler EB et al (1998) Malignant meningioma: an indication for initial aggressive surgery and adjuvant radiotherapy. J Neurooncol 37:177–188

Eddleman CS, Liu JK (2007) Optic nerve sheath meningioma: current diagnosis and treatment. Neurosurg Focus 23:E4

Estall V, Eaton D, Burton KE, Jefferies SJ, Jena R, Burnet NG (2010a) Intensity-modulated radiotherapy plan optimisation for skull base lesions: practical class solutions for dose escalation. Clin Oncol (R Coll Radiol) 22(4): 313–320

Estall V, Fairfoul J, Jena R, Jefferies SJ, Burton KE, Burnet NG (2010b) Skull base meningioma: Comparison of intensity modulated radiotherapy planning techniques using the moduleaf micro-multileaf collimator and helical tomotherapy. Clin Oncol (R Coll Radiol) 22(3):179–184

Eustacchio S, Trummer M, Fuchs I, Schrottner O, Sutter B, Pendl G (2002) Preservation of cranial nerve function following Gamma Knife radiosurgery for benign skull base meningiomas: experience in 121 patients with follow-up of 5 to 9.8 years. Acta Neurochir Suppl 84:71–76

Flickinger JC (1989) An integrated logistic formula for prediction of complications from radiosurgery. Int J Radiat Oncol Biol Phys 17:879–885

Frighetto L, De Salles AA, Behnke E et al (2003) Image-guided frameless stereotactic biopsy sampling of parasellar lesions. Technical note. J Neurosurg 98:920–925

Gabibov GA, Blinkov SM, Tcherekayev VA (1988) The management of optic nerve meningiomas and gliomas. J Neurosurg 68:889–893

Glaholm J, Bloom HJ, Crow JH (1990) The role of radiotherapy in the management of intracranial meningiomas: the Royal

Marsden Hospital experience with 186 patients. Int J Radiat Oncol Biol Phys 18:755–761

Goldsmith BJ, Wara WM, Wilson CB et al (1994) Postoperative irradiation for subtotally resected meningiomas. a retrospective analysis of 140 patients treated from 1967 to 1990. J Neurosurg 80:195–201

Hakim R, Alexander E 3rd, Loeffler JS et al (1998) Results of linear accelerator-based radiosurgery for intracranial meningiomas. Neurosurgery 42:446–453, Discussion 453–444

Harris AE, Lee JY, Omalu B et al (2003) The effect of radiosurgery during management of aggressive meningiomas. Surg Neurol 60:298–305, Discussion 305

Hasegawa T, Kida Y, Yoshimoto M, Koike J, Iizuka H, Ishii D (2007) Long-term outcomes of Gamma Knife surgery for cavernous sinus meningiomas. J Neurosurg 107:745–751

Huffmann BC, Reinacher PC, Gilsbach JM (2005) Gamma knife surgery for atypical meningiomas. J Neurosurg 102(Suppl): 283–286

Hug EB, Devries A, Thornton AF et al (2000) Management of atypical and malignant meningiomas: role of high-dose, 3D-conformal radiation therapy. J Neurooncol 48:151–160

Iwai Y, Yamanaka K, Ishiguro T (2003) Gamma knife radiosurgery for the treatment of cavernous sinus meningiomas. Neurosurgery 52:517–524, Discussion 523–514

Jaaskelainen J, Haltia M, Servo A (1986) Atypical and anaplastic meningiomas: radiology, surgery, radiotherapy, and outcome. Surg Neurol 25:233–242

Johnson WD, Loredo LN, Slater JD (2008) Surgery and radiotherapy: complementary tools in the management of benign intracranial tumors. Neurosurg Focus 24:E2

Kamada K, Todo T, Masutani Y et al (2005) Combined use of tractography-integrated functional neuronavigation and direct fiber stimulation. J Neurosurg 102:664–672

Kennerdell JS, Maroon JC, Malton M, Warren FA (1988) The management of optic nerve sheath meningiomas. Am J Ophthalmol 106:450–457

Kjellberg RN, Davis KR, Lyons S et al (1983) Bragg peak proton beam therapy for arteriovenous malformation of the brain. Clin Neurosurg 31:248–290

Kleihues P, Louis DN, Scheithauer BW et al (2002) The WHO classification of tumors of the nervous system. J Neuropathol Exp Neurol 61:215–225, Discussion 226–219

Kobayashi T, Kida Y, Mori Y (2001) Long-term results of stereotactic gamma radiosurgery of meningiomas. Surg Neurol 55:325–331

Kokubo M, Shibamoto Y, Takahashi JA, Sasai K, Oya N, Hashimoto N, Hiraoka M (2000) Efficacy of conventional radiotherapy for recurrent meningioma. J Neurooncol 48(1):51–5

Kondziolka D, Lunsford LD (1992) Radiosurgery of meningiomas. Neurosurg Clin N Am 3:219–230

Kondziolka D, Levy EI, Niranjan A et al (1999) Long-term outcomes after meningiomas radiosurgery: physician and patient perspectives. J Neurosurg 91:44–50

Kondziolka D, Nathoo N, Flickinger JC et al (2003) Long-term results after radiosurgery for benign intracranial tumors. Neurosurgery 53:815–821, Discussion 821–812

Kupersmith MJ, Warren FA, Newall J et al (1987) Irradiation of meningiomas of the intracranial anterior visual pathway. Ann Neurol 21:131–137

Leber KA, Bergloff J, Pendl G (1998) Dose-response tolerance of the visual pathways and cranial nerves of the cavernous sinus to stereotactic radiosurgery. J Neurosurg 88:43–50

Lee JY, Niranjan A, McInerney J et al (2002) Stereotactic radiosurgery providing long-term tumor control of cavernous sinus meningiomas. J Neurosurg 97:65–72

Lee JY, Kondziolka D, Flickinger JC, Lunsford LD (2007) Radiosurgery for intracranial meningiomas. Prog Neurol Surg 20:142–149

Leksell L (1983) Stereotactic radiosurgery. J Neurol Neurosurg Psychiatry 46:797–803

Mahmood A, Caccamo DV, Tomecek FJ et al (1993) Atypical and malignant meningiomas: a clinicopathological review. Neurosurgery 33:955–963

Marks LB, Spencer DP (1991) The influence of volume on the tolerance of the brain to radiosurgery. J Neurosurg 75:177–180

Maruyama K, Shin M, Kurita H, Kawahara N, Morita A, Kirino T (2004) Proposed treatment strategy for cavernous sinus meningiomas: a prospective study. Neurosurgery 55:1068–1075

Mattozo CA, De Salles AA, Klement IA, Gorgulho A, McArthur D, Ford JM, Agazaryan N, Kelly DF, Selch MT (2007) Stereotactic radiation treatment for recurrent nonbenign meningiomas. J Neurosurg 106(5):846–854

Milker-Zabel S, Zabel A, Schulz-Ertner D et al (2005) Fractionated stereotactic radiotherapy in patients with benign or atypical intracranial meningioma: long-term experience and prognostic factors. Int J Radiat Oncol Biol Phys 61:809–816

Milker-Zabel S, Zabel-du Bois A, Huber P, Schlegel W, Debus J (2007) Intensity-modulated radiotherapy for complex-shaped meningioma of the skull base: long-term experience of a single institution. Int J Radiat Oncol Biol Phys 68:858–863

Milosevic MF, Frost PJ, Laperriere NJ et al (1996) Radiotherapy for atypical or malignant intracranial meningioma. Int J Radiat Oncol Biol Phys 34:817–822

Natarajan SK, Sekhar LN, Schessel D, Morita A (2007) Petroclival meningiomas: multimodality treatment and outcomes at long-term follow-up. Neurosurgery 60:965–979, Discussion 79–81

Nicolato A, Foroni R, Alessandrini F et al (2002) The role of Gamma Knife radiosurgery in the management of cavernous sinus meningiomas. Int J Radiat Oncol Biol Phys 53:992–1000

Nutting C, Brada M, Brazil L et al (1999) Radiotherapy in the treatment of benign meningiomas of the skull base. J Neurosurg 90:823–827

O'Sullivan MG, van Loveren HR, Tew JM Jr (1997) The surgical resectability of meningiomas of the cavernous sinus. Neurosurgery 40:238–244, Discussion 245–237

Ojemann SG, Sneed PK, Larson DA et al (2000) Radiosurgery for malignant meningioma: results in 22 patients. J Neurosurg 93(Suppl 3):62–67

Palma L, Celli P, Franco C et al (1997) Long-term prognosis for atypical and malignant meningiomas: a study of 71 surgical cases. J Neurosurg 86:793–800

Park CK, Jung HW, Kim JE, Paek SH, Kim DG (2006) The selection of the optimal therapeutic strategy for petroclival meningiomas. Surg Neurol 66:160–165, Discussion 5–6

Patil CG, Hoang S, Borchers DJ 3rd et al (2008) Predictors of peritumoral edema after stereotactic radiosurgery of

supratentorial meningiomas. Neurosurgery 63:435–440, Discussion 40–42
Perry A, Scheithauer BW, Stafford SL et al (1999) "Malignancy" in meningiomas: a clinicopathologic study of 116 patients, with grading implications. Cancer 85:2046–2056
Pirzkall A, Debus J, Haering P et al (2003) Intensity modulated radiotherapy (IMRT) for recurrent, residual, or untreated skull-base meningiomas: preliminary clinical experience. Int J Radiat Oncol Biol Phys 55:362–372
Pollock BE, Stafford SL, Utter A et al (2003) Stereotactic radiosurgery provides equivalent tumor control to Simpson Grade 1 resection for patients with small- to medium-size meningiomas. Int J Radiat Oncol Biol Phys 55: 1000–1005
Pourel N, Auque J, Bracard S et al (2001) Efficacy of external fractionated radiation therapy in the treatment of meningiomas: a 20-year experience. Radiother Oncol 61: 65–70
Ramina R, Neto MC, Fernandes YB, Silva EB, Mattei TA, Aguiar PH (2008) Surgical removal of small petroclival meningiomas. Acta Neurochir (Wien) 150:431–438, Discussion 8–9
Reinert M, Babey M, Curschmann J, Vajtai I, Seiler RW, Mariani L (2006) Morbidity in 201 patients with small sized meningioma treated by microsurgery. Acta Neurochir (Wien) 148:1257–1265, Discussion 66
Roche PH, Pellet W, Fuentes S, Thomassin JM, Regis J (2003) Gamma knife radiosurgical management of petroclival meningiomas results and indications. Acta Neurochir (Wien) 145:883–888, Discussion 8
Rohde V, Spangenberg P, Mayfrank L et al (2005) Advanced neuronavigation in skull base tumors and vascular lesions. Minim Invasive Neurosurg 48:13–18
Rohringer M, Sutherland GR, Louw DF et al (1989) Incidence and clinicopathological features of meningioma. J Neurosurg 71:665–672
Romanelli P, Wowra B, Muacevic A (2007) Multisession CyberKnife radiosurgery for optic nerve sheath meningiomas. Neurosurg Focus 23:E11
Sekhar LN, Swamy NK, Jaiswal V et al (1994) Surgical excision of meningiomas involving the clivus: preoperative and intraoperative features as predictors of postoperative functional deterioration. J Neurosurg 81:860–868
Selch MT, Ahn E, Laskari A et al (2004) Stereotactic radiotherapy for treatment of cavernous sinus meningiomas. Int J Radiat Oncol Biol Phys 59:101–111
Shafron DH, Friedman WA, Buatti JM et al (1999) Linac radiosurgery for benign meningiomas. Int J Radiat Oncol Biol Phys 43:321–327
Simpson D (1957) The recurrence of intracranial meningiomas after surgical treatment. J Neurochem 20:22–39
Soyuer S, Chang EL, Selek U et al (2004) Radiotherapy after surgery for benign cerebral meningioma. Radiother Oncol 71:85–90
Spiegelmann R, Nissim O, Menhel J et al (2002) Linear accelerator radiosurgery for meningiomas in and around the cavernous sinus. Neurosurgery 51:1373–1379, Discussion 1379–1380
Stafford SL, Pollock BE, Foote RL et al (2001) Meningioma radiosurgery: tumor control, outcomes, and complications among 190 consecutive patients. Neurosurgery 49:1029–1037, Discussion 1037–1028
Stafford SL, Pollock BE, Leavitt JA et al (2003) A study on the radiation tolerance of the optic nerves and chiasm after stereotactic radiosurgery. Int J Radiat Oncol Biol Phys 55:1177–1181
Subach BR, Lunsford LD, Kondziolka D, Maitz AH, Flickinger JC (1998) Management of petroclival meningiomas by stereotactic radiosurgery. Neurosurgery 42:437–443, Discussion 43–45
Tishler RB, Loeffler JS, Lunsford LD et al (1993) Tolerance of cranial nerves of the cavernous sinus to radiosurgery. Int J Radiat Oncol Biol Phys 27:215–221
Torres RC, Frighetto L, De Salles AA et al (2003) Radiosurgery and stereotactic radiotherapy for intracranial meningiomas. Neurosurg Focus 14:e5
Torres RC, De Salles AA, Frighetto L et al (2004) Long-term follow-up using Linac radiosurgery and stereotactic radiotherapy as a minimally invasive treatment for intracranial meningiomas. Radiosurgery 5:115–123
Turbin RE, Thompson CR, Kennerdell JS, Cockerham KP, Kupersmith MJ (2002) A long-term visual outcome comparison in patients with optic nerve sheath meningioma managed with observation, surgery, radiotherapy, or surgery and radiotherapy. Ophthalmology 109:890–900
Vernimmen FJ, Harris JK, Wilson JA et al (2001) Stereotactic proton beam therapy of skull base meningiomas. Int J Radiat Oncol Biol Phys 49:99–105
Wara WM, Sheline GE, Newman H et al (1975) Radiation therapy of meningiomas. Am J Roentgenol Radium Ther Nucl Med 123:453–458
Ware ML, Larson DA, Sneed PK et al (2004) Surgical resection and permanent brachytherapy for recurrent atypical and malignant meningioma. Neurosurgery 54:55–63, Discussion 63–54
Wilson CB (1996) Cavernous sinus meningiomas. Surg Neurol 46:191–192
Yang S, Law M, Zagzag D et al (2003) Dynamic contrast-enhanced perfusion MR imaging measurements of endothelial permeability: differentiation between atypical and typical meningiomas. Am J Neuroradiol 24: 1554–1559

9 Acoustic Neuromas

Yves Lazorthes, Jean Sabatier, Jean-Albert Lotterie, F. Loubes, Pierre-Yves Borius, Emmanuelle Cassol, P. Duthill, Isabelle Berry, and Igor Latorzeff

9.1 Introduction and History

Vestibular schwannoma (VS) is a benign neoplasm of Schwann cell origin. It occurs predominantly on the vestibular division of the eighth cranial nerve at the transition with oligodendroglia and at or within the internal auditory meatus. Rarely, tumors arise from cochlear division of the VIII nerve. This slow-growing tumor can become rather large without symptoms other than tinnitus, hearing loss, and/or unsteadiness. Modern neuroimaging permits early-stage tumor diagnosis. The evolution of VS surgical therapy is the illustration of the history of modern neurosurgery.

The initial treatment for acoustic neuromas has successively focused on

(a) *Palliation*: intracapsular tumor debulking (H. Cushing, last publication in 1932; overall mortality = 7.7%)
(b) *Cure*: the first total removal was achieved by W. Dandy in 1925. In his last 41 cases, mortality decreased to 2.4% (Dandy 1941)
(c) *Preservation of the facial nerve*: H. Olivecrona introduced the concept (20% facial nerve recovery), but the mortality rate increased to 23% (Olivecrona 1967)

During the microsurgical era (1960s and 1970s), the operative mortality fell by 50%, successful total removal increased by nearly 85%, and facial nerve prevention occurred in about 80% of patients. The microsurgical approaches are suboccipital (Rand and Kurze 1965; Rhoton 1974) and translabyrinthine (House 1979). Yasargil (1977) pioneered the technique in optimizing the preservation of brainstem vascular supply and nerve function.

Due to the advent of many technological advances, the contemporary era is focused on cranial nerve preservation. Reduced tumor size at diagnosis, multidisciplinary neuro-otological management, improved anesthesia, and intraoperative nerve monitoring are just a few of the modern advances. The global result of these advances includes a dramatic reduction of operative mortality (1%) and a total tumor removal range of 95%. Facial nerve preservation is considered feasible for all small tumors (Koos I and II), but not significantly decreased with large tumors. A functional hearing preservation rate of 40% after total removal was reported (Samii 1997). The postoperative complications (CSF leak meningitis, vascular accident, lower cranial nerve deficit) are still a risk.

The first publication reporting the results of VS radiosurgery appears in the 1980s (Noren et al. 1993; Kamerer et al. 1988). During this era, with the advance of microsurgery, the use of radiosurgery was controversial and critics stated that patients would be at risk of recurrence and late malignancy. In 1991, a consensus conference (NIH consensus statement) concluded that surgical resection was the treatment of choice for most patients with VS, but more research is needed regarding the risks and benefits of alternative management strategies.

The long-term and cumulative radiosurgical experience has refuted all these claims and provides increasing data demonstrating that stereotactic radiosurgery is a less invasive and more functionally conservative technique (Pollock et al. 1998; Lundsford et al. 2005; Regis et al. 2002, 2004, 2008).

Y. Lazorthes (✉), J. Sabatier, J.-A. Lotterie, F. Loubes, P.-Y. Borius, E. Cassol, P. Duthil, I. Berry, and I. Latorzeff
Department of Neurosurgery, Regional Center of Stereotactic Radiosurgery, 1 Avenue Jean Pouhlès, TSA 50032, Toulouse, Midi-Pyrénées 31059, France
e-mail: ylazorth@cict.fr

A.A.F. De Salles et al. (eds.), *Shaped Beam Radiosurgery*,
DOI: 10.1007/978-3-642-11151-8_9, © Springer-Verlag Berlin Heidelberg 2011

9.2 Goals and Radiosurgical Effects

The primary objective in treating acoustic neuromas is tumor growth control, verified by long-term post radiosurgical imaging with volume measurements. Frequently, the tumor volume does not decrease during the first year and early growth of the VS (a few mm) can be observed. The incidence of this transient expansion occurs frequently: from 3–5% (Régis and Roche 2008) up to 74% (Nagano et al. 2008). In general and at long-term neuroimaging (3–5 years), the tumor growth control is 98% (Regis et al. 2008).

The secondary objective concerning neurological outcomes stemming from acoustic neuroma treatments is the preservation of motor/sensory facial functions and hearing function (when preoperatively functional). The results depend largely on the tumor size (Koos et al. 1976) and the extension into the internal auditory canal. A temporary deficit can be observed between the sixth and eighteenth month during the transient expansion of the tumor.

The neurosurgeon has to inform the patient about the rationale for the treatment, his place in the management strategy, the expected results and the specific risks compared to the natural history of untreated tumors and the other surgical alternatives. The radiobiological effects of radiosurgery include tumor blood vessel destruction and damage to individual tumor cells (perhaps dose-dependant) leading to the inability of the tumor cells to go through mitosis. For slow-growth tumors like schwannomas that act like late responding tissue, tumor cells do not die until they attempt cell division apoptose.

The risk of developing facial and/or trigeminal and/or acoustic neuropathies following acoustic neuroma radiosurgery is significantly correlated with the marginal doses prescribed (minimum tumor dose) and the length of cranial nerve irradiated (diameter of the VS) since the cochleo-vestibulo-facial bundle lies along the capsule of the tumor and the cisternal part of trigeminal nerve is in close relationship in a Koos III tumors (Flickinger et al. 1996; Niranjan et al. 2008). Neuropathy of the trigeminal nerve has been reported with doses minimums of 13 Gy or less. This risk increases for patients with medical history of facial nerve motor deficit (posttraumatic, post surgical for previous VS resection and specialty patients with a previous a frigore facial palsy).

9.3 Indications

Acoustic neuromas must be managed by multidisciplinary teams that are able to propose all microsurgical and radiosurgical alternatives in order to provide higher probability of functional preservation and good quality of life. Concerning the large tumors deforming the brainstem and shifting the fourth ventricle (Koos stage IV), the first-line treatment remains microsurgery. However, there is a strong tendency to promote a combined approach starting with a microsurgical stage with large intracapsular debulking followed 3–6 months later by a radiosurgical stage. Concerning the small- and mid-sized tumors (Koos I, II and III), with a maximum diameter of 30 mm, radiosurgery now represents the first-line management, especially in young patients with few symptoms (Lundsford et al. 2005; Regis et al. 2004, 2008).

Summary of the trigeminal and facial (House and Brackman: grade ≥ 3) deficits and the acoustic nerve preservation (Gardner and Roberston: grades 1 and 2) reported in the radiosurgery literature:

References	(*n*) Pts	Volume (cc)	Follow-up (months)	Volume control (%)	VII deficit %	V deficit %	VIII preservation %
Prasad et al. (2000)	153	ND	12–120	?	2	3.2	40
Regis et al. (2004)	1,000		36–132		1.3	0.6	60
Flickinger et al. (2004)	313	1.1	24	98	0	4.4	78 (from pre-RDS useful hearing)
Hasegawa et al. (2005)	301	5.6	93	92	<1	2	ND
Lunsford et al. (2005)	829	2.5	≥5 years	98	1	2,7	50–77
Friedman et al. (2006)	390	2.2	40	90	4.4	3.6	
Chopra et al. (2007)	216	1.3	68	98			71

9.4 Shaped Beam Radiosurgery: A Multidisciplinary Approach

9.4.1 Background and Rationale

Stereotactic radiosurgery is a multidisciplinary neuroanatomic-based and image-guided technique. To be perfectly aware of the normal microanatomy of the cerebellopontine angle (cerebellopontine cistern and the contents), and to know all the anatomical variations (rotation of the nerve VII–VIII complex, A.I.C.A. loops, internal acoustic meatus dimensions) are all prerequisites. Different authors have contributed to improve this basic knowledge (Matsumo and Rhoton 1988; Yasargil et al. 2002; Lescanne et al. 2008). Integrating the lessons from microsurgical management and the pathology of VS tumors is an independent professional background. The classification concerning tumor grading by size proposed in 1976 by N.T. Koos is still the volume reference. However, M. Samii has improved the precision of this classification in function of the tumor extension (or origin) in the internal acoustic meatus. This sub-grading is interesting for radiosurgery concerning the relationship with a fragile structure: the cochlea.

The distortions of the CPA cistern contents associated with the growth patterns of large tumors (Koos III and IV) have been described (Sampath and Rini 2000). The facial nerve is stretched over the surface of the VS capsule, most common with the most frequent course around the anterosuperior pole of the tumor. Often the facial nerve is distorted upward and closely applied to the trigeminal nerve. The least common course is around lower part of the tumor.

The trigeminal nerve is in the upper part of the tumor. The contact and distortion start at the root entry zone and can involve all the cisternal portions of the fifth nerve. The cochlear nerve usually is found in the midpoint or below the tumor. Occasionally, the cochleo-vestibulo-facial bundle can be completely invested by the VS. The anatomical data are a valuable guide for the image planning, but there are no strict guidelines and optimal neuroimaging modalities are important in order to identify anatomical structures.

9.4.2 Technical Considerations

Acoustic neuromas tend to have an irregular surface contour and a variable extension in the IAC. They are in close relationship with highly functional and fragile surrounding structures of the cranial nerves of the CPA cistern and also brainstem in the Koos III grade. When a high and single dose is delivered in a single session, the safety is based on high spatial accuracy. Novalis® Radiosurgery provides us with an optimal dose fall-off. Accurate 3D image planning and dose planning require high-resolution image planning in all three anatomical planes. CT-imaging ensures stereotactic accuracy and permits correction of any MRI distortions (Regis et al. 2002). Radiosurgery is an exclusively image-guided technique (no immediate control of the effect is possible), and so it requires a strict quality control of the steps of the procedure. In managing the radiosurgical treatment of acoustic neuromas, sparring of the surrounding structures is critically important and requires high conformality and high selectivity of the dose delivery technique. While many centers have not embraced frameless procedures as accurate for radiosurgery of VS, including the senior author of this chapter, there is a growing body of evidence supporting that the improved precision of frameless radiosurgery leads to better accuracy of such treatments as an alternative to frame-based. (Please see Sect. 3.1, Chap. 3 in this book for additional information on this topic.)

Optimal planning is related to high conformality and the ability to confine the selected treatment to the 3D volumetric targets. This technical objective is dependent on the MRI imaging technique. High selectivity is defined as the ability to restrict dose to surrounding tissue outside the tumor target volume. This technical objective is optimized by shaped beam radiosurgery.

9.4.3 Imaging Protocol

The radiological phase quality is critical; imaging modalities and their acquisition parameters always require special attention, particularly for VS. The contribution of each imaging modality (MRI and CT) is complementary. The objectives and technical requirements for sequence selection are (1) perfect delineation of the exact tumor contrast enhancement and avoid any overestimating of the tumor volume, (2) precise identification of the surrounding brainstem and cranial nerves and vessels (V and VII and VIII) during their path in the CPA cisterna and in the internal auditory canal (IAC), and (3) delineating the exact expansion of the tumor at the fundus of the IAC and its relationship with the intrapetrous neuro-otologic structures (cochlea, labyrinth and facial nerve). In practice, the image planning is realized with iPlan® RT image and is based on the registration of a non-stereotactic MRI with a CT scan systematically performed in stereotactic conditions in order to limit inaccuracies.

9.4.4 The Preoperative Non-stereotactic MRI

Magnetic resonance imaging is performed a few days or weeks before the radiosurgical procedure. The acquisition parameters are optimized in order to optimize the limitation of distortions: volumetric (T2-CISS) injected and non-injected.

T1-weighted volumetric MRI pulse sequences (3DT1) enable iPlan segmentation (automatic and manual) of the organs at risk (brainstem, medulla oblongata, and visual pathways) and subsequent contouring of the tumor. This sequence is useful to show the interface with brainstem in Koos III and is more sensitive to magnetic field heterogeneity, inducing frequent distortions detected along the *Z*-axis. This sequence is more sensitive to magnetic field heterogeneity, inducing frequent distortions detected along the *Z*-axis. Other disadvantages are a global overestimation of the target volume and an enhancement of surrounding structures like arachnoid hyperhemia and vessels.

Steady-state (CISS) T2-weighted volumetric pulse sequences (3DT2) minimize partial volume effects and distortions. The injection of gadolinium corrects the limits of non-injected CISS, and in practice, high-resolution 0.5 mm, 3–3DT2-axial sequences (like CISS with Siemens, Fiesta with GE) are performed with and without contrast. The non-injected CISS allows us to visualize the small tumors (Koos I and II), the CPA cistern contents (nerve and vessels), and the limits between the tumor capsule and the cerebrospinal fluid, but no visualization of nerves in close contact. The injected CISS improves the visualization of the interfaces between tumor, nerves and brainstem and also of the intracanalicular extension. Fat saturation pulse sequence is complementary in post-microsurgery conditions.

9.4.5 The Stereotactic CT Scan

The images are acquired with a fiducial system attached to the Brainlab frame. Parameters of the acquisition are those used for high-resolution petrous bone investigations (slice thickness = 0.5 mm, placed edge to edge, with and without injection, in bony windows). The complementary advantages are (1) very low distortion, (2) reference to check the MRI distortion (fusion CT/MRI), (3) accurate visualization and correction of the exact limits of the intracanalicular extension of the acoustic neuroma on the MRI sequences (the tumor extension in the IAC is compared with the limits of the bony canal, as displayed in the CT bone window), and (4) a better application of the exact volume of the tumor as a compromise between the overestimated volumes of T1 3D GADO and T2-CISS sequences.

9.4.6 Frame Application: Specific Requirements

Minimize the pain and discomfort related to the frame application (explanation of procedure, premedication, intravenous perfusion of analgesic drug, careful intradermic and subcutaneous local anesthesia). Take into account the constraints related to imaging and planning (reliable fixation of the frame to the head, but perfect symmetry is not crucial). The frame must be aligned with the orbito-meatal line, sufficiently low in order to cover the entire tumor area of the skull base and the surrounding critical structures (including the optic pathways).

9.4.7 Image Planning with iPlan® RT Image

The steps for planning are:

(a) Localization of CT scan stereotactic images in the stereotactic space. Assign the appropriate Brainlab CT scan localizer and proceed to complete automatic localization. Properly localized slices must cover all the radiosurgical area. It is recommended to only ignore slices without localization information at the beginning or at the end of the data set.

(b) Image fusion (MRI on stereotactic CT scan) (modify range function), before conducting an automatic fusion and after to visually verify the perfect accuracy of the image registration (spy glass) on a full screen image.

(c) Identification and segmentation of the anatomical structures (Figs. 9.1 and 9.2). Segmentation of the organ at risk structures +++ iPlan® RT image automatic segmentation can under no circumstances replace the neurosurgeon's and neuroradiologist's knowledge of the regional anatomy and its pathological variations with the tumor expansion. All automatically segmented structures must be reviewed, and if necessary, corrected manually (e.g., brush, eraser, etc.).

For acoustic neuromas, the brain stem and medulla structures are corrected slice after slice, on axial and coronal 3DT1 MRI views for a Koos III tumor. The visualization of the interface pons-tumor is better with

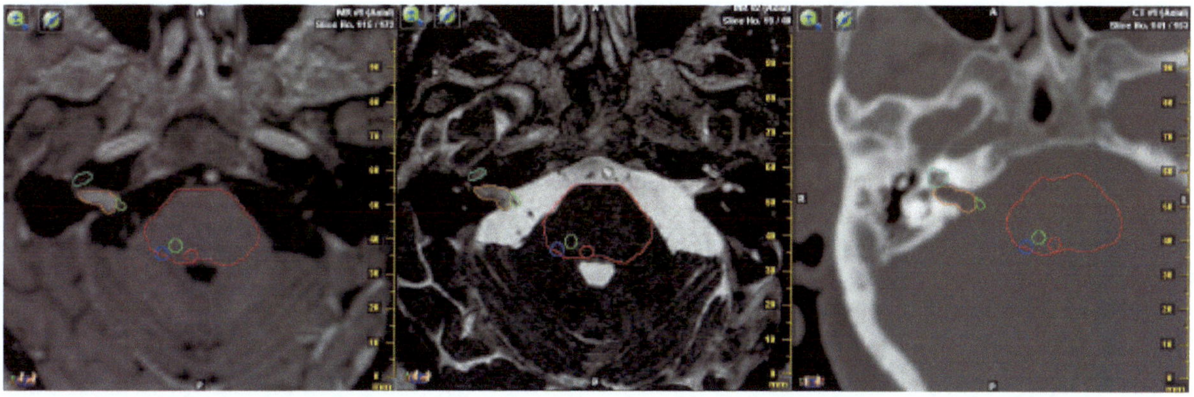

Fig. 9.1 Tumor and OAR segmentation (*left*: 3DT1 MRI, *middle*: 3D steady state T2 (CISS), *right*: CT)

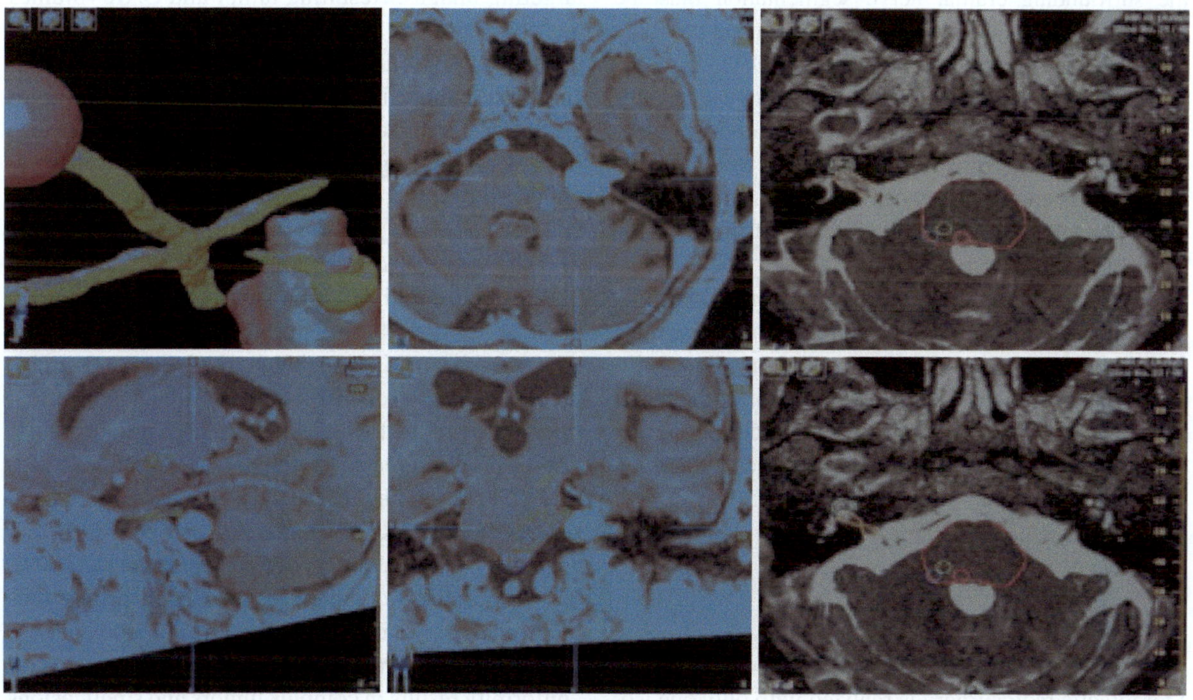

Fig. 9.2 Automatic segmentation of OARs and TV, represented with KOOS II (*left* and *middle part*) and KOOS I VS (*right part*)

3DT2 injected CISS. Chiasma and optic tracts are verified and corrected with axial and coronal 3D MRI images, but optic nerve corrections must be done on axial CT scan images. All the other OARs, and especially the surrounding cranial nerves, are not automatically segmented and must be manually created (add new object).

First the facial and cochleovestibular nerves are usually well visualized in small and middle tumors (Koos I and II) at the emergence and in cisterna. The cisternal portion definition could be poor, but the enhancement of the tumor improves this delineation. For stage III tumors, it is possible to reduce by 1 mm the anterior pole of the tumor (object manipulation/shrink object option) in order to reduce irradiation in the most frequent situation of the VII–VIII bundle. Concerning hearing preservation, Linskey (2008) strongly recommends the following during planning: (1) a prescription dose 3D conformality so that the ventral cochlear nucleus (VCN) receives ≤ 9 Gy, and that the basal turn of the cochlea receives the lowest possible dose ≤ 5 Gy and (2) also exclusion of the dura mater of the anterior border of the IAC. Concerning the trigeminal nerve, the emergency (pons entry zone) and the cisternal part is always identifiable for the three initial stages of the tumor on axial view of 3DT2-CISS MRI. In practice, complementary manual corrections of the surrounding cranial nerve segmentation must be done after tumor delineation. The cochlea and vestibule are segmented on bone window CT scan.

In this step, the object is manually drawn slice after slice on 3DT2-CISS MRI axial views. To start the segmentation, the interpolation function can be used in the four or eight contiguous slices tab, but in order to avoid errors, ensure to review the final object in all of the original slices concerned.

The image planning of acoustic neuromas in its cisternal part and particularly in its intracanalicular must be carefully visualized and corrected on a bone window CT scan. There is an overestimation of the target volume with 3D MRI images. In practice, the intracanalicular part of the VS must fit perfectly the bony IAC and meatus.

9.4.8 Dose Planning

Stereotactic radiosurgery is realized with only one isocenter and corresponding shaped beams optimizing homogeneity of the dose distribution within the target volume and conformal dose planning. Once the contouring stage on the stereotactic computed tomography fused with previously obtained MR images is performed, the next part of the process is to proceed to the dosimetry planning. Although the details of radiosurgical treatment techniques differ somewhat from system to system, the basic paradigm is inclusive. So we are going to provide a detailed description of our technique for a typical radiosurgical procedure at the University of Toulouse, France.

The goal of planning is to provide a highly conformal dose distribution using BrainSCAN® or iPlan® RT Dose; two Novalis Radiosurgery dedicated treatment planning software platforms (Brainlab AG, Feldkirchen, Germany).

9.4.9 Management of Dose Distribution Inside the Target Volume (TV)

The patient's tumor and OAR critical structures (i.e., brainstem, facial and trigeminal nerves, cochlea, medulla oblongata, optic apparatus and cortex) were contoured in 1 mm slices on the original radiosurgical targeting images. Resulting tumor and OAR volumes are coupled with the original radiosurgery plans to generate dose-volume histograms. Stereotactic radiosurgery planning is realized with only one isocenter even if the target volume has a complex shape because of the leaf-painting function included in the software, which allows the physician model targeting coverage and normal tissue preservation.

The Novalis Radiosurgery 6 MeV accelerator uses a 3 mm micro-multileaf collimator. The beam arrangement is performed with shaped beams in a dynamic conformal arc (DCA) technique in order to optimize homogeneity at every 10° of arc. This plan generates a steep dose gradient which allows a high dose of radiation to be delivered to the tumor with minimal exposure to surrounding tissue. The intensity-modulated radiotherapy (IMRT) technique is also permitted but, as shown in a recent article by Wiggenraad et al. (2009), based on a direct comparison with DCA, it only provides physicists with a better conformity index in concave tumors whereas DCA seems to produce better conformity results in complex tumors and small lesions (Fig. 9.3).

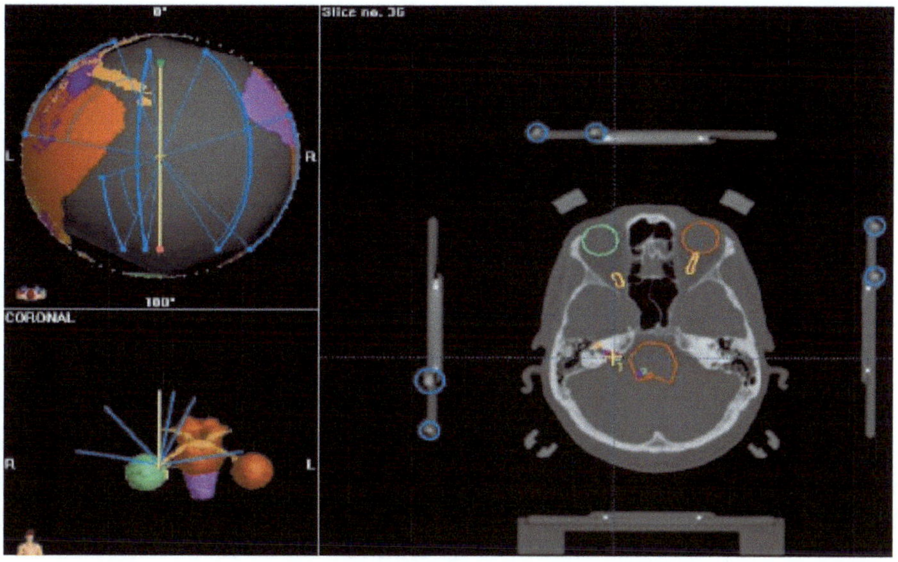

Fig. 9.3 Beam arrangement with six DCA, single isocenter, covering TV of a KOOS grade II right vestibular schwannoma

9.4.10 Conformity Index

The evaluation checks for optimizing treatments are: (1) visual inspection of the dose distribution in various planes and (2) inspection of the dose volume histogram, but they do not fully quantify the conformity of dose distributions (Feuvret 2006; Wagner et al. 2003). A goal of stereotactic radiosurgery (SRS) is to achieve optimal dose–volume conformity (i.e., to limit the prescription dose to a volume closely coincident with the target volume) (Feuvret 2006; Beegle et al. 2007; Friedmann and Foote 2003). The conformity index is a tool for scoring a given plan or for evaluating different treatment plans for the same patient. In our daily practice, the goal for dose prescription is to be as close as possible to the 100% referenced prescribed dose encompassing the total tumor volume.

Taking into account OAR proximity, especially the brainstem, the conformity index has to sometimes be adapted and adjusted to critical structure anatomy. Historically, linear accelerators have been considered to have less dose conformality compared to Gamma Knife (GK) (Hazard et al. 2009). Since its inception, however, linear accelerator-based radiosurgery has increased in sophistication. Nowadays, single isocenter dynamic conformal arc techniques with a micro-multileaf collimator are able to achieve equivalent conformality, but with superior homogeneity compared to multiple isocenters (Solberg et al. 2001).

Using the method of isodose surface selection, Hazard showed that the conformity index of linear accelerator-based SRS is comparable to the reported conformity index for gamma knife SRS. Thus, using the method described by Wagner et al. (2003), a conformity index, a dose gradient index, and a conformity/gradient index were used for each patient by using point measurements from the target and total volume on dose-volume histogram curves. These indices can only be used to compare different stereotactic plans. Unfortunately, the conformity index, gradient index, and conformity/gradient index have no effect on local control because they have no significant effect on outcomes after radiosurgery for VS, according to Beegle et al. (2007), in the modern 3D planning and dose prescription practice. They found, like others authors (Foote et al. 2001; Flickinger et al. 2004), that tumor volume and delivered dose are the most important treatment factors correlated to the risk of facial numbness or facial weakness.

9.5 Radiosurgery

The published experience involving the use of LINAC-based radiosurgery for the treatment of VS is relatively limited compared to the GK literature. Nevertheless, the dose prescription for vestibular schwannomas is well referenced (Friedmann and Foote 2003; Flickinger

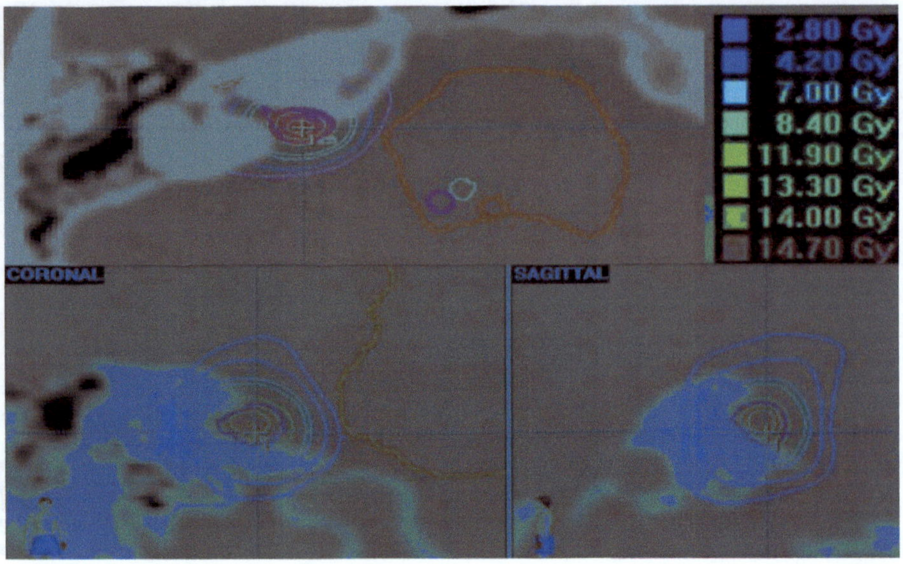

Fig. 9.4 Planning dosimetry for 12 Gy surrounding TV on the 86% isodose level representing 14 Gy isocenter dose prescription delivered with DCA

et al. 2004; Chopra et al. 2007). A single dose of 12 Gy on the standard prescription isodose (80–90% with a LINAC, with a treatment plan normalized to 100% for the maximum dose) is delivered to the tumor volume. The marginal dose selection then has to be adapted such that at least 95% of the volume is covered by the prescription isodose with respect to OAR constraints. We plan to deliver less than 12 Gy as the maximum dose to the brainstem. In some cases, a maximum dose point in the brainstem over 12 Gy may be tolerated if the volume receiving 12 Gy is below 1 cm^3.

Concerning the cochlea, the prescription varies if hearing preservation is mandatory or not. The maximum tolerated dose should be less than 5 Gy to allow preservation. When drawn on targeting images, the facial and trigeminal nerves dose delivered to these two critical structures can be reported. The dose distribution is influenced by the tumor volume (VS) and the proximity or not of the trigeminal root. As reported by different studies (Foote et al. 2001; Regis et al. 2004, 2008; Chopra et al. 2007), the respect of marginal dose of 12 Gy is most likely to yield long-term tumor control without causing cranial neuropathy (Fig. 9.4).

9.6 Fractionation

In addition, stereotactic radiotherapy (SRT) has been used as an alternative management for VS (Maire et al. 1995). This method is proposed as a way of exploiting the precision of stereotactic radiation delivery to minimize the dose to normal brain, while using lower fractionated doses in an effort to minimize complications (Maire et al. 1995; Meijer et al. 2003). The stereotactic head frame is replaced by re-locatable mask. Different studies have tried to address the issue between the two treatment options. Andrews et al. (2001) compared the results in patients treated using Gamma Knife radiosurgery with those patients treated using fractionated stereotactic radiotherapy with a re-locatable mask. Sixty-nine patients were treated using the Gamma Knife, and 56 patients were treated using SRT. Tumor control rates were high (97%) for sporadic tumors in both groups. Cranial nerve morbidities were comparably low in both groups, with the exception of functional hearing preservation, which was 2.5-fold higher in patients who had received SRT. This last result may now be even improved with modern linear accelerator-based radiosurgery with dynamic conformal arc dosimetry planning. Stereotactic radiotherapy has gained widespread adoption in recent year, though some radiosurgery practitioners still believe that optimal results can be achieved using highly conformal single fraction radiosurgery, while sparing the patient the inconvenience of a prolonged treatment course.

9.7 Follow-Up and Conclusion

Tumor growth control of acoustic schwannomas must be verified by long-term imaging with volume measurements. Minimum follow-up is 3 years, not only for

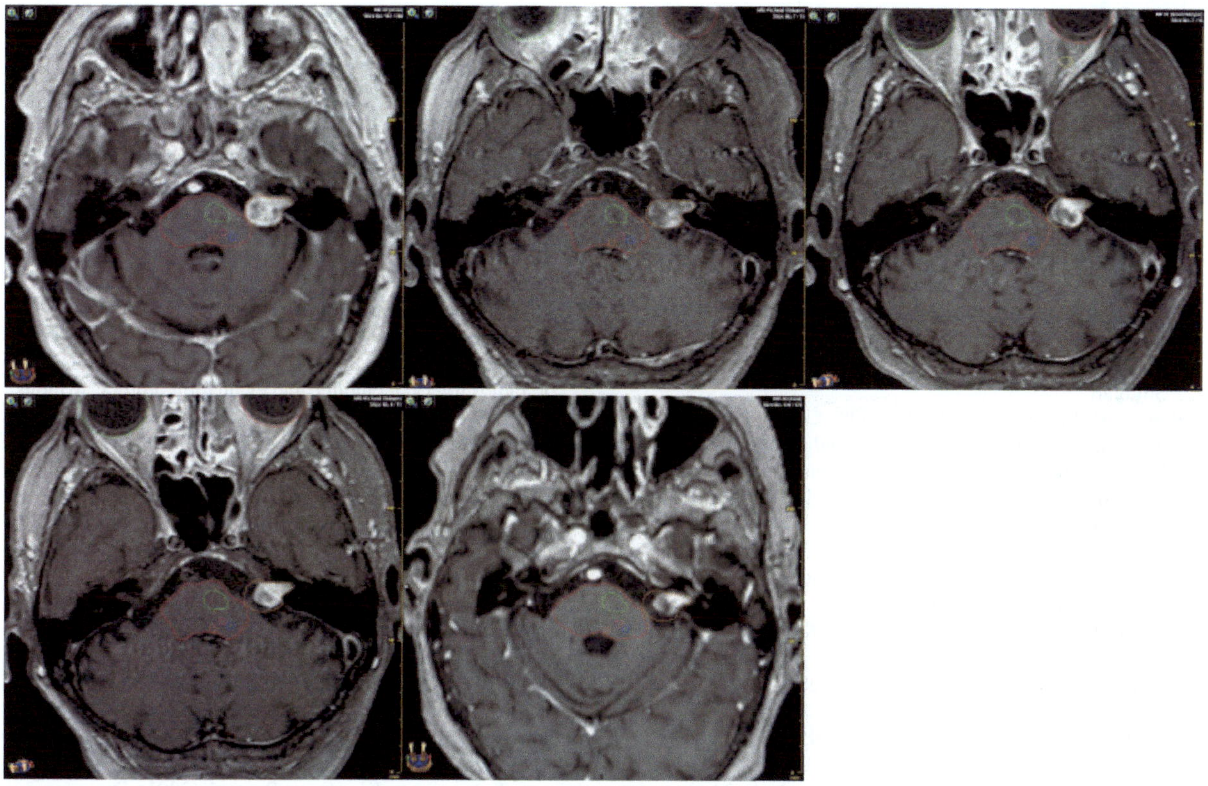

Fig. 9.5 MRI follow-up at 0, 6, 12, 18 and 24 month

tumor control, but also for cranial nerve preservation. In practice, we recommend conducting a neurological evaluation and an MRI (3D-T1 and T2 sequences) every 6 months during the first 2 years post-treatment and then repeating every year until 5 years of follow-up have been reached (Fig. 9.5).

In conclusion, radiosurgery is no longer just an alternative treatment option and must be considered as a first-line defense for most patients with a newly diagnosed acoustic neuromas of small or medium size (KOOS I, II and III).

References

Andrews DW, Suarez O, Goldman HW et al (2001) Stereotactic radiosurgery and fractionated stereotactic radiotherapy for the treatment of acoustic schwannomas: comparative observations of 125 patients treated at one institution. Int J Radiat Oncol Biol Phys 50:1265–1278

Beegle RD, Friedman WA, Bova FJ (2007) Effect of treatment plan quality on outcomes after radiosurgery for vestibular schwannoma. J Neurosurg 107:913–916

Chopra R, Kondziola D, Nirajan A, Lunford LD, Flickinger JC (2007) Long-term follow-up of acoustic schwannoma radiosurgery with marginal doses of 12 to 13 Gy. Int J Radiat Oncol Biol Phys 68(3):845–851

Cushing H (1932) Intracranial tumors. Notes upon a series of 2,000 verified cases with surgical mortality pertaining thereto. Charles C Thomas, Springfield, IL

Dandy WE (1941) Results of removal of acoustic tumors by the unilateral approach. AMA Arch Surg 42:1026–1043

Feuvret L, Noel G, Mazeron JJ, Bey P (2006) Conformity index:a review. Int J Radiat Oncol Biol Phys 64(2):333–342

Flickinger JC, Kondzialka D, Lunsford LD (1996) Dose and diameter relationships for facial trigeminal and acoustic neuropathies following acoustic neuroma radiosurgery. Radiother Oncol 41:215–219

Flickinger JC, Kondziolka D, Niranjan A, Maitz A, Voynov G, Lunsford LD (2004) Acoustic neuroma radiosurgery with marginal tumor doses of 12 to 13 Gy. Int J Radiat Oncol Biol Phys 60:225–230

Foote KD, Friedman WA, Buatti JM et al (2001) Analysis of risk factors associated with radiosurgery for vestibular schwannoma. J Neurosurg 95:440–449

Friedmann WA, Foote KD (2003) Linear accelerator–based radiosurgery for vestibular schwannoma. Neurosurg Focus 14(5):e2

Friedman WA, Bradshaw P, Myers A, Boua FJ (2006) Linear accelerator radiosurgery for vestibular schwannomas. J Neurosurg 105(5):655–6

Hasegawa T, Kida Y, Kobayashi T, Yoshimoto M, Mori Y, Yoshida J (2005) Long-term outcomes in patients with vestibular schwannomas treated using gamma knife surgery: 10 year follow-up. J Neurosurg 102:10–16

Hazard LJ, Wang B, Skidmore TB, Chern S-S, Salter YBJ, Jensen RL, Shrieve DC (2009) Conformity of linac-based stereotactic radiosurgery using dynamic conformal arcs and micro-multileaf collimator. Int J Radiat Oncol Biol Phys 73(2):562–570

House WF (1979) Translabyrinthine approach. In: House WF, Luetje CM (eds) Acoustic tumors. University Park Press, Baltimore, MD, pp 43–87

Kamerer DB, Lunsford LD, Moller M (1988) Gamma Knife: an alternative treatment for acoustic neuromas. Ann Oto Rhinol Laryn 97:631–635

Koos WT, Spetzler RF, Böck FW, Salah S (1976) Microsurgery of cerebello-pontine angle tumors. In: Koos WT, Spetzler RF, Bock FW (eds) Clinical microneurosurgery. Georg, Stuttgart

Lescanne E, Francois P, Velut S (2008) Cerebellopontine cistern: microanatomy applied to vestibular schwannomas. In: Regis J, Roche PH (eds) Modern management of acoustic neuroma, vol 21, Progress in Neurological Surgery. Karger, Basel, pp 43–53

Linskey ME (2008) Hearing preservation in vestibular schwannoma stereotactic radiosurgery: what really matters? J Neurosurg 109(Suppl):129–136)

Lundsford LD, Niranja A, Flickinger JC, Maitz A, Kondziolka A (2005) Radiosurgery of vestibular schwannomas: summary of experience in 829 cases. J Neurosurg 102(Suppl): 195–199

Maire JP, Caudry M, Darrouzet V et al (1995) Fractionated radiation therapy in the treatment of stage III and IV cerebellopontine angle neurinomas: long-term results in 24 cases. Int J Radiat Oncol Biol Phys 32:1137–1143

Matsumo M, Rhoton Al (1988) Microsurgery anatomy of the posterior fossa cistern. Neurosurgery 23:58–80

Meijer OWN, Vandertop WP, Baayen JC, Slotman BJ (2003) Single-fraction vs. fractionated linac-based stereotactic radiosurgery for vestibular schwannoma: a single-institution study. Int J Radiat Oncol Biol Phys 56(5):1390–1396

Nagano O, Higuchi Y, Serizawa T, Ono J, Matsuda S, Yamakimi I, Saeki N (2008) Transient expansion of vestibular schwannoma following stereotactic radiosurgery. J Neurosurg 109:811–816

Niranjan A, Flickinger JC (2008) Radiobiology, principle and technique of radiosurgery. In: Regis J, Roche PH (eds) Modern management of acoustic neuromas, vol 21, Progress in Neurological Surgery. Karger, Basel, pp 32–42

Noren G, Greitz D, Hirsch A, Lax I (1993) Gamma-knife in acoustic tumors. Acta Neurochir Suppl 58:104–107

Olivecrona H (1967) Acoustic tumors. J Neurosurg 26:6–13

Pollock BE, Lunsford LD, Noren G (1998) Vestibular schwannoma management in the next century: a radiosurgical perspective. Neurosurgery 43(3):475–483

Prasad D, Steiner M, Steiner L (2000) Gamma surgery for vestibular schwannoma. J Neurosurg 92:745–759

Rand R, Kurze T (1965) Micro-neurosurgical resection of acoustic tumors by a transmeatal posterior fossa approach. Bull Los Angeles Neurol Soc 30:17–20

Régis J, Roche PH (eds) (2008) Modern management of acoustic neuromas, vol 21, Progress in Neurological Surgery. Karger, Basel, pp 32–42

Regis J, Roche PH, Delsentin C, Soumare O, Thomassin JM, Pellet W (2002) Stereotactic radiosurgery for vestibular schwannomas. In: Pollock BE (ed) Contemporary stereotactic radiosurgery: technique and evaluation. Futura, Armonk, pp 181–212

Regis J, Delfanti C, Roche PH, Thomassin JM, Pellet W (2004) Functional outcomes of radiosurgical treatment of vestibular schwannomas: 1000 successive cases and review of the literature. Neurochirurgie 50:301–311

Rhoton Al (1974) Microsurgery of the internal acoustic meatus. Surg Neurol 2:311–318

Samii M, Matthies C (1997) Management of 1000 vestibular schwannomas (acoustic neuromas): the facial nerve preservation and restitution of function. Neurosurgery 40:684–694

Sampath P, Rini D, Long DM (2000) Microanatomical in the cerebellopontine angle associated with vestibular schwannomas: a retrospective study of 1006 consecutive cases. J Neurosurg 92:70–78

Solberg T, Boedeker KL, Fogg R et al (2001) Dynamic arc radiosurgery field shaping: a comparison with static field conformal and noncoplanar circular arcs. Int J Radiat Oncol Biol Phys 49:1481–1491

Wagner TH, Bova FJ, Friedman WA, Buatti JM, Bouchet LG, Meeks SL (2003) A simple and reliable index for scoring rival stereotactic radiosurgery plans. Int J Radiat Oncol Biol Phys 57:1141–1149

Wiggenraad RG, Petoukhova AL, Versluis L, Van Santvoort JPC (2009) Stereotactic radiotherapy of intracranial tumors: a comparison of intensity-modulated radiotherapy and dynamic conformal arc. Int J Radiat Oncol Biol Phys 74(4):1018–1026; Int J Radiat Oncol Biol Phys (2006) 64:333–342

Yasargil MG, Smith RD, Gasser JC (1977) Microsurgical approach to acoustic neuromas. Adv Tech Stand Neurosurg 4:93–129

Yasargil MG, Lescanne E, Velut S, Lefrancq T, Destrieux C (2002) The internal acoustic meatus. J Neurosurg 97: 1014–1017

10 Pituitary Adenomas

Winston W. Lien and Joseph C. Chen

10.1 Introduction

Pituitary adenomas represent the most common neoplasms near the sella turcica and constitute approximately 10–12% of all intracranial tumors (Seegenschmiedt 2008; Sanno et al. 2003). Pituitary tumors are classified as microadenomas or macroadenomas based on size, with microadenomas defined as <10 mm in diameter and macroadenomas being ≥10 mm in diameter (Knisely and Sperduto 2008). Pituitary adenomas are also divided into two broad categories: functioning (67%) and non-functioning (33%). Functioning adenomas can be further subdivided by which hormone is secreted: prolactin (28% of all pituitary adenomas), growth hormone (23%), ACTH (8%), and others (such as TSH-producing and gonadotropin-producing, 7%; Committee of Brain Tumor Registry of Japan 2000; Thapar et al. 1997). Management of pituitary adenomas can include observation, medical management, surgical management, and radiation therapy.

10.2 Clinical Presentation

Pituitary adenomas commonly present with endocrine abnormalities due to either hypersecretion or, less commonly, hormonal insufficiency caused by compression of the gland or pituitary stalk. Possible endocrinological presentations include Cushing's disease, galactorrhea, amenorrhea, impotence, acromegaly, hyperthyroidism, and hypopituitarism. In addition to endocrinopathies, adenomas can cause symptoms through local mass effect. As pituitary tumors grow, they can extend laterally into the cavernous sinus causing diplopia or facial sensory deficits. Superior tumor extension can cause compression of the optic nerves, resulting in bitemporal hemianopsia or bitemporal superior quadrantanopsia.

10.3 General Management Principles

If asymptomatic, non-functioning microadenomas can be observed, while surgery is generally recommended for the treatment of macroadenomas. Surgical techniques can include transsphenoidal resection as well as various approaches from above the skull base including pterional, supraorbital, and subfrontal methods.

For prolactinomas, medical management is usually the preferred initial intervention. Bromocriptine and cabergoline are dopamine agonists that can lower prolactin levels and induce tumor shrinkage. As tumor response is typically quite rapid, initial medical management is reasonable even in cases with significant mass effect. Accordingly, pharmacologic management remains the standard of care for prolactinomas with surgery and radiation usually reserved for cases of refractory tumors or intolerance to medication (Shomali 2008).

Surgical methods for management of these tumors are well developed and represent the mainstay of treatment for corticotropic (ACTH), somatotropic (GH), and thyrotropic (TSH) pituitary adenomas.

W.W. Lien
Department of Radiation Oncology, Southern California Permanente Medical Group, Los Angeles, CA 90027, USA

J.C. Chen (✉)
Department of Neurosurgery, Southern California Permanente Medical Group, Los Angeles, CA 90027, USA
e-mail: joseph.c.chen@kp.org

A.A.F. De Salles et al. (eds.), *Shaped Beam Radiosurgery*,
DOI: 10.1007/978-3-642-11151-8_10, © Springer-Verlag Berlin Heidelberg 2011

Surgery also remains the preferred means of initial management for functioning, non-prolactin-secreting adenomas as response to medical management is inconsistent.

Surgery, when successful, can result in rapid correction of pituitary endocrinopathies in functioning adenomas and relieve symptoms from mass effect in patients with non-functioning macroadenomas. In some instances, surgery may not attain the goals of long-term endocrinologic remission or eradication of tumor. In these cases, adjuvant radiation is usually recommended. This is especially true in cases of recurrent tumors or unresectable cases involving the cavernous sinus. All candidates for treatment should have a full endocrinologic evaluation and formal visual field testing. In this chapter, methods as well as perioperative care issues will be discussed in the context of LINAC treatment methods with Novalis® Radiosurgery (Brainlab AG, Feldkirchen, Germany).

10.4 Radiation for Non-functioning Pituitary Adenomas

Approximately one-third of pituitary adenomas are non-functioning or null-cell adenomas and are quite common in the general population with an incidence of approximately 20% (Radhakrishnan et al. 1995; Annegers et al. 1981). The general indications for treatment of non-functioning adenomas are diameter greater than 1 cm (macroadenomas) or symptomatic compression of surrounding neural structures, most typically the optic chiasm. In such instances, surgery is generally the preferred initial treatment as it can immediately address mass effect and endocrine abnormalities. Surgery, however, may result in incomplete resection of tumor, particularly in cases of fibrous tumors or in situations where tumor invades the cavernous sinus (Greenman et al. 2003). The decision whether or not to deliver postoperative radiation should be based upon the amount of residual disease, the patient's age (elderly patients tend to have slowly progressive tumors), invasion of the cavernous sinus, dural invasion, or aggressive appearing histology (Greenman et al. 2003; Meij et al. 2002; Laws et al. 1982). Reported control rates following transsphenoidal resection are approximately 50–80% (Laws et al. 1982; Chandler et al. 1987; Friedman et al. 1989). Immediate salvage radiation can be considered for patients with macroscopic residual disease. Conversely, in patients with minimal amounts of residual disease, patients may be closely followed with serial imaging.

Historically, the most common radiation technique for treatment of pituitary adenomas was conventional fractionated radiotherapy (CRT) and achieved reasonable success with approximately 90% of cases controlled at 10 years (Grigsby et al. 1989; McCollough et al. 1991; Brada et al. 1993; Tsang et al. 1994; Zierhut et al. 1995; Breen et al. 1998; Gittoes et al. 1998; Sasaki et al. 2000; Woollons et al. 2000; Table 10.1). Fractionated treatment over a 5–6 week period usually consisted of two-parallel laterally opposed beams, with or without an additional anterior beam, focused on the pituitary sella. The advantages of CRT included its simplicity of setup, good long-term safety data, and proven efficacy. However, CRT fell out of favor due to its imprecision, inconvenience to the patient, and inability to reduce dose to critical structures.

Leksell (1951) initially described the technique of stereotactic radiosurgery in 1951 utilizing a proton source mounted to a stereotactic frame. In 1968, the

Table 10.1 Conventional radiation therapy (CRT) for non-functioning pituitary adenomas

References	Patients	Median follow-up (years)	Control rate (%)
Grigsby et al. (1989)	121	11.7	90
McCollough et al. (1991)	105	7.8	95
Brada et al. (1993)	411	10.8	94
Tsang et al. (1994)	160	8.7	87
Zierhut et al. (1995)	138	6.5	95
Breen et al. (1998)	120	9	87.5
Gittoes et al. (1998)	126	7.5	93
Sasaki et al. (2000)	91	8.2	93
Woollons et al. (2000)	50	5	72

first patient with pituitary adenoma was treated with radiosurgery (Backlund 1969). Betti et al. (1991) were the first to describe LINAC-based stereotactic radiosurgery as an alternative to Gamma Knife treatments. Since that time, the technology has been refined rapidly, and current technology is able to achieve an accuracy of 0.60±0.36 mm (Rahimian et al. 2004).

LINAC-based devices, such as Novalis radiosurgery, utilize a collimated X-ray beam with the patient placed in a fixed, stereotactically defined position as the beam rotates around the target. The treatment couch is rotated into various positions, allowing for multiple, non-coplanar arcs to treat the target. This allows a high dose of radiation to be delivered to the point of intersection of the arcs with a sharp dose gradient outside of the target, thereby minimizing dose to the remaining normal tissues. Advances, such as multileaf collimators (MLCs) and intensity-modulated radiation therapy/radiosurgery (IMRT/IMRS), have allowed further improvements in dose definition and beam shaping. Additionally, image-guided radiotherapy (IGRT) has allowed for less uncertainty in the treatment of tumors near critical structures. Image guidance, even with frameless techniques, has reduced translational errors to 0.31±0.26 mm and rotational errors to 0.26±0.23 degrees for Novalis radiosurgery (Wurm et al. 2008).

With the widespread use of stereotactic radiosurgery, single fraction treatments for pituitary adenomas have increased. Results with SRS are excellent, with control rates in excess of 90% (Lim et al. 1998; Witt et al. 1998; Izawa et al. 2000; Feigl et al. 2002; Sheehan et al. 2002; Wowra and Stummer 2002; Petrovich et al. 2003; Pollock and Carpenter 2003; Losa et al. 2004; Iwai et al. 2005; Mingione et al. 2006; Table 10.2). Although these control rates are comparable to CRT, stereotactic techniques have been widely adopted due to their ability to safely treat in a single fraction and to reduce dose to critical normal structures. SRS, however, is unable to treat lesions that are close to or involving the optic chiasm or optic nerves. These techniques have continued to improve due to advancements in patient immobilization, image co-registration, and three-dimensional treatment planning (Brada et al. 2004).

While the data regarding fractionated stereotactic radiotherapy (fSRT) is relatively immature, with median follow-up periods of less than 5 years, early results are promising with over 90% control at 3 years. Complication rates are low and are comparable to those reported with conventional radiotherapy (Mitsumori et al. 1998; Milker-Zabel et al. 2001; Paek et al. 2005; Colin et al. 2005; Minniti et al. 2006; Table 10.3). These excellent control rates must be interpreted with caution, as pituitary adenomas are relatively slow growing and changes may not be apparent early in the disease course. As fSRT is commonly reserved for more difficult cases, such as tumors involving the optic chiasm, long-term results may be inferior to SRS data due to selection bias.

Table 10.2 Radiosurgery (SRS) for non-functioning pituitary adenomas

References	Patients	Median follow-up (months)	Control rate (%)
Lim et al. (1998)	22	26	92
Witt et al. (1998)	24	32	94
Izawa et al. (2000)	23	6	91
Feigl et al. (2002)	61	55	94
Sheehan et al. (2002)	42	31	97
Wowra and Stummer (2002)	45	55	93
Petrovich et al. (2003)	56	36	94
Pollock and Carpenter (2003)	33	43	97
Losa et al. (2004)	56	41	88
Iwai et al. (2005)	34	60	93
Mingione et al. (2006)	100	45	92

Table 10.3 Fractionated stereotactic radiotherapy (fSRT) for non-functioning pituitary adenomas

References	Patients	Median follow-up (years)	Control rate (%)
Mitsumori et al. (1998)	30	2.2	86
Milker-Zabel et al. (2001)	68	3.2	93
Paek et al. (2005)	68	2.5	98
Colin et al. (2005)	110	4	99
Minniti et al. (2006)	92	2.8	98

The literature does not suggest any significant clinical differences between SRS and fSRT for either functioning or non-functioning adenomas. Some data, however, suggests that normalization of hormonal function is achieved more rapidly with SRS as compared to fractionated treatments (Mitsumori et al. 1998). The indications for each technique vary and will be outlined later in this chapter.

10.5 Radiation for Functioning Pituitary Adenomas

Prolactinomas represent the most common functioning pituitary adenoma and comprise 28% of functioning adenomas (Committee of Brain Tumor Registry of Japan 2000; Thapar et al. 1997). As prolactinomas respond well to medical intervention, radiation and surgery are less frequently employed when compared to the other functioning adenomas. Nevertheless, surgical interventions should be considered in patients who have intolerable side effects from medication or in tumors that are resistant to medication. The criterion for defining endocrinologic remission for prolactinomas is fairly consistent throughout the literature. Most studies define remission as having normal serum prolactin levels. While results are relatively variable, it can be expected that approximately 50% of patients will have endocrinologic remission at 10 years following fractionated radiation (Tsagarakis et al. 1991; Littley et al. 1991; Williams et al. 1994; Wallace and Holdaway 1995; Tsang et al. 1996; Ozgen et al. 1999; Table 10.4). For radiosurgery, the rates of endocrinologic remission vary widely with reported remission rates ranging from 15 to 68% (Levy et al. 1991; Kim et al. 1999; Mokry et al. 1999; Landolt and Lomax 2000; Zhang et al. 2000; Choi et al. 2003; Table 10.4). According to a review of the literature by Brada and Jankowska (2008), 26% of patients have normalization of prolactin levels while 55% of patients experience a decrease in serum prolactin levels with reported times to hormonal response ranging from 5 to 41 months.

Table 10.4 Radiation for prolactin-secreting pituitary adenomas

References	Patients	Median follow-up (years)	Endocrinologic control rate (%)
Conventional radiation			
Tsagarakis et al. (1991)	36	8.5	50
Littley et al. (1991)	58	10	50 (predicted)
Williams et al. (1994)	28	Not stated	29
Wallace and Holdaway (1995)	25	4	33
Tsang et al. (1996)	64	10	25
Ozgen et al. (1999)	106	Not stated	58
Radiosurgery			
Levy et al. (1991)	20	Not stated	60
Kim et al. (1999)	18	2.3	17
Mokry et al. (1999)	21	2.6	68
Landolt and Lomax (2000)	20	2.4	55
Zhang et al. (2000)	128	2.8	53
Choi et al. (2003)	21	3.5	24

Adrenocorticotropic hormone (ACTH)-secreting adenomas result in excess cortisol production leading to Cushing's disease and make up 8% of functioning adenomas (Committee of Brain Tumor Registry of Japan 2000; Thapar et al. 1997). In cases where neurosurgical intervention is unsuccessful, it is generally accepted that radiation should be administered postoperatively. In contrast to prolactinomas, there has been much debate as to the criteria that should be used to define endocrinologic control of Cushing's. The most commonly used test is a 24-h urine-free cortisol. Other tests that have been used include serum ACTH, low-dose dexamethasone suppression test, and serum cortisol or salivary cortisol. Many studies, unfortunately, do not state their criterion for endocrinologic "cure" and report that hormone normalization usually takes about 1–2 years. In general, one would expect about 60% of patients to achieve endocrinologic remission following either conventional radiation or SRS (Witt et al. 1998; Sheehan et al. 2000, 2002; Tsang et al. 1996; Levy et al. 1991; Brada and Jankowska 2008; Nagesser et al. 2000; Howlett et al. 1989; Estrada et al. 1997; Laws and Vance 1999; Table 10.5). This is supported by Nagesser et al. (2000) who report a 64% endocrinologic cure rate utilizing a

Table 10.5 Radiation for Cushing's disease

References	Patients	Median follow-up (years)	Endocrinologic control rate (%)
Conventional radiation			
Howlett et al. (1989)	21	9.5	57
Tsang et al. (1996)	29	10	53
Estrada et al. (1997)	30	3.5	83
Nagesser et al. (2000)	86	21	64
Radiosurgery			
Levy et al. (1991)	64	Not stated	86
Witt et al. (1998)	25	2.7	28
Laws and Vance (1999)	50	Not stated	58
Sheehan et al. (2000)	43	3.7	63
Kobayashi et al. (2002)	20	5.3	35

Table 10.6 Radiation for acromegaly

References	Patients	Median follow-up (years)	Endocrinologic control rate (%)
Conventional radiation			
Eastman et al. (1992)	87	20	89
Tsang et al. (1996)	52	10	46
Thalassinos et al. (1998)	46	7.6	55
Biermasz et al. (2000)	40	10.3	76
Radiosurgery			
Hayashi et al. (1999)	22	1.3	41
Laws and Vance (1999)	56	NR	25
Zhang et al. (2000)	68	2.8	96
Pollock et al. (2002)	26	3.5	42
Attanasio et al. (2003)	30	3.8	30

low-dose dexamethasone suppression test after a median follow-up of 21 years.

Growth hormone (GH)-secreting tumors, which may cause acromegaly, are less common than prolactin-secreting pituitary adenomas and represent 23% of hormonal active tumors (Committee of Brain Tumor Registry of Japan 2000; Thapar et al. 1997). In addition to surgery and radiation, somatostatin analogs can be used to decrease levels of GH and insulin-like growth factor-1 (IGF-1). Landolt et al. (2000) postulated that medical therapy may decrease the metabolic rate of the tumor, thus rendering it more resistant to radiation treatment. Hence, if radiation is planned, medical therapy should be stopped at least 2 weeks prior to treatment. Postoperative radiation therapy should be considered for patients with basal GH levels >5 mcg/L (Varia et al. 2007). While no data suggests that fractionated treatment is superior to SRS, median follow-up is longer for conventional techniques with long-term endocrinologic control rates of 55–90% at 10 years (Tsang et al. 1996; Zhang et al. 2000; Laws and Vance 1999; Eastman et al. 1992; Thalassinos et al. 1998; Biermasz et al. 2000; Hayashi et al. 1999; Pollock et al. 2002; Attanasio et al. 2003; Table 10.6). Cure is defined by most authors as basal GH <5 mcg/L or <1 mcg/L with glucose load and normal IGF-1 levels.

10.6 Methods

High-quality imaging is critical for the treatment of pituitary adenomas. Since these tumors are most often treated in the postoperative setting, normal gland as well as scar and postsurgical debris, including the fat used for repair, may result in a complicated imaging picture. Newer MRI methods, such as dynamic contrast-enhanced sequences, may be useful in delineating the location of residual adenoma, particularly for smaller lesions (Friedman et al. 2007; Yoon et al. 2001). In addition, high-resolution CT imaging used for fiducial localization may be helpful in determining the lateral borders of the tumor. Recently, a functional imaging modality, ^{11}C-methionine positron emission tomography (PET), has been reported as being useful for delineating adenoma target volumes for radiosurgery planning (Levivier et al. 2004). ^{11}C-methionine PET has also been shown to accurately predict endocrinologic response of pituitary adenomas (Muhr 2006). Comparison of multiple imaging modalities is often needed in order to outline a reasonable treatment volume. Following MRI or functional imaging, CT planning is performed with the patient in a localizable position with an immobilization device. For single fraction SRS treatments, a stereotactic head frame can be applied to the patient under local anesthesia. Alternatively, noninvasive immobilization can be employed with use of thermoplastic mask in concert with high-resolution image-guided patient positioning as exemplified by the ExacTrac® X-Ray (Brainlab AG, Feldkirchen, Germany) system. At our facility, we perform the vast majority of radiosurgery procedures using the frameless method both for single or multi-fraction treatments. Immobilization and reproducibility are of paramount importance given the delicate nature of the structures in proximity to the pituitary gland. Patient positioning should be reproducible with errors of <1 mm for single fraction treatments. After CT planning, the images are exported to software capable of fusing the CT images to the previously acquired MRI series. The target volume and normal intracranial structures are contoured and correlated between the CT and MRI images. Pituitary adenomas have been treated with a wide variety of doses, fractionation schedules, and conformities. Small tumors located at sufficient distance from the optic chiasm can typically be treated with single fraction methods using forward treatment planning. As tumor size increases and the distance between the optic structures and tumor surface decreases, there is a greater likelihood that inverse treatment planning methods and fractionation are necessary in order to minimize the risk of injury to the optic apparatus. For single fraction radiosurgery, the goal of treatment should include coverage of the complete tumor volume to a dose of at least 12 Gy while limiting the dose to the optic chiasm to a maximum of 8–10 Gy (Tishler et al. 1993). Non-functioning pituitary adenomas appear to require a lower dose for control (Lim et al. 1998; Izawa et al. 2000; Landolt and Lomax 2000) with most institutions treating to a peripheral dose of 13–15 Gy (Laws et al. 2004). For functioning adenomas, some investigators have found that hormone normalization correlates with factors such as treatment isodose, maximal dose, margin dose, and absence of hormone-suppressive medication (Mokry et al. 1999; Landolt and Lomax 2000; Hayashi et al. 1999). As such, most advocate delivery of higher doses (20–30 Gy) in order to more rapidly normalize hormone levels (Laws et al. 2004). At our institution, we have typically used 45–50 Gy in 25–30 fractions for large tumors involving the optic nerve and chiasm. In these cases, we limit the optic structures to doses less than 2 Gy/day. In order to determine the optimal radiosurgery treatment plan, it is useful to categorize these lesions based on factors such as size and distance from the optic chiasm. Table 10.7 is shown below with general guidelines that our institution has utilized to aid in determining the most appropriate treatment course for patients.

Table 10.7 Radiosurgical classification of pituitary adenomas using LINAC

Class 1	
Tumor volume ≤5 mL	Single fraction radiosurgery
Tumor ≥3 mm from optic chiasm	
Class 2	
Tumor volume >5 mL	Single fraction radiosurgery or fractionated stereotactic radiosurgery with prescription isodose line of 80%
Tumor ≥3 mm from optic chiasm	
Class 3	
Tumor <3 mm from optic chiasm	Fractionated stereotactic radiosurgery with prescription isodose line of 80–95%
Class 4[a]	
Tumor in contact with optic chiasm	Fractionated stereotactic radiosurgery with prescription isodose line of 95%
Class 5[a]	
Tumor engulfing optic chiasm	Fractionated stereotactic radiosurgery with prescription isodose line of >95%

[a]*Note*: In practice, Class 4 and 5 tumors would be treated in a similar manner

10.7 Case Illustrations

Case 1. A 59-year-old female who presented with acromegaly, including changes in her jaw, hands, and feet. Imaging showed a pituitary mass >1 cm. She was initially treated with octreotide. IGF-1 levels decreased but did not normalize. She underwent transsphenoidal resection of her pituitary tumor with pathologic confirmation of pituitary adenoma. As postoperative IGF-1 levels were persistently elevated, she was treated with single fraction SRS using ten conformal static beams with Novalis radiosurgery. Given a 4-mm distance between the residual tumor and optic chiasm and treatment volume of 1.65 cc, she was categorized as a Class 1 patient. Twenty-four gray was prescribed to the 80% isodose line with treatment volume including the tumor periphery. Following radiosurgery, the patient's IGF-1 levels slowly normalized. Five years after radiosurgery, IGF-1 levels remain normal with the patient receiving monthly octreotide injections. Her endocrine function is otherwise normal, and she has not required treatment for hypopituitarism (Figs. 10.1–10.4).

Case 2. A 66-year-old male who presented with blurry vision and diplopia. Imaging revealed a large mass within the sella with invasion of the suprasellar cistern, sphenoid sinus, and right cavernous sinus. Laboratory studies were normal with the exception of hypogonadism with an LH of <0.1 mIU/mL. The patient underwent transsphenoidal resection with pathologic confirmation of pituitary adenoma. On postoperative imaging, residual tumor was noted involving the optic chiasm bilaterally (Class 4). Treatment volume was 8.46 cc. Postoperative fractionated SRT with five-dynamic conformal arcs was delivered to a total dose of 46.8 Gy (1.8 Gy/day) prescribed to the 90% isodose line. The patient is clinically stable 5 years after treatment with no tumor progression. His vision remains intact, and he does not currently require endocrine replacement (Figs. 10.5–10.7).

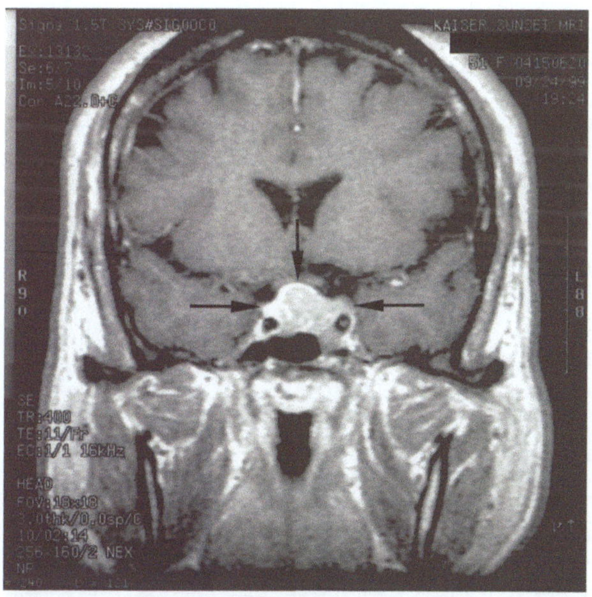

Fig. 10.1 Fifty-nine-year-old female with functioning adenoma causing acromegaly. The black arrows show the preoperative close relationship between the tumor and the optic quiasm. The patient underwent a transsphenoidal resection of the mass

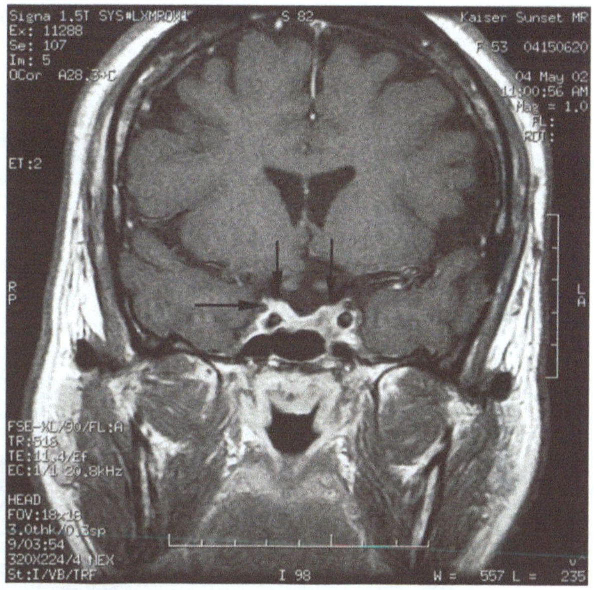

Fig. 10.2 Pituitary mass (*black arrows*) following 4 years of medical therapy

10.8 Discussion

Radiation therapy, either SRS or fSRT, is an effective treatment for pituitary adenomas that are not cured by medical management or surgery alone. While stereotactic techniques represent state-of-the-art technology, conventional radiotherapeutic techniques have demonstrated good long-term control with minimal morbidity. Stereotactic techniques are clearly superior to conventional treatments in minimizing radiation dose to normal brain tissue and to critical intracranial structures. Longer follow-up and more experience will determine if stereotactic techniques truly offer clinical benefit in terms of reducing late toxicities or increasing efficacy of treatment.

Hypopituitarism is the most common late complication of radiotherapy with 0–40% of patients

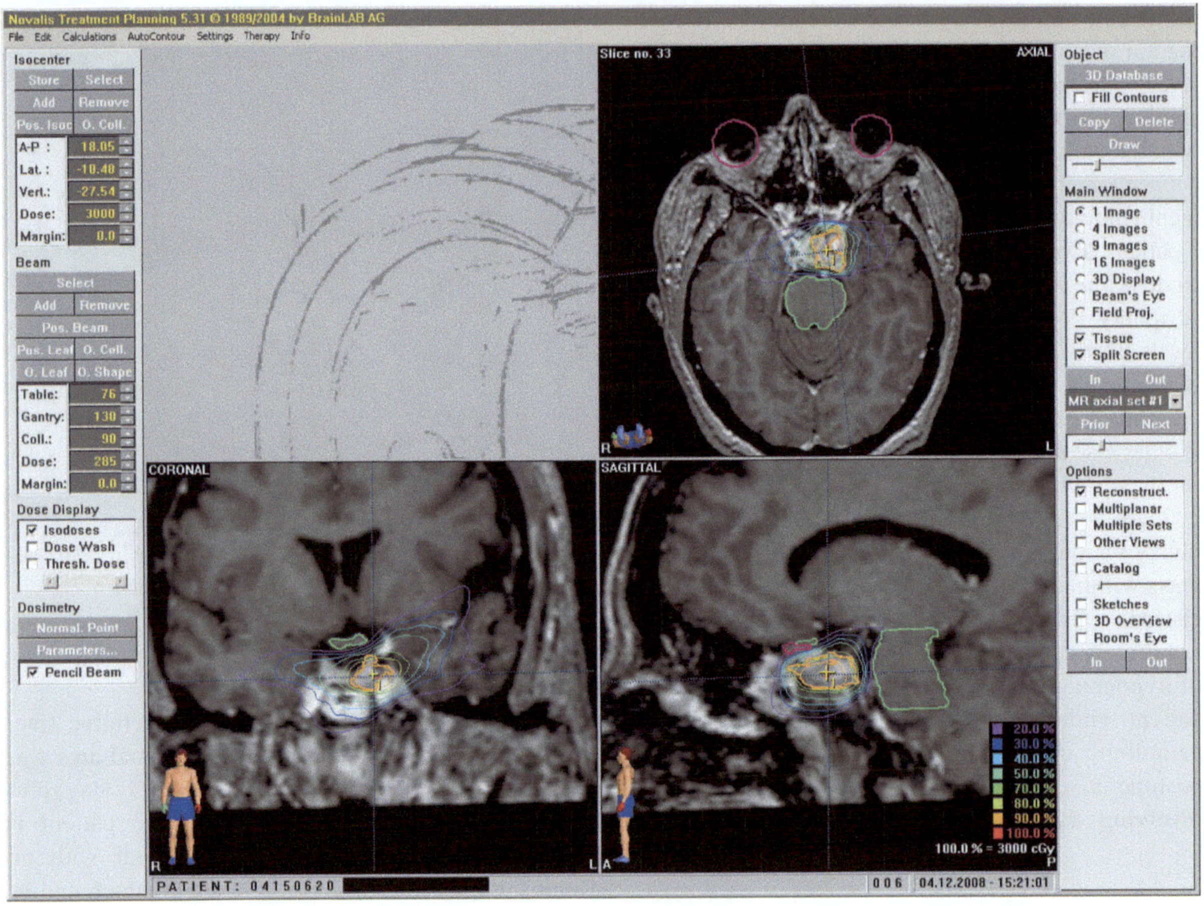

Fig. 10.3 Single fraction stereotactic radiosurgery for residual pituitary mass. Class 1 patient (treatment volume 1.65 cc and 4 mm distance from optic chiasm). Treated to 24 Gy prescribed to the 80% isodose line

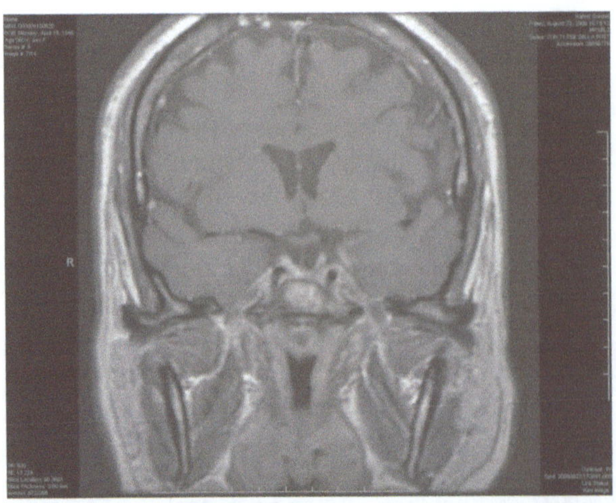

Fig. 10.4 Five years following radiosurgery. IGF-1 levels are normal on monthly octreotide

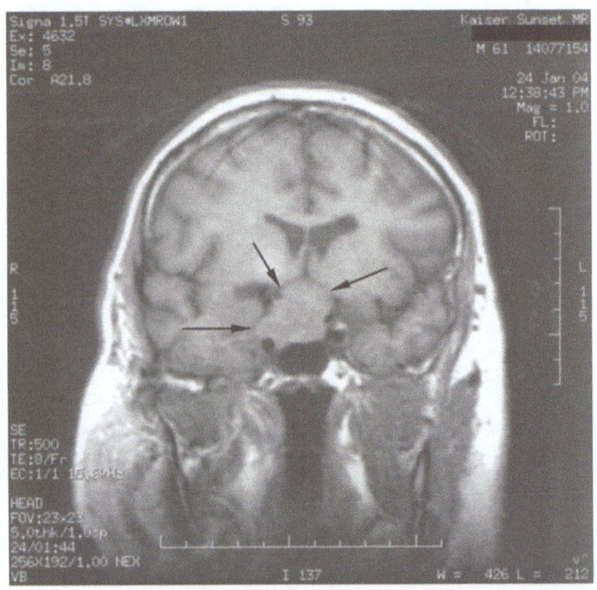

Fig. 10.5 Sixty-six-year-old male with large pituitary macroadenoma (*black arrows*) causing visual disturbances with invasion of the suprasellar cistern, sphenoid sinus and right cavernous sinus

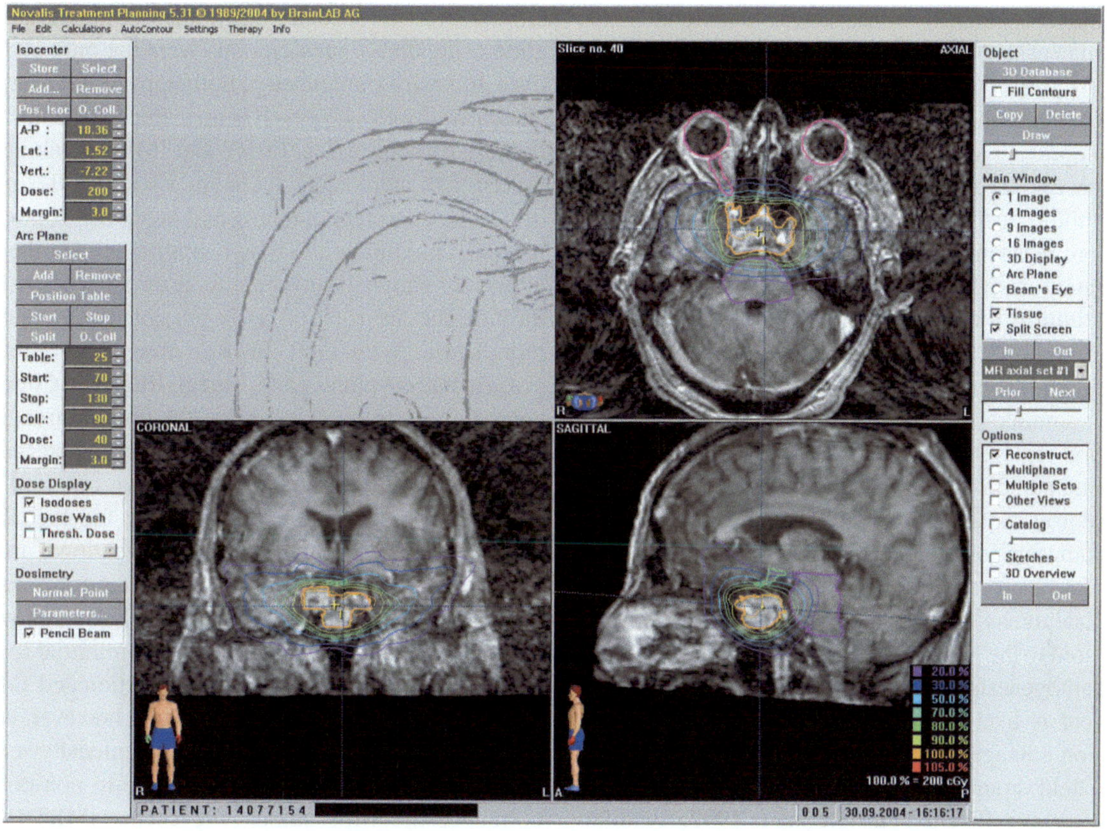

Fig. 10.6 Treated with surgical decompression followed by fractionated stereotactic radiotherapy. Class 4 patient (tumor pushing on optic chiasm). Treated to 46.8 Gy (1.8 Gy/day) prescribed to the 90% isodose line

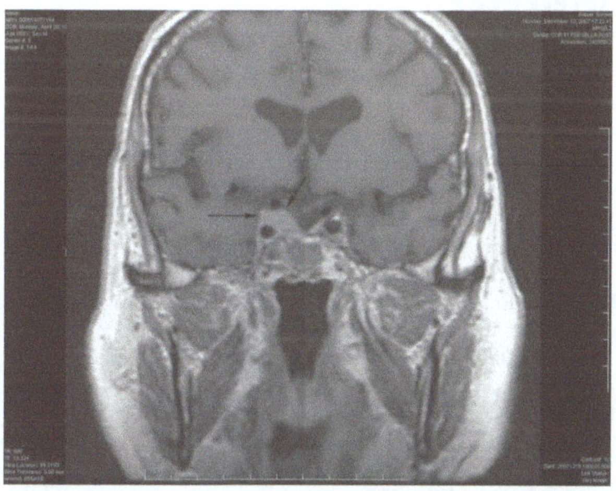

Fig. 10.7 Five years following fSRT with stable MRI findings and no significant radiation related morbidity. The black arrows point to the supra sellar extension of the tumor in close relationship with the optic apparatus and right cavernous sinus

developing long-term hormonal deficiencies (Pollock and Carpenter 2003; Laws and Vance 1999; Laws et al. 2004). With longer follow-up, however, the incidence of hypopituitarism may be much higher. Höybye et al. (2001) report deficiencies in one or more of the LH/FSH, TSH, and ACTH axes in 75% of patients and note that many patients continued to manifest hormone deficiencies more than 10 years after radiation. Though the reported rates of hypopituitarism are higher with conventional RT (20–40%) as compared to SRS (0–30%), this could simply be due to the longer follow-up time in the conventionally treated patients (Lim et al. 1998; Witt et al. 1998; Izawa et al. 2000; Feigl et al. 2002; Sheehan et al. 2002; Wowra and Stummer 2002; Petrovich et al. 2003; Pollock and Carpenter 2003; Losa et al. 2004; Iwai et al. 2005; Mingione et al. 2006).

SRS or fractionated radiation-induced optic neuritis is relatively rare with the reported incidence between

1% and 5% (Sasaki et al. 2000; Backlund 1969; Rahimian et al. 2004; Izawa et al. 2000; Petrovich et al. 2003). Laws et al. (2004) reviewed 34 studies with 1,567 patients and found only a 1% incidence of damage to optic nerves or the optic chiasm. The other cranial nerves in the cavernous sinus, including the oculomotor, trochlear, trigeminal, and abducens nerves, are more resistant to radiation damage with complication rates of <1% (Laws et al. 2004). Parenchymal brain injury following radiosurgery is also quite uncommon with incidence of brain necrosis or inflammation reported as <1% (Becker et al. 2002). The areas most commonly affected are the hypothalamic and temporal regions.

Some authors have also reported an increased rate of cerebrovascular accidents (CVA) in patients treated with radiation for pituitary adenomas. Brada reported a 4.1-fold increase in CVAs in 334 patients with pituitary adenomas treated with surgery and radiation compared to the general population (Brada et al. 2002). The pathogenesis of CVA development is not entirely clear but is likely a combination of hypopituitarism, radiation damage, and surgery. While it is known that large field cranial radiation in children results in long-term cognitive deficits (Donahue 1992; Syndikus et al. 1994), there is no clear evidence of neurocognitive dysfunction in adults radiated to small cranial fields.

Finally, though radiation therapy can cure pituitary adenomas, it can also induce secondary tumors. Meningiomas are the most common radiation-induced brain tumors followed by astrocytomas. The cumulative risk of secondary brain tumors following conventional three-field radiotherapy as reported by Minniti is 2.4% at 20 years (Minniti et al. 2005).

10.9 Future Considerations

The use of radiosurgery for pituitary tumors has been well established. With the arrival of mature image-guided techniques, highly precise frameless treatments are now possible which offer equivalent accuracy while improving patient comfort compared to traditional frame-based techniques. Even with advances in image guidance, it is sometimes difficult to treat tumors to an adequate dose without exceeding normal tissue tolerances. This is especially true in cases in which tumors are large, irregularly shaped, or very close to critical structures. Historically, altering dose fractionation or treatment prescriptions were the only alternatives. Intensity-modulated radiotherapy or radiosurgery (IMRT or IMRS), however, is now able to be employed in these difficult cases. IMRT and IMRS combine the precision of stereotactic techniques with the flexibility of inverse treatment planning and computer-controlled intensity modulation. Though traditional arc therapy allows for simple beam shaping, dose cannot be varied through the arc rotation as is possible with intensity modulation. With IMRT/IMRS, dose constraints are given to target volumes and critical structures. Complex computer algorithms determine the optimal treatment techniques to best satisfy the physician determined dose constraints. Multiple authors have reported that IMRS can improve dose conformality for irregularly shaped lesions compared to more conventional arcs or fixed fields (Pirzkall et al. 2003; Jensen et al. 2008). An early report by Mackley et al. (2007) has shown a progression-free survival of 97% with minimal toxicities in short-term follow-up using fractionated IMRT. The long-term advantage of IMRT has, however, yet to be established. There is concern that intensity-modulated treatment increases integral dose to non-critical normal tissues. Most authors suggest that IMRT/IMRS is not necessary for small spherical lesions though larger, irregular lesions may benefit from this newer technology.

References

Annegers JF, Schoenberg BS, Okazak H, Kurland LT (1981) Epidemiologic study of primary intracranial neoplasms. Arch Neurol 38:217–219

Attanasio R, Epaminonda P, Motti E, Giugni E, Ventrella L, Cozzi R, Farabola M, Loli P, Beck-Peccoz P, Arosio M (2003) Gamma-knife radiosurgery in acromegaly: a 4-year follow-up study. J Clin Endocrinol Metab 88(7): 3105–3112

Backlund EO (1969) Stereotactic treatment of craniopharyngiomas. In: Hamberger CA, Wersäll J (eds) Nobel symposium 10: disorders of the skull base region. Almqvist and Wiksell, Stockholm, pp 237–244

Becker G, Kocher M, Kortmann RD, Paulsen F, Jeremic B, Müller RP, Bamberg M (2002) Radiation therapy in the multimodal treatment approach of pituitary adenoma. Strahlenther Onkol 178(4):173–186

Betti OO, Galmarini D, Derechinsky V (1991) Radiosurgery with a linear accelerator. Methodological aspects. Stereotact Funct Neurosurg 57(1–2):87–98

Biermasz NR, Dulken HV, Roelfsema F (2000) Postoperative radiotherapy in acromegaly is effective in reducing GH concentration to safe levels. Clin Endocrinol (Oxf) 53(3): 321–327

Brada M, Jankowska P (2008) Radiotherapy for pituitary adenomas. Endocrinol Metab Clin North Am 37(1):263–275

Brada M, Rajan B, Traish D, Ashley S, Holmes-Sellors PJ, Nussey S, Uttley D (1993) The long-term efficacy of conservative surgery and radiotherapy in the control of pituitary adenomas. Clin Endocrinol (Oxf) 38(6):571–578

Brada M, Ashley S, Ford D, Traish D, Burchell L, Rajan B (2002) Cerebrovascular mortality in patients with pituitary adenoma. Clin Endocrinol (Oxf) 57(6):713–717

Brada M, Ajithkumar TV, Minniti G (2004) Radiosurgery for pituitary adenomas. Clin Endocrinol 61:531–543

Breen P, Flickinger JC, Kondziolka D, Martinez AJ (1998) Radiotherapy for nonfunctional pituitary adenoma: analysis of long-term tumor control. J Neurosurg 89(6):933–938

Chandler WF, Schteingart DE, Lloyd RV, McKeever PE, Ibarra-Perez G (1987) Surgical treatment of Cushing's disease. J Neurosurg 66:204–212

Choi JY, Chang JH, Chang JW, Ha Y, Park YG, Chung SS (2003) Radiological and hormonal responses of functioning pituitary adenomas after gamma knife radiosurgery. Yonsei Med J 44(4):602–607

Colin P, Jovenin N, Delemer B, Caron J, Grulet H, Hecart AC, Lukas C, Bazin A, Bernard MH, Scherpereel B, Peruzzi P, Nakib I, Redon C, Rousseaux P (2005) Treatment of pituitary adenomas by fractionated stereotactic radiotherapy: a prospective study of 110 patients. Int J Radiat Oncol Biol Phys 62(2):333–341

Committee of Brain Tumor Registry of Japan (2000) Report of brain tumor registry of Japan (10th edn.). Neurol Med Chir 40(Suppl):5–11

Donahue B (1992) Short- and long-term complications of radiation therapy for pediatric brain tumors. Pediatr Neurosurg 18(4):207–217

Eastman RC, Gorden P, Glatstein E, Roth J (1992) Radiation therapy of acromegaly. Endocrinol Metab Clin North Am 21(3):693–712

Estrada J, Boronat M, Mielgo M, Magallón R, Millan I, Díez S, Lucas T, Barceló B (1997) The long-term outcome of pituitary irradiation after unsuccessful transsphenoidal surgery in Cushing's disease. N Engl J Med 336(3):172–177

Feigl GC, Bonelli CM, Berghold A, Mokry M (2002) Effects of gamma knife radiosurgery of pituitary adenomas on pituitary function. J Neurosurg 97(5 Suppl):415–421

Friedman RB, Oldfield EH, Nieman LK, Chrousos GP, Doppman JL, Cutler GB, Loriaux DL (1989) Repeat transsphenoidal surgery for Cushing's disease. J Neurosurg 71:520–527

Friedman TC, Zuckerbraun E, Lee ML, Kabil MS, Shahinian H (2007) Dynamic pituitary MRI has high sensitivity and specificity for the diagnosis of mild Cushing's syndrome and should be part of the initial workup. Horm Metab Res 39(6):451–456

Gittoes NJ, Bates AS, Tse W, Bullivant B, Sheppard MC, Clayton RN, Stewart PM (1998) Radiotherapy for non-function pituitary tumours. Clin Endocrinol (Oxf) 48(3): 331–337

Greenman Y, Ouaknine G, Veschev I, Reider-Groswasser II, Segev Y, Stern N (2003) Postoperative surveillance of clinically non-functional pituitary macroadenomas: markers of tumor quiescence and regrowth. Clin Endocrinol 58: 763–769

Grigsby PW, Simpson JR, Emami BN, Fineberg BB, Schwartz HG (1989) Prognostic factors and results of surgery and postoperative irradiation in the management of pituitary adenomas. Int J Radiat Oncol Biol Phys 16(6):1411–1417

Hayashi M, Izawa M, Hiyama H, Nakamura S, Atsuchi S, Sato H, Nakaya K, Sasaki K, Ochiai T, Kubo O, Hori T, Takakura K (1999) Gamma Knife radiosurgery for pituitary adenomas. Stereotact Funct Neurosurg 72(Suppl 1):111–118

Howlett TA, Plowman PN, Wass JA, Rees LH, Jones AE, Besser GM (1989) Megavoltage pituitary irradiation in the management of Cushing's disease and Nelson's syndrome: long-term follow-up. Clin Endocrinol (Oxf) 31(3):309–323

Höybye C, Grenbäck E, Rähn T, Degerblad M, Thorén M, Hulting AL (2001) Adrenocorticotropic hormone-producing pituitary tumors: 12- to 22-year follow-up after treatment with stereotactic radiosurgery. Neurosurgery 49(2): 284–291

Iwai Y, Yamanaka K, Yoshioka K (2005) Radiosurgery for nonfunctioning pituitary adenomas. Neurosurgery 56(4):699–705, discussion 699–705

Izawa M, Hayashi M, Nakaya K, Satoh H, Ochiai T, Hori T, Takakura K (2000) Gamma knife radiosurgery for pituitary adenomas. J Neurosurg 93(Suppl 3):19–22

Jensen RL, Wendland MM, Chern SS, Shrieve DC (2008) Novalis intensity-modulated radiosurgery: methods for pre-treatment planning. Neurosurgery 62(5 Suppl):A2–A9

Kim SH, Huh R, Chang JW, Park YG, Chung SS (1999) Gamma Knife radiosurgery for functioning pituitary adenomas. Stereotact Funct Neurosurg 72(Suppl 1):101–110

Knisely JPS, Sperduto PW (2008) Pituitary and pituitary region tumors: fractionated radiation therapy perspective. In: Chin L, Regine W (eds) Principles and practice of stereotactic radiosurgery. Springer, New York, pp 317–326

Kobayashi T, Kida Y, Mori Y (2002) Gamma knife radiosurgery in the treatment of Cushing disease: long-term results. J Neurosurg 97(5 Suppl):422–428

Landolt AM, Lomax N (2000) Gamma knife radiosurgery for prolactinomas. J Neurosurg 93(Suppl 3):14–18

Landolt AM, Haller D, Lomax N, Scheib S, Schubiger O, Siegfried J, Wellis G (2000) Octreotide may act as a radioprotective agent in acromegaly. J Clin Endocrinol Metab 85(3):1287–1289

Laws ER Jr, Vance ML (1999) Radiosurgery for pituitary tumors and craniopharyngiomas. Neurosurg Clin N Am 10(2):327–336

Laws ER, Ebersold MJ, Piepgras DG (1982) The results of transsphenoidal surgery in specific clinical entities. In: Laws ER, Randall R, Kern EB, Abboud CF (eds) Management of pituitary adenomas and related lesions with emphasis on transsphenoidal microsurgery. Appleton-Century-Crofts, New York, pp 277–305

Laws ER, Sheehan JP, Sheehan JM, Jagnathan J, Jane JA Jr, Oskouian R (2004) Stereotactic radiosurgery for pituitary adenomas: a review of the literature. J Neurooncol 69(1–3): 257–272

Leksell L (1951) The stereotaxic method and radiosurgery of the brain. Acta Chir Scand 102:316–319

Levivier M, Massager N, Wikler D, Lorenzoni J, Ruiz S, Devriendt D, David P, Desmedt F, Simon S, Van Houtte P, Brotchi J, Goldman S (2004) Use of stereotactic PET images in dosimetry planning of radiosurgery for brain tumors: clinical experience and proposed classification. J Nucl Med 45(7):1146–1154

Levy RP, Fabrikant JI, Frankel KA, Phillips MH, Lyman JT, Lawrence JH, Tobias CA (1991) Heavy-charged-particle radiosurgery of the pituitary gland: clinical results of 840 patients. Stereotact Funct Neurosurg 57(1–2):22–35

Lim YL, Leem W, Kim TS, Rhee BA, Kim GK (1998) Four years' experiences in the treatment of pituitary adenomas with gamma knife radiosurgery. Stereotact Funct Neurosurg 70(Suppl 1):95–109

Littley MD, Shalet SM, Reid H, Beardwell CG, Sutton ML (1991) The effect of external pituitary irradiation on elevated serum prolactin levels in patients with pituitary macroadenomas. Q J Med 81(296):985–998

Losa M, Valle M, Mortini P, Franzin A, da Passano CF, Cenzato M, Bianchi S, Picozzi P, Giovanelli M (2004) Gamma knife surgery for treatment of residual nonfunctioning pituitary adenomas after surgical debulking. J Neurosurg 100(3): 438–444

Mackley HB, Reddy CA, Lee SY, Harnisch GA, Mayberg MR, Hamrahian AH, Suh JH (2007) Intensity-modulated radiotherapy for pituitary adenomas: the preliminary report of the Cleveland Clinic experience. Int J Radiat Oncol Biol Phys 67(1):232–239

McCollough WM, Marcus RB Jr, Rhoton AL Jr, Ballinger WE, Million RR (1991) Long-term follow-up of radiotherapy for pituitary adenoma: the absence of late recurrence after greater than or equal to 4500 cGy. Int J Radiat Oncol Biol Phys 21(3):607–614

Meij BP, Lopes MB, Ellegala DB, Alden TD, Laws ER (2002) The long-term significance of microscopic dural invasion in 354 patients with pituitary adenomas treated with transsphenoidal surgery. J Neurosurg 39:437–444

Milker-Zabel S, Debus J, Thilmann C, Schlegel W, Wannenmacher M (2001) Fractionated stereotactically guided radiotherapy and radiosurgery in the treatment of functional and nonfunctional adenomas of the pituitary gland. Int J Radiat Oncol Biol Phys 50(5):1279–1286

Mingione V, Yen CP, Vance ML, Steiner M, Sheehan J, Laws ER, Steiner L (2006) Gamma surgery in the treatment of nonsecretory pituitary macroadenoma. J Neurosurg 104(6): 876–883

Minniti G, Traish D, Ashley S, Gonsalves A, Brada M (2005) Risk of second brain tumor after conservative surgery and radiotherapy for pituitary adenoma: update after an additional 10 years. Clin Endocrinol Metab 90(2):800–804

Minniti G, Traish D, Ashley S, Gonsalves A, Brada M (2006) Fractionated stereotactic conformal radiotherapy for secreting and nonsecreting pituitary adenomas. Clin Endocrinol (Oxf) 64(5):542–548

Mitsumori M, Shrieve DC, Alexander E III, Kaiser UB, Richardson GE, Black PM, Loeffler JS (1998) Initial clinical results of LINAC-based stereotactic radiosurgery and stereotactic radiotherapy for pituitary adenomas. Int J Radiat Oncol Biol Phys 42(3):573–580

Mokry M, Ramschak-Schwarzer S, Simbrunner J, Ganz JC, Pendl G (1999) A six year experience with the postoperative radiosurgical management of pituitary adenomas. Stereotact Funct Neurosurg 72(Suppl 1):88–100

Muhr C (2006) Positron emission tomography in acromegaly and other pituitary adenoma patients. Neuroendocrinology 83(3–4):205–210

Nagesser SK, van Seters AP, Kievit J, Hermans J, van Dulken H, Krans HM, van de Velde CJ (2000) Treatment of pituitary-dependent Cushing's syndrome: long-term results of unilateral adrenalectomy followed by external pituitary irradiation compared to transsphenoidal pituitary surgery. Clin Endocrinol (Oxf) 52(4):427–435

Ozgen T, Oruckaptan HH, Ozcan OE, Acikgoz B (1999) Prolactin secreting pituitary adenomas: analysis of 429 surgically treated patients, effect of adjuvant treatment modalities and review of the literature. Acta Neurochir (Wien) 141(12):1287–1294

Paek SH, Downes MB, Bednarz G, Keane WM, Werner-Wasik M, Curran WJ Jr, Andrews DW (2005) Integration of surgery with fractionated stereotactic radiotherapy for treatment of nonfunctioning pituitary macroadenomas. Int J Radiat Oncol Biol Phys 61(3):795–808

Petrovich Z, Yu C, Giannotta SL, Zee CS, Apuzzo ML (2003) Gamma knife radiosurgery for pituitary adenoma: early results. Neurosurgery 53(1):51–59, Discussion 59–61

Pirzkall A, Debus J, Haering P, Rhein B, Grosser KH, Höss A, Wannenmacher M (2003) Intensity modulated radiotherapy (IMRT) for recurrent, residual, or untreated skull-base meningiomas: preliminary clinical experience. Int J Radiat Oncol Biol Phys 55(2):362–372

Pollock BE, Carpenter PC (2003) Stereotactic radiosurgery as an alternative to fractionated radiotherapy for patients with recurrent or residual nonfunctioning pituitary adenomas. Neurosurgery 53(5):1086–1091, Discussion 1091–1094

Pollock BE, Nippoldt TB, Stafford SL, Foote RL, Abboud CF (2002) Results of stereotactic radiosurgery in patients with hormone-producing pituitary adenomas: factors associated with endocrine normalization. J Neurosurg 97(3): 525–530

Radhakrishnan K, Mokri B, Parisi JE, O'Fallon WM, Sunku J, Kurland LT (1995) The trends in incidence of primary brain tumors in the population of Rochester, Minnesota. Ann Neurol 37:67–73

Rahimian J, Chen JC, Rao AA, Girvigian MR, Miller MJ, Greathouse HE (2004) Geometrical accuracy of the Novalis stereotactic radiosurgery system for trigeminal neuralgia. J Neurosurg 101(3 Suppl):351–355

Sanno N, Teramoto A, Osamura RY, Horvath E, Kovacs K, Lloyd RV, Scheithauer BW (2003) Pathology of pituitary tumors. Neurosurg Clin N Am 14:25–39

Sasaki R, Murakami M, Okamoto Y, Kono K, Yoden E, Nakajima T, Nabeshima S, Kuroda Y (2000) The efficacy of conventional radiation therapy in the management of pituitary adenoma. Int J Radiat Oncol Biol Phys 47(5):1337–1345

Seegenschmiedt MH (2008) Radiotherapy of nonmalignant diseases. In: Halperin EC, Perez CA, Brady LW (eds) Perez and Brady's principles and practice of radiation oncology, 5th edn. Lippincott Williams & Wilkins, Philadelphia, pp 1936–1937

Sheehan JM, Vance ML, Sheehan JP, Ellegala DB, Laws ER Jr (2000) Radiosurgery for Cushing's disease after failed transsphenoidal surgery. J Neurosurg 93(5):738–742

Sheehan JP, Kondziolka D, Flickinger J, Lunsford LD (2002) Radiosurgery for residual or recurrent nonfunctioning pituitary adenoma. J Neurosurg 97(5 Suppl):408–414

Shomali ME (2008) Pituitary and pituitary region tumors: medical therapy perspective. In: Chin L, Regine W (eds) Principles and practice of stereotactic radiosurgery. Springer, New York, pp 327–331

Syndikus I, Tait D, Ashley S, Jannoun L (1994) Long-term follow-up of young children with brain tumors after irradiation. Int J Radiat Oncol Biol Phys 30(4):781–787

Thalassinos NC, Tsagarakis S, Ioannides G, Tzavara I, Papavasiliou C (1998) Megavoltage pituitary irradiation lowers but seldom leads to safe GH levels in acromegaly: a long-term follow-up study. Eur J Endocrinol 138(2): 160–163

Thapar K, Kovacs K, Laws ER (1997) Pituitary tumors. In: Black P, Loeffler J (eds) Cancer of the nervous system. Blackwell, Cambridge, pp 106–127

Tishler RB, Loeffler JS, Lunsford LD, Duma C, Alexander E III, Kooy HM, Flickinger JC (1993) Tolerance of cranial nerves of the cavernous sinus to radiosurgery. Int J Radiat Oncol Biol Phys 27(2):215–221

Tsagarakis S, Grossman A, Plowman PN, Jones AE, Touzel R, Rees LH, Wass JA, Besser GM (1991) Megavoltage pituitary irradiation in the management of prolactinomas: long-term follow-up. Clin Endocrinol 34(5):399–406

Tsang RW, Brierley JD, Panzarella T, Gospodarowicz MK, Sutcliffe SB, Simpson WJ (1994) Radiation therapy for pituitary adenoma: treatment outcome and prognostic factors. Int J Radiat Oncol Biol Phys 30(3):557–565

Tsang RW, Brierley JD, Panzarella T, Gospodarowicz MK, Sutcliffe SB, Simpson WJ (1996) Role of radiation therapy in clinical hormonally-active pituitary adenomas. Radiother Oncol 41(1):45–53

Varia MA, Ewend MG, Sharpless J, Morris DE (2007) Pituitary tumors. In: Gunderson LL, Tepper JE (eds) Clinical radiation oncology, 2nd edn. Elsevier Churchill Livingstone, Philadelphia, pp 567–589

Wallace EA, Holdaway IM (1995) Treatment of macroprolactinomas at Auckland Hospital 1975–91. NZ Med J 108(994):50–52

Williams M, van Seters AP, Hermans J, Leer JW (1994) Evaluation of the effects of radiotherapy on macroprolactinomas using the decline rate of serum prolactin levels as a dynamic parameter. Clin Oncol 6(2):102–109

Witt TC, Kondziolka D, Flickinger JC, Lunsford LD (1998) Gamma Knife radiosurgery for pituitary tumors. In: Lunsford LD, Kondziolka D, Flickinger JC (eds) Progress in neurological surgery, vol 14. Karger, Basel, pp 114–127

Woollons AC, Hunn MK, Rajapakse YR, Toomath R, Hamilton DA, Conaglen JV, Balakrishnan V (2000) Non-functioning pituitary adenomas: indications for postoperative radiotherapy. Clin Endocrinol (Oxf) 53(6):713–717

Wowra B, Stummer W (2002) Efficacy of gamma knife radiosurgery for nonfunctioning pituitary adenomas: a quantitative follow-up with magnetic resonance imaging-based volumetric analysis. J Neurosurg 97(5 Suppl):429–432

Wurm RE, Erbel S, Schwenkert I, Gum F, Agaoglu D, Schild R, Schlenger L, Scheffler D, Brock M, Budach V (2008) Novalis frameless image-guided noninvasive radiosurgery: initial experience. Neurosurgery 62(5 Suppl):A11–A17, discussion A17–A18

Yoon PH, Kim DI, Jeon P, Lee SI, Lee SK, Kim SH (2001) Pituitary adenomas: early postoperative MR imaging after transsphenoidal resection. Am J Neuroradiol 22(6): 1097–1104

Zhang N, Pan L, Dai J, Wang B, Wang E, Zhang W, Cai P (2000) Gamma Knife radiosurgery as a primary surgical treatment for hypersecreting pituitary adenomas. Stereotact Funct Neurosurg 75(2–3):123–128

Zierhut D, Flentje M, Adolph J, Erdmann J, Raue F, Wannenmacher M (1995) External radiotherapy of pituitary adenomas. Int J Radiat Oncol Biol Phys 33(2):307–314

Craniopharyngiomas

11

Michael Selch

Craniopharyngiomas are histologically benign parasellar tumors derived from proliferation of vestigial remnants of Rathke's pouch. The tumor is typically composed of anastomosing trabeculae of epithelial cells associated with an epithelial lined cyst (Ghatak et al. 1971; Petito et al. 1976). The latter may be composed of a single layer of cells or a stratified squamous epithelium. Tumor cells closely resemble the squamous components of normal skin and may be arranged in one of two distinctive morphologic patterns. The most common appearance is the adamantinomatous variant. Tumor tissue recapitulates the fetal tooth bud and resembles the adamantinoma/ameloblastoma arising in the jaw of adults. This variant is virtually always cystic and calcified. A less common variant is the papillary squamous craniopharyngioma. This variant occurs almost exclusively in adults and is rarely calcified. Approximately one-half of papillary tumors are cystic (Crotty et al. 1995). There appears to be no difference in control of these two variants by radiotherapy.

Purely intrasellar craniopharyngioma is unusual. In a combined experience with 92 children, tumor was confined to the sella in four patients (Hoffman et al. 1992; Thomsett et al. 1980). More commonly, the tumor is partially or entirely suprasellar. Suprasellar craniopharyngioma may extend in either a prechiasmatic direction and impinge on the optic apparatus or in a retrochiasmatic direction and compress the third ventricle. Either route of extension has implications for stereotactic irradiation. Given the local growth pattern, the clinical presentation of craniopharyngioma is dominated by visual and endocrine disturbances.

The initial management of craniopharyngioma remains controversial. There are strong advocates for either aggressive surgery aimed at gross total resection or minimally invasive surgery followed by adjunctive radiotherapy (Wisoff 2008). Recent non-randomized trials from the Children's Hospital of Philadelphia and Washington University demonstrate superior 10-year local control rates with less than total tumor removal combined with conventional external beam radiotherapy compared to attempted total resection alone. In the Philadelphia experience, control rate after combined therapy was 84% compared to 42% after aggressive surgery (Stripp et al. 2004). Respective control rates in the Washington University series were 100 and 32% (Lin et al. 2008). In neither series was there a significant difference in long-term overall survival rate, attesting to the impact of salvage therapies upon local recurrence. In both centers, the ultimate local control rate following "upfront" radiotherapy equaled that following radiotherapy administered for recurrence after initial aggressive surgery. It must be recognized, however, that patients managed with initial aggressive surgery alone are exposed to the morbidities of surgery as well as any local tumor failure. In a small longitudinal study, Merchant et al. (2002) demonstrated greater loss of full scale IQ following aggressive surgery (−10 points) compared to minimal surgery plus radiotherapy (−1.25 points; $p<0.06$) after a 72-month follow-up. In the Philadelphia experience, the incidence of diabetes insipidus was 88% in the aggressive surgical group compared to 65% in the combined modality therapy group ($p=0.03$). The respective incidences of diabetes insipidus in the Washington University experience were 93 and 59% ($p=0.04$).

Despite these apparent advantages of minimally invasive surgery and radiotherapy, efforts must be made to

M. Selch
Department of Radiation Oncology, David Geffen School of Medicine at UCLA, 200 UCLA Medical Plaza, Suite B265, Los Angeles, CA 90095, USA
e-mail: mselch@mednet.ucla.edu

A.A.F. De Salles et al. (eds.), *Shaped Beam Radiosurgery*,
DOI: 10.1007/978-3-642-11151-8_11, © Springer-Verlag Berlin Heidelberg 2011

limit the volume of central nervous system exposed to ionizing irradiation. In a larger prospective trial, Merchant et al. (2006) analyzed predictors of cognitive decline following modern conformal radiotherapy for pediatric craniopharyngioma. Patients received 54–55.8 Gy to a volume including the gross tumor plus an additional 1 cm. margin for the clinical target volume and 0.3–0.5 cm. for the planning target volume. After a median follow-up of 36 months, the most significant factors associated with longitudinal cognitive decline were the volume of supratentorial brain receiving >45 Gy ($p=0.029$) and the volume of temporal lobe receiving >45 Gy ($p=0.046$).

Stereotactic irradiation provides a method for delivering an effective tumor dose for craniopharyngioma while vastly decreasing the volume of parenchyma exposed to high dose. Both stereotactic radiosurgery (SRS) and stereotactic radiotherapy (SRT) have been used for craniopharyngioma. The utility of SRS for this tumor is limited by the proximity of the lesion to the optic apparatus and the pituitary stalk. The threshold tolerance of the optic apparatus to SRS has been estimated to be 8–10 Gy with a steep increase in optic neuropathy beyond this range. According to Tischler et al. (1993), there were no episodes of optic neuropathy when the maximum SRS dose to the chiasm was <8 Gy compared to an incidence of 25% above 8 Gy. Leber et al. (1998) reported no optic neuropathy below 10 Gy compared to an incidence of 27% between 10 and 15 Gy and 76% above 15 Gy. SRS volume constraints have not been established for the optic apparatus. For this reason, the maximum allowable dose to any region of the optic apparatus in the setting of SRS is 8 Gy at UCLA. Given the growth pattern of craniopharyngioma, the physician electing SRS for treatment is often faced with accepting a risk of permanent optic injury or selectively reducing the dose to that portion of the tumor in proximity to the chiasm and risking local relapse.

The proximity of craniopharyngioma to the pituitary infundibulum represents another potential factor limiting the application of SRS. Fiegl et al. (2002) reported that the median pituitary stalk dose associated with SRS-induced endocrinopathy was 7.7 Gy compared to 5.5 Gy for those without posttreatment hormonal deterioration in a series of 92 patients with pituitary adenoma.

There is extensive gamma-knife SRS experience for treatment of craniopharyngioma (Barajas et al. 2002; Chung et al. 1998, 2000; Kobayashi et al. 2000, 2005; Mokry 1999; Prasad et al. 1995; Ulfarsson et al. 2002). Use of multiple isocenters is routine in this experience. The marginal dose is prescribed at the 50–60% isodose line, resulting in a large degree of target dose inhomogeneity. SRS investigators do not describe the margin of normal tissue included within the treatment isodose. Prescribed marginal tumor dose varies from 11.5 to 14 Gy. Although Ulfarsson et al. (2002) suggested a marginal dose of 6 Gy controlled craniopharyngioma, most investigators concur that minimum marginal doses >10 Gy are necessary. Given the accepted tolerance of the optic apparatus to SRS, it is not surprising that selective reduction of dose below the nominal prescription dose is commonplace for the portion of tumor impinging upon the chiasm. SRS investigators frequently restrict the optic apparatus and a small rim of tumor to the 30% isodose line (Barajas et al. 2002). In a further attempt to restrict dose to the optic apparatus, many SRS investigators include only the solid component of tumor in the treatment volume and exclude the cystic component. With selective dose reduction and irradiation of only the solid portion of tumor, local tumor relapse rates following gamma-knife SRS vary from 10 to 56% and cyst enlargement rates vary from 0 to 67% (Table 11.1). Local relapse rates following SRS treatment of a volume including

Table 11.1 Results of stereotactic radiosurgery for craniopharyngioma

Series	# Pts	Margin (mm)	GTV	Marginal dose (Gy)	% Progression	
					Cyst	Solid
Chung et al. (2000)	31	?	S+C	12	10	13
Kobayashi et al. (2000)	33	?	S+C	12.8	7	8
Mokry (1999)	23	?	S	12	0	56
Prasad et al. (1995)	8	?	S	12	25	12
Ulfarsson et al. (2002)	21	?	S	3–25	67	33
Barajas et al. (2002)	10	?	S	14	10	10
Kobayashi et al. (2005)	98	?	S+C	11.5	9	11

GTV gross tumor volume, *S* solid component, *C* cystic component both cystic and solid components are 13–20% and cyst enlargement rates vary from 10 to 24%. The largest experience with SRS for craniopharyngioma was reported by Kobayashi et al. (2005). In a series of 98 patients, mean tumor size and volume were 18.8 mm and 3.5 cc, respectively. The gross tumor volume included the cystic and solid components and was treated with a mean of 4.5 isocenters. Marginal tumor dose was 11.5 Gy, and the optic chiasm/nerve dose was <10.7 Gy. After a mean 66-month follow-up, tumor progression was documented in 20%. Cyst enlargement accounted for 45% of all tumor progressions. Solid tumor regrowth or new lesions occurred in 55% of the relapsing patients. Visual injury occurred in 3%. In a prior report, this group delivered a marginal tumor dose of 12.8 Gy and optic apparatus doses <12 Gy (Kobayashi et al. 2000). Visual injury was reported in 6% and tumor progression in 15%. The results indicate the challenge of delivering an effective SRS dose for craniopharyngioma while avoiding serious visual morbidity.

The use of SRS at UCLA for craniopharyngioma is restricted to the rare solid tumor with minimal residual disease after decompressive surgery located several millimeters from both the optic apparatus and infundibulum. In this unusual setting, the prescribed dose is 14–16 Gy, depending upon the maximum dose to the chiasm and pituitary stalk (Fig. 11.1). Specifics concerning margins and treatment planning are identical to the following discussion of SRT.

SRT represents a more flexible option for craniopharyngioma and in many centers, including UCLA, has become the radiotherapeutic treatment of choice for this tumor (Combs et al. 2007; Minniti et al. 2007). SRT exploits the biologic advantage of dose fractionation for normal tissue while maintaining the physical advantage inherent in the steep dose falloff. SRT can be used even for tumors abutting the optic

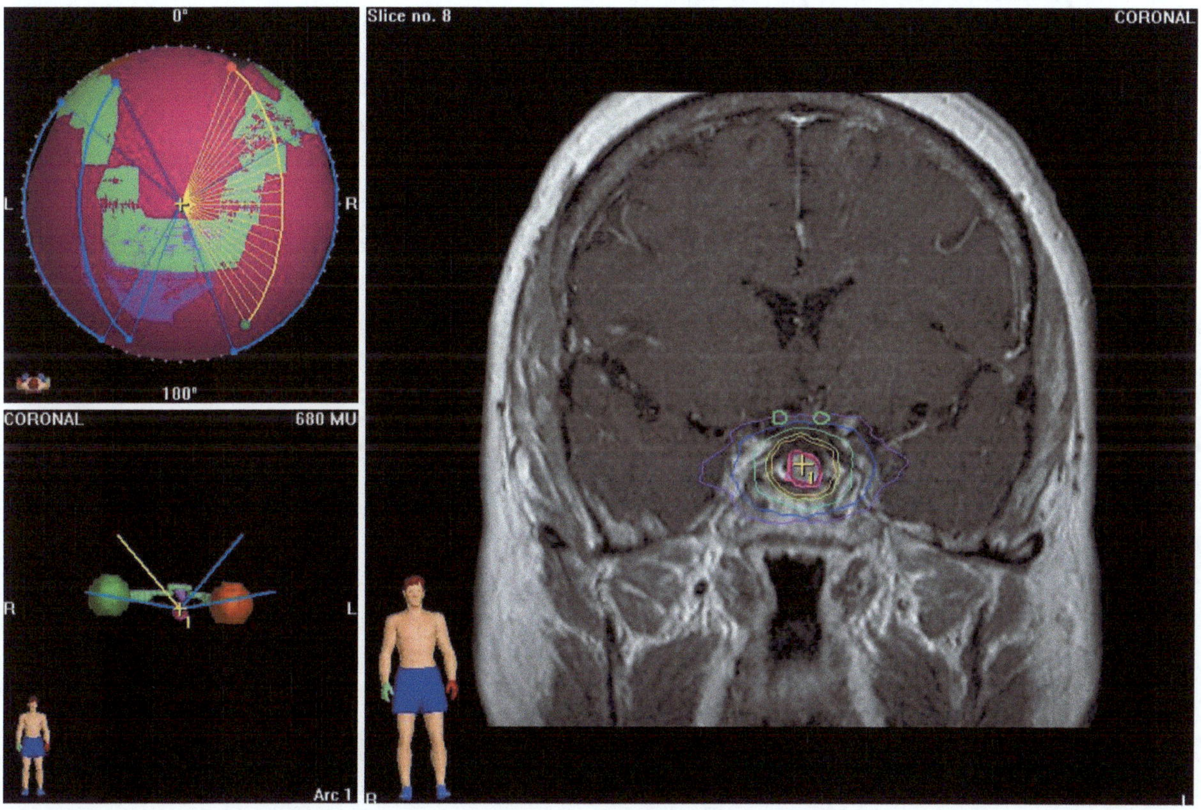

Fig. 11.1 Coronal T1-weighted contrast-enhanced MRI demonstrating isodose distribution for 13-mm residual solid craniopharyngioma. The target plus a 3-mm margin was included within the 90% isodose line (*yellow*) and received a dose of 16 Gy (tumor maximum 17.78 Gy). The overlying chiasm received a maximum dose of 4.4 Gy. The target was irradiated with four dynamic arcs

chiasm/nerve since the total dose required to control craniopharyngioma is well within the tolerance of the optic apparatus. Parsons et al. (1994) retrospectively reviewed the incidence of optic neuropathy following conventional radiotherapy for head and neck cancer. Among those treated with daily fractions of <1.8 Gy, the respective incidences of optic nerve injury associated with total doses <59 Gy were 0/87 and 5/61 after >59 Gy. For patients treated with >1.8 Gy fractions, the respective incidences of optic neuropathy were 0/8 and 10/25.

At UCLA, all patients with craniopharyngioma undergo cyst decompression and/or minimally invasive transnasal surgery for immediate symptom palliation. Adjuvant SRT is offered to all patients except in the rare setting of residual tumor <3 cm in greatest dimension located several millimeters from the optic apparatus. Patients receiving SRT are immobilized with a custom-fitted thermoplastic face mask (Fig. 11.2). This approach has replaced the Gill-Thomas-Cosman (GTC) frame previously used at UCLA. The precision of daily patient positioning using these relocatable systems has been evaluated. Using the GTC system, random repositioning deviations in the anterior–posterior, medial–lateral, and superior–inferior dimensions have varied from −0.039 to 0.6 mm, −0.113 to 0.7 mm, and 0.06 to 0.7 mm, respectively (Burton et al. 2002; Cohen et al. 1995; Solberg et al. 1999). Using the GTC frame, the overall deviation vector varies from 0.468 to 1.2 mm. Using the thermoplastic mask system, random deviations in the three major axes vary from 0.6 to 0.7 mm, 0.6 to 1.1 mm, and 0.6 to 0.8 mm, respectively (Alheit et al. 2001; Fuss et al. 2004; Kumar et al. 2005). The overall deviation vector varies from 1.58 to 2.1 mm. According to Burton et al. (2002), 97% of all displacement vectors are <2.5 mm using a GTC frame. With the mask system, 95% of vectors are <3.3 mm.

SRS and SRT are delivered at UCLA by a dedicated 6 MV linear accelerator (Clinac 600SR, Varian Associates, Palo Alto, CA). In the literature, isocenter deviations of accelerators dedicated to stereotactic irradiation vary from 0.06 to 1.17 mm (Gibbs et al. 1992).

For dosimetry planning, all patients undergo non-contrast-enhanced CT with 1.5 mm axial slice thickness and contrast-enhanced MRI with 2–3 mm slice thickness. The CT scan is performed with the stereotactic fiducial system attached to the immobilization apparatus. Flickinger et al. (1996) have demonstrated a significant reduction in cranial nerve morbidity among acoustic neuroma patients receiving SRS who were planned with MRI compared to reformatted CT. CT and MRI data sets are co-registered for treatment planning to eliminate the impact of image distortion inherent in MRI and improve the geometric fidelity of target delineation (Kooy et al. 1994a, b; Poetker et al. 2005). Cohen et al. (1995) demonstrated a significant reduction in

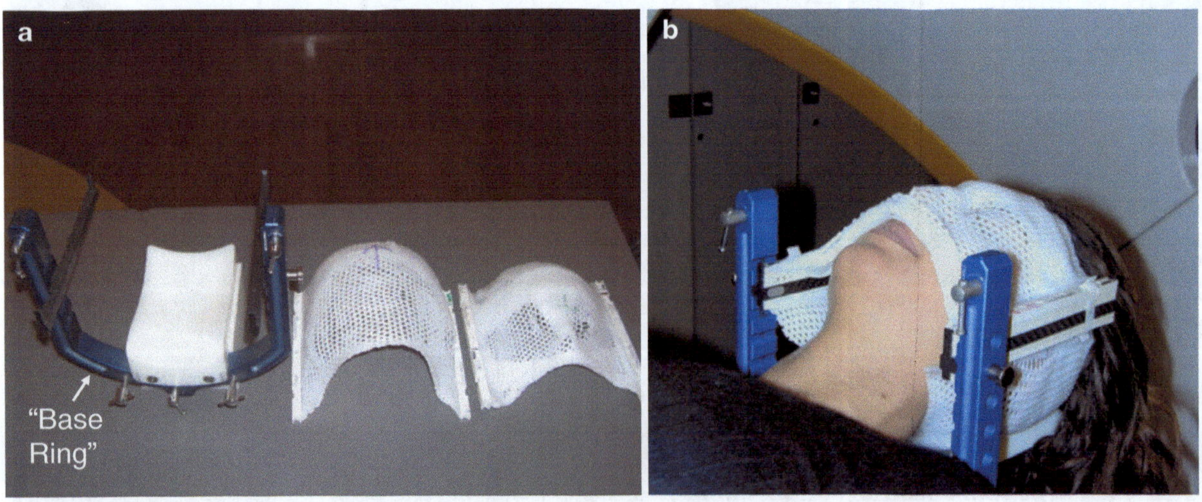

Fig. 11.2 (**a**) Components of the relocatable thermoplastic face mask immobilization system used at UCLA for SRT. (**b**) Face mask in place for patient treatment

mean error for co-registered MRI compared to use of a fiducial MRI alone. The mean three-dimensional error for co-registered MRI was 2.08 mm compared to 4.13 mm for a fiducial scan ($p<0.005$). Individual errors were reduced in all three axes: anterior–posterior 2.92 to 1.1 mm ($p=0.001$); medial–lateral 1.25 to 0.83 mm ($p<0.05$); and superior–inferior 1.98 to 0.94 mm ($p<0.03$).

The GTV is determined by the neurosurgeon and radiation oncologist using the enhanced axial, coronal, and sagittal MRI. Both the cystic and solid components are included in the GTV (Fig. 11.3). The margin of normal tissue added to account for microscopic tumor extension (CTV) and geometric uncertainties (PTV) is controversial. Histopathologic analysis of craniopharyngioma typically reveals occult tumor extension no more than 1 mm from either cystic or solid tumor components (Bartlett 1971; Kobayashi et al. 1981). The CTV margin must also accommodate possible cyst expansion during a 5–6 week course of SRT. The PTV margin must account for systematic and random errors associated with imaging, patient relocation, and accelerator/couch isocentricity. A useful formula for determining the PTV has been proposed by Kumar et al. (2005): 2 × standard deviation of the distribution of systematic error + 0.7 × average of the standard deviation of the distribution of the random error. According to this approach, adding approximately a 3-mm PTV margin to the CTV ensures that >95% of target is encompassed by the treatment isodose line. There has been no systematic study of PTV margins and the failure pattern of craniopharyngioma following SRT. At UCLA, margins of 3–5 mm are utilized for the solid component and 5–8 mm for the cystic component (Fig. 11.4). Combs et al. (2007) employ a 2-mm margin. Minniti et al. (2007) use a 5-mm margin if the patient is immobilized by a GTC frame and 8 mm if a mask system is used.

Dose conformality is assured by use of a micro-multileaf collimator (mMLC) as part of the Novalis® Radiosurgery system (Brainlab AG, Feldkirchen, Germany). The current UCLA mMLC consists of 26 pairs of individually motorized leaves varying in width from 3 to 5.5 mm (Fig. 11.5). The next generation mMLC consists of 60 pairs of leaves varying in width from 2.5 to 5 mm. Use of fixed diameter circular beam collimation has been abandoned for treatment of craniopharyngioma. Isodosimetric comparisons demonstrate a

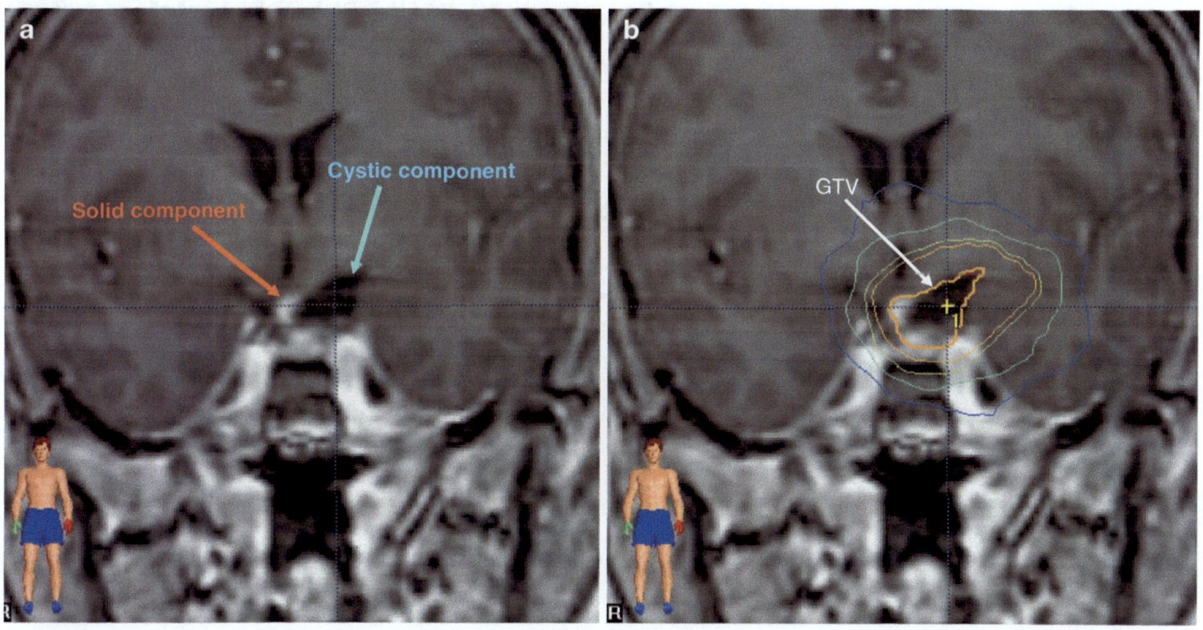

Fig. 11.3 (**a**) Coronal T1-weighted MRI demonstrating residual cystic and solid components of craniopharyngioma. (**b**) Coronal T1-weighted MRI of the same patient demonstrating GTV incorporating both cystic and solid components. Also displayed are SRT isodose lines (90% *yellow*; 80% *green*; 50% *light blue*; 30% *dark blue*) and margin added to the GTV. Treatment was prescribed to the 90% isodose line

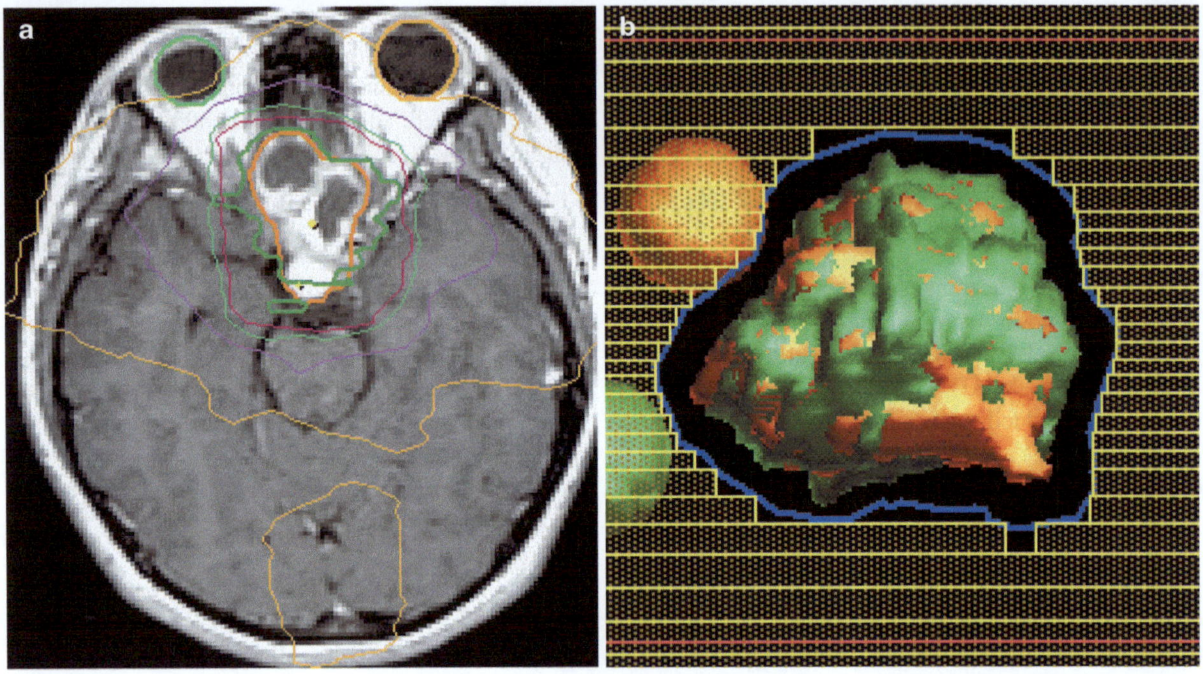

Fig. 11.4 (**a**) Axial T1-weighted contrast-enhanced MRI demonstrating cystic and solid craniopharyngioma GTV, treatment isodose lines (90% *red*; 80% *green*; 50% *purple*; 20% *yellow*) and margin added to GTV. The target received 50.4 Gy prescribed at 90% (maximum dose 56 Gy). Maximum dose to the optic nerves was 51.5 Gy. (**b**) Conformal field shaping using the mMLC

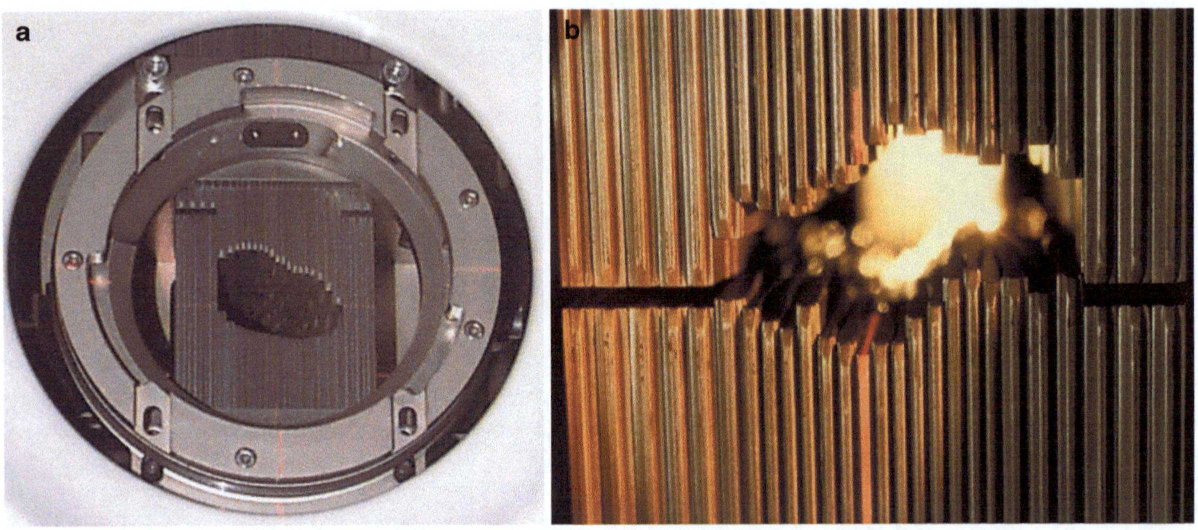

Fig. 11.5 (**a, b**) Patient's eye view of the Novalis Radiosurgery mMLC used for conformal stereotactic irradiation. The leaf widths are 3, 4.5, and 5.5 mm

significant conformality advantage for multiple isocenter dosimetry typical of a gamma-knife compared to use of a spherical collimator, albeit at the cost of dose inhomogeneity (Plowman and Doughty 1999). In a modeling study, the dose conformality advantage of multiple isocenter planning was associated with a reduced risk of normal tissue injury (Smith et al. 1998). The conformality of a linear accelerator treatment plan can be markedly improved by use of an mMLC (Shiu et al. 1997). Leaf width <3 mm results in conformality superior to devices with >5-mm leaf width (Monk et al. 2003). Dynamically altering the shape of an mMLC-collimated field during arc SRT results in further conformality improvement compared to static conformal beams (Perks et al. 2003; Solberg et al. 2001). At UCLA, craniopharyngiomas are typically irradiated with 4–6 dynamic arcs. A sagittal arc (i.e., table angle 0° or 180°) should be avoided due to unnecessary dose to the thyroid and mediastinal structures with this particular beam arrangement (Shepherd et al. 1997).

All targets are irradiated with a single isocenter with dose prescribed at the 90–95% isodose line which encompasses the PTV. The result is a dose distribution with a minimal gradient between tumor minimum and maximum dose and a homogeneity index of 1.05–1.11. The impact of target dose inhomogeneity on outcome following stereotactic irradiation is controversial. Nedzi et al. (1991) reported that target dose inhomogeneity >5–10 Gy was the most significant multivariate predictor of morbidity following SRS for a variety of cranial lesions.

Dose selection for craniopharyngioma is guided by historical results with conventional radiotherapy. Patients typically receive 50.4 Gy prescribed at the 90–95% isodose line in 1.8 Gy daily increments. The tumor maximum varies from 53 to 56 Gy. Dose constraints for the optic apparatus are a maximum dose of <52 Gy with daily fraction size <2 Gy. It is recognized that other investigators permit optic apparatus dose <54 Gy in the setting of SRT. There are no specific dose constraints for the temporal lobe or infundibulum. Varlotto et al. (2002) have questioned the use of 50–55 Gy for craniopharyngioma. They demonstrated a significant correlation of local control with prescribed dose in a series of 24 patients treated with conventional radiotherapy. After a median follow-up of 12 years, the 15-year progression-free survival was 100% for those receiving >60 Gy compared to 34% in the group receiving <57 Gy. Complications were also related to dose. The authors concluded that survival free of any adverse effect (complication or local relapse) was optimized with dose between 55 and 63 Gy. This series is noteworthy given the long follow-up and a documented local relapse 14 years after irradiation. The follow-up in this series exceeds that of all current SRT reports.

Routine mid-course CT/MRI is not done at UCLA. Repeat imaging is obtained only if symptoms progress, suggesting cyst expansion. Merchant et al. (2002) reported three patients required replanning based upon results of routine mid-course imaging during conventional radiotherapy.

Table 11.2 displays the outcome of SRT for craniopharyngioma. Tarbell et al. (1996) first published results of SRT for craniopharyngioma. Patients were immobilized with a GTC frame. Targets were irradiated with a single isocenter and circular collimation. Marginal tumor dose was 50.4–54 Gy prescribed at the 90–95% isodose line. The investigators do not specify the margin of normal tissue included within the prescription isodose. There were no local or marginal tumor relapses after a median 15-month follow-up. There was one cyst enlargement during SRT and two transient enlargements 7–8 months after treatment that resolved without intervention. No patient suffered visual or endocrine deficits due to SRT.

In a preliminary experience with 16 patients at UCLA, median tumor size and volume were 2.8 cm and 7.7 cc, respectively (Selch et al. 2002). Tumor abutted or compressed the optic chiasm in all cases. After a median 28-month follow-up, 3-year overall survival rate was 93%. The 3-year freedom from solid tumor growth and cyst expansion were 94% and 81%, respectively. Imaging response of craniopharyngioma

Table 11.2 Results of stereotactic radiation therapy for craniopharyngioma

Series	# Pts	Margin (mm)	GTV	Marginal dose (Gy)	% Progression	
					Cyst	Solid
Tarbell et al. (1996)	21	?	S+C	50.4	14	0
Selch et al. (2002)	16	3–8	S+C	50.4	20	13
Combs et al. (2007)	40	2	S+C	46.8	10	0
Minniti et al. (2007)	39	5–8	S+C	47.5	30	5

GTV gross tumor volume, *S* solid component, *C* cystic component

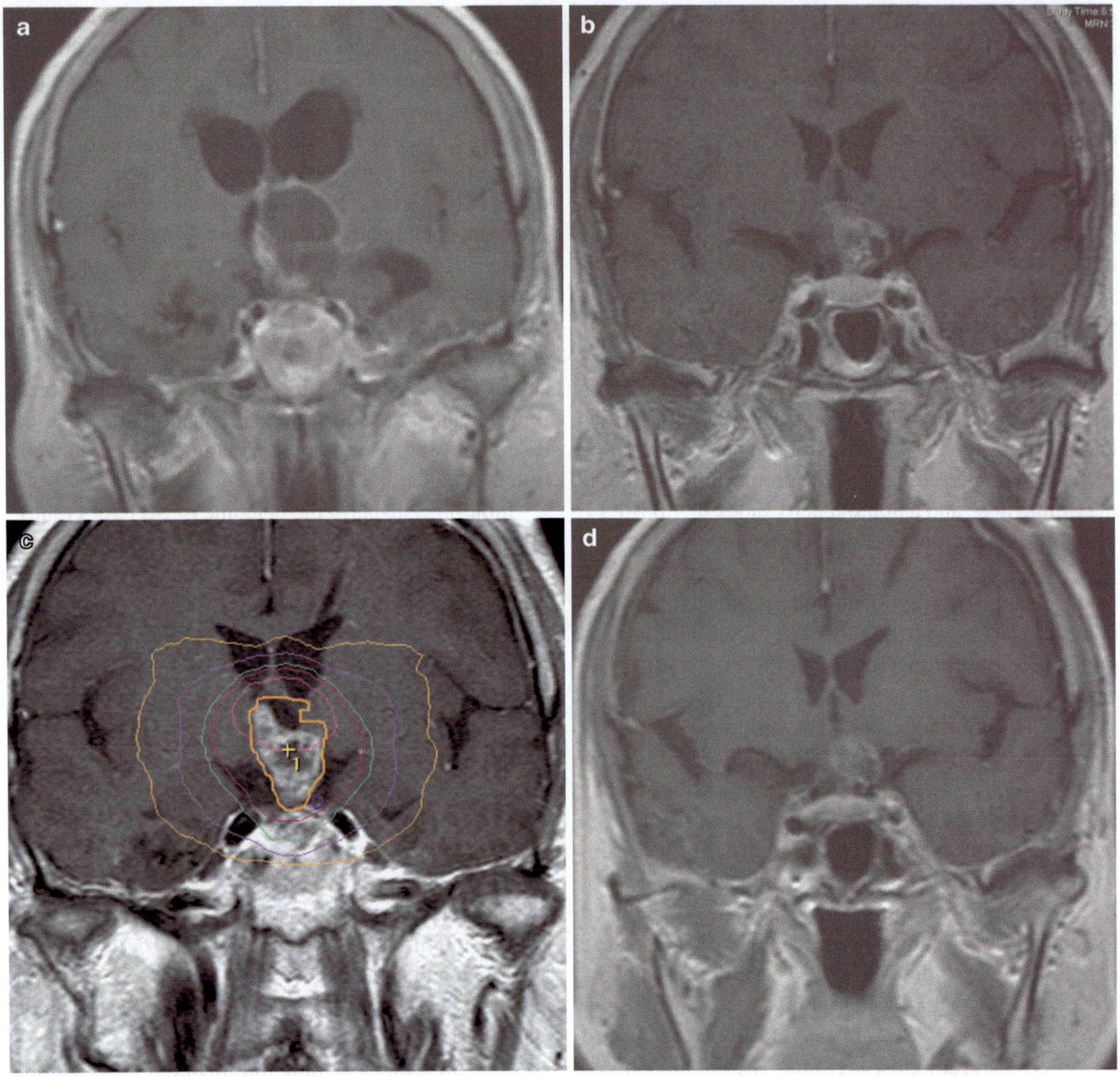

Fig. 11.6 (**a**) Pre-decompression coronal T1-weighted MRI of a craniopharyngioma in a 47-year-old man. (**b**) Coronal T1-weighted MRI following transnasal cyst aspiration demonstrating residual tumor. (**c**) Coronal T1-weighted MRI demonstrating isodose distribution for SRT (95% *pink*; 90% *red*; 80% *green*; 50% *purple*; 20% *yellow*). The target received 48.6 Gy prescribed at the 90% isodose line. (**d**) Six-month follow-up coronal T1-weighted MRI demonstrating interval response of the residual tumor

occurred in 50% of cases (Figs. 11.6 and 11.7) Growth of the solid component occurred in two patients – one during SRT and one at 40 months. Cyst expansion occurred in three patients between one and 6 months after treatment. Cyst aspiration was required in two patients, and cyst enlargement spontaneously resolved in the remaining patient.

Larger experiences with SRT have been reported by investigators in Heidelberg and London. Combs et al. (2007) treated 40 patients, including 6 children, immobilized with a face mask system. The GTV included both cystic and solid components. The median PTV volume was 20.7 cc. Not all patients had co-registered CT–MRI for dosimetry planning. The median tumor

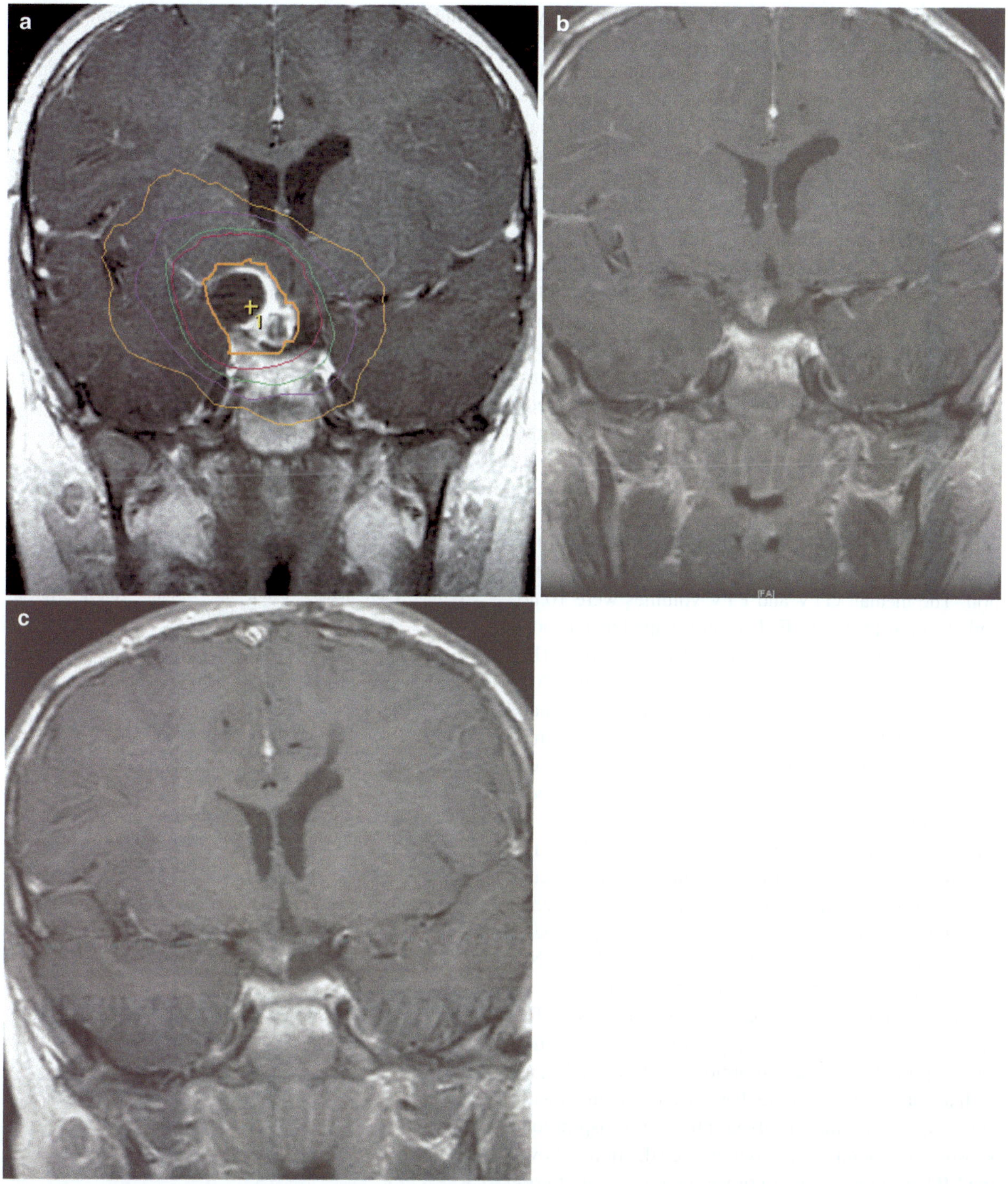

Fig. 11.7 (**a**) Coronal T1-weighted MRI demonstrating isodose distribution (90% *red*; 80% *green*; 50% *purple*; 20% *yellow*) for residual cystic and solid craniopharyngioma in a 40-year-old woman. The target received 49.6 Gy prescribed at 90% (tumor maximum 55 Gy). The maximum dose to the optic chiasm was 52.3 Gy. (**b**) Follow-up MRI at 12 months. (**c**) Follow-up MRI at 24 months

maximum dose was 52.2 Gy (range 50.4–57.6 Gy), and the 90% isodose line encompassed the PTV. Conformality was assured with a 5-mm leaf width mMLC. After a 98-month follow-up, the progression-free survival was 100%. Complete response was documented in 10%, partial tumor response in 63%, and 27% of tumors were unchanged. There was no difference in local control between tumors irradiated immediately after minimally invasive surgery or at the time of documented progression. Cyst expansion occurred in one patient during SRT and 3 months after completion of treatment in two other patients. The authors cautioned that immediate surgical intervention for cyst expansion is not required in an otherwise asymptomatic patient. One expanded cyst spontaneously resolved. New hormone deficiency occurred in one of eight patients with normal function prior to SRT.

Minniti et al. (2007) reported results of SRT for 39 patients, including 19 children, immobilized with a GTC frame. The GTV included both cystic and solid tumor components and all had CT–MRI co-registration. The median GTV and PTV volumes were 10 cc and 36 cc, respectively. Fields were shaped by customized blocks in 32 cases and an mMLC in 7 cases. The target received an isocenter dose of 50 Gy with the 95% isodose line encompassing the PTV. After a median 40-month follow-up, 3- and 5-year progression-free survival rates were 97 and 92%. Two tumors progressed at 8 and 41 months after SRT. There was no difference in outcome between pediatric and adult patients. There was a total of 12 cyst enlargement: 7 during SRT and 5 occurring within 8 months of completing treatment. The authors do not consider cyst expansion as a manifestation of tumor progression, an opinion in agreement with Combs et al. and the approach at UCLA. No patient developed visual morbidity due to SRT.

Serious morbidity has been unusual after SRT for craniopharyngioma. Optic apparatus injury has not been reported. All visual morbidities in our series, as well as that in the literature, have been associated with cyst expansion and resolved after cyst aspiration. Prospective longitudinal cognitive evaluation following SRT is not available to prove the reduction of normal tissue exposure in SRT is associated with an improved functional outcome. No second malignancies have been reported following either SRS or SRT for craniopharyngiomas. There are case reports of malignant glioma occurring after conventional radiotherapy for craniopharyngioma (Krazinger et al. 2001; Rittinger et al. 2003). Mean latency from irradiation to induction of glioma in these cases is 10.7 years. There are also case reports of transformation to malignant peripheral nerve sheath tumor and secondary gliomas and sarcomas following SRS for vestibular schwannoma (Balasubramaniam et al. 2007; Koh et al. 2007; Shamisa et al. 2001; Shin et al. 2002). Latency in these cases varies from 7 to 16 years after SRS. The latencies in these experiences are longer than the follow-up duration of reported SRS and SRT series. Given the survival rates typical of irradiated craniopharyngioma patients, prolonged follow-up will be required to establish the ultimate safety of stereotactic approaches to this tumor.

References

Alheit H, Dornfeld S, Dawel M et al (2001) Patient position reproducibility in fractionated stereotactically guided conformal radiotherapy using the Brainlab mask system. Strahlenther Onkol 177(5):264–268

Balasubramaniam A, Shannon P, Hodaie M et al (2007) Glioblastoma multiforme after stereotactic radiotherapy for acoustic neuroma: case report and review of the literature. Neuro Oncol 9:447–453

Barajas MA, Ramirez-Guzman G, Rodriquez-Vazquez C et al (2002) Multimodal management of craniopharyngiomas: neuroendoscopy, microsurgery and radiosurgery. J Neurosurg 97(Suppl 5):607–609

Bartlett JR (1971) Craniopharyngiomas: an analysis of some aspects of symptomatology, radiology and histology. Brain 94:725–732

Burton KE, Thomas SJ, Whitney D et al (2002) Accuracy of a relocatable stereotactic radiotherapy head frame evaluated by use of a depth helmet. Clin Oncol 14:31–39

Chung WY, Pan HC, Guo WY et al (1998) Protection of visual pathway in gamma knife radiosurgery for craniopharyngioma. Stereotact Funct Neurosurg 70(Suppl 1):139–151

Chung WY, Pan DH, Shiau CY et al (2000) Gamma knife radiosurgery for craniopharyngiomas. J Neurosurg 93(Suppl 3):47–56

Cohen DS, Lustgarten JH, Miller E et al (1995) Effects of coregistration of MR to CT images on MR stereotactic accuracy. J Neurosurg 82:772–779

Combs SE, Thilmann C, Huber PE et al (2007) Achievement of long-term local control in patients with craniopharyngiomas using high precision stereotactic radiotherapy. Cancer 109:2308–2314

Crotty TB, Scheithauer BW, Young WF et al (1995) Papillary craniopharyngioma: a clinicopathological study of 48 cases. J Neurosurg 83:206–214

Fiegl GC, Bonelli CM, Berghold A et al (2002) Effects of gamma knife radiosurgery of pituitary adenomas on pituitary function. J Neurosurg 97(Suppl 5):415–421

Flickinger JC, Knodziolka D, Pollock BE et al (1996) Evolution of technique for vestibular schwannoma radiosurgery and effect on outcome. Int J Radiat Oncol Biol Phys 36:275–280

Fuss M, Salter BJ, Cheek D et al (2004) Repositioning accuracy of a commercially available thermoplastic mask system. Radiother Oncol 71:339–345

Ghatak NR, Hirano A, Zimmerman HM et al (1971) Ultrastructure of a craniopharyngioma. Cancer 27: 1465–1475

Gibbs FA, Buechler D, Leavitt DD et al (1992) Measurement of mechanical accuracy of isocenter in conventional linear-accelerator-based radiosurgery. Int J Radiat Oncol Biol Phys 25:117–122

Hoffman HJ, DeSilva M, Humphreys RP et al (1992) Aggressive surgical management of craniopharyngiomas in childhood. J Neurosurg 76:47–52

Kobayashi T, Kageyama N, Yoshida J et al (1981) Pathologic and clinical basis of the indications for treatment of craniopharyngiomas. Neurol Med Chir (Tokyo) 21:39–47

Kobayashi T, Kida Y, Mori Y (2000) Effects and prognostic factors in the treatment of craniopharyngiomas by gamma knife. In: Knodziolka D (ed) Radiosurgery 1999, vol 3. Karger, Basel, pp 192–204

Kobayashi T, Kida Y, Mori Y et al (2005) Long-term results of gamma-knife surgery for the treatment of craniopharyngioma in 98 consecutive cases. J Neurosurg 103(6 Suppl Pediatrics):482–488

Koh ES, Millar BA, Menard C et al (2007) Fractionated stereotactic radiotherapy for acoustic neuroma. Single institution experience at the Princess Margaret Hospital. Cancer 109:1203–1210

Kooy HM, van Herk M, Barnes PD et al (1994a) Image fusion for stereotactic radiotherapy and radiosurgery treatment planning. Int J Radiat Oncol Biol Phys 28:1229–1234

Kooy HM, Dunbar SF, Tarbell NJ et al (1994b) Adaptation and verification of the relocatable Gill-Thomas-Cosman frame in stereotactic radiotherapy. Int J Radiat Oncol Biol Phys 30:685–691

Krazinger M, Jones N, Rittinger O et al (2001) Malignant glioma as a secondary malignant neoplasm after radiation therapy for craniopharyngioma: a report of a case and review of the literature. Onkologie 1:66–72

Kumar S, Burke K, Nalder C et al (2005) Treatment accuracy of fractionated stereotactic radiotherapy. Radiother Oncol 74: 53–59

Leber KA, Bergloff J, Pendl G (1998) Dose-response tolerance of the visual pathways and cranial nerves of the cavernous sinus to stereotactic radiosurgery. J Neurosurg 88: 43–50

Lin LL, El Naqa I, Leonard JR et al (2008) Long-term outcome in children treated for craniopharyngioma with and without radiotherapy. J Neurosurg Pediatr 1:126–130

Merchant TE, Kiehna EN, Sanford RA et al (2002) Craniopharyngioma: the St. Jude Children's Research Hospital Experience 1984–2001. Int J Radiat Oncol Biol Phys 53:533–542

Merchant TE, Kiehna EN, Kun LE et al (2006) Phase II trial of conformal radiation therapy for pediatric patients with craniopharyngioma and correlation of surgical factors and radiation dosimetry with change in cognitive function. J Neurosurg 104(2 Suppl Pediatrics):94–102

Minniti G, Saran F, Traish D et al (2007) Fractionated stereotactic conformal radiotherapy following conservative surgery in the control of craniopharyngiomas. Radiother Oncol 82:90–95

Mokry M (1999) Craniopharyngiomas: a six year experience with gamma knife radiosurgery. Stereotact Funct Neurosurg 72:S140–S149

Monk JE, Perks JR, Doughty D et al (2003) Comparison of a micro-multileaf collimator with a 5-mm-leaf-width collimator for intracranial stereotactic radiotherapy. Int J Radiat Oncol Biol Phys 57:1443–1449

Nedzi LA, Kooy HM, Alexander E et al (1991) Variables associated with the development of complications from radiosurgery of intracranial tumors. Int J Radiat Oncol Biol Phys 21:591–599

Parsons JT, Bova FJ, Fitzgerald CR et al (1994) Radiation optic neuropathy after megavoltage external beam irradiation: analysis of time-dose factors. Int J Radiat Oncol Biol Phys 30:755–763

Perks JR, St. George EJ, El Hamri K et al (2003) Stereotactic radiosurgery XVI: isodosimetric comparison of photon stereotactic radiosurgery techniques (gamma knife vs. micro-multileaf collimator linear accelerator) for acoustic neuroma-and potential clinical importance. Int J Radiat Oncol Biol Phys 57:1450–1459

Petito CK, DiGirolami U, Earle KM (1976) Craniopharyngioma: a clinical and pathological review. Cancer 37:1944–1952

Plowman PN, Doughty D (1999) Stereotactic radiosurgery, X: clinical isodosimetry of gamma knife versus linear accelerator X-knife for pituitary and acoustic tumors. Clin Oncol 11:321–329

Poetker DM, Jursinic PA, Runge-Samuelson CL et al (2005) Distortion of magnetic resonance images used in gamma knife radiosurgery treatment planning: implications for acoustic neuroma outcome. Otol Neurotol 26:1220–1228

Prasad D, Steiner M, Steiner L (1995) Gamma knife surgery for craniopharyngioma. Acta Neurochir 134:167–176

Rittinger O, Kranzinger M, Jones R et al (2003) Malignant astrocytoma arising 10 years after combined treatment of craniopharyngioma. J Pediatr Endocrinol Metab 16:97–101

Selch MT, DeSalles AAF, Wade M et al (2002) Initial clinical results of stereotactic radiotherapy for the treatment of craniopharyngiomas. Technol Cancer Res Treat 1:51–59

Shamisa A, Bance M, Nag S et al (2001) Glioblastoma multiforme occurring in a patient treated with gamma knife surgery. Case report and review of the literature. J Neurosurg 94:816–821

Shepherd SF, Childs PJ, Graham JD et al (1997) Whole body dose from linear accelerator-based stereotactic radiotherapy. Int J Radiat Oncol Biol Phys 38:7657–7665

Shin M, Ueki K, Kurita H et al (2002) Malignant transformation of a vestibular schwannoma after gamma knife radiosurgery. Lancet 360:309–310

Shiu AS, Kooy HM, Ewton JR et al (1997) Comparison of miniature multileaf collimation (MMLC) with circular collimation for stereotactic treatment. Int J Radiat Oncol Biol Phys 37:679–688

Smith V, Verhey L, Serago C (1998) Comparison of radiosurgery treatment modalities based on complication and control probabilities. Int J Radiat Oncol Biol Phys 40:507–513

Solberg TD, Ford JM, Medin P et al (1999) Reproducibility of frame positioning for fractionated stereotactic radiosurgery. J Radiosurg 2:57–64

Solberg TD, Boedeker KL, Fogg R et al (2001) Dynamic arc radiosurgery field shaping: a comparison with static field conformal and noncoplanar circular arcs. Int J Radiat Oncol Biol Phys 49:1481–1491

Stripp DCH, Maity A, Janss AJ et al (2004) Surgery with or without radiation therapy in the management of craniopharyngiomas in children and young adults. Int J Radiat Oncol Biol Phys 58:714–720

Tarbell NJ, Scott RM, Goumnerova LC et al (1996) Craniopharyngioma: preliminary results of stereotactic radiation therapy. In: Kondziolka D (ed) Radiosurgery 1995, vol 1. Karger, Basel, pp 75–82

Thomsett MJ, Conte FA, Kaplan SL (1980) Endocrine and neurologic outcome in childhood craniopharyngiomas: review of effect of treatment in 42 patients. J Pediatr 97: 728–735

Tischler RB, Loeffler JS, Lunsford LD et al (1993) Tolerance of cranial nerves of the cavernous sinus to radiosurgery. Int J Radiat Oncol Biol Phys 27:215–221

Ulfarsson E, Lindquist C, Roberts M et al (2002) Gamma knife radiosurgery for patients with craniopharyngiomas: long-term results in the first Swedish patients. J Neurosurg 97(Suppl 5):613–622

Varlotto JM, Flickinger JC, Kondziolka D et al (2002) External beam irradiation of craniopharyngiomas: long-term analysis of tumor control and morbidity. Int J Radiat Oncol Biol Phys 54:492–499

Wisoff J (2008) Craniopharyngioma. J Neurosurg Pediatr 1:124–125

12 Management of Brain Metastases

Naren Ramakrishna

12.1 Introduction

Brain metastases are among the most feared complications of cancer. Improved systemic therapy has resulted in improved survival for patients with metastatic cancer and a rise in incidence of brain metastases, often as a sole site of failure. In this setting, both the efficacy and toxicity of brain metastasis treatment are of even greater importance. While treatment paradigms remain controversial, recent survival and neurocognitive outcomes data have led to a greater emphasis on stereotactic radiosurgery (SRS), and a diminished use of whole-brain radiotherapy both in the initial and recurrent setting. SRS has also proven to be a viable alternative to surgical resection among select patients. As the number of patients and the number of lesions and sessions per patient increases, the comfort and logistics of treatment are of increasing importance. The emergence of image-guided frameless radiosurgery has provided a robust technique for safe and effective treatment of brain metastases with improved patient comfort and treatment logistics.

Brain metastases may develop in approximately 40–50% of patients with systemic cancer (Zimm et al. 1981) and are clinically evident in approximately 15% (Schouten et al. 2002). In the USA, the annual incidence of brain metastases is over 170,000, comprising over 40% of intracranial tumors (Wen 1997). The majority of patients are symptomatic and approximately 20–40% may eventually die of complications related to their brain disease.

The treatment of brain metastases is among the most controversial areas in oncology. The principal objectives of treatment of brain metastases are to palliate neurological symptoms and achieve tumor control while minimizing toxicity. The choice of therapy is influenced by many factors including (1) tumor histology, size, number, and location of lesions; (2) the presence or absence of neurological symptoms; (3) extracranial disease status, expected survival, age, and performance status; (4) prior treatment history; and (5) expected toxicities of treatment. Optimum therapy requires multidisciplinary collaboration to facilitate treatment which minimizes the risk of neurological death and symptomatic progression, while balancing the expected benefits of therapy against the risks of treatment-related toxicity.

While brain metastases most commonly occur in the presence of progressive extracranial disease, with improved systemic therapies, a greater proportion of patients present with brain metastases with controlled extracranial disease at the time of their CNS diagnosis (Bendell et al. 2003). Furthermore, the CNS may remain a site of repeated relapse. This pattern of presentation and potential relapse in the setting of controlled extracranial disease poses a great challenge to existing conventions regarding sequencing and/or combining the modalities of surgery, SRS, and WBRT.

12.2 Whole-Brain Radiotherapy

Whole-brain radiotherapy (WBRT) has played a central role in brain metastases therapy for over five decades. Early randomized trial data demonstrated a survival

N. Ramakrishna
Department of Radiation Oncology, MD Anderson Cancer Center Orlando, 1400 S. Orange Ave, Orlando, FL 32806, USA
e-mail: naren.ramakrishna@orhs.org

A.A.F. De Salles et al. (eds.), *Shaped Beam Radiosurgery*,
DOI: 10.1007/978-3-642-11151-8_12, © Springer-Verlag Berlin Heidelberg 2011

benefit for brain metastases patients treated with WBRT compared to supportive care only (Chao et al. 1954). In addition to a survival benefit, WBRT provides effective palliation of neurological symptoms (Coia 1992; Cairncross et al. 1980), with durable improvement, or stability of neurological symptoms observed in approximately 70–90% of patients (Coia 1992; Cairncross et al. 1980). For patients presenting with cranial nerve deficits, approximately 40% may have an improvement with WBRT (Cairncross et al. 1980).

A wide range of WBRT dose-fractionation schedules ranging from 2,000 cGy in 5 fractions to 4,000 cGy in 20 fractions have been compared for efficacy and toxicity in two randomized trials conducted by the RTOG (Gelber et al. 1981). While no significant difference in median survival or duration of symptom palliation was observed among the various schedules, symptomatic relief occurred sooner in patients treated with larger fractions. Further shortened WBRT courses such as 1,000 cGy in a single fraction or 1,200 cGy in two fractions achieve survival and palliative benefits similar to more extended fractionation schemes, but are associated with unacceptable acute toxicity and are therefore not used (Borgelt et al. 1981). The current standard therapy of 3,000 cGy in ten 300 cGy fractions over 2 weeks represents a balance between the prompt palliation of larger fractions with the decreased acute side effects of more extended fractionation. While 3,000 cGy in ten fractions may be appropriate for patients with expected survivals of less than 6 months, the dose-fractionation schedule should be individualized and in patients who may be long-term survivors, or in those in whom concurrent chemotherapy or targeted therapy is used, a more extended dose fractionation, such as 3,750 cGy in 250 cGy fractions or 4,000 cGy in 200 cGy fractions, may be more appropriate as it may decrease the risk of neurocognitive sequelae (Schultheiss et al. 1995).

A major concern with WBRT is the risk of injury to functional brain tissue. The toxicity of WBRT may be divided into acute, early-delayed, and late effects (Sheline et al. 1980). The most debilitating acute and early-delayed effects include fatigue and somnolence, which can be profound. They may arise within the first week of therapy and persist for weeks or months (Cross and Glantz 2003). Other prominent acute and early-delayed effects of WBRT include hair-loss, skin erythema, loss of taste, and decreased appetite. While the acute and early-delayed effects are generally reversible, the late effects are generally permanent and may be progressive. Potential late effects of particular concern are radiation-related leukoencephalopathy and necrosis, which may manifest clinically as significant neurologic or neurocognitive dysfunction (Cross and Glantz 2003).

The potential for significant neurocognitive dysfunction following WBRT is of substantial concern, particularly for patients with extended survival. The actual risk of WBRT-induced neurocognitive dysfunction is difficult to characterize accurately as most brain metastases patients do not survive sufficiently long to realize the gamut of potential cognitive late effects. In addition, there is vast heterogeneity in potential contributing factors such as chemotherapy treatments, radiation dose fractionation, pretreatment neurocognitive status, age, and tumor-related paraneoplastic and direct effects. DeAngelis and colleagues described 12 cases of progressive dementia which developed at a median of 14 months following treatment with WBRT alone or surgery + WBRT. All patients displayed cortical atrophy and also developed urinary incontinence and ataxia – seven patients died of these complications with no evidence of tumor recurrence. Their treatment was done with relatively large fraction sizes ranging from 300 to 600 cGy and total doses of 2,500–3,900 cGy (DeAngelis et al. 1989). Other factors which may increase the risk of late radiation toxicity from whole-brain radiotherapy include age, extent of disease, diabetes mellitus, concomitant chemotherapy (Cross and Glantz 2003; Crossen et al. 1994), and multiple sclerosis (Murphy et al. 2003).

Following surgical resection of a solitary brain metastasis, postoperative WBRT has frequently been employed with the rationale that both local and distant brain failure (DBF) may be improved. A randomized trial by Patchell et al. (1998) examined the effects of postoperative WBRT for patients with a surgically resected solitary brain metastasis. In this study, 95 patients were randomized to either WBRT or no further treatment following complete resection of a solitary brain metastasis. The addition of WBRT decreased the risk of local recurrence (10 vs. 47%, $p<0.01$), distant brain failure (14 vs. 37%, $p<0.01$), and risk of neurological death (14 vs. 44%, $p<0.03$). While no significant difference in overall survival was found, the higher risk of neurological death observed with surgery alone has been suggested as a justification for combined therapy in this group of patients. The impact, however, of the elevated risk of local or distant brain failure on quality of life (QOL) compared to the toxicity from the addition of WBRT, particularly in patients with long expected survival, remains unclear, especially when other low morbidity salvage therapies such as SRS may be effective. The possibility that WBRT may be omitted in select patients, particularly those undergoing radiosurgery for limited brain metastatic disease, is discussed further below.

12.3 Surgery

Surgery has been essential for treatment of brain metastases with symptomatic mass effect, and/or to establish a histological diagnosis. In addition to its palliative benefit, retrospective data support a benefit to survival among appropriately selected brain metastasis patients (Lagerwaard et al. 1999). Three prospective, randomized trials evaluated the survival benefit of surgery in patients with single brain metastases. In a study reported by Patchell et al. (1990), 48 patients were randomly assigned to either surgery followed by WBRT versus WBRT alone. Patients treated with surgery together with WBRT displayed improved local control (20 vs. 52%, $p<0.02$), increased median duration of functional independence (38 vs. 8 weeks; $p<0.005$), and longer overall survival (40 vs. 15 weeks; $p<0.01$). A second randomized study evaluating the same treatment groups was conducted by Noordijk and colleagues. Among the 63 patients randomized, those receiving both surgery and WBRT demonstrated increased survival (median 10 vs. 6 months; $p=0.04$) and functionally independent survival (7.5 vs. 3.5 months; $p=0.06$) versus patients treated with WBRT alone (Noordijk et al. 1994). Improved overall survival was noted only among patients with stable or absent extracranial disease; patients with progressive extracranial disease displayed a median survival of only 5 months irrespective of the treatment. In contrast to the two studies above, a third randomized study reported by Mintz et al. (1996) reported no difference in either survival or functionally independent survival with the addition of surgery to WBRT. In comparison to the two prior studies, a greater proportion of patients with active extracranial disease and low performance status were included in the study population. In addition, CT was used for brain staging and may have missed additional lesions detectable on MRI. Taken together, these data strongly support consideration of surgical resection among patients with a single metastasis and stable or absent extracranial disease.

For patients with multiple brain metastases, the role of surgery remains controversial, with data limited to retrospective series. Bindal et al. (1993) reported on a series of 56 patients who underwent resection of multiple lesions: the 30 patients who had all of their brain metastases resected displayed improved survival compared to the 26 patients who had resection of only some of the lesions (MS 14 vs. 6 months). The authors also compared the survival of the patients with resection of all metastasis with a group of 26 patients matched for diagnosis of the primary lesion and systemic disease status which had been submitted to resection of a single brain metastasis. A more recent retrospective study by Iwadate and colleagues also reported favorable survival following surgical resection for patients with multiple metastases provided that the unresected tumors were of a small size. Among patients with multiple metastases who underwent surgical resection, those with unresected tumors less than 2 cm achieved a median survival of 12.4 months, versus 4.5 months for those with unresected tumors greater than 2 cm; the patients with a single metastasis who underwent resection achieved a median survival of 9 months (Iwadate et al. 2000). In contrast to these findings, Hazuka et al. (1993) reported a median survival of only 5 months among a group of 18 patients who underwent resection of multiple metastases versus 11 months for 28 patients who underwent resection of a single lesion. In this study however, only 1 of 18 patients underwent complete resection of all metastases in the multiple metastasis group, likely accounting for the relatively poor survival in that group. In addition to residual tumor size and complete resection of all lesions, patient performance status and other prognostic parameters may also have a significant impact on outcome. In a retrospective study by Pollock et al. (2003) evaluating outcomes of aggressive surgical resection or radiosurgery for patients with multiple metastases, those patients undergoing treatment who belonged to RTOG recursive partitioning analysis (RPA) class I displayed the greatest median survival (19 months) versus those in RPA class II (13 months) and RPA class III (8 months). These results also compared favorably to expected median survival by RPA class (Gaspar et al. 1997). While the data from these retrospective studies is encouraging, the impact of selection bias on the overall outcomes could be significant and the quality of life (QOL) implications of surgery-related adverse effects are not well characterized in this setting. In many clinical settings, a decision must be made between surgery and SRS, discussed further below.

12.4 Stereotactic Radiosurgery

SRS has come to play an increasingly important role in the management of brain metastases, and may present a viable alternative to surgery, WBRT, or both. SRS involves the precise delivery of a single intense dose of focused radiation to one or more tumor masses with rapid dose falloff beyond the tumor margin. Tumors may be targeted for treatment with the aid of a minimally invasive stereotactic frame (Leksell 1951; Tsai et al. 1991), or using X-ray image guidance together with mask immobilization (Verellen et al. 2003), a technique referred to as frameless radiosurgery (FRS). The precise dose localization and shaping achieved with radiosurgery minimize the treatment-related injury that may result from normal tissue irradiation. Overall, SRS for brain metastases is thought to have a local control rate of approximately 85%; local control is optimal with doses greater than or equal to 1,800 cGy (Boyd and Mehta 1999; Shiau et al. 1997). SRS has the potential for noninvasive local tumor control while allowing targeting of multiple lesions.

Treatment-related adverse effects using SRS depend on multiple factors including tumor size, location, radiosurgery dose, and prior treatment. The RTOG performed an SRS phase I dose escalation study to determine the maximum tolerated SRS dose (MTD) in patients previously irradiated for either a recurrent primary brain tumor or recurrent single metastasis (Shaw et al. 2000). A total of 156 patients were enrolled and treatment was delivered by either linac-based or Gamma-knife radiosurgery. Dose was escalated in 3 Gy increments such that grade 3–5 toxicity at 3 months following SRS remained <20%. For tumors 3–4 cm in diameter, the MTD was 15 Gy, for those 2–3 cm in diameter the MTD was 18 Gy, and for those <2 cm the MTD was 24 Gy. On multivariate analysis, increased dose, worsening KPS, and increasing tumor diameter were associated with higher risk of grade 3–5 neurotoxicity. The actuarial incidence of radionecrosis at 12 months post SRS was 8%, and at 24 months, was 11%. While this study has been widely utilized as a guide for treatment dose, a number of parameters bear noting. In this trial, SRS for single recurrent brain metastases was performed >3 months following WBRT. Also, patients were ineligible for the study if any systemic therapy were planned within 3 months. Consideration for dose reduction, particularly for larger lesions, would be warranted if the interval from WBRT is short, or if cytotoxic systemic therapy is planned.

While surgical resection is expected to provide superior palliation for large tumors, or those with symptomatic mass effect, SRS has been proposed as an alternative to surgery for patients with single small- to medium-sized lesions without symptomatic mass effect. A recent retrospective series by O'Neill et al. (2003) from Mayo Clinic evaluated outcomes for patients with solitary brain metastases <35 mm without symptomatic mass effect treated with either surgery or radiosurgery. No difference in 1-year survival was noted between treatment arms; Cox multivariate analysis identified performance status as a significant prognostic factor for survival. While there was no difference in survival noted between arms, a significant improvement in local control was observed in the SRS group where no local recurrence was observed (0/26) versus 15% (11/74) in the surgery arm ($p=0.020$). The overall recurrence rates including distant brain failure were not significantly different: 29% in the SRS arm and 30% in the surgery arm; the use of salvage WBRT following surgery or SRS was not significantly different between the groups, 82% among the surgery patients and 96% of the SRS patients ($p=0.172$).

While there have been no randomized trials directly comparing surgery to SRS, several studies have evaluated whether SRS combined with WBRT results in similar outcomes to surgery + WBRT for patients with a solitary brain metastasis. Auchter and colleagues performed a multi-institutional retrospective review of outcomes for patients undergoing SRS + WBRT. To adjust for the bias of treating smaller or unresectable lesions, the 122 patients selected for analysis were those with a solitary brain metastasis deemed surgically resectable who instead underwent treatment with SRS followed by WBRT. The median survival following SRS + WBRT treatment was 1.1 years, comparing favorably to the expected survival for similar patients treated with surgery and WBRT (Patchell et al. 1990, 1998; Auchter et al. 1996). Of note, the overall local control rate of 86% within the SRS volume, and 22% outside the SRS volume was comparable to that observed in the first Patchell study in the arm receiving surgery + WBRT (Patchell et al. 1990). Taken together, these data strongly support the adoption of SRS in lieu of surgery for selected tumors <3.5 cm and without symptomatic mass effect.

For patients with multiple brain metastases, the appropriate sequencing and combination of modalities remain controversial. Patients with multiple (2–4) brain metastases were treated with WBRT alone in the past. These patients are now more likely to receive WBRT and upfront SRS based on the rationale that SRS should improve local tumor control and potentially survival, if extracranial disease is controlled. Early data to support this view was reported in a single institution randomized trial by Kondziolka and colleagues which evaluated WBRT alone versus WBRT + SRS for patients with 2–4 lesions <2.5 cm in size. Study accrual was terminated at 60% (27 patients) following interim evaluation that revealed a significant improvement in local control with combined treatment. Patients receiving both SRS and WBRT had a local recurrence rate at 1 year of only 8% versus 100% for those receiving WBRT alone. The median time to local recurrence was 6 months for WBRT alone, and 36 months following WBRT + SRS ($p=0.00005$). Despite the substantial difference in local control, no significant difference in survival was observed between either treatment group (Kondziolka et al. 1999).

To determine if WBRT + SRS was associated with a survival benefit versus WBRT alone, the RTOG conducted a study in 333 patients with 1–3 brain metastases. Patients were randomized to WBRT+SRS or WBRT alone and the primary endpoint was overall survival (Andrews et al 2004). The 1-year local control rate was increased for the combined treatment group (82 vs. 71%, $p=0.01$), a smaller improvement than that observed in the Kondziolka study above (Kondziolka et al. 1999). While no significant difference in overall or cause-specific survival was observed for the entire treatment group, several subgroups were identified which showed benefit from combined treatment. Patients with a solitary metastasis treated in the combined arm achieved a median survival of 6.9 versus 4.5 months ($p=0.04$), a magnitude of difference quite similar to the results observed in the first Patchell randomized trial comparing surgery + WBRT with WBRT alone (Patchell et al. 1990). In addition, patients in RPA Class I, age <50, or those with squamous or non-small cell histology showed significant survival benefit from combined treatment. Patients undergoing combined treatment were more likely to have stable or improved performance status at 3 months (50 vs. 33%, $p=0.02$) and 6 months (43 vs. 27%, $p=0.03$) posttreatment. These results suggest that combining WBRT + SRS may confer a survival benefit limited to select patients, while the probability of maintaining a stable or increased performance status may be a more general benefit of combined treatment.

The capacity of SRS to achieve local control of multiple intracranial tumors has prompted examination of whether initial treatment with SRS may allow WBRT to be deferred or eliminated for patients with a single or multiple metastases. Aoyama and colleagues reported the results of the JROSG 99-1 randomized trial evaluating SRS alone versus SRS plus WBRT for 132 patients with 1–4 brain metastases (Aoyama et al. 2006). The primary endpoint was survival, and patients were stratified by number of metastases, extracranial disease status, and primary site. The SRS margin dose was reduced by 30% for the combined treatment group relative to the MTDs from the RTOG 90-05 dose escalation study (Shaw et al. 2000) in order to decrease the risk of toxicity. No difference in overall survival, neurologic survival, or functional preservation was observed between the treatment groups. As expected, the risk of developing distant brain failure was higher in the SRS alone arm versus the combined treatment arm (63.7 vs. 41.5%, $p=0.03$). In addition, the 12 month local control was greater for combined treatment than for SRS alone (88.7 vs. 72.5%, $p=0.02$). While the patients in the SRS alone arm required salvage more frequently (44 vs. 17%), the majority of salvage was with SRS alone; WBRT was used for salvage in only 16% of patients randomized to the SRS alone arm. These study findings show that the use of SRS alone for patients with 1–4 brain metastases may not compromise survival, but does result in increased risk of distant and local brain failure which can usually be salvaged with additional SRS. Since brain recurrence can be symptomatic, when SRS alone is used, careful clinical and radiographic follow-up to detect brain failure is warranted.

The choice of deferring initial WBRT and treating with SRS alone upfront must take into consideration the risk of increasing distant brain failure (DBF). The impact of early DBF versus the morbidity of WBRT on

QOL is not well understood. In a study aimed at determining the rate and impact of early DBF occurring after SRS alone, Regine et al. (2002) prospectively assessed the recurrence pattern and symptomatic effects of recurrence in 36 patients treated with SRS alone. They found that 71% of patients displayed symptomatic recurrence, of which 59% had an associated neurological deficit. The overall rate of symptomatic recurrence was 80% in patients with active disease limited to the brain only, versus 35% for patients with active extracranial disease ($p=0.03$), likely a result of patients dying prior to recurrence among those with active extracranial disease.

A comprehensive neurocognitive assessment of patients treated with WBRT was performed as part of the phase III trial PCI-P120-9801 evaluating the radiosensitizer motexafin gadolinium. This revealed that patients with better than median local and distant tumor control displayed significantly improved preservation of executive and fine motor function relative to patients with less than median response to treatment (Li et al. 2007). These results support the notion that optimizing local and distant brain tumor control is an essential facet of preserving neurocognitive function.

An important recent study on the effect of treatment on neurocognitive function by Chang and colleagues at MD Anderson Cancer Center randomized patients to SRS plus WBRT versus SRS alone, with patients stratified by histology, RTOG RPA class, and number of brain metastases. The primary endpoint of neurocognitive function was measured using a revised Hopkins Verbal Learning Test. The trial was stopped after accrual of 58 patients as patients randomly assigned to the combined SRS + WBRT arm had a higher >96% probability of a significant decline in learning and memory function (52%) at 4 months compared with patients receiving SRS alone (24%). Patients receiving combined treatment had a higher probability of freedom from CNS recurrence at 1 year (73%) versus patients in the SRS alone arm (27%, $p=0.0003$; Chang et al. 2009). Further follow-up may clarify if the benefit to neurocognitive function observed at 4 months is maintained at later time points despite the increased risk of DBF.

Another context in which there has been great interest in substituting SRS for WBRT is following surgical resection of a brain metastasis. The local control reported following surgery alone in Patchell's trial of surgery alone versus surgery + WBRT was 54% (Patchell et al. 1998). The addition of WBRT increased local control to 90% ($p<0.01$) but resulted in no significant improvement in overall survival. Multiple retrospective studies have demonstrated that postoperative SRS boost in lieu of WBRT is associated with high local control and acceptable toxicity (Soltys et al. 2008; Iwai et al. 2008; Kim et al. 2006; Mathieu et al. 2008; Jagannathan et al. 2009). Table 12.1 summarizes results from recent studies utilizing radiosurgical boost following surgical resection.

The local control outcomes of resection cavity boosts range between 73% and 94% and a variety of treatment-related factors may influence outcome. Soltys et al. (2008) reported that while target volume did not relate to outcome, less conformal plans were associated with improved local control, with the least conformal quartile of plans demonstrating 100% local control versus 63% for the most conformal quartile, suggesting that imprecise delineation of the cavity margin might benefit from less steep dose falloff. The addition of a 1–2 mm margin around the resection cavity edge has been proposed to address the spatial uncertainty in cavity delineation (Soltys et al. 2008;

Table 12.1 Outcomes for SRS to the resection cavity following surgical resection of a brain metastasis

References	# Pts	WBRT	Margin dose: range (Gy)/ median (Gy)	Target size: median (cc)/ range (cc)	Median FU (months)	Local control
Soltys et al. (2008)	72	No	18.6/15–30	9.8/0.1–66.8	8.1	79% at 12 months
Iwai et al. (2008)	21	No	17/13–23	10.7/3.4–23.3	21.6	82% at 12 months
Jagannathan et al. (2009)	47	11/47	19/6–22	10.5/1.75–34.45	11	94% at 14 months
Kim et al. (2006)[a]	79	79/79	18/8–24	>15	NS	94.9%
Mathieu et al. (2008)	40	10/40	16/11–20	9.1/0.6–39.9	13	73% at 13 months

[a]SRS to resection cavity for surgical resection following WBRT failure

Iwai et al. 2008; Mathieu et al. 2008) and in response to pathologic findings of tumor cell infiltration beyond the discrete tumor margin (Baumert et al. 2006). Iwai and colleagues found that local control improved with doses of >18 Gy ($p=0.03$) and also noted an increased risk of meningeal carcinomatosis for posterior fossa lesions ($p=0.05$), while observing meningeal carcinomatosis in 24% of their patients overall. In contrast, Kim et al. (2006) observed development of meningeal carcinomatosis in only 5.1% of patients with no increase for posterior fossa locations; the patient population in this study had all previously received WBRT and underwent surgical salvage followed by SRS boost to the resection cavity.

Another clinical setting well suited for SRS is the treatment of post-WBRT failures. The use of WBRT re-treatment, typically with total doses of 2,000–2,500 cGy in 200 cGy fractions, is associated with significant morbidity and a posttreatment median survival of only 3.5–5 months (Coia 1992; Cooper et al. 1990). Re-irradiation of <5 brain metastases is best accomplished with SRS which has far less toxicity than WBRT re-treatment, and improved disease control versus systemic treatments (Noel et al. 2001; Alexander et al. 1995).

The optimal treatment of multiple brain metastases (>4) remains controversial with some investigators recommending SRS for >4 metastases only in the setting of controlled extracranial disease based on the poor expected survival of such patients (Cho et al. 2000). Bhatnagar et al. (2006) reported a retrospective review of 205 patients who underwent radiosurgery for treatment of four or more metastases in the initial or re-irradiation setting. In this study, radiosurgery was used following WBRT failure in 38% of patients, with WBRT in 46% of patients and as a sole treatment modality in 17% of patients. The median overall survival was 8 months and median time to brain progression 9 months. Multivariate analysis of prognostic factors for survival identified total volume of metastases, rather than total number was predictive for survival. Additional prognostic factors for survival were age, margin dose, and RPA class. For local control, the only significant prognostic factor was total treatment volume; no impact was noted for number of lesions, age, or RPA class (Bhatnagar et al. 2006). Subsequent analysis by recursive partitioning identified a favorable subgroup consisting of 43% of patients with median survival of 13 months who had <7 tumors and <7 cc of cumulative tumor volume, versus 6 months median survival for the remaining patients (Bhatnagar et al. 2007). These data support the increased use of radiosurgery for treatment of select patients with recurrent brain metastases and >4 lesions.

12.5 Frameless Radiosurgery

While the reliable immobilization and target localization accuracy of invasive frame-based SRS have established the technique as a historical gold standard, the use of invasive frames is associated with significant disadvantages including patient discomfort, risk of injury from fracture or infection, and logistical hurdles for treatment. Head frames may also shift relative to the patient, compromising treatment accuracy, and potentially resulting in injury (Ott 1998). These shortcomings are of even greater detriment in the setting of multiple metastases treatment or multiple treatment sessions.

The development of image-guided stereotactic localization methods using either optical image guidance (Ryken et al. 2001), or stereoscopic X-ray imaging (Verellen et al. 2003) has provided a foundation for frameless radiosurgical treatment (Verellen et al. 2008). One such image-guided system, the ExacTrac® X-Ray (Brainlab AG, Feldkirchen, Germany), utilizes dual floor-mounted kV X-ray tubes which project onto ceiling mounted amorphous silicon detectors and generate stereoscopic oblique images through machine isocenter (Verellen et al. 2003). The system creates an image fusion of the kV X-ray images with a digital reconstructed radiograph (DRR) library generated at the time of simulation and generates a predicted position shift to place the patient such that the target is coincident with the planning isocenter. An infrared tracking system is used to verify relative shifts and to provide initial patient position.

Both phantom-based end-to-end tests and clinical validation have demonstrated overall system accuracy within tolerances appropriate for radiosurgery (Lamba et al. 2009; Solberg et al. 2008; Ramakrishna et al. 2010). As with all types of stereotactic radiosurgery, a systematic adherence to strict quality assurance and physician/physicist supervision is essential for adequate treatment.

As expected based on the tests of clinical quality assurance, the early clinical results of frameless radiosurgery (FRS) for brain metastases utilizing the Novalis® Radiosurgery system are consistent with the results observed with frame-based radiosurgery treatment. Chen and colleagues reported on 54 patients treated with FRS and report a 6-month actuarial control rate of 88% (Chen et al. 2009). Breneman et al. (2009) note local control rates of 90, 80, 78, and 78% at 6, 12, 18, and 24 months. Among the advantages of the frameless radiosurgery system is the ability to perform intensity-modulated radiosurgery (IMRS), a technique not usually logistically possible with invasive-frame-based treatment, due to the time needed for dosimetric quality assurance. Further studies should clarify the potential benefits of this approach in reducing the risk of radiation necrosis and/or for radiosurgical dose escalation.

12.6 Treatment Guidelines and Conclusions

The treatment of brain metastases remains highly controversial. The emergence of SRS as a safe and effective modality for local control of brain metastases has led to its widespread adoption and use, often in lieu of WBRT. The advent of frameless radiosurgery allows for improved treatment logistics, greater options for treatment planning, and improved patient comfort.

General guidelines for treatment may be divided between patients with good prognosis (controlled extracranial disease/good expected survival/limited medical comorbidities) versus poor prognosis patients (uncontrolled extracranial disease/poor expected survival/high medical comorbidities). Treatment may be further stratified by number and pattern of metastases, and the presence of symptomatic mass effect (Table 12.2). In general, for patients with good prognosis and <4 metastases, SRS or surgery is appropriate initial management, with the selection based on the size and symptomatic mass effect of lesions. WBRT may be added if there is concern for local control either as a result of radioresistant histology, radiosurgical dose reduction due to tumor size or location, or after surgery if tumor dissemination is suspected. For poor prognosis patients and for those with >4 lesions, WBRT may be more appropriate in initial management, though palliative SRS treatment may be reasonable in contexts where duration of treatment is critical.

Table 12.2 Initial management of brain metastatic disease

Number of metastases	Prognosis: good versus poor[a]	Symptomatic mass effect/ size >4 cm	Primary treatment	(±)Additional treatment[b]	Comments
1	Good	No	SRS	NT versus WB	S for pathology
		Yes	S	SRS versus WB	
	Poor	No	WB versus SRS		Palliative SRS if short duration of treatment critical
		Yes	S versus WB	SRS	
2–4	Good	No	SRS	NT versus WB	
		Yes	S+SRS	WB versus SRS	S only for critical symptomatic lesions
	Poor	No	SRS versus WB		
		Yes	WB		
>4	Good	No	WB versus SRS	SRS versus WB	
		Yes	WB	SRS	
	Poor	No	WB		
		Yes	WB		
Diffuse/LMD	All	NA	WB		

NT no treatment, *S* surgery, *SRS* stereotactic radiosurgery, *WB* whole-brain radiotherapy

[a]Good prognosis patients: those without progressive extracranial disease/limited medical comorbidities/long expected survival. Poor prognosis patients: those with progressive extracranial disease/significant medical comorbidities/short expected survival

[b]Select additional treatments based on clinical/prognostic considerations

All treatment decisions should be individualized and involve multidisciplinary collaboration between neurosurgeons, medical and radiation oncologists to take into consideration the many complexities of managing both the oncologic and neurologic manifestations of metastatic cancer.

References

Alexander E III et al (1995) Stereotactic radiosurgery for the definitive, noninvasive treatment of brain metastases. J Natl Cancer Inst 87(1):34–40

Andrews DW et al (2004) Whole brain radiation therapy with or without stereotactic radiosurgery boost for patients with one to three brain metastases: phase III results of the RTOG 9508 randomised trial. Lancet 363(9422):1665–1672

Aoyama H et al (2006) Stereotactic radiosurgery plus whole-brain radiation therapy vs stereotactic radiosurgery alone for treatment of brain metastases: a randomized controlled trial. JAMA 295(21):2483–2491

Auchter RM et al (1996) A multiinstitutional outcome and prognostic factor analysis of radiosurgery for resectable single brain metastasis. Int J Radiat Oncol Biol Phys 35(1):27–35

Baumert BG et al (2006) A pathology-based substrate for target definition in radiosurgery of brain metastases. Int J Radiat Oncol Biol Phys 66(1):187–194

Bendell JC et al (2003) Central nervous system metastases in women who receive trastuzumab-based therapy for metastatic breast carcinoma. Cancer 97(12):2972–2977

Bhatnagar AK et al (2006) Stereotactic radiosurgery for four or more intracranial metastases. Int J Radiat Oncol Biol Phys 64(3):898–903

Bhatnagar AK et al (2007) Recursive partitioning analysis of prognostic factors for patients with four or more intracranial metastases treated with radiosurgery. Technol Cancer Res Treat 6(3):153–160

Bindal RK et al (1993) Surgical treatment of multiple brain metastases. J Neurosurg 79(2):210–216

Borgelt B et al (1981) Ultra-rapid high dose irradiation schedules for the palliation of brain metastases: final results of the first two studies by the Radiation Therapy Oncology Group. Int J Radiat Oncol Biol Phys 7(12):1633–1638

Boyd TS, Mehta MP (1999) Stereotactic radiosurgery for brain metastases. Oncol (Huntingt) 13(10):1397–1409, discussion, 1409–1410, 1413

Breneman JC et al (2009) Frameless image-guided intracranial stereotactic radiosurgery: clinical outcomes for brain metastases. Int J Radiat Oncol Biol Phys 74(3):702–706

Cairncross JG, Kim JH, Posner JB (1980) Radiation therapy for brain metastases. Ann Neurol 7(6):529–541

Chang EL et al (2009) Neurocognition in patients with brain metastases treated with radiosurgery or radiosurgery plus whole-brain irradiation: a randomised controlled trial. Lancet Oncol 10(11):1037–1044

Chao J, Phillips R, Nickson J (1954) Roentgen ray therapy of cerebral metastases. Cancer 7:682–689

Chen JC et al (2009) Control of brain metastases using frameless image-guided radiosurgery. Neurosurg Focus 27(6):E6

Cho KH et al (2000) The role of radiosurgery for multiple brain metastases. Neurosurg Focus 9(2):e2

Coia LR (1992) The role of radiation therapy in the treatment of brain metastases. Int J Radiat Oncol Biol Phys 23(1): 229–238

Cooper JS, Steinfeld AD, Lerch IA (1990) Cerebral metastases: value of reirradiation in selected patients. Radiology 174(3 Pt 1):883–885

Cross NE, Glantz MJ (2003) Neurologic complications of radiation therapy. Neurol Clin 21(1):249–277

Crossen JR et al (1994) Neurobehavioral sequelae of cranial irradiation in adults: a review of radiation-induced encephalopathy. J Clin Oncol 12(3):627–642

DeAngelis LM, Delattre JY, Posner JB (1989) Radiation-induced dementia in patients cured of brain metastases. Neurology 39(6):789–796

Gaspar L et al (1997) Recursive partitioning analysis (RPA) of prognostic factors in three Radiation Therapy Oncology Group (RTOG) brain metastases trials. Int J Radiat Oncol Biol Phys 37(4):745–751

Gelber RD et al (1981) Equivalence of radiation schedules for the palliative treatment of brain metastases in patients with favorable prognosis. Cancer 48(8):1749–1753

Hazuka MB et al (1993) Multiple brain metastases are associated with poor survival in patients treated with surgery and radiotherapy. J Clin Oncol 11(2):369–373

Iwadate Y, Namba H, Yamaura A (2000) Significance of surgical resection for the treatment of multiple brain metastases. Anticancer Res 20(1B):573–577

Iwai Y, Yamanaka K, Yasui T (2008) Boost radiosurgery for treatment of brain metastases after surgical resections. Surg Neurol 69(2):181–186, discussion 186

Jagannathan J et al (2009) Gamma Knife radiosurgery to the surgical cavity following resection of brain metastases. J Neurosurg 111(3):431–438

Kim PK et al (2006) Gamma Knife surgery targeting the resection cavity of brain metastasis that has progressed after whole-brain radiotherapy. J Neurosurg 105(Suppl):75–78

Kondziolka D et al (1999) Stereotactic radiosurgery plus whole brain radiotherapy versus radiotherapy alone for patients with multiple brain metastases. Int J Radiat Oncol Biol Phys 45(2):427–434

Lagerwaard FJ et al (1999) Identification of prognostic factors in patients with brain metastases: a review of 1292 patients. Int J Radiat Oncol Biol Phys 43(4):795–803

Lamba M, Breneman JC, Warnick RE (2009) Evaluation of image-guided positioning for frameless intracranial radiosurgery. Int J Radiat Oncol Biol Phys 74(3):913–919

Leksell L (1951) The stereotaxic method and radiosurgery of the brain. Acta Chir Scand 102(4):316–319

Li J et al (2007) Regression after whole-brain radiation therapy for brain metastases correlates with survival and improved neurocognitive function. J Clin Oncol 25(10):1260–1266

Mathieu D et al (2008) Tumor bed radiosurgery after resection of cerebral metastases. Neurosurgery 62(4):817–823

Mintz AH et al (1996) A randomized trial to assess the efficacy of surgery in addition to radiotherapy in patients with a single cerebral metastasis. Cancer 78(7):1470–1476

Murphy CB et al (2003) Clinical exacerbation of multiple sclerosis following radiotherapy. Arch Neurol 60(2):273–275

Noel G et al (2001) Radiosurgery for re-irradiation of brain metastasis: results in 54 patients. Radiother Oncol 60(1): 61–67

Noordijk EM et al (1994) The choice of treatment of single brain metastasis should be based on extracranial tumor activity and age. Int J Radiat Oncol Biol Phys 29(4):711–717
O'Neill BP et al (2003) A comparison of surgical resection and stereotactic radiosurgery in the treatment of solitary brain metastases. Int J Radiat Oncol Biol Phys 55(5): 1169–1176
Ott K (1998) An algorithm for the empirical determination of intracranial stereotactic targets. Stereotact Funct Neurosurg 71(1):29–35
Patchell RA et al (1990) A randomized trial of surgery in the treatment of single metastases to the brain. N Engl J Med 322(8):494–500
Patchell RA et al (1998) Postoperative radiotherapy in the treatment of single metastases to the brain: a randomized trial. JAMA 280(17):1485–1489
Pollock BE, Brown PD, Foote RL, Stafford SL, Schomberg PJ, Neurooncol J (2003) Properly selected patients with multiple brain metastases may benefit from aggressive treatment of their intracranial disease. 61(1):73–80.
Ramakrishna N et al (2010) A clinical comparison of patient setup and intra-fraction motion using frame-based radiosurgery versus a frameless image-guided radiosurgery system for intracranial lesions. Radiother Oncol 95(1): 109–115
Regine WF et al (2002) Risk of symptomatic brain tumor recurrence and neurologic deficit after radiosurgery alone in patients with newly diagnosed brain metastases: results and implications. Int J Radiat Oncol Biol Phys 52(2):333–338
Ryken TC et al (2001) Initial clinical experience with frameless stereotactic radiosurgery: analysis of accuracy and feasibility. Int J Radiat Oncol Biol Phys 51(4):1152–1158
Schouten LJ et al (2002) Incidence of brain metastases in a cohort of patients with carcinoma of the breast, colon, kidney, and lung and melanoma. Cancer 94(10):2698–2705
Schultheiss TE et al (1995) Radiation response of the central nervous system. Int J Radiat Oncol Biol Phys 31(5): 1093–1112
Shaw E et al (2000) Single dose radiosurgical treatment of recurrent previously irradiated primary brain tumors and brain metastases: final report of RTOG protocol 90–05. Int J Radiat Oncol Biol Phys 47(2):291–298
Sheline GE, Wara WM, Smith V (1980) Therapeutic irradiation and brain injury. Int J Radiat Oncol Biol Phys 6(9): 1215–1228
Shiau CY et al (1997) Radiosurgery for brain metastases: relationship of dose and pattern of enhancement to local control. Int J Radiat Oncol Biol Phys 37(2):375–383
Solberg TD et al (2008) Quality assurance of immobilization and target localization systems for frameless stereotactic cranial and extracranial hypofractionated radiotherapy. Int J Radiat Oncol Biol Phys 71(1 Suppl):S131–S135
Soltys SG et al (2008) Stereotactic radiosurgery of the postoperative resection cavity for brain metastases. Int J Radiat Oncol Biol Phys 70(1):187–193
Tsai JS et al (1991) Quality assurance in stereotactic radiosurgery using a standard linear accelerator. Int J Radiat Oncol Biol Phys 21(3):737–748
Verellen D et al (2003) Quality assurance of a system for improved target localization and patient set-up that combines real-time infrared tracking and stereoscopic X-ray imaging. Radiother Oncol 67(1):129–141
Verellen D et al (2008) An overview of volumetric imaging technologies and their quality assurance for IGRT. Acta Oncol 47(7):1271–1278
Wen PY (1997) Diagnosis and management of brain tumors. In: Black P, Loeffler J (eds) Cancer of the nervous system. Blackwell, Cambridge, pp 106–127
Zimm S et al (1981) Intracerebral metastases in solid-tumor patients: natural history and results of treatment. Cancer 48(2):384–394

Recurrent Malignant Gliomas

13

Changhu Chen

13.1 Introduction

Malignant gliomas are the most common brain tumor in adults. Each year, more than 14,000 new cases are diagnosed in the USA. Glioblastomas account for approximately 60–70% of malignant gliomas, anaplastic astrocytomas for 10–15%, and anaplastic oligodendrogliomas, anaplastic oligoastrocytomas, and less common tumors such as anaplastic ependymomas and anaplastic gangliogliomas account for the rest (Primary Brain Tumors in the United States Statistical Report 2007–2008).

The standard therapy for newly diagnosed malignant gliomas involves surgical resection, when feasible, and radiotherapy with chemotherapy. Postoperative radiation therapy (RT), 60 Gy in 30 fractions, concurrent with temozolomide followed by adjuvant temozolomide chemotherapy has become the standard treatment since the publication of the results from the randomized trial by the European Organization for Research and Treatment of Cancer (EORTC) and National Cancer Institute of Canada (NCIC; Stupp et al. 2005). The current standard of care for patients with newly diagnosed anaplastic astrocytoma is surgical resection followed by RT (60 Gy in 30 fractions), with or without concomitant and adjuvant carmustine. Temozolomide has been widely used in patients with anaplastic astrocytoma (Stupp et al. 2006; Schiff 2007). After surgical resection, radiation, and chemotherapy, malignant gliomas eventually recur in a vast majority of patients (Stupp et al. 2005; Filippini et al. 2008). Malignant gliomas infiltrate deeply into normal brain tissue. Tumor cells are found in the area of edema far away from the main tumor mass (Burger et al. 1983; Fisher and Buffler 2005). However, clinically, most malignant gliomas recur within 2 cm of the primary tumor location (Hess et al. 1994; Wong et al. 1999).

There is no standard treatment for recurrent malignant gliomas. For the subset of patients able to undergo additional surgery at the time of recurrence, the carmustine-impregnated wafer implantation improves median survival by an average of 8 weeks (Brem et al. 1995). A variety of salvage chemotherapy agents/regimens have been used in this setting with limited benefit (Butowski et al. 2006). As the recurrent tumor is usually localized, re-irradiation seems logical for the patients who cannot undergo further surgery and the patients with gross residual tumors after surgical resection. Patients with a recurrent malignant glioma usually have received a full dose of radiation (60 Gy) in their initial treatment. Initial radiation port routinely covers areas of edema with generous margins. Re-irradiation has been done in a more focal fashion, usually with a stereotactic technique. There have been no prospective trials in the re-irradiation setting and a variety of radiation doses, fractionation, as well as concurrent systematic agents have been used. Re-irradiation is not the treatment choice for all recurrent malignant gliomas; rather, it appears to benefit only a selected group of patients.

C. Chen
Department of Radiation Oncology, University of Colorado Denver, 1665 Aurora Court, Suite 1032, Aurora, CO 80045, USA
e-mail: changhu.chen@ucdenver.edu

A.A.F. De Salles et al. (eds.), *Shaped Beam Radiosurgery*,
DOI: 10.1007/978-3-642-11151-8_13,

13.2 SRS and FSRT for Recurrent Malignant Gliomas

In an attempt to spare brain tissue and critical structures in the re-irradiation setting for recurrent malignant gliomas, stereotactic radiosurgery (SRS) and fractionated stereotactic radiotherapy (FSRT) have been used. SRS is a form of stereotactically localized, high-dose radiation, generally administered with a Gamma Knife® (Elekta, Stockholm, Sweden), Cyberknife® (Accuray, Sunnyvale, CA), or a specially adapted linear accelerator such as the Novalis® Radiosurgery system (Brainlab AG, Feldkirchen, Germany). Gamma Knife radiosurgery is usually administered as a single fraction, whereas Brainlab or other linear accelerator-based radiosurgery may be fractionated. SRS is defined here in this chapter as single fraction high-dose stereotactic radiosurgery, and FSRT stereotactically localized radiation therapy delivered in more than one fraction.

SRS tends to be used for lesions ≤4 cm in the largest diameter. Some SRS series are listed in Table 13.1. The median survival time from SRS was approximately 10–13 months. It seems that SRS is associated with high rates of radionecrosis and re-operation, in the range of 22–24%. In a series reported from Korea, SRS significantly prolonged survival as a salvage treatment in patients with recurrent glioblastoma when compared with a historic control group (23 vs. 12 months; $p < 0.0001$; Kong et al. 2007). It should be noted that those were the patients treated at the first sign of recurrence on brain MRI. All patients were with a recurrent lesion <3 cm in maximum dimension.

FSRT may be used for lesion >4 cm in size or for lesions near critical structures and not suitable for SRS. Several studies have shown that FSRT is safe and effective (Shaw et al. 1993; Cho et al. 1999; Hudes et al. 1999; Shepherd et al. 1997; Glass et al. 1997; Lederman et al. 2000; Wurm et al. 2006). Cho et al. compared SRS (a median dose of 17 Gy) with FSRT at 2.5 Gy/day to a median dose of 37.5 Gy. Survival rates between the two groups were comparable, but the patients who received FSRT experienced fewer late complications – radionecrosis (Cho et al. 1999). There has been no prospective trial to compare these two stereotactic modalities, and only a few patients underwent further surgical intervention with ultimate pathologic confirmation of radionecrosis. For series showed in Table 13.2, the median survival was reported to be 7–12 months after FSRT for patients with recurrent malignant gliomas.

13.2.1 Target Definition

In a re-irradiation setting, the target (gross tumor volume, GTV) is a contrast-enhancing lesion on T1-weighted MRI. Figure 13.1 demonstrates a contrast-enhancing lesion in the left temporal lobe (left) and the target outlined (right). Margins given around the target volumes

Table 13.1 SRS for recurrent malignant gliomas

References	Modality	No. of patients	Median tumor volume (ml)	Median dose (Gy)	Median survival (months)	Toxicity
Kong et al. (2007)	SRS	65 GBM 49 grade 3 gliomas	10.6	16	13 for GBM 26 for grade 3 gliomas	Radionecrosis on MRI 19.3%
Shrieve et al. (1995)	SRS	86 GBM	10	13	10.2	22% re-operation
Combs et al. (2005)	SRS	32 GBM	10	15	10	None
Kondziolka et al. (1997)	SRS	19 GBM 23 AA	6	15	30 for GBM 31 for AA	22% re-operation
Cho et al. (1999)	SRS	27 GBM 19 grade 3 Gliomas	30	17	11	22% re-operation

Table 13.2 FSRT for recurrent malignant gliomas

References	Modality	No. of patients	Median tumor volume (cc)	Dose range (Gy)	Fraction size/schedule	Median survival (months)	Toxicity
Schwer et al. (2008)	FSRT+gefitinib	15	41.3	18–36	6–12 Gy, daily	10.3	No DLT
Cho et al. (1999)	FSRT/SRS	25	25	37.5	2.5 Gy, daily	12	Re-operation on 3 pts – all with tumor
Hudes et al. (1999)	FSRT	20	12.7	24–35	3–3.5 Gy, daily	10.5	No grade 3 toxicity, no re-operation due to toxicity, 25% re-operation due to tumor progression
Shepherd et al. (1997)	FSRT	29	24	20–50	5 Gy, daily	11	No dose-limiting acute toxicity, re-operation 6% for radiation necrosis
Glass et al. (1997)	FSRT+CDDP	20	14	42	3–6 Gy, twice/week	13.75	25% re-operation for tumor progression and necrosis, 40% tumor progression, 55% stable
Lederman et al. (2000)	FSRT+taxol	88	32.8	24	4–9 Gy, weekly	7	11% re-operation for expanding mass, 49% radiographic progression, 40% stable
Wurm et al. (2006)	FSRT+topotecan	25	16.5	25–30	5–6 Gy, daily	14.5	12% grade 2 late toxicity, no re-operation

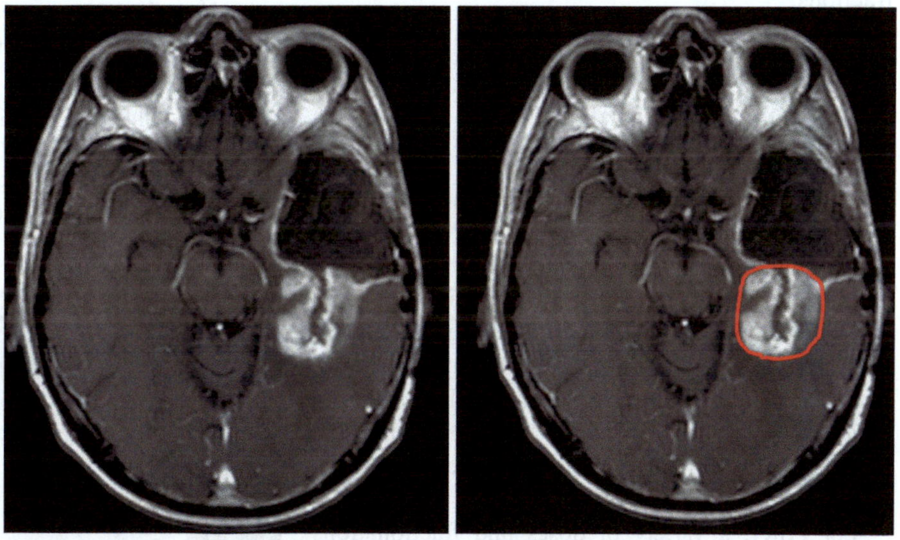

Fig. 13.1 Delineation of gross tumor volume (GTV)

(GTV) varied across the reports. No margin is usually given when SRS is performed with a rigid head frame (Schwer et al. 2009). A margin of 1–3 mm is given for FSRT, and an even more generous margin of 5–10 mm may be given if the fraction size of FSRT is close to conventional fractionation such as 2–2.5 Gy per fraction.

GTV or GTV with a margin should be adequately covered with a desirable isodose line (>95% of the target volumes be covered with a specified isodose), and the dose falloff should be as fast as possible (Shaw et al. 1993). When the target is near a critical structure such as the brain stem or optic chiasm, tumor

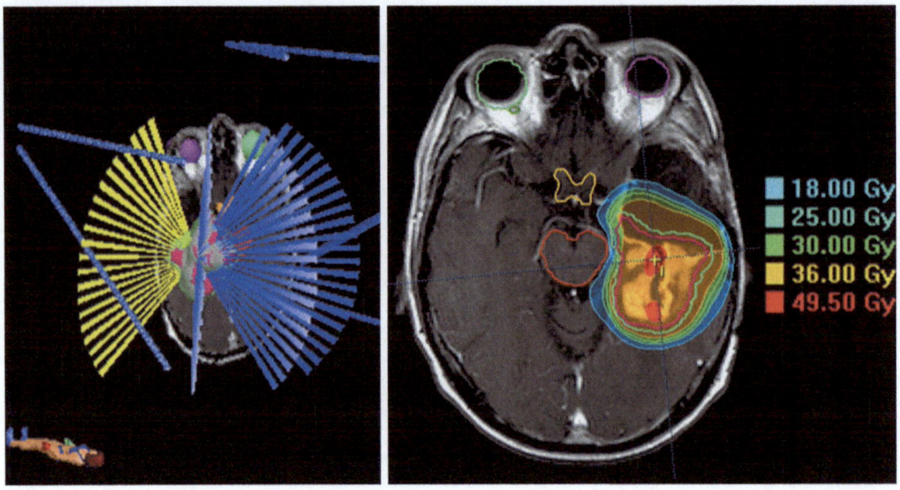

Fig. 13.2 No margin was added to the gross tumor volume by the brainstem (*dark magenta*) to avoid overdosing the brainstem. Eighteen gray isodose line curved around the brainstem

coverage may need to be compromised in order to spare these structures. Figure 13.2 shows that the GTV (dark magenta) + 2 mm margin (light green) is adequately covered by the 36 Gy isodose line in a FSRT plan, but the coverage is somewhat compromised to avoid overdosing the brain stem. The dose distributions curved around the brainstem, the maximum dose to the brain stem remained <18 Gy in three fractions.

13.2.2 Dose Decision

RTOG 9005 trial determined the maximum tolerated re-irradiation doses of single fraction radiosurgery after an initial median radiation dose of 60 Gy were 24 Gy, 18 Gy, and 15 Gy for tumors <20 mm, 21–30 mm, and 31–40 mm in maximum diameter, respectively. Unacceptable CNS toxicity was more likely in patients with larger tumors. The actuarial incidence of radionecrosis was 5%, 8%, 9%, and 11% at 6 months, 12 months, 18 months, and 24 months, respectively, following radiosurgery.

For FSRT, a variety of doses and fractionations were reported (Table 13.2). A recent phase I study showed that a total dose of 36 Gy in three fractions was well tolerated in patients who received a median dose of 60 Gy in the past. Recurrent tumors up to 6 cm in the largest diameter were treated (Schwer et al. 2008). However, further prospective study is warranted in this setting.

13.2.3 Immobilization

A rigid head frame is routinely used in SRS for immobilization. A neurosurgeon is usually teamed up to perform the procedure. Once a head frame is placed, CT simulation is then performed. The accuracy of a rigid head frame for immobilization is considered to be within 1–2 mm. Recently emerged frameless image-guided positioning appeared adequate for patient immobilization for intracranial radiosurgery (Lamba et al. 2009).

In FSRT, a plastic mask is usually used for immobilization and reproducing the head position for multiple fractions. Figure 13.3 shows a Brainlab mask made for a patient who was going to receive FSRT. The

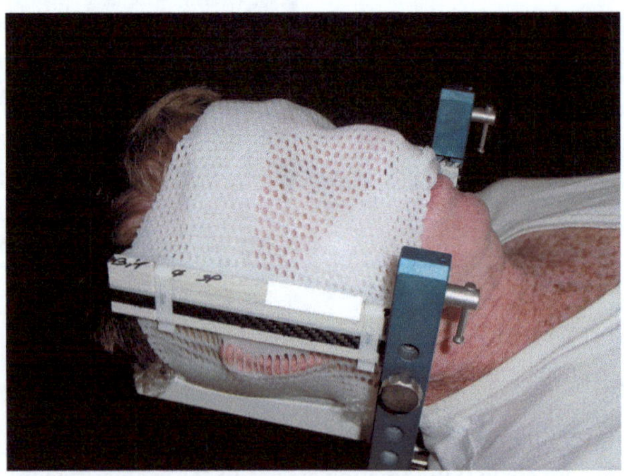

Fig. 13.3 Brainlab mask for immobilization for FSRT

accuracy of a removable plastic mask, such as a Brainlab mask, is within 1–3 mm.

A treatment planning brain MRI with gadolinium contrast is mandatory for target delineation for either SRS or FSRT. It is advantageous to have a thin-cut brain MRI (slice thickness 2–3 mm), especially when a small lesion is been treated. The MRI images are fused with simulation CT images for contouring the target volume and critical structures.

13.2.4 Case Illustration

A 53-year-old man presented with a 2-month history of headaches, memory loss, and visual hallucination. A brain MRI revealed a 5 × 10 cm rim-enhancing mass in the right frontal lobe with severe mass effect. The patient was taken to the operating room and underwent a craniotomy and resection of the tumor. Pathology revealed a glioblastoma multiforme. Postoperative brain MRI showed postsurgical changes with enhancing tissue present along the posterior aspect of the surgical bed extending into the right frontal lobe and corpus callosum. The patient was treated with postoperative radiation therapy with concurrent temozolomide chemotherapy at 75 mg/m^2/day followed by adjuvant temozolomide chemotherapy at 200 mg/m^2 5 days every 28 days. The radiation therapy was delivered with three-dimensional technique. An initial 46 Gy in 2 Gy fractions covered the T2 abnormality with a 2 cm margin. A 14 Gy boost in 2 Gy fractions was given to the surgical cavity and residual enhancement on T1-weighted MRI with 1.0 cm margin. The patient received a total dose of 60 Gy over 6 weeks.

Five months after the radiation therapy was completed, there was evidence of tumor recurrence at the posterior aspect of the surgical cavity. His adjuvant temozolomide chemotherapy was changed to 7 days on and 7 days off dosing schedule. Radiographically, the recurrent tumor progressed during the next 4 months of intensified temozolomide chemotherapy.

The patient was subsequently enrolled on a phase I FSRT dose escalation trial (Schwer et al. 2008). He received gefitinib, an epidermal growth factor receptor inhibitor, at 100 mg daily, and FSRT to a total dose of 30 Gy in three fractions over 3 consecutive days. Figure 13.4 shows the FSRT plan.

After the re-irradiation with FSRT, he was followed with monthly clinic visits and brain MRIs at 1 month and 3 months after FSRT, then once every 3 months. Five months after the FSRT re-irradiation, the patient developed evidence of disease progression on brain MRIs with an enlarging T1-enhancing lesion and dramatically increasing T2 abnormality (Fig. 13.5). He also developed grade 2 headaches. He had no focal neurological deficit. The patient underwent a second surgical resection of the presumed progressive tumor. The pathology demonstrated extensive radionecrosis with scattered tumor cells (Fig. 13.6a). It was clear that the enhancing lesion on the brain MRI was not a progressive tumor. The patient did well after the second surgery. Further brain MRIs up to 12 months after FSRT re-irradiation revealed stable postoperative changes on the T1-weighted imaging and the T2 abnormality had gradually improved. The patient died 27 months after FSRT, 40 months after the initial diagnosis.

13.3 Discussion

SRS has been reported to be well tolerated in patients with a recurrent malignant glioma. RTOG 90-05 was a large phase I trial designed to determine the maximum tolerated dose (MTD) of single fraction radiosurgery in patients with recurrent, previously irradiated primary brain tumors and brain metastases. The MTD was 24 Gy for tumors <20 mm, 18 Gy for tumors of 21–30 mm, and 15 Gy for tumors of 31–40 mm in maximum diameter. Doses were prescribed to the 50–90% isodose line. All patients with a recurrent primary tumor received a median of 60 Gy of prior radiation. The actuarial incidence of radionecrosis was 11% at 24 months following radiosurgery. SRS also seems to benefit only a selected group of patients. Shrieve reported that a median dose of 13 Gy (range, 6–20 Gy) prescribed to a 50–100% isodose line of patients with a recurrent glioblastoma with a median volume of 10.1 cm^3 (range 2.2–83 cm^3) resulted in a median actuarial survival of 10.2 months, with survivals of 12 and 24 months being 45% and 19%. A younger age and a smaller tumor volume were predictive of a better outcome. Twenty-two percent of the patients required re-operation after SRS (Shrieve et al. 1995). Kong et al. treated patients with a recurrent malignant gliomas <3 cm in maximum

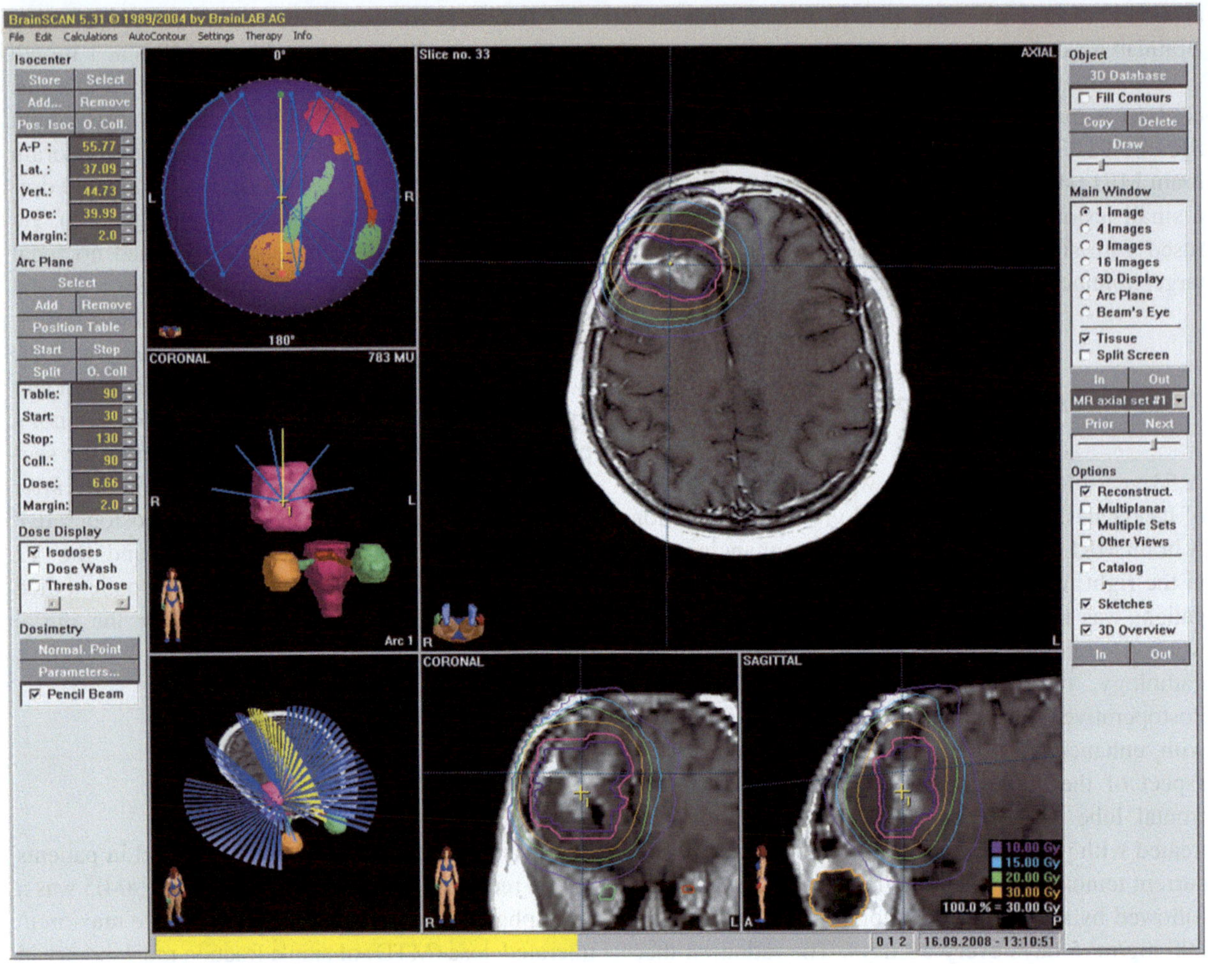

Fig. 13.4 A FSRT plan – 30 Gy isodose line (*brown*) adequately covers the GTV (*purple*) plus 2 mm margin (*dark magenta*)

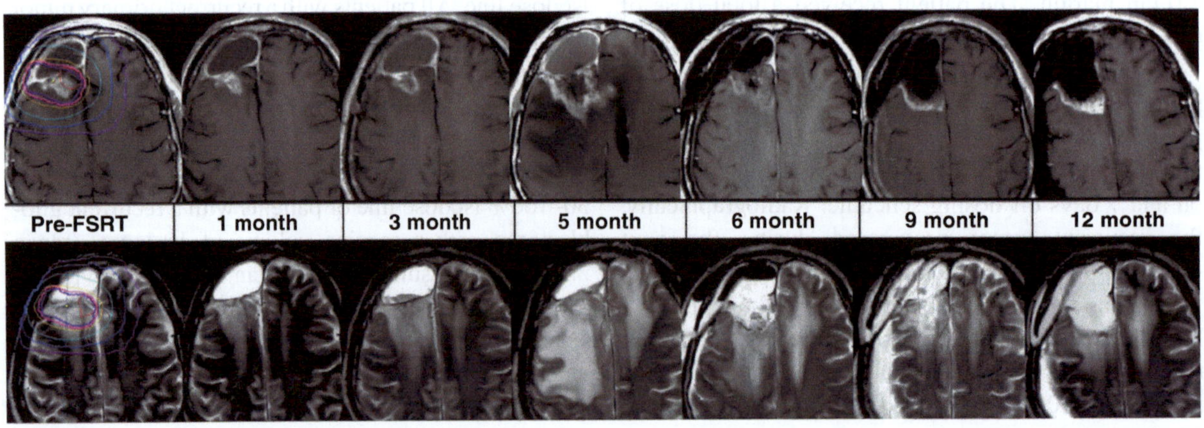

Fig. 13.5 T1 and T2 MRI images from one patient (at pre-FSRT and 1, 3, 5, 6, 9, and 12 months after treatment). Patient underwent surgical resection between the 5- and 6-month scans

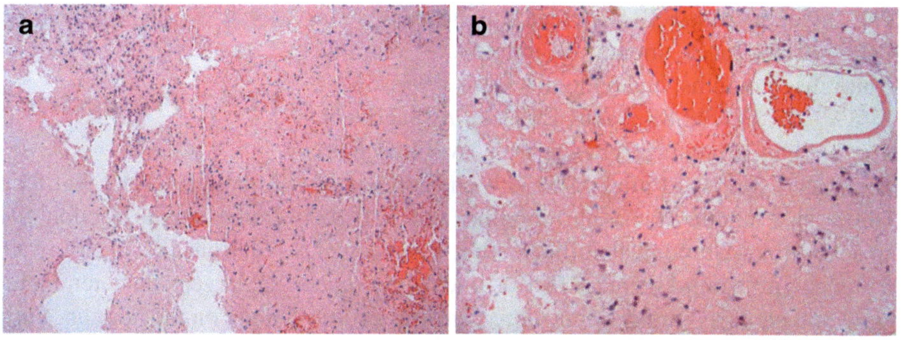

Fig. 13.6 Pathologic specimens from two patients who underwent surgical resection after FSRT: (**a**) severe radiation-induced tissue necrosis with scattered tumor cells (H&E 100×) and (**b**) characteristic vascular fibrinoid necrosis seen with therapy-induced necrosis (H&E 200×)

dimension. The median marginal dose of 16 Gy (range 12–50 Gy) was given to the 50% isodose line (range 24.3–96.2%) with a Gamma Knife or 80% isodose line with a linear accelerator. Compared with a historic control group, SRS significantly prolonged survival as a salvage treatment in patients with recurrent glioblastomas (23 vs. 12 months; $p<0.0001$). Radiation-induced necrosis was observed in 22 of 114 patients.

For FSRT, a wide range of dose and fractionation have been used. FSRT has been generally used for large lesions or the ones close to critical structures. FSRT has been reported to be well tolerated in patients with a recurrent malignant glioma who received a full dose of partial brain radiation with conventional fraction of 1.8–2 Gy. A median survival of 7–12 months was reported from mostly single institutional experiences. The re-operation rate and rate of radionecrosis associated with FSRT may be lower than that with single fraction SRS (Cho et al. 1999). However, there has been no prospective comparison.

Most reported FRST doses and fractions were from single institution empirical practice. There is a need for prospective studies in this respect to determine a maximum tolerated FSRT dose and fractionation. The design of such a trial will likely be complex. Different doses and fractions, sizes of recurrent tumors, and even tumor locations need to be taken into consideration. There has been a small phase I dose escalation trial reported from the University of Colorado Denver in patients with a recurrent malignant glioma who received a median dose of 60 Gy in 1.8–2 Gy per fraction in the past. Recurrent malignant gliomas up to 6 cm in the largest diameter were treated with FSRT (it was called SRS in the original publication using the ASTRO-endorsed SRS definition) in combination with an EGFR inhibitor gefitinib. FSRT was delivered in three fractions over 3 consecutive days. The FSRT dose was escalated from 18 to 36 Gy. There was no dose-limiting toxicity (DLT) reported. The DLT was defined in this small prospective study as ≥grade 3 toxicity using Common Terminology Criteria for Adverse Events v3.0 (CTCAE; Schwer et al. 2008). Thirty-six gray in three fractions is being tested in a further trial combined with another biologic targeted agent.

Brain MRI has been used routinely in the follow-up of patients with brain tumors. Prominent postradiation MRI changes were observed in the setting of re-irradiation. Schwer et al. quantified the changes of T1 enhancement and T2 abnormality in the follow-up brain MRIs in patients who received re-irradiation in the form of FSRT for recurrent malignant gliomas. Seventy-seven MRI datasets were studied. Brain MRI images were uploaded onto Brain SCAN® Version 5.31 SRS treatment planning system (Brainlab AG, Feldkirchen, Germany). Post-contrast T1 (T1C) and T2 abnormalities were outlined on each MRI slice, and the abnormal T1C and T2 signal volumes were then calculated by the iPlan® (Brainlab AG, Feldkirchen, Germany) and plotted against time from treatment (Fig. 13.7).

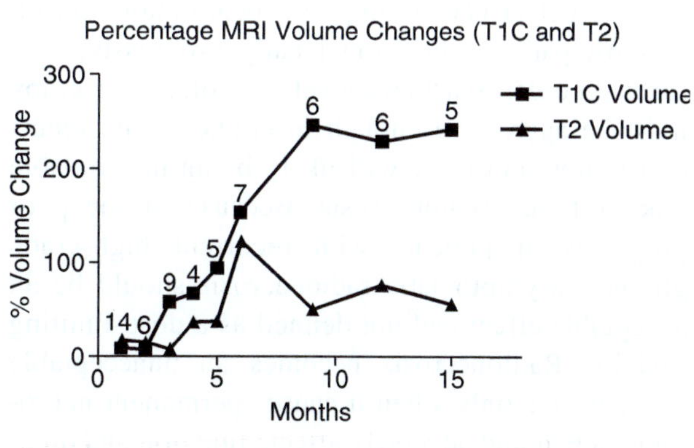

Fig. 13.7 Percentage Increases in T1C and T2 MRI volumes. The number of available studies analyzed at each time point is indicated above the graph

The median post-FSRT percentage increases in T1C volume at 1 month, 2 months, 3 months, 4 months, 5 months, and 6 months were 8.9%, 6.9%, 57.3%, 65.8%, 92.8%, and 152.2%, respectively. The median percentage change in T2 volume likewise trended upward after SRS with an increase of 18.0% at 1 month, 36.5% at 4 months, and 122.2% at 6 months. Although it is likely that a subset of patients with a rapid increase in T1C and T2 volume experienced early tumor recurrence, an interesting pattern emerged in patients who survived more than a few months after FSRT. Overall survival was significantly increased in the patients with the most dramatic (i.e., >90% or 150%) increase in T1C volume within 6 months of FSRT. It was speculated that the most dramatic T1C volume increase following the FSRT and EGFR inhibition, in this report, was the result of a vigorous treatment response rather than tumor progression (Schwer et al. 2009).

It should be noted that the RTOG central nervous system toxicity criteria define clinically or radiographically suspected radionecrosis and histologically proven radionecrosis at the time of an operation as grade 4 toxicity (Shaw et al. 2000), whereas the CTCAE version 3 defines asymptomatic CNS necrosis with only radiographic findings as grade 1 toxicity. Grade 2 CNS necrosis is defined as symptomatic, but not interfering with activities of daily living (ADL). Grade 3 CNS necrosis is symptomatic and interferes with ADL. Grade 4 CNS necrosis is defined as life-threatening and requires operative intervention (available at http://ctep.cancer.gov/forms/CTCAEv3.pdf, accessed September 20, 2008). In patients with malignant gliomas, especially in those with a recurrent malignant glioma, there is a clear need to improve local tumor control, as most patients die from locally progressive diseases. In order to achieve local control, radiotherapy must be aggressive enough to eradicate the recurrent tumor, and there will likely be an unavoidable risk of tissue radionecrosis. Because of the poor prognosis of patients with recurrent high-grade gliomas, asymptomatic radionecrosis should be an acceptable effect and not defined as a dose-limiting toxicity. Radionecrosis becomes an unacceptable consequence only when it causes permanent neurologic deficit and adversely affects function and quality of life (Shepherd et al. 1997).

13.4 Future Directions

13.4.1 Prospective Clinical Trials

Although RTOG 90-05 determined the maximum tolerated single fraction SRS doses in patients with a recurrent previously irradiated brain tumor <4 cm in the largest diameter, there has been no further efficacy study on the horizon. Further phase II and III prospective trials are needed to confirm the toxicity and efficacy. In the FSRT re-irradiation setting, large-scale phase I trial is needed to find an appropriate dose and fractionation schedule. With further phase II or III trial, the ultimate goal is to establish guidelines in this setting. In reality, clinical trials of this kind are unlikely to happen in the foreseeable future. At the time a malignant glioma recurs, the main issue is still local tumor control. Re-irradiation in the form of SRS or FSRT needs to be evaluated in a systematic fashion in prospective clinical trials.

13.4.2 Patient Selection

SRS or FSRT is beneficial to some. Patients with small recurrent tumors and good performance status fare better after re-irradiation. There is a tendency on the neuro-oncology side that patients with a recurrent malignant glioma exhaust all potential chemotherapy regimens before they are referred for re-irradiation. A recurrent tumor may be better treated with re-irradiation in the form of SRS or FSRT when it is small and at the first sign of recurrence.

13.4.3 Systemic Agents for Radiosensitization

After SRS or FSRT, local tumor progression is still a problem. In RTOG 90-05 study, with up to 1-year follow-up posttreatment, 40% of patients had local tumor progression within the radiosurgical target volume as their first site of failure. The same results were observed in FSRT (Combs et al. 2005). Improved local tumor control is warranted. Systemic agents have been used with FSRT as radiosensitizer. Biologic agents have been emerging in the brain tumor treatment. Combining re-irradiation with a systemic agent or biologic agent may increase radiation efficacy, and potentially increase local tumor control. On the other hand, malignant gliomas are infiltrative disease, an effective systemic agent or biologic agent can potentially treat microscopic disease infiltrating beyond the re-irradiation volume.

References

Brem H, Piantadosi S, Burger PC et al (1995) Placebo-controlled trial of safety and efficacy of intraoperative controlled delivery by biodegradable polymers of chemotherapy for recurrent gliomas: the polymer-brain tumor treatment group. Lancet 345:1008–1012

Burger PC, Dubois PJ, Schold SC et al (1983) Computerized tomographic and pathologic studies of the untreated, quiescent and recurrent glioblastoma multiforme. J Neurosurg 58:159–169

Butowski NA, Sneed PK, Chang SM (2006) Diagnosis and treatment of recurrent high-grade astrocytoma. J Clin Oncol 24:1273–1280

Cho KH, Hall WA, Gerbi BJ et al (1999) Single dose versus fractionated stereotactic radiotherapy for recurrent high-grade gliomas. Int J Radiat Oncol Biol Phys 45:1133–1141

Combs SE, Widmer V, Thilmann C et al (2005) Stereotactic radiosurgery (SRS): treatment option for recurrent glioblastoma multiforme (GBM). Cancer 104:2168–2173

Filippini G, Falcone C, Boiardi A et al (2008) Prognostic factors for survival in 676 consecutive patients with newly diagnosed primary glioblastoma. Neuro Oncol 10:79–87

Fisher PG, Buffler PA (2005) Malignant gliomas in 2005: where to go from here? JAMA 293:615–617

Glass J, Silverman CL, Axelrod R et al (1997) Fractionated stereotactic radiosurgery with cis-platinum radiosensitization in the treatment of recurrent, progressive, or persistent malignant astrocytoma. Am J Clin Oncol 20:226–229

Hess CF, Schaaf JC, Kortmann RD et al (1994) Malignant glioma: patterns of failure following individually tailored limited volume irradiation. Radiother Oncol 30:146–149

Hudes RS, Corn BW, Werner-Wasik M et al (1999) A Phase I dose escalation study of hypofractionated stereotactic radiosurgery as salvage therapy for persistent or recurrent malignant glioma. Int J Radiat Oncol Biol Phys 43:293–298

Kondziolka D, Flickinger JC, Bissonette DJ et al (1997) Survival benefit of stereotactic radiosurgery for patients with malignant glial neoplasms. Neurosurgery 41:776–783

Kong D, Lee J, Park K et al (2007) Efficiency of stereotactic radiosurgery as a salvage treatment for recurrent malignant gliomas. Cancer 112:2046–2051

Lamba M, Breneman JC, Warnick RE (2009) Evaluation of image-guided positioning for frameless intracranial radiosurgery. Int J Radiat Oncol Biol Phys 1(74):913–919

Lederman G, Wronski M, Arbit E et al (2000) Treatment of recurrent glioblastoma multiforme using fractionated stereotactic radiosurgery and concurrent paclitaxel. Am J Clin Oncol 23:155–159

Primary Brain Tumors in the United States Statistical Report (2007–2008) http://www.cbtrus.org/reports/2007–2008/2007 report.pdf (accessed September 18, 2008)

Schiff D (2007) Temozolomide and radiation in low-grade and anaplastic gliomas: temoradiation. Cancer Invest 25(8): 776–784

Schwer AL, Damek DM, Kavanagh BD et al (2008) A phase I dose-escalation study of fractionated stereotactic radiosurgery in combination with gefitinib in patients with recurrent malignant gliomas. Int J Radiat Oncol Biol Phys 70: 993–1001

Schwer A, Kavanagh B, McCammon R et al (2009) Radiographic and histopathologic observations after combined EGFR inhibition and hypofractionated stereotactic radiosurgery in Patients with recurrent malignant gliomas. Int J Radiat Oncol Biol Phys 73:1352–1357

Shaw E, Kline R, Gillin M et al (1993) Radiation Therapy Oncology Group: radiosurgery quality assurance guidelines. Int J Radiat Oncol Biol Phys 27:1231–1239

Shaw E, Scott C, Souhami L et al (2000) Single dose radiosurgical treatment of recurrent previously irradiated primary brain tumors and brain metastases: final report of RTOG protocol 90-05. Int J Radiat Oncol Biol Phys 47:291–298

Shepherd SF, Laing RW, Cosgrove VP et al (1997) Hypofractionated stereotactic radiosurgery in the management of recurrent glioma. Int J Radiat Oncol Biol Phys 37:393–398

Shrieve DC, Alexander E III, Wen PY et al (1995) Comparison of stereotactic radiosurgery and brachytherapy in the treatment of recurrent glioblastoma multiforme. Neurosurgery 36:275–282

Stupp R, Mason WP, van den Bent MJ et al (2005) Radiotherapy plus concomitant and adjuvant temozolomide for glioblastoma. N Engl J Med 352:987–996

Stupp R, Hegi ME, van den Bent MJ et al (2006) Changing paradigms – an update on the multidisciplinary management of malignant glioma. Oncologist 11(2):165–180

Wong ET, Hess KR, Gleason MJ et al (1999) Outcomes and prognostic factors in recurrent glioma patients enrolled onto Phase II clinical trials. J Clin Oncol 17:2572–2579

Wurm RE, Kuczer DA, Schlenger L et al (2006) Hypofractionated stereotactic radiosurgery combined with topotecan in recurrent malignant glioma. Int J Radiat Oncol Biol Phys 66 (Suppl 4):S26–S32

14 Hypofractionated Shaped Beam Radiosurgery for Cranial and Spinal Chordomas

Moon-Jun Sohn, Dong-Joon Lee, and C. Jin Whang

14.1 Introduction

Chordomas are rare, malignant tumors that account for between 1 and 4% of all malignant spinal tumors and can occur anywhere between the clivus and the coccyx. The majority of chordomas are found in the rostral (skull base 25–35%) and caudal (sacrococcygeal, 50%) regions, but around 15% of chordomas occur in the mobile spine. Histologically, chordomas present as a lobular arrangement of cells with a mucinous matrix and tend to grow in cords, irregular bands or pseudoacinar forms. Chordomas occur about twice as frequently in males as in females and are predominantly found in adults and the elderly (Cohen-Gadol and Al-Mefty 2008; Pamir and Ozduman 2008; McMaster et al. 2001).

Chordomas are challenging to treat both because of their histology and invasive nature which frequently results in them infiltrating or surrounding critical structures such as the optic nerve, spinal cord, or brainstem (Lanzino et al. 2001). If left untreated, these tumors grow uncontrollably and thus surgical resection with adjuvant radiotherapy (RT) was usually considered the best treatment. However, complete and total surgical resection is very challenging and subsequent regrowth is frequently accompanied by some metastases (3–48%) (Arnautovic and Al-Mefty 2001). Until recently, eventual morbidity was usually inevitable due to local disease progression, partly because chordomas have a very high postsurgical recurrence rate even when apparent total surgical resection is achieved (Arnautovic and Al-Mefty 2001; Crockard et al. 2001). Final prognosis is dependent upon a range of factors including the age of the patient at onset, general health, history of surgery, and the extent of resection, the degree of adjuvant radiotherapy used, and the level of cytogenetic abnormalities (Pamir and Ozduman 2008; Lanzino et al. 2001; Tai et al. 2000). Key factors for success in treating chordomas include ensuring that the optimum dose and dose fraction are used with an appropriate clinical protocol and maintaining a regular pattern of follow-up examinations with aggressive retreatment of any signs of recurrence (Tai et al. 2000; Pamir et al. 2004). In the following section, we present a brief review of current literature, a summary of treatment options, historical outcomes, and case studies.

14.2 Brief History of the Application

Until very recently, surgical excision has been regarded as the most effective treatment, especially when accompanied by some form of postoperative adjuvant therapy due to the high potential for postsurgical recurrence (Pamir and Ozduman 2008; Pamir et al. 2004; Tai et al. 1995). The results of chemotherapy have been discouraging and thus radiation has been seen as the most effective and appropriate adjuvant treatment modality (Tai et al. 1995, 2000; Pamir et al. 2004). A historical review of the literature shows the use of conventional RT is limited by the tolerance of the surrounding critical organs and consequently suboptimal levels of radiation have had to be used resulting in poor outcomes (Pamir and Ozduman 2008; Tai et al. 1995). However, recent technical advances and improved protocols have

M.-J. Sohn (✉), D.-J. Lee, and C.J. Whang
Department of Neurosurgery, Novalis Radiosurgery Center, Inje University Ilsan Paik Hospital, 2240 Daehwa-dong, Ilsan Seo-Gu, Goyang, Gyeonggi Province, Korea
e-mail: mjsohn@paik.ac.kr

A.A.F. De Salles et al. (eds.), *Shaped Beam Radiosurgery*,
DOI: 10.1007/978-3-642-11151-8_14, © Springer-Verlag Berlin Heidelberg 2011

shown promising results and allowed the clinically effective targeting of chordomas. In the following section, we present a brief historical review of the various treatments that have been applied to chordoma.

14.2.1 Surgery with Adjuvant Support

Complete and total surgical resection offers the best clinical outcomes and prognosis, but it is technically very challenging as chordomas are outgrowths of the notochord. Even where radical resection is achieved, it must be supported by adjuvant treatment (Sekhar et al. 2001). Reports of radical resection for cranial-base chordoma range from 12 to 71.6% and the extent of surgery and degree of adjuvant treatment show a strong correlation with extended durable local control (Table 14.1; Sekhar et al. 2001; Gay et al. 1995; Colli and Al-Mefty 2001; Tamaki et al. 2001; Tzortzidis et al. 2006; Cho et al. 2008). Gay et al. (1995) observed a 5-year recurrence-free survival (RFS) rate of 65% for cranial-base chordoma in 67% of patients who underwent either total or near-total resection. However, for comparison, the overall 5-year RFS in chondrosarcoma patients was 90%. Colli and Al-Mefty (2001) reported 5-year RFS rates of 51% with surgery in 45% of cranial-base chordoma patients that had radical resection. Tamaki et al. (2001) reported surgical experience with 17 patients with cranial chordomas. Total or near-total resection was achieved in 30% of the group (5/17) overall, however, the majority of these cases (4 patients) were treated post-1990 using improved surgical techniques. In the patients treated after 1990, the 5-year RFS rate increased from 51% (overall) to 77% (post-1990) in line with the frequency of total or near-total resections. To summarize, surgical resection was always accompanied by some form of adjuvant radiotherapy or radiosurgery with long-term survival rates and improved quality of life being essentially determined by two main factors: the degree of resection and the level of adjuvant radiotherapy.

14.2.2 Conventional RT

Conventional RT is seen as the adjuvant treatment of choice; however, there is still some debate on the role and clinical effect of conventional RT in the treatment of chordomas (Table 14.2; Fuller and Bloom 1988; Romero et al. 1993; Catton et al. 1996). The correlation between increased disease-free survival rates and radiation dose is often highlighted in the literature with 5-year progression-free survival rates ranging from 15 to 70% and higher doses generally resulting in better outcomes. Fuller and Bloom (1988) suggested that better tumor control was associated with high doses (>55 Gy) and this was further supported by Romero et al. (1993) who reported that the progression-free interval was higher in patients who received doses of more than 48 Gy than in those who received less than

Table 14.1 Literature reviews for surgery with adjuvant treatment for skull-base chordomas

References	No	Surgical outcome (TR%/STR%/PR%)	Adjuvant Tx	5-year RFS (%)
Gay et al. (1995)	29	40/14/6 (67/23/10)	GK (20 Gy)/proton (50–75 CGE)/EBRT (50–60 Gy)	65
Colli and Al-Mefty (2001)	53	31/18/12 (49.2/28.6/22.2)	25 Proton/8 RT/17 no RT/3 Prev. RT (90.9/19.4/38.5/0% at 4-year RFS)	50.7
Tamaki et al. (2001)	17	5/9/3 (30/53/18)	13 C-RT (40–69 Gy, 50.8 Gy) 2 combined SRS (10–12 Gy)	51
Tzortzidis et al. (2006)	74	53/21 (71.6/28.4)	Proton/RS/EBRT (38/43/19%) 26 Reop (GTR) (35%)	41
Cho et al. (2008)	19	3/11/5 (15.8/57.9/26.3)	10 RT (50–70 Gy)/1 GK 19 Gy/3 RT+GK (15–16 Gy) 6 Reop	40

No number of patients, *TR* total or near-total resection, *STR* subtotal resection, *PR* partial resection, *Tx* treatment, *Reop* reoperation, *RFS* recurrence-free survival

Table 14.2 Conventional photon RT for cranial and spinal chordomas

References	No	Total dose (Gy)	Fx dose	Local progression (median)	5-year PFS (%)
Fuller and Bloom (1988)	25	55 (45–65) 60–65 (30–70)	1.5–1.7 1.6–1.7	<50 Gy vs. >55 Gy (19 vs. 45 months, $p=0.016$)	33
Romero et al.(1993)	18	50 (30–65)	–	<40 Gy vs. >48 Gy (31 vs. 0% at 5 PFS, $p=0.04$)	17
Catton et al. (1996)	45	50 (25–60)	2 Gy×25 8 Gy×3 3–4 Gy×11	<50 Gy vs. >50 Gy (no differences in PFS)	23

Fx fractionated, *PFS* progression-free survival

40 Gy (Romero et al. 1993). Catton et al. (1996) suggested that although his data showed no meaningful difference between <50 Gy and >50 Gy in terms of clinical effectiveness, doses of over 60 Gy would result in better outcomes. Conventional RT had little curative effect because the radiation doses used were insufficient but worked well as a palliative treatment although the options for re-treatment were limited due to the risk of radiation injury to adjacent normal tissue. Because of these limitations, the role of surgery has been emphasized; however, with improved means of delivering high-dose RT, it is anticipated that better clinical outcomes can be achieved without the need to perform technically challenging invasive procedures.

14.2.3 Gamma Knife Radiosurgery®

The results of recent studies into the treatment of chordomas using Gamma Knife surgery (GKS) have been encouraging, especially where small tumors are concerned (Table 14.3). Muthukumar et al. (1998) reported positive clinical results in early experiences at the University of Pittsburgh with GKS using 12–20 Gy, marginal dose (average 18 Gy) in nine chordoma patients with tumors of less than 30 cm^3. Martin et al. (2007) analyzed long-term follow-up results from the same institute for patients with mean tumors volumes of 9.8 cm^3 and marginal doses of 10.5–25 Gy (median dose of 16 Gy) and reported overall local tumor control of 62% at 5 years. Krishnan et al. (2005) reported encouraging results for 25 chordomas using GKS, (range 10–20 Gy, median marginal dose of 15 Gy). When analyzing the data for the 18 typical chordomas they treated, they achieved 42% local tumor control with less than 15 Gy at the margins and 63% local tumor control at four years with >15 Gy (marginal dose). Three of the patients required retreatment at 3 years and ten experienced complications (34%), but all those who experienced complications had been previously treated with EBRT. This indicates that 15 Gy at the tumor margins is safe and that the higher doses resulted in more positive clinical outcomes. Hasegawa et al. (2007) also concluded that a marginal dose of 15 Gy was the minimum required to achieve durable tumor control and with repeated treatments, they were eventually able to achieve 72% local tumor control.

When reporting their data, they focused mainly on the size of the tumor as being a key indicator for

Table 14.3 Gamma Knife radiosurgery for skull-base chordomas

References	No	TV (range)	Marginal dose (range)	Combined Tx	5-year LC rate (%)	5-year RFS (%)
Krishnan et al. (2005)	25	14.4 ml, (0.65–65.1)	15 Gy (10–20)	19 EBRT 50.4 Gy	52	67
Martin et al. (2007)	18	9.8 ml, (0.08–22)	16 Gy (10.5–25)	15 FRT 65 Gy 7 PBRT 75 CGE	62.9	–
Hasegawa et al. (2007)	27	19.7 ml, (0.4–94.3)	14 Gy (9–20)	7 reop. 14 repeated SRS	76	42

TV target volume (median), *Tx* treatment, *LC* local control, *RFS* recurrence-free survival successful outcomes. However, further review shows that smaller tumors were subjected to higher doses and, as has been reported elsewhere, this would also impact positively on clinical outcomes. In summary, a mean or median marginal dose of at least 15 Gy (range 10–12 Gy to 20–25 Gy) has been shown to achieve local tumor control even though the actual dose used varied according to tumor location, volume, and previous history of RT. Our review of the literature suggests that doses of greater than 18–20 Gy in a single session appear to be optimal for durable local tumor control.

14.3 Brief Summary of the Current Literature Results

Significant improvement in radiation-related technologies, radiosurgical techniques, and clinical protocols has led to better dose delivery, dose distribution, and planning (Knisely and Linskey 2006; Debus et al. 2000). As more sophisticated image-guided and 3D conformal planning systems are developed and commercialized for proton beam systems or advanced photon SRS/SRT, we may well see further improvements in the performance of radiosurgery for the treatment of chordoma. Below we have briefly reviewed the main advances in photon and particle beam therapies and the improved clinical results they have delivered (Tables 14.4 and 14.5).

14.4 Advances in LINAC-Based Stereotactic RT/RS

The need for higher doses and concern about complications have resulted in the development of advanced technologies such as beam shaping, intensity modulation, and image-guided stereotactic radiosurgery (IG-SRS) capable of more precise and conformal dose distributions. Knisely and Linskey (2006) reviewed the various radiosurgical modalities including Gamma Knife, proton beam, and advanced photon stereotactic radiosurgery and discussed the clinical outcomes achieved and compared them to conventional radiation treatment. They point out that effective targeting and dose escalation can be achieved using stereotactic techniques and intensity-modulated radiotherapy with

Table 14.4 Advanced LINAC radiosurgery/therapies for cranial and spinal chordomas

References	No	TV (range)	Marginal dose (Gy)	Dose/fraction	5-year LC rate (%)	5-year RFS (%)
Debus et al. (2000)	37	56 ml (17–215)	66.6 Gy	1.8 Gy × 37 Fx	50	–
Chang et al. (2001)	10	14.4 ml (0.65–65.1)	19.4 Gy at 93% IDL	18–24 Gy in 1–3 Fx	–	80% at 3 years
Gwak et al. (2005)	7	18.8 ml (10.4–31.5)	35 Gy at 82% IDL	21–43.6 Gy in 3–5 Fx	–	–
Present series	9	16.2 ml (0.8–35.7)	32 Gy at 80% IDL	32–40 Gy in 4–5 Fx	–	–

TV target volume (median), *Tx* treatment, *IDL* isodose line, *LC* local control, *RFS* recurrence-free survival

Table 14.5 Proton beam RT: particle beam RT for cranial and spinal chordomas

References	No	TV (range)	Target dose (CGE)	Dose per fraction (CGE)	5-year LC rate (%)	5-year PFS (%)
Hug et al. (1995, 1999, 2001)	14	–	74.6	1.8–2.0	53	53
	33		70.7	1.8	92	79
	53		68	1.8–1.92	–	64
Schulz-Ertner et al. (2002)	24	18.8 ml (10.4–31.5)	60 GyE (carbon ion)	3	90 (2 years)	83 (2 years)
Igaki et al. (2004)	13	27.4 ml (3.3–88.4)	72 (PR + photon)	2.0–3.5	46	42.2
Noel et al. (2005)	100	23 ml (1–125)	67 (PR + photon)	1.8–2.0	53.8 (4 years)	–
Weber et al. (2005)	18	16.4 ml (1.8–48.1)	74 (proton)	1.8–2.0	87.5 (3 years)	–

TV target volume (median), *PR* proton beam RT, *LC* local control, *PFS* progression-free survival multileaf collimators and advanced inverse 3D dose planning to spare critical structures while delivering relatively high conformal doses. Debus et al. (2000) reported successful outcomes from FSRT on 45 skull-base chordomas and chondrosarcomas between 1990 and 1997 using 3D conformal treatment planning. The total target doses were 66.6 Gy and 64.9 Gy, respectively, and they achieved a 5-year local control rate of 50% for 37 chordomas (100% for 8 chondrosarcomas).

Robotic arm-mounted LINAC SRS with the CyberKnife® (Accuray, Inc., Sunnyvale, CA) has been reported as achieving good results using a hypofractionated regimen. Chang et al. (2001) treated 10 chordomas (8 cranial base and 2 cervical lesions) with a mean dose of 19.4 Gy (range 18–24 Gy) and a maximum intratumoral dose of 27 Gy (range 24.1–33.1 Gy) at the 70–80% IDL in 1–3 fractions. There were no radiation-induced complications at an average of 4 years follow-up; however, two patients showed recurrent tumors and were retreated with combined surgery and RS. Gwak et al. (2005) also reported on seven chordomas and two chondrosarcomas with total tumor dose range of 21–43.6 Gy delivered in up to five fractions and concluded that treatment was effective over the 27-month follow-up. They experienced only one case of asymptomatic recurrence and two cases of radiation-induced myelopathy. Overall, the literature shows that using advanced precision radiosurgery in a hypofractionated regime can achieve effective tumor control with minimal risk of collateral damage. However, follow-up is still required to confirm the long-term efficacy of this treatment modality.

14.5 Charged Particle Radiation Therapies

It has been established that charged particle irradiation with proton, carbon, and heavy ions is both biologically effective and has advantages over conventional radiotherapy due to the sharp dose distribution (Bragg peak effect) which can allow better targeting of tumors.

Early experience with proton beam therapy and combined photon–proton RT resulted in significantly better outcomes than previously recorded with photon RT, and local tumor control rates of 73–76% at 5 years were achieved using between 65 and 83 GyE (Munzenrider and Liebsch 1999; Hug et al. 1995, 1999; Hug 2001; Noel et al. 2001). Recently, it has been reported that proton-only beam treatments resulted in improved tumor dose homogeneity and had less impact on adjacent critical organs as compared to combined photon–proton beam treatments (Noel et al. 2005; Feuvret et al. 2007). This was further supported by Pamir et al. (2004) who also found that 70 Gy provided adequate control for most patients and were associated with improved long-term survival rates. Spot-scanning proton radiation therapy is reportedly an improved adjuvant modality that offers high rates of tumor control in skull-base chordomas. Weber et al. (2005) obtained a 3-year local control rate of 87.5% from 28 patients with chordomas treated with 74 CGE. These results suggest that spot scanning is also an efficient and safe treatment for chordomas.

Other particle beam therapies such as carbon ion, heavy ions have been reported to produce positive clinical results over conventional photon RT (Igaki et al. 2004; Schulz-Ertner et al. 2002). However, long-term follow-up is required and dose-escalation trials are being conducted. Although positive results can be achieved with particle beam RT, the high costs and limited availability of treatment limit its use.

With the benefit of sophisticated software, precision targeting systems, and improved protocols, advanced photon-based radiosurgery or radiotherapy is able to achieve similar dose distribution and clinical outcomes as particle beam therapies at much lower cost and with greater accessibility. Further advances in radiosurgical techniques and our improved understanding of radiation biology should continue to deliver improved results in the form of better tumor control and reduced risk of normal tissue damage.

14.6 Outlining the Lesion: Defining the Target

The effective coverage and targeting of chordomas are key factors for success in treating them. For this reason, and to ensure that we sacrifice as little normal tissue as possible and minimize the irradiation of vital organs, defining the target is of critical importance. The first step is to obtain quality CT and MRI images and fuse these together to provide a coherent visualization of the tumor to enable the identification of critical structures such as the clival target, optic nerve, brainstem, and spinal cord or target.

Once the relevant organs and critical structures adjacent to the tumor have been outlined, an inverse treatment planning approach should be used to determine the optimum balance of tumor coverage with minimum normal tissue sacrifice and/or irradiation of critical structures. By carefully modeling, reviewing, and remodeling the effects of irradiation, it is possible to determine the most appropriate and effective dose, fractionation protocol, and system mode that should be used. Until recently, it was common to leave a relatively large margin to allow for positioning uncertainty and interfractional/intrafractional error. However, with the advent of high-precision intensity-modulated IG-SRS systems and hypofractionated treatment schedules, margins can be significantly reduced and this has a direct impact on clinical outcomes as better tumor coverage is directly correlated with positive clinical outcomes. Wherever possible, repositioning error should be less than a millimeter and always reduced to an absolute minimum.

14.7 Dose Decision

The radiation dose and treatment mode should be determined based on a combination of factors including the proximity of the tumor to critical structures, the size and shape of the tumor, and the radiation tolerance of surrounding tissues. The potential for undesirable effects limits the radiation volume and dose fractions that can be tolerated by the CNS and optimum dosing may not be possible because of proximity to critical dose-limiting structures such as the brainstem, optic nerve, etc. Wherever possible, both high conformity and selectivity should be used. For spinal chordomas, however, it may be better to accept a reduced level of selectivity and sacrifice some normal tissue, such as muscle, to achieve better tumor coverage.

For spinal chordoma, intensity-modulated radiosurgery (IMRS) with the higher dosages it allows can deliver better clinical outcomes, albeit with substantially greater volumes of normal tissue receiving raised doses of radiation. For cranial chordoma, the use of a more selective treatment mode such as the dynamic conformal arc on a Novalis® Radiosurgery System (Brainlab AG, Feldkirchen, Germany) can help reduce normal tissue damage while achieving maximum tumor coverage. In cases where the tumor is located far enough away from critical structures, however, a conformal beam mode will provide better conformity and selectivity with lower external beam doses.

14.8 Targeting Issues

To define target coverage and adequate dose delivery, DVH (dose-volume histogram) analysis of both the tumor and critical structures should be conducted and dosimetric decisions made based on the conformity index, tumor coverage, and extent of normal tissue irradiation.

For the purposes of target definition, GTV may be considered equivalent to CTV at authors' institute. The use of treatment mode varies depending on the locations of the tumors.

Dose planning for a patient with spinal chordoma was shown in Fig. 14.1. We were able to achieve 98% tumor coverage at the 80% IDL with only 10% normal tissue irradiation and successfully avoid the esophagus and trachea using IMRS and a hypofractionated dose

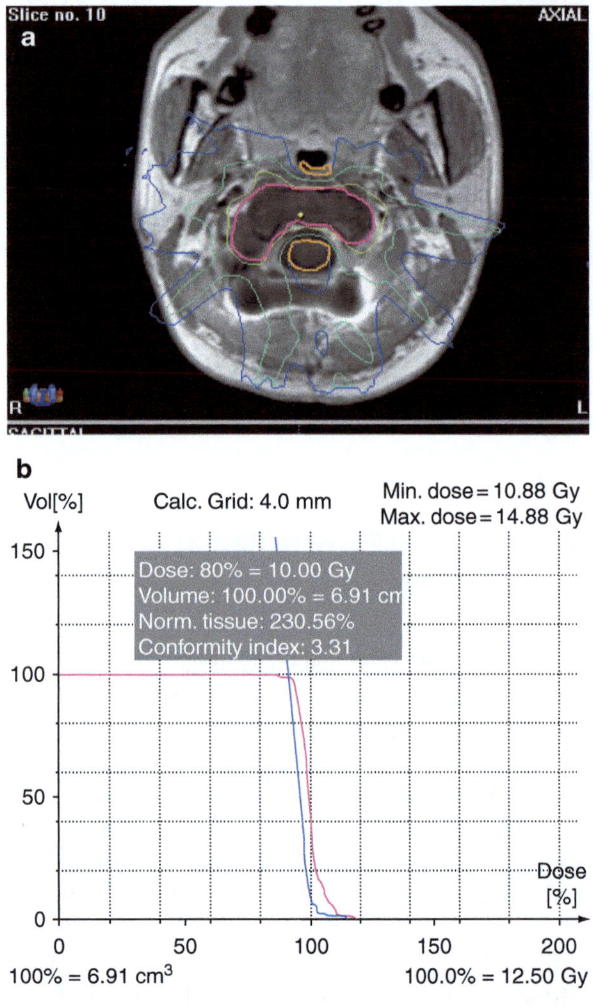

Fig. 14.1 Dose planning for a patient with spinal chordoma

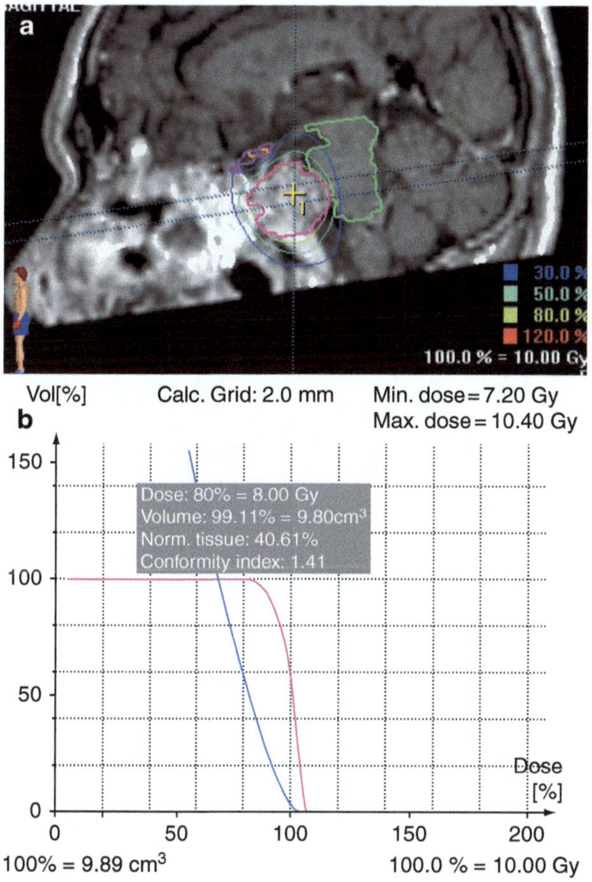

Fig. 14.2 DVH analysis for a patient with clival chordoma using dynamic arc shows

regimen, 8 Gy×4. The histogram shows complete target coverage at the 80% isodose line with a conformity index of 3.31. Note the increased conformity index as a result of using IMRS, thus helping to avoid undesirable irradiation of critical organs.

Figure 14.2 showed DVH analysis for a patient with clival chordoma using dynamic arc. This shows greater than 98% tumor coverage at the 80% IDL with 9% irradiation of normal tissue. This approach showed better conformity with a higher concentration of radiation focused on the target than when the dynamic arc mode was used.

14.9 Case Illustrations

Case 1. A 47-year-old male patient with clival chordoma underwent biopsy of the lesion to confirm the diagnosis. He underwent hypofractionated radiosurgery as the primary treatment modality. We prescribed hypofractionated scheme of 8 Gy×5. A year after radiosurgery, the tumor was completely resolved as shown in Fig. 14.3.

Case 2. A 63-year-old male patient presented with sacral chordoma. He had previously undergone two radical resections, but the tumor eventually recurred. We treated the recurrent tumor with hypofractionated stereotactic irradiation (8 Gy×4) with intensity modulation. Without the option of SRS, we would have had no choice but to conduct a third radical resection of the recurrent lesion. After radiosurgery, the lesion gradually reduced in size over a period of 24 months (Fig. 14.4).

14.10 Discussion

A review of current literature and our own clinical experience strongly suggest that chordomas are best treated aggressively with high BED and maximum tumor coverage (Pamir et al. 2004; Tai et al. 1995; Chang et al. 2001; Gwak et al. 2005). The use of lower doses or reduced tumor coverage may prove counterproductive by failing to achieve effective tumor control while limiting future treatment options. Pamir and Ozduman (2008) have reported that radiation doses of 70 Gy are adequate to provide lasting tumor control (especially for chondrosarcomas) and aggressive tumor resection is related to improved survival rates due to decompression of the neutral elements and usually provides symptomatic relief. The average survival period for untreated chordomas is only 28 months from the onset of symptoms; however, studies show that both radical resection and high-dose radiation, in particular proton beam therapy, usually result in improved long-term survival rates although most tumors recur with time (Colli and Al-Mefty 2001; Tzortzidis et al. 2006; Hug et al. 1999; Hug 2001). Pamir and Ozduman (2008) also found that poor prognostic factors were age (<5 years), subtotal resection, and cytogenetic abnormalities. Patients with chondroid chordomas showed better prognosis than those with chordomas. Tumors in adult patients with sacrococcygeal and vertebral chordomas were most likely to metastasize. The location of the metastases varied and they could occur almost anywhere, even in the lungs, fat tissue graft sites, and other distal sites; however, the most common sites were in bone or skin tissue. Metastases were rarely encountered immediately after

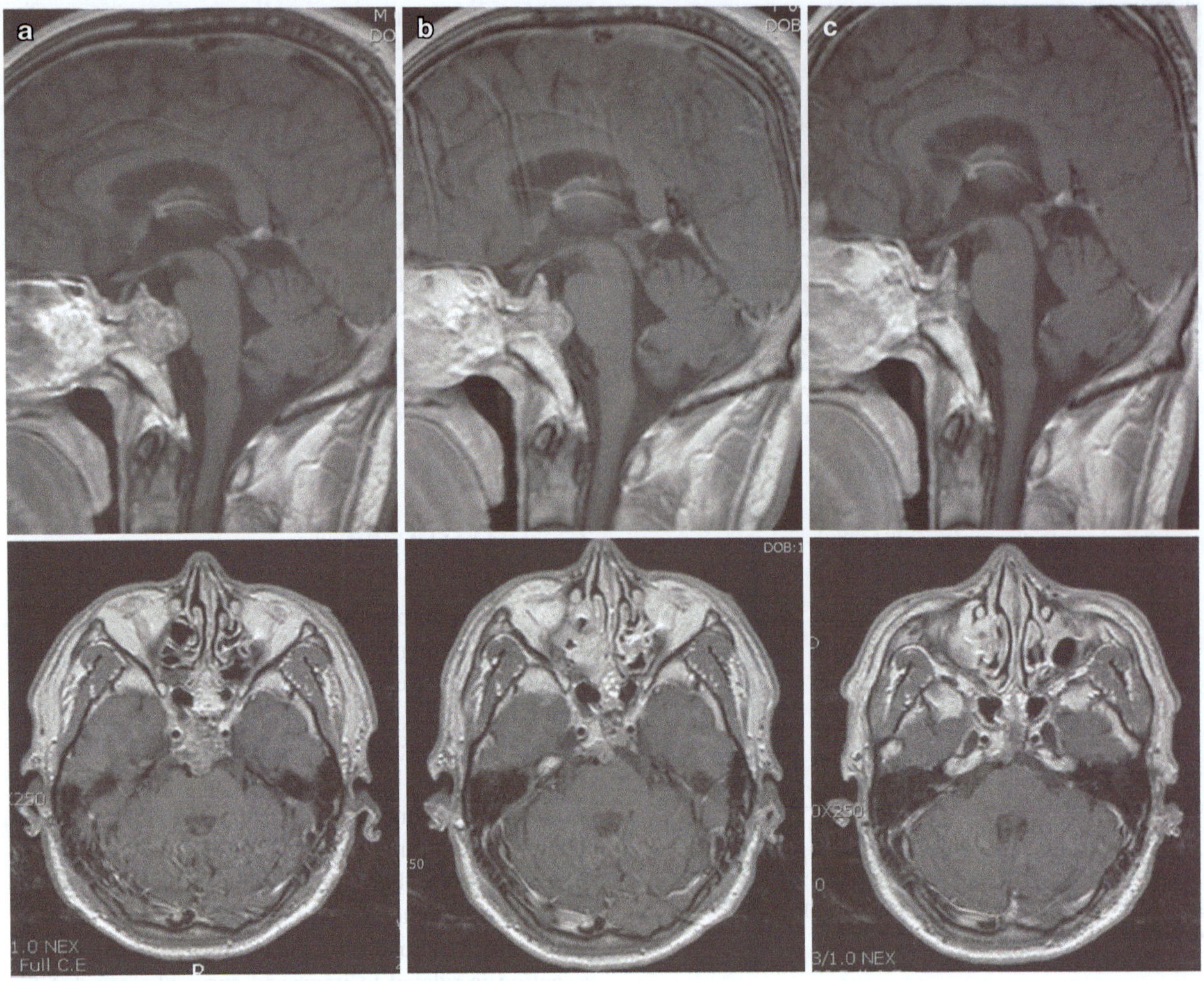

Fig. 14.3 MR images show tumor before and after surgery. Following treatment, the tumor is reduced in volume to a point where its presence has no clinical impact. (**a**) Prior to the treatment, the mass of the clival chordoma can be seen compressing the brainstem. (**b**) At 6 months after Tx, the tumor is significantly smaller. (**c**) One year after treatment, the tumor is insignificant in size

initial diagnosis but were relatively common along the operative route following resection with reports of metastases due to seeding running as high as 7.3%.

The avoidance of complications is a major factor in treatment planning. The most commonly reported complications are endocrine dysfunction, and temporal lobe, brain stem or spinal cord injury accompanied by visual loss, hearing loss, and/or memory impairment and myelopathy. A review of the literature indicates between 26 and 84% endocrine dysfunction after proton beam therapy, 8–20% visual complications, and 2.2–13% temporal lobe complication within 5-years of treatment (Pamir and Ozduman 2008; Gwak et al. 2005; Hug et al. 1999; Debus et al. 1997). Complications are most common 14–45 months after treatment and increase with time. Risk factors include higher doses than 50 CGE to the pituitary axis and higher than 70 CGE to the pituitary gland. Krishnan et al. (2005) reported radiation-related complications such as cranial nerve deficits, radiation necrosis, and pituitary dysfunction; all of the patients that suffered complications had had previous radiation treatment.

The use of advanced radiosurgical technology and protocols has also been correlated with high levels of tumor control and decreased toxicity in a substantial number of cancers.

Although long-term follow-up is still required, our experience shows that high BED's and high levels of

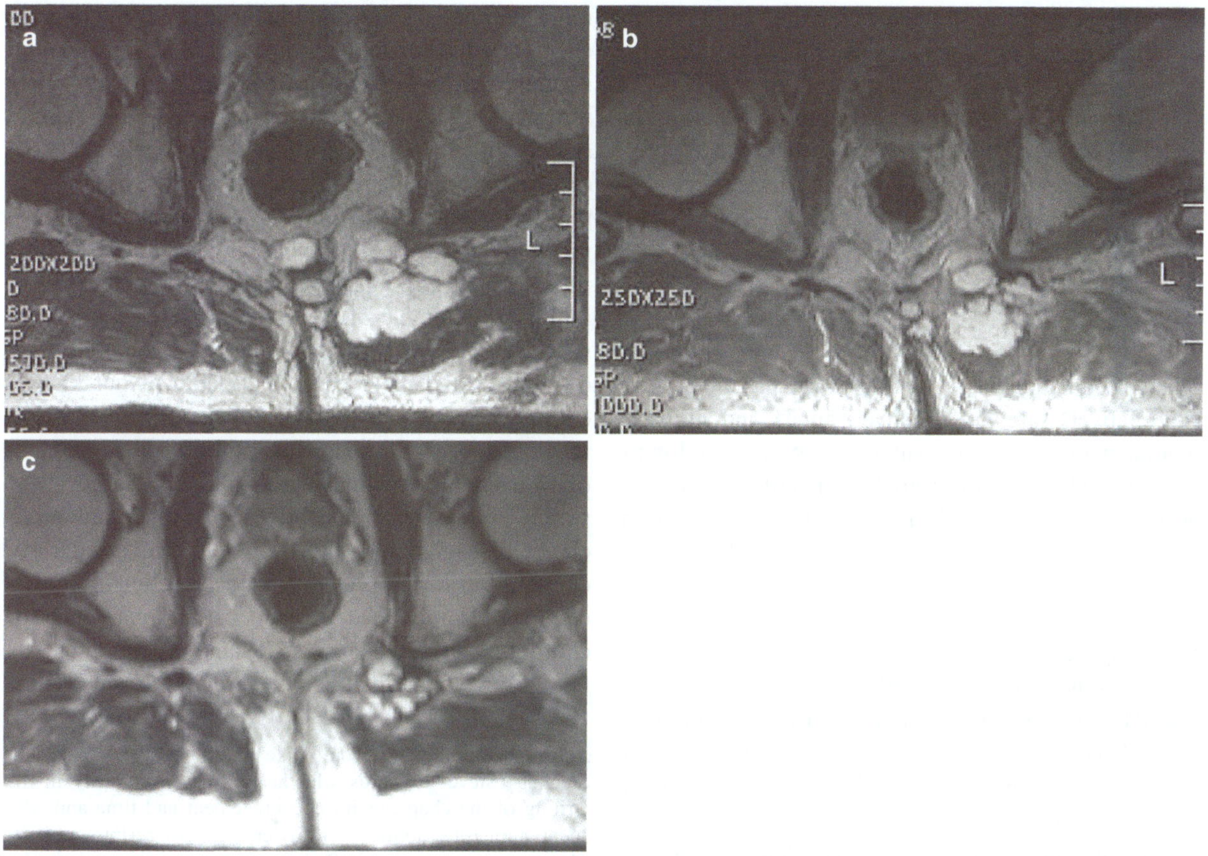

Fig. 14.4 Images above show the recurrent sacral chordoma (**a**: pre-radiosurgical MRI). Follow-up MRI at 12 and 24 months post-SRS reveals that serial changes of the tumors (**b** and **c**) which tumor is effectively controlled over time

tumor coverage results in better clinical outcomes and that by leveraging our knowledge of anatomy, modern technical advances such as intensity modulation, and recently developed protocols, BEDs of up to 83 Gy $\alpha/\beta=5$, can be used resulting in the best possible clinical outcomes while minimizing the negative impact on surrounding critical organs and normal tissue.

Chordomas can be effectively controlled in various ways. Highly targeted, conformal, high-dose radiosurgery is probably the most effective treatment available at this time (Muthukumar et al. 1998; Martin et al. 2007; Krishnan et al. 2005; Hasegawa et al. 2007; Knisely and Linskey 2006; Debus et al. 2000; Chang et al. 2001; Gwak et al. 2005). Care must be taken to select the most appropriate system, mode, dose, and clinical protocol, but by taking into account all these factors, chordoma can be effectively controlled and patients can benefit from extended, symptom-free life span. The results that we have achieved using IG-SRS compare favorably with the results achieved with heavy beam particle therapy and proton therapy. When treating chordomas, conservative dose planning and/or concerns about damaging adjacent critical structures may result in suboptimal doses being used. The tolerance of normal tissue to radiation varies according to its structure. While it is important not to underestimate the potential for damage to surrounding critical organs, it is equally important to recognize that the use of suboptimal doses may not have the desired clinical impact and may limit future treatment options. If suboptimal doses must be used, careful follow-up should be conducted and the use of a booster dose considered.

In summary, when it is not possible to apply the desired maximum BED because of the location, proximity to critical organs, or size of the tumor, it is especially important to observe and monitor regression and consider re-treatment not only when there are signs of regrowth but also when the tumor has reduced in size.

When the tumor has stopped regressing and GTV is sufficiently reduced, a window of opportunity may be present for aggressive re-treatment without unacceptable damage to surrounding normal tissue resulting in greatly improved clinical outcomes and longer progression-free survival rates.

14.11 Conclusion

Shaped beam radiosurgery using Novalis Radiosurgery is a relatively safe and effective primary and adjuvant treatment modality for cranial and spinal chordomas and can, when carefully applied, result in extended progression-free survival and local tumor control. High radiation doses of >83 and up to 104 Gy (BED $\alpha/\beta=5$), administered as a single dose or by a hypofractionated protocol on tumors of smaller volume resulted in achieving better local control. For larger tumors, the prognosis is less certain and surgical resection followed by SRS may be required to achieve the optimum clinical outcome. Based on current research and our own clinical experience, it would seem that a number of factors contribute to a positive clinical outcome.

An early diagnosis helps a great deal as this also usually also means smaller tumor volumes. The avoidance of repeated surgical intervention may help as it reduces surgical morbidity and the likelihood of seeding. Low-dose and/or large-scale radiation therapy may prove counterproductive by limiting future available treatment options. Targeted, high conformity, high-dose radiosurgery with a high degree of tumor coverage results in better clinical outcomes.

The use of a relevant visualization and treatment planning protocol can contribute significantly to dose planning and therefore clinical outcomes.

14.12 Future Directions

Since IGSRS is a relatively young field of medicine, the potential for improvements in protocols, technology, and our understanding of the clinical applications of radiation are excellent. In terms of the technology, we can expect improvements in software and hardware, providing better anatomical data, and simpler more automated setup and treatment. Image data management will probably be improved, and visualization systems will probably be integrated to provide better information on the effects of a particular dose regime and treatment modality, thus enabling better clinical decisions to be made. Multi-mode systems are currently being developed as are systems that will allow a much greater degree of positioning accuracy and take into account irregular movements allowing for the improved treatment of the lungs and other mobile tissue. New clinical protocols are continually being developed, and the breadth and depth of our knowledge of the clinical uses of SRS make this a very exciting field to be working in. Not so long ago the treatment of even small chordomas without invasive surgery was simply not an option, today it may be the treatment of choice, especially for those that are diagnosed early enough. Further improvements in our clinical knowledge will surely lead to even better treatments for chordomas using advanced SRS and probably help us in treating other equally challenging tumors as well.

Acknowledgments I would like to offer special thanks to Stephen (Steve) Edwards who helped me enormously in the writing of the chapter with encouragement and time and who spent numerous hours poring over the manuscript with me. Thanks are also due to Ms. Park Tae Hyun, (Jennie; student who is studying in Marine biology BSc course at the University of St. Adrews, UK) for her secretarial support and data organization which was particularly helpful.

References

Arnautovic K, Al-Mefty O (2001) Surgical seeding of chordomas. Neurosurg Focus 10:E7

Catton C, Sullivan B, Bell R, Laperriere N, Cummings B, Fornasier V, Wunder J (1996) Chordoma: long-term follow-up after radical photon irradiation. Radiother Oncol 41: 67–70

Chang SD, Martin DP, Lee E, Adler JR (2001) Stereotactic radiosurgery and hypofractionated stereotactic radiotherapy for residual or recurrent cranial base and cervical chordomas. Neurosurg Focus 10:E5

Cho YH, Kim JH, Khang SK, Lee JK, Kim CJ (2008) Chordomas and chondrosarcomas of the skull base: comparative analysis of clinical results in 30 patients. Neurosurg Rev 31: 35–43

Cohen-Gadol AA, Al-Mefty O (2008) Skull base tumors. In: Bernstein M, Berger MS (eds) Neuro-oncology. The essentials, 2nd edn. Thieme, New York, pp 327–329

Colli B, Al-Mefty O (2001) Chordomas of the skull base: follow-up review and prognostic factors. Neurosurg Focus 10:E1

Crockard HA, Steel T, Plowman N, Singh A, Crossman J, Revesz T, Holton JL, Cheeseman A (2001) A multidisciplinary team approach to skull base chordomas. J Neurosurg 95:175–183

Debus J, Hug EB, Liebsch NJ, O'Farrel D, Finkelstein D, Efird J, Mnzenrider JE (1997) Brainstem tolerance to conformal radiotherapy of skull base tumors. Int J Radiat Oncol Biol Phys 39:967–975

Debus J, Schulz-Ertner D, Schad L, Essig M, Rhein B, Thillmann CO, Wannenmacher M (2000) Stereotactic fractionated radiotherapy for chordomas and chondrosarcomas of the skull base. Int J Radiat Oncol Biol Phys 47:591–596

Feuvret L, Noel G, Weber D et al (2007) A treatment planning comparison of combined photon–proton beams versus proton beams – only for the treatment of skull base tumors. Int J Radiat Oncol Biol Phys 69(3):944–954

Fuller DB, Bloom JG (1988) Radiotherapy for chordoma. Int J Radiat Oncol Biol Phys 15:331–339

Gay E, Sekhar LN, Rubinstein E, Wright DC, Sen C, Janecka I, Snyderman CH (1995) Chordomas and chondrosarcomas of the cranial base: results and follow-up of 60 patients. Neurosurgery 36:887–897

Gwak HS, Yoo HJ, Youn SM, Chang U, Lee DH, Yoo SY, Rhee CH (2005) Hypofractionated stereotactic radiation therapy for skull base and upper cervical chordoma and chondrosarcoma: preliminary results. Stereotact Funct Neurosurg 83: 233–243

Hasegawa T, Ishii D, Kida Y, Yoshimoto M, Koike J, Iizuka H (2007) Gamma Knife surgery for skull base chordomas and chondrosarcomas. J Neurosurg 107:752–757

Hug EB (2001) Review of skull base chordomas: prognostic factors and long-term results of proton-beam radiotherapy. Neurosurg Focus 10:E11

Hug EB, Fitzek MN, Liebsch NJ, Munzenrider JE (1995) Locally challenging osteo- and chondrogenic tumors of the axial skeleton: Results of combined proton and photon radiation therapy using three-dimensional treatment planning. Int J Radiat Oncol Biol Phys 31:467–476

Hug EB, Loredo LN, Slater JD, Devries A, Grove RI, Schaefer RA, Rosenberg AE, Slater JM (1999) Proton radiation therapy for chordomas and chondrosarcomas of the skull base. J Neurosurg 91:432–439

Igaki H, Tokuuye K, Okumura T, Sugahara S, Kagei K, Hata M, Ohara K, Hashimoto T, Tsuboi K, Takano S, Matsumura A, Akine Y (2004) Clinical results of proton beam therapy for skull base chordoma. Int Radiat Oncol Biol Phys 60: 1120–1126

Knisely JPS, Linskey ME (2006) Less common indications for stereotactic radiosurgery or fractionated radiotherapy for patients with benign brain tumors. Neurosurg Clin N Am 17:149–167

Krishnan S, Foote RL, Brown PD, Pollock BE, Link MJ, Garces YI (2005) Radiosurgery for cranial base chordomas and chondrosarcomas. Neurosurgery 56:777–784

Lanzino G, Dumont AS, Lopes BS, Laws ER (2001) Skull base chordomas: overview of disease, management options, and outcome. Neurosurg Focus 10:E12

Martin JJ, Niranjan A, Kondziolka D, Flickinger JC, Lozanne KA, Lunsford LD (2007) Radiosurgery for chordomas and chondrosarcoma of the skull base. J Neurosurg 107: 758–764

McMaster ML, Goldstein AM, Bromley CM, Ishibe N, Parry DM (2001) Chordoma: incidence and survival patterns in the United States. 1973–1995. Cancer Causes Control 12: 1–11

Munzenrider J, Liebsch N (1999) Proton therapy for tumors of the skull base. Strahlenther Onkol 175:57–63

Muthukumar N, Kondziolka D, Lunsford LD, Flickinger JC (1998) Stereotactic radiosurgery for chordoma and chondrosarcoma: further experiences. Int J Radiat Oncol Biol Phys 41:387–392

Noel G, Habrand JL, Mammar H, Pontvert D, Haie-Meder C, Hasboun D, Moisson P, Ferrand R, Beaudre A, Boisserie G, Gaboriaud G, Mazal A, Kerody K, Schlienger M, Mazeron JJ (2001) Combination of photon and proton radiation therapy for chordomas and chondrosarcomas of the skull base: the centre de protontherapie d'Orsay experience. Int J Radiat Oncol Biol Phys 52:392–398

Noel G, Feuvret L, Calugaru V, Dhermain F, Mammar H, Haie-Meder C, Pontvert D, Hasboun D, Ferrand R, Nauray C, Boisserie G, Beaudre A, Gaboriaud G, Mazal A, Habrand JL, Mazeron JJ (2005) Chordomas of the base of the skull and upper cervical spine: one hundred patients irradiated by a 3D conformal technique combining photon and proton beams. Acta Oncol 44:700–708

Pamir MN, Ozduman K (2008) Tumor-biology and current treatment of skull-base chordomas. In: Pickard J (ed) Advances and technical standards in neurosurgery, vol 3. Springer, Austria, pp 35–129

Pamir MN, Kilic T, Ture U, Ozek MM (2004) Multimodality management of 26 skull-base chordomas with 4-year mean follow-up: experience at a single institution. Acta Neurochir (Wien) 146:343–354

Romero J, Cardenes H, la Torre A, Valcarcel F, Magallon R, Regueiro C, Aragon G (1993) Chordoma: results of radiation therapy in eighteen patients. Radiother Oncol 29: 27–32

Schulz-Ertner D, Haberer T, Jakel O, Thilmann C, Kramer M, Enghardt W, Kraft G, Wannenmacher M, Debus J (2002) Radiotherapy for chordomas and low-grade chondrosarcomas of the skull base with carbon ions. Int J Radiat Oncol Biol Phys 53:36–42

Sekhar LN, Pranatartiharan R, Chanda A, Wright DC (2001) Chordomas and chondrosarcomas of the skull base: results and complications of surgical management. Neurosurg Focus 10:E2

Tai PT, Craighead P, Bagdon F (1995) Optimization of radiotherapy for patients with cranial chordoma. A review of dose-response ratios for photons techniques. Cancer 75: 749–756

Tai PT, Craighead P, Liem SK, Jo BH, Stitt L, Tonita J (2000) Management issues in chordoma: a case series. Clin Oncol 12:80–86

Tamaki N, Nagashima T, Ehara K, Motooka Y, Barua KK (2001) Surgical approaches and strategies for skull base chordomas. Neurosurg Focus 10:E9

Tzortzidis F, Elahi F, Wright D, Natarajan SK, Sekhar LN (2006) Patient outcome at long-term follow-up after aggressive microsurgical resection of cranial base chordomas. Neurosurgery 59:230–237

Weber DC, Rutz HP, Pedroni ES, Bolsi A, Timmermann B, Verwey J, Lomax AJ, Goitein G (2005) Results of spot-scanning proton radiation therapy for chordoma and chondrosarcoma of the skull base: the Paul Scherrer institut experience. Int J Radiat Oncol Biol Phys 63:401–409

Unusual Skull Based Tumors Addressed with Single Dose or Fractionated Shaped Beam Stereotactic Radiation

15

Edward Melian, John Leonetti, Douglas Anderson, Vikram Prabhu, and Anil Sethi

15.1 Introduction

Stereotactic radiation is a reasonable approach for a multitude of rare tumors of the skull base. These tumors are infrequently resected completely without substantial morbidity. Examples of such tumors are paragangliomas, recurrent cancer of the nasopharynx, esthesioneuroblastoma, recurrent salivary gland carcinoma, and rhabdomyosarcoma in the orbit. Due to their rarity, there are no large series of tumors treated with shaped beam radiosurgery presented herein.

15.2 Paragangliomas

Paragangliomas of the head and neck are highly vascular tumors of neural crest origin that arise at the bifurcation of the carotid or more superiorly in the infratemporal region (glomus vagale), the jugular bulb (glomus jugulare), or in the middle ear (glomus tympanicum). Cervical tumors are usually amenable to surgical excision, but the larger glomus tumors of the temporal bone are more difficult to treat surgically (Boedeker et al. 2005). Complete surgical excision can be curative but is often associated with significant morbidity to the lower cranial nerves. Radiotherapy has been used for many years with clinical results approaching and, at times, surpassing those of surgical excision. Recent patient series by Hinerman et al. (2001) and Foote et al. (2002) are available for the use of conventional fractionated radiation and stereotactic radiosurgery, respectively. A review of the use of radiation for these head and neck paragangliomas by Mendenhall et al. (2001) is also available. While not obtaining marked radiographic responses, radiation is able to prevent most lesions from progressing. The local control rates for external beam radiotherapy range from 70% to 100% with long-term complication rates of 4–20%. Gamma Knife® (Elekta, Stockholm, Sweden) series show control rates close to 100% and minimal morbidity, but with only short-term follow-up. Tumor shrinkage occurs in a minority of patients (Krych et al. 2006; Saringer et al. 2002). A small series of five patients (4 de novo 1 recurrent) treated with a LINAC based system had two local recurrences, both within 4 years of treatment (Feigenberg et al. 2002).

E. Melian (✉) and V. Prabhu
Department of Radiation Oncology, Loyola University Medical Center, 2160 S First Ave, Maywood, IL 60153, USA and Department of Neurological Surgery, Loyola University Medical Center, Maywood, IL 60153, USA
e-mail: emelian@lumc.edu

J. Leonetti
Department of Otolaryngology, Loyola University Medical Center, Maywood, IL 60153, USA

D. Anderson
Department of Neurological Surgery, Loyola University Medical Center, Maywood, IL 60153, USA

A. Sethi
Department of Radiation Oncology, Loyola University Medical Center, 2160 S First Ave, Maywood, IL 60153, USA

15.2.1 Illustrative Case

A 63-year-old woman with a paraganglioma involving much of the temporal bone presented with intractable pain. She presented with hearing loss over 10 years when the diagnosis was made. Eight years after the diagnosis, she developed significant medically refractory

A.A.F. De Salles et al. (eds.), *Shaped Beam Radiosurgery*,
DOI: 10.1007/978-3-642-11151-8_15, © Springer-Verlag Berlin Heidelberg 2011

facial pain. The decision to treat with stereotactic radiation was based on the extent of the lesion and comorbidities. Due to the volume of the lesion and the superior extent, a 6-week course of intensity-modulated fractionated stereotactic radiotherapy was offered. A thermoplastic mask was made for immobilization. CT was obtained with mask and localizer. All CT and previously obtained narrow sliced MRI data were downloaded to the treatment planning computer. CT and MR images were fused, and tumor was delineated. A 3 mm expansion was made for the PTV. An 11 field intensity-modulated plan was created to deliver 50.4 Gy in 28 fractions to the PTV and 56 Gy in 28 fractions to the GTV. A pseudo structure was created on the treatment plan to push dose away from the adjacent brainstem and brain. As pain relief was part of the treatment goal, it was allowed a buildup of dose in the tumor center of 64 Gy (Fig. 15.1). The treatment was delivered with daily orthogonal images for isocenter verification with the ExacTrac® X-Ray positioning system (Brainlab AG, Feldkirchen, Germany).

Pain initially worsened during first few weeks of radiotherapy, but then began to decrease. Her narcotic requirements decreased and her functional capacity

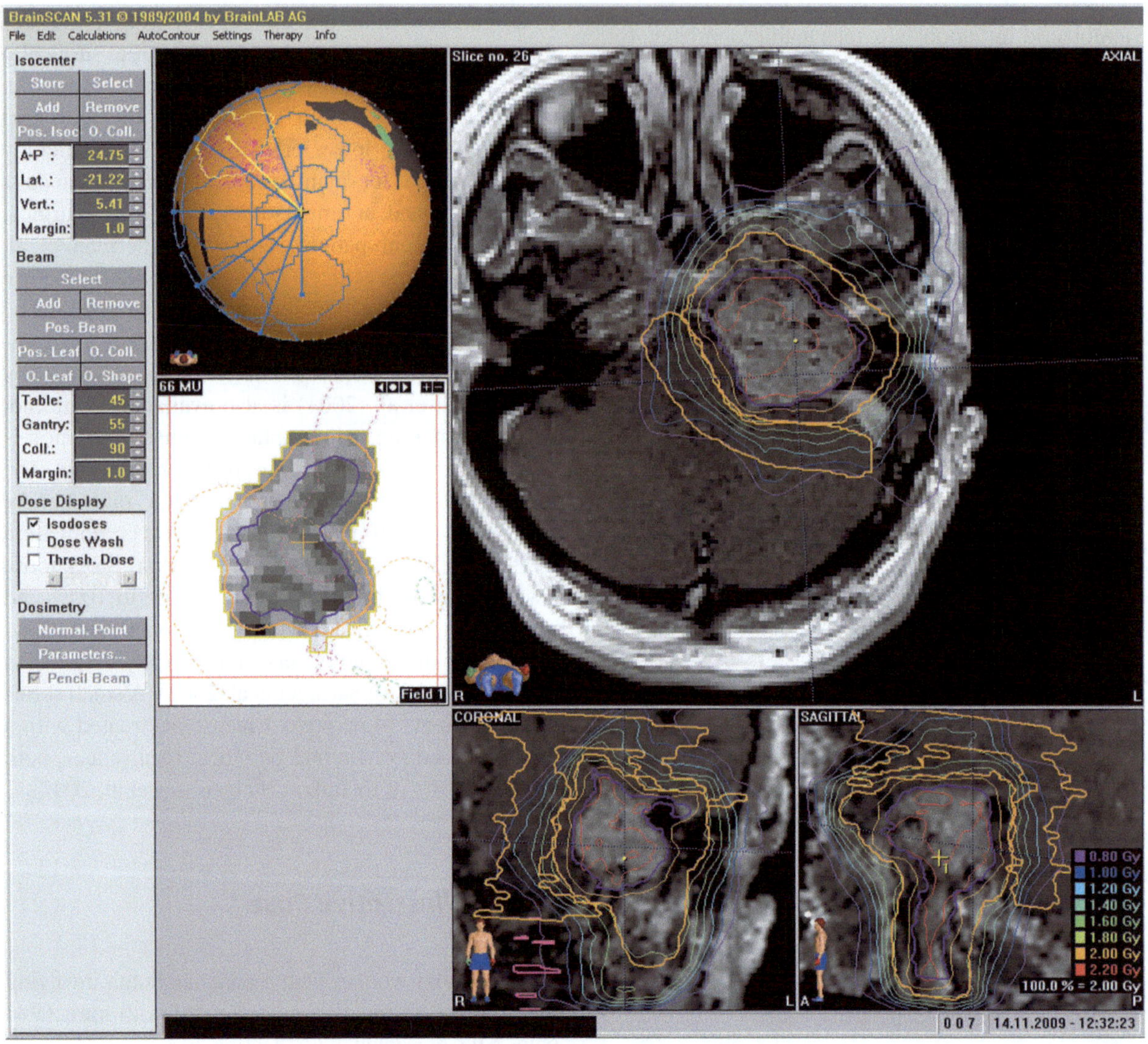

Fig. 15.1 Beam arrangement and isodose curves for de novo paraganglioma. Beams are distributed over the left hemisphere. A pseudo structure was created to push dose away from the brainstem and brain

improved. At 6 months posttreatment, she continues to have some pain but now tolerable with narcotic dose decreased by 80%. Follow-up MR scans showed minimal, if any, change in the lesion.

15.3 Recurrence of Nasopharyngeal Carcinoma

Local recurrence of nasopharyngeal carcinoma is a difficult clinical dilemma. While surgery can be effective for localized early recurrence, it is rarely used in more extensive disease (Hao et al. 2008). There is a growing body of literature on the use of single dose radiosurgery and fractionated stereotactic radiotherapy for salvage with results dependent mostly on local extension and volume of tumor at recurrence (Chua et al. 2007, 2009; O'Donell et al. 2008; Leung et al. 2009; Wu et al. 2007; Benfari et al. 2008). Large lesions are associated with poorer control rates and greater complication rates. (Chua et al. 2009). Often times, the tolerance dose to the optic chiasm and optic nerves has already been used during the initial course of treatment for the patient.

15.3.1 *Illustrative Case*

The patient presented with an intracranial recurrence of nasopharyngeal carcinoma 7 years following definitive chemo-radiotherapy. Initial treatment delivered dose to the optic chiasm and optic nerves to near tolerance. The patient clinically had already a sixth nerve palsy and facial pain. The medial edge of the recurrent tumor abutted the sella turcica. PET was useful in delineating the medial extent of tumor. The CT, PET, and MRI were used for optimal target delineation. The gross lesion with 3 mm PTV was targeted in this recurrent palliative setting. Ten shaped beams delivered with intensity modulation allowed decrease of dose to the optic nerves and chiasm (Fig. 15.2).

The patient experienced complete response to treatment and remained locally controlled at the left skull base over 2 years later, when he developed contralateral pain and was found to have progression in the contralateral nasopharynx extending to the right cavernous sinus, necessitating further treatment. As tolerance doses were not exceeded during the second treatment, it was possible to treat the contralateral side. At this third treatment, considering the distance from chiasm greater and his cranial nerve deficits in need of palliation, the scheme of 25 Gy in five fractions was chosen. Again, the patient experienced resolution of symptoms and radiographic response. MRI 1 year later showed continued control of both lesions.

15.4 Esthesioneuroblastomas

Esthesioneuroblastomas are midline lesions which present somewhat insidiously with loss of smell and taste with or without nasal congestion. They originate from the olfactory epithelium in the region of the cribriform plate and upper nasal cavity. As fractionated radiotherapy alone controls about a third of the lesions treated (Benfari et al. 2008), the surgery and postoperative radiotherapy provide local control for about two thirds of the lesions treated (Broich et al. 1997; Dulguerov et al. 2001; Loy et al. 2006). A small series of patients treated with endoscopic resection and postoperative radiosurgery showed acceptable in field control in a short follow-up, however with marginal failures (Unger et al. 2005). A recent surgical meta-analysis supports the use of endoscopic resection over open resection (Devaiah and Andreoli 2009), although this remains controversial (Levine 2009).

15.4.1 *Illustrative Case*

Herein is an example of a recurrent tumor along the anterior falx treated with radiosurgery. This lesion was found on surveillance MRI and was not symptomatic. The patient presented in 1998 with nasal congestion. Imaging disclosed a cribriform plate lesion. Craniofacial resection led to the histological diagnosis of Esthesioneuroblastoma. Surgery was followed by 60 Gy conventional radiotherapy. In 2004, recurrence in the cervical region led to further radiation therapy. She received bilateral fields with 64 Gy in 32 fractions, as well as concurrent cisplatinum chemotherapy. She developed esophageal fibrosis with consequent mild dysphagia, responding well to dilation. In 2006, recurrence measuring $1.5 \times 0.7 \times 1.5$ cm anterior falx

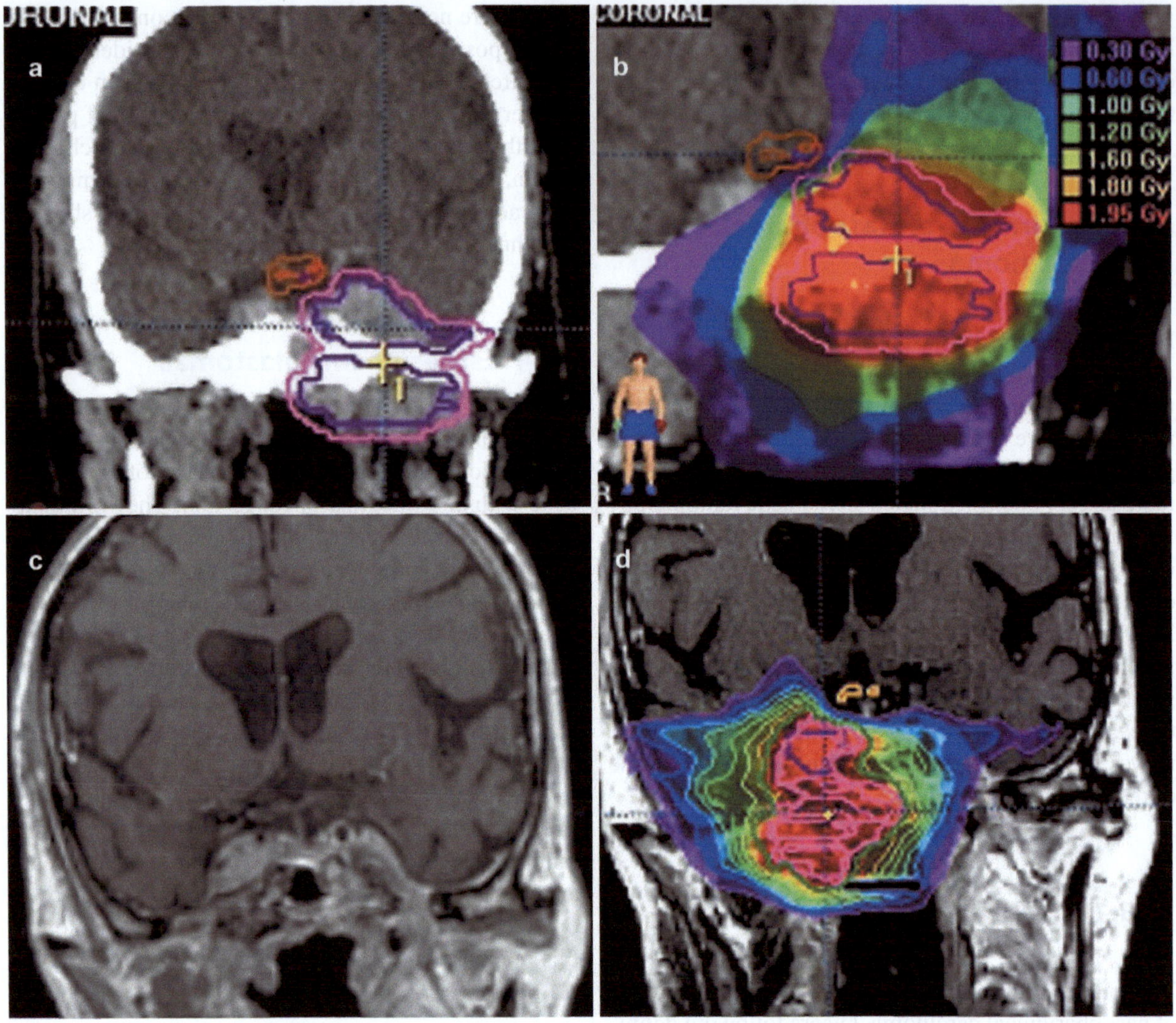

Fig. 15.2 Recurrent nasopharynx carcinoma (**a**) pre treatment, (**b**) treatment plan isodoses [May 2006] carving out region of optic nerves, and (**c**) August 2008 with tumor locally controlled but with contralateral recurrence, (**d**) treatment of contralateral disease

cerebri was detected on follow-up MRI. This recurrence was treated with stereotactic radiosurgery using a conformal beam approach. Such small lesions derive little, if any, benefit from intensity modulation planning.

The Brainlab Stereotactic head-frame was placed by the Neurosurgical team under local anesthetic and intravenous morphine. CT scan was obtained in the Brainlab localizer frame. CT and previously obtained thin sliced MRI scans were merged with the image fusion software. Axial and coronal MRI T1 with contrast images were used to delineate the target volume. A 12 shaped beam single isocenter plan was created to deliver 20 Gy to the 80% isodose at the periphery of the lesion. Coverage at 20 Gy was 100%, and conformality index was 1.8. She received her radiosurgery in the summer of 2006.

Nine months later, she developed some evidence of radionecrosis in the adjacent brain, symptomatic with headache. MRI T1godolinium-enhanced showed the area of breakdown of the blood–brain barrier and edema (Fig. 15.3). This was managed with steroids. In 2009, she developed an asymptomatic distant recurrence along the lateral convexity which was treated with surgery. She remained locally controlled in the anterior falx site.

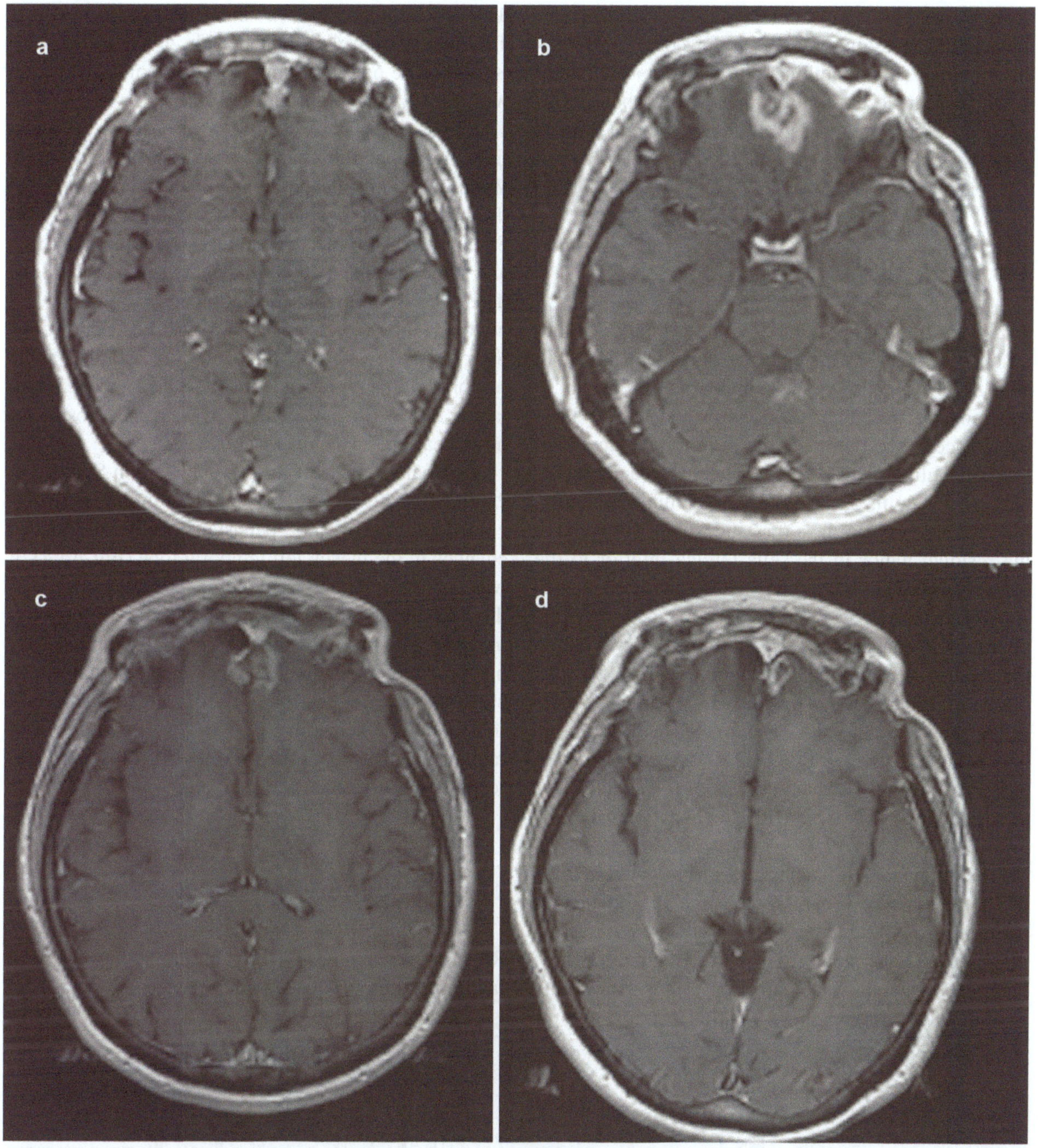

Fig. 15.3 (**a**) Pretreatment of recurrence, (**b**) post treatment necrosis at 9 months, (**c**) improvement of necrotic region at 13 months post treatment and (**d**) at 36 months post treatment with resolution of edema and injury

15.5 Adenoid Cystic Carcinomas

Adenoid cystic carcinomas are rare tumors of the upper aerodigestive tract which originate in minor and major salivary glands. They have a tendency to spread along nerves and have been noted to track the nerves back to the skull base (Barrett and Speight 2009; Hanna et al. 2007). Five-year survival can still be good even with temporal bone involvement (Leonetti et al. 2008); however, survival does not plateau and continues to decline even 15 years posttreatment. The standar treatment for these lesion is surgery followed by local radiation therapy. This combination yields approximately 80% 10-year local control rates with about 60% 10-year disease-free survival due to distant failure (Gomez et al. 2008; Chen et al. 2006).

15.5.1 Illustrative Case

A 29-year-old man presented with a primary adenoid cystic carcinoma of the right parotid gland in 1998. Resection was followed by radiotherapy 60 Gy in 30 fractions. In December 2002, he was found to have recurrence in the region of the sella turcica and right base of skull. This was treated with stereotactic radiotherapy 45 Gy in 25 fractions to a volume including the optic nerves. A radiosurgery boost was delivered to the residual tumor in the sella turcica inferior to the optic chiasm. This was done with the Radionics® radiosurgery system. It was felt to have reached the optic chiasmal tolerance dose. He developed low volume metastatic disease in the liver and lung which was just observed. Progression in the mid-clival region, inferior to the recurrence in 2002, was treated with radiosurgery using the Novalis® Radiosurgery system (Brainlab AG, Feldkirchen, Germany) in 2006. It was delivered 22 Gy to the 87% isodose with excellent control of the lesion.

The dominant liver metastasis was resected in 2007 as the lesion was progressing, while the other sites were relatively stable. In December 2007, he developed diplopia secondary to a sixth nerve palsy. There was progression in the left cavernous sinus. He was not a candidate for further surgery in this location, and the data on chemotherapy was not felt to be compelling. This progression was treated with 20 Gy to the 80% isodose. The optic chiasm maximum point pixel dose was 4.8 Gy. The right and left optic nerves received 1.5 Gy and 5.0 Gy, respectively. In order to keep this tight border at the chiasm, shaped beam was used. Within 2 months, the patient experienced resolution of the diplopia and regained lateral motion of the left eye. Since then, he has needed palliative radiotherapy to rib and spine lesions in 2008. In the late summer 2008, he developed symptomatic radiation necrosis in the left medial temporal lobe, leading to headache only. Steroids resolved the headache and radiographic response of the region of necrosis. Steroids were maintained in low dose, leading to avascular necrosis of a hip 1 year later. His hip was replaced.

Ophthalmoplegia of the left appeared in September 2009. MRI showed recurrence of the tumor in the left cavernous sinus and persistent radiation-induced changes in the mesial left temporal lobe (Fig. 15.4). It was not felt prudent to retreat this area due to previous dose received, progression within the high dose volume, and the presence of radiation injury already. He has been recommended to begin a bevacizumab-based chemotherapy regime after the hip surgery. This case illustrates the versatility of the novel techniques of radiation delivery and the protracted evolution of this resilient disease.

15.6 Rhabdomyosarcomas

Rhabdomyosarcomas of the orbit are among the most favorable of the soft tissue sarcomas in children. There is excellent long-term local control and survival (Crist

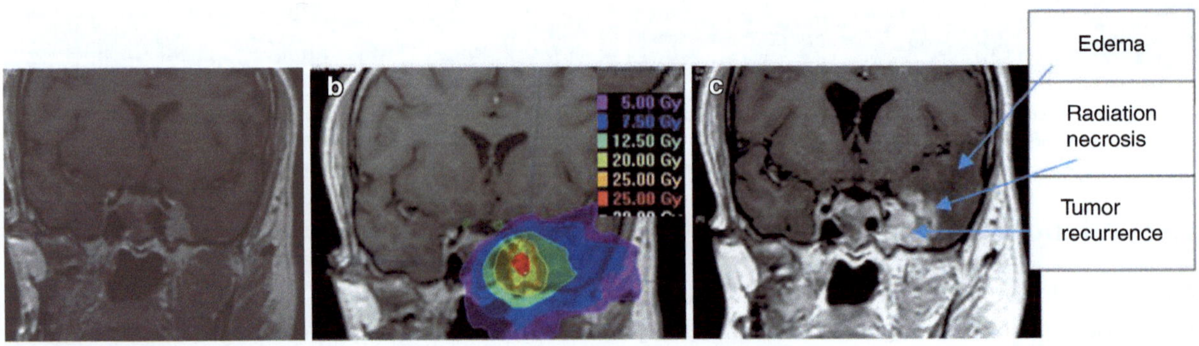

Fig. 15.4 (**a**) Left cavernous sinus recurrence, (**b**) shaped beam radiosurgery planning, and (**c**) radiation induced changes in the mesial temporal lobe

et al. 1995, 2001; Koscielniak et al. 1999; Rodary et al. 1988). Treatment with surgery which would involve loss of the eye is no longer acceptable as the results of radiation and chemotherapy are excellent (Crist et al. 2001; Meazza et al. 2006; Flamant et al. 1998). Conventional radiation can lead however to long-term difficulties with dry eye and changes in bone growth with consequent disfigurement. Stereotactic delivery with tight conformal fields and daily online image guidance to confirm setup allow for avoidance of these undesirable side effects. Stereotactic radiotherapy has been used in a limited number of patients with success (Combs et al. 2007).

15.6.1 Illustrative Case

A 33-month-old boy presented with left eye exophthalmos and ptosis. Ophthalmic exam under anesthesia found normal ocular mobility, normal intraocular pressures, and equally reactive pupils. Both upper and lower lids were noted to be edematous. MRI in 2007 disclosed a 2.1×1.6×1.1 cm mass in the anterosuperior aspect of the left orbit displacing the globe inferiorly (Fig. 15.5). It was contiguous with the left superior rectus muscle and the levator palpebrae superioris muscle. The optic nerve was encased. A fat plane separated the lesion from the lachrymal gland. Rhabdomyosarcoma of the orbit became the working diagnosis.

Excision biopsy of a density adherent to the medial portion of the orbit lesion led to dissection of the superior oblique tendon with a small amount of tumor left on the tendon to preserve function. Hematoxylin and eosin staining showed a small round blue cell tumor.

Based on the preliminary pathology, he had metastatic work-up with CT scan of chest under anesthesia, removal of surgical drain, left subclavian port placement, lumbar puncture, and bilateral bone marrow aspiration and biopsy. A bone scan was also done. These tests confirmed disease limited to the orbit. Once pathology confirmed diagnosis, he was started on vincristine/dactinomycin/cyclophosphamide (VAC) chemotherapy with the diagnosis of embryonic rhabdomyosarcoma Stage I Clinical Group III. He received a total of three cycles of the chemotherapy prior to being sent for radiotherapy to the original tumor bed.

Pre-stereotactic radiotherapy MRI of 2 months later showed resolution of the pre-chemotherapy mass. Minimal heterogeneous T2 signal and enhancement were seen in surgical bed. A thin sliced series was requested as well for use for image fusion for the stereotactic radiotherapy planning.

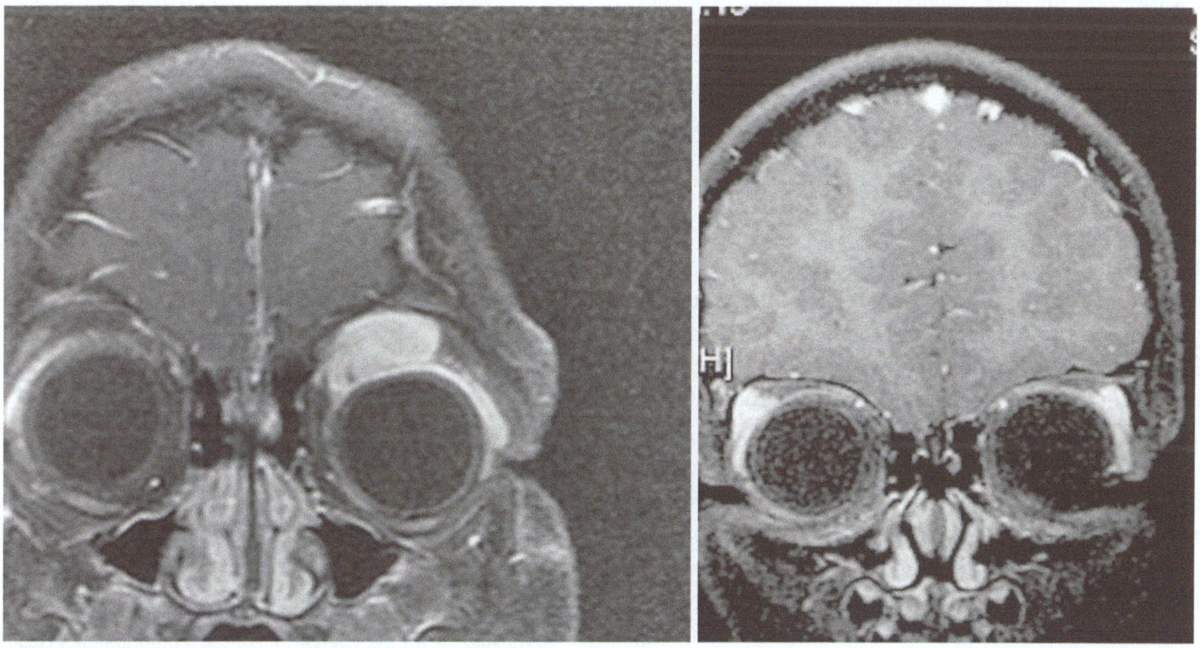

Fig. 15.5 Orbital rhabdomyosarcoma in 3-year-old boy at diagnosis and 18 months post subtotal surgery, chemotherapy, and radiotherapy

Due to his young age, simulation and treatment were done under anesthesia provided by a pediatric anesthesiologist. A mask immobilization was created by our simulation team. Care was taken to keep his head position slightly extended to help maintain his airway. Simulation CT was obtained in the immobilization mask. The pre-chemotherapy and post-chemotherapy MRIs were fused to the treatment planning CT. A target was created by noting the original tumor bed expanding the CTV while respecting barriers such as the bony roof of the orbit which did not appear to be violated by tumor. It was not felt that the lens could be spared; however, the dose was reduced to the lachrymal gland. Lachrymal gland tolerance per Children's Oncology group is 41.4 Gy while we wished to give 45 Gy in 25 fractions to the target. A plan was created using 12 non-coplanar shaped fields. As the size of the lesion was small, any advantage gained by intensity modulation was minimal; to minimize the child's time under anesthesia, the plan was without intensity modulation.

The stereotactic radiotherapy region was stable on serial follow-up scans for 14 months. Imaging 18 months later was reported normal. Ophthalmological follow-up confirmed 20/20 vision bilaterally, full ocular motion, and a very mild enophthalmos.

The use of the shaped beam therapy has helped maintain this child with a moist and useful eye. In addition, by limiting the high dose volume irradiated, it may also decrease the risk of a second malignancy (Spunt et al. 2001).

15.7 Conclusion

In each of these five illustrative cases, there is evidence of tumor response to radiation. The choice to use single dose or fractionated treatment was based upon lesion volume, proximity to optic nerves, optic chiasm, retina, and, to a lesser extent, tumor histology. Local control is possible for these rare and difficulty histology. Failures are most likely out of the field secondary to imaging limitations. Despite some failures, patients received benefit from the stereotactic radiation. These anecdotal case reports suggest value of stereotactic radiotherapy and the rationale for its application.

The radiation therapy benefit is well known for rhabdomyosarcomas, recurrent nasopharyngeal carcinoma, and de novo paraganglioma. There is less information on the treatment of recurrent esthesioneuroblastoma; however, the experience with de novo treatment of esthesioneuroblastoma makes it a reasonable treatment option in the recurrence setting. The role of dose escalation in the resilient adenoid cystic carcinoma is well known. Palliation of symptoms and delayed progression help maintain good quality of life. This report offers guidelines where reports of large series are not available.

References

Barrett AW, Speight PM (2009) Perineural invasion in adenoid cystic carcinoma of the salivary glands: a valid prognostic indicator? Oral Oncol 45(11):936–940

Benfari G, Fusconi M, Ciofalo A et al (2008) Radiotherapy alone for local tumour control in esthesioneuroblastoma. Acta Otorhinolaryngol Ital 28(6):292–297

Boedeker CC, Ridder GJ, Schipper J (2005) Paragangliomas of the head and neck: diagnosis and treatment. Fam Cancer 4:55–59

Broich G, Pagliari A, Ottaviani F (1997) Esthesioneuroblastoma: a general review of the cases published since the discovery of the tumour in 1924. Anticancer Res 17:2683–2706

Chen AM, Bucci MK, Weinberg V et al (2006) Adenoid cystic carcinoma of the head and neck treated by surgery with or without postoperative radiation therapy: prognostic features of recurrence. Int J Radiat Oncol Biol Phys 66(1):152–159

Chua DT, Wei WI, Sham JS et al (2007) Stereotactic radiosurgery versus gold grain implantation in salvaging local failures of nasopharyngeal carcinoma. Int J Radiat Oncol Biol Phys 69(2):469–474

Chua DT, Hung KW, Lee V et al (2009) Validation of a prognostic scoring system for locally recurrent nasopharyngeal carcinoma treated by stereotactic radiosurgery. BMC Cancer 9:131

Combs SE, Behnisch W, Kulozik AE et al (2007) Intensity modulated radiotherapy (IMRT) and fractionated stereotactic radiotherapy (FSRT) for children with head-and-neck-rhabdomyosarcoma. BMC Cancer 7:177

Crist W, Gehan EA, Ragab AH et al (1995) The third intergroup rhabdomyosarcoma study. J Clin Oncol 13:610–630

Crist W, Anderson JR, Meza JL et al (2001) Intergroup rhabdomyosarcoma study-IV: results for patients with nonmetastatic disease. J Clin Oncol 19:3091–3102

Devaiah AK, Andreoli MT (2009) Treatment of esthesioneuroblastoma: a 16-year meta-analysis of 361 patients. Laryngoscope 119(7):1412–1416

Dulguerov P, Allal AS, Calcaterra TC (2001) Esthesioneuroblastoma: a meta-analysis and review. Lancet Oncol 2:683–690

Feigenberg SJ, Mendenhall WM, Hinerman RW (2002) Radiosurgery for paraganglioma of the temporal bone. Head Neck 24(4):384–389

Flamant F, Rodary C, Rey A et al (1998) Treatment of non-metastatic rhabdomyosarcomas in childhood and adolescence. Results of the second study of the international society of paediatric oncology: MMT84. Eur J Cancer 34:1050–1062

Foote RL, Pollock BE, Gorman DA et al (2002) Glomus jugulare tumor: tumor control and complications after stereotactic radiosurgery. Head Neck 24:332–338

Gomez DR, Hoppe BS, Wolden SL et al (2008) Outcomes and prognostic variables in adenoid cystic carcinoma of the head and neck: a recent experience. Int J Radiat Oncol Biol Phys 70(5):1365–1372

Hanna E, Vural E, Prokopakis E et al (2007) The sensitivity and specificity of high-resolution imaging in evaluating perineural spread of adenoid cystic carcinoma to the skull base. Arch Otolaryngol Head Neck Surg 133(6):541

Hao SP, Tsang NM, Chang KP, Hsu YS et al (2008) Nasopharyngectomy for recurrent nasopharyngeal carcinoma: a review of 53 patients and prognostic factors. Acta Otolaryngol 128:473–481

Hinerman RW, Mendenhall WM, Amdur RJ et al (2001) Definitive radiotherapy in the management of chemodectomas arising in the temporal bone, carotid body and glomus vagale. Head Neck 23:363–371

Koscielniak E, Harms D, Henze G et al (1999) Results of treatment for soft tissue sarcoma in childhood and adolescence: a final report of the German cooperative soft tissue sarcoma study CWS-86. J Clin Oncol 17:3706–3719

Krych AJ, Foote RL, Brown PD, Garces YI, Link MJ (2006) Long-term results of irradiation for paraganglioma. Int J Radiat Oncol Biol Phys 65(4):1063–1066

Leonetti JP, Marzo SJ, Agarwal N (2008) Adenoid cystic carcinoma of the parotid gland with temporal bone invasion. Otol Neurotol 29(4):545–548

Leung TW, Victy Y, Wong W et al (2009) Stereotactic radiotherapy for locally recurrent nasopharyngeal carcinoma. Int J Radiat Oncol Biol Phys 75(3):734–741

Levine PA (2009) Would Dr. Ogura approve of endoscopic resection of esthesioneuroblastomas? An analysis of endoscopic resection data versus that of craniofacial resection. Laryngoscope 119:3–7

Loy AH, Reibel JF, Read PW et al (2006) Esthesioneuroblastoma: continued follow-up of a single institution's experience. Arch Otolaryngol Head Neck Surg 132(2):134–138

Meazza C, Ferrari A, Casanova M et al (2006) Rhabdomyosarcoma of the head and neck region: experience at the pediatric unit of the Istituto Nazionale Tumori, Milan. J Otolaryngol 35(1):53–59

Mendenhall WM, Hinerman RW, Amdur RJ et al (2001) Treatment of paragangliomas with radiation therapy. Otolaryng Clin N Am 34(5):1007–1020

O'Donell HE, Plowman PN, Khaira MK et al (2008) PET scanning and Gamma Knife H radiosurgery in the early diagnosis and salvage "cure" of locally recurrent nasopharyngeal carcinoma. Br J Radiol 81:26–30

Rodary C, Rey A, Olive D et al (1988) Prognostic factors in 281 children with nonmetastatic rhabdomyosarcoma (RMS) at diagnosis. Med Pediatr Oncol 16:71–77

Saringer W, Kitz K, Czerny C et al (2002) Paragangliomas of the temporal bone: results of different treatment modalities in 53 patients. Acta Neurochir 144(12):1255–1264, Discussion 1264

Spunt SH, Meza JL, Anderson JR et al (2001) Second malignant neoplasms (SMN) in children treated for rhabdomyosarcoma: a report from the intergroup rhabdomyosarcoma studies (IRS) I–IV. Children's Oncology Group Soft Tissue Sarcoma Committee, Arcadia

Unger F, Haselsberger K, Walch C, Stammberger H, Papaefthymiou G (2005) Combined endoscopic surgery and radiosurgery as treatment modality for olfactory neuroblastoma (esthesioneuroblastoma). Acta Neurochir (Wien) 147:595–602

Wu SX, Chua DT, Deng ML et al (2007) Outcome of fractionated stereotactic radiotherapy for 90 patients with locally persistent and recurrent nasopharyngeal carcinoma. Int J Radiat Oncol Biol Phys 69(3):761–769

Skull-Base Malignant Tumors

16

Yoshimasa Mori

16.1 Background

Skull base malignant tumors are challenging situations because they often involve critical structures, including cranial nerves. This study reports the treatment results of Novalis® Radiosurgery (Brainlab AG, Feldkirchen, Germany) fractionated stereotactic radiotherapy (SRT) for skull base metastases from other visceral carcinomas, and skull base recurrence of head and neck malignant tumors. Novalis stereotactic radiotherapy can give high dose to the tumors sparing normal structures. As Novalis Radiosurgery has an X-ray image analysis system (ExacTrac® X-Ray, Brainlab AG, Feldkirchen, Germany) to correct patient position before each treatment session, skull base lesions are exactly targeted after localization of skull base bone structures. SRT has the radiobiologic advantage of conventional fractionation in addition to the mechanical precision of stereotactic devices.

16.2 Materials and Methods

We treated 24 patients with malignant skull base tumors, including 8 cases of metastases (metastasis group, Tables 16.1 and 16.2) and 16 cases of recurrent tumors of malignant head and neck tumors (recurrent head and neck tumor group, Tables 16.3 and 16.4) in the skull base. In the metastasis group, no patient had undergone radiation therapy at skull base tumor site before. In the recurrent head and neck tumor group, the recurrent tumor site was inside the field of the prior conventional external-beam radiation therapy (EBRT) in 8 patients among 16. Eighteen patients including all eight with metastases and ten with recurrent head and neck tumors had neurological symptoms with cranial nerve involvement including visual disturbance, extraocular muscle movement disorders, facial dysesthesia, hoarseness, and so on.

16.3 Stereotactic Radiotherapy Technique

The Novalis Radiosurgery system consists of several stereotactic components. Infrared passive reflectors attached noninvasively to the patient's body surface were used for primary positioning of the target close to the isocenter of a linear accelerator (LINAC). Radiographic image guidance was used for fine positioning adjustments based on internal anatomy, such as the skull base bony structures. The infrared guidance is also used to monitor external patient motion during treatment. The infrared positioning system consists of a pair of cameras in the radiosurgery room that emit and detect infrared radiation reflected from markers placed on the patient's body surface. Data are disseminated to yield real-time positional information. Translation and rotation in all three major axes (six dimensions) are displayed on multiple monitors. The treatment couch is mechanically driven to automatically position the patient near the isocenter, based on information derived from the infrared positioning to determine the position of the head relative to the isocenter. The radiographs are digitally transferred to a computer where they are compared with digitally reconstructed radiography (DRR) generated from a pretreatment computerized tomography scan. DRR represents the position of a perfectly

Y. Mori
Nagoya Radiosurgery Center, Nagoya Kyoritsu Hospital,
1–172 Hokke, Nakagawa, Nagoya, Aichi 454–0933, Japan
e-mail: ymori@kaikou.or.jp

A.A.F. De Salles et al. (eds.), *Shaped Beam Radiosurgery*,
DOI: 10.1007/978-3-642-11151-8_16, © Springer-Verlag Berlin Heidelberg 2011

Table 16.1 Cases of Novalis stereotactic radiotherapy for metastatic skull base tumors

Case	Age/sex	Primary carcinoma	Location of tumor	Vol. (ml)	Cranial nerve signs	Prior RTx[a]	Total dose (Gy)	Fraction
1	63/M	Prostate	Parasellar	112	V, VI, VII, IX–XI	(–)	30	10
2	55/F	Hepatoma	Sphenoid–maxillary	71	III, V	(–)	35	10
3	38/M	Renal cell	Middle fossa	49	VII	(–)	40	10
4	74/M	Nasal melanoma	Maxillary	112	III	(–)	50	10
5	47/F	Breast	Middle fossa	49	II	(–)	35	10
6	54/M	Cholangiocellular	Parasellar	45	II, V	(–)	36	12
7	38/M	Carcinoid	Parasellar	63	III, V	(–)	30	10
8	57/F	Breast	Middle fossa	54	II	(–)	36	12

[a]RTx: conventional external-beam radiation therapy

Table 16.2 Results of Novalis stereotactic radiotherapy for metastatic skull base tumors

Case	Follow-up (months)	Local result	Cranial nerve signs	Survival	Remarks
1	12	PR	Improved	Alive	Pain was relieved
2	9	PR	Improved	Dead	Died from primary heopatoma
3	8	PR	Improved	Alive	
4	11	PR	Improved	Alive	Lung metastasis developed (4 months)
5	10	PR	Unchanged	Alive	Brain metastasis was treated by Gamma Knife
6	13	PG NC	Unchanged	Alive	Repeat Novalis SRT was done for relapse
7	6	PR	Improved	Alive	
8	2	PR	Unchanged	Alive	

SRT stereotactic radiotherapy, *PR* partial remission, *NC* unchanged, *PG* progression

aligned patient. Radiographs and DRR are fused automatically to determine if any patient positioning adjustments are necessary, and the treatment couch is moved to reposition the patient appropriately. After shifts have been applied, a pair of radiographs are exposed to confirm patient positioning. A thermoplastic shell on the head and neck through shoulder minimizes the patient's movement during treatment (Fig. 16.1).

16.3.1 Dose Planning

Twenty-four tumors were treated by Novalis Radiosurgery SRT with non-coplanar conformal multi-beam or coplanar intensity-modulated multi-beam with 30– 54 Gy (at 100% isodose) in 10–18 fractions (Tables 16.1 and 16.3). If the treatment site had been covered by the previous EBRT the total dose was reduced. The tumors were covered by 90–95% isodose.

16.3.2 Methods of Evaluation

The effects of Novalis Radiosurgery SRT were evaluated based mainly on changes of tumor size on MRI taken every 2–3 months after treatment. A 4-grade system was devised: complete response (CR, tumor disappearance), partial response (PR, >30% tumor diameter reduction), no change (NC, <30% reduction and <20% tumor enlargement), and progression (PG,

Table 16.3 Cases of Novalis stereotactic radiotherapy for skull base recurrence of malignant head and neck tumors

Case	Age/sex	Diagnosis[a]	Location of tumor	Vol. (ml)	Cranial nerve signs	Prior RTx[b]	Total dose (Gy)	Fraction
9	36/M	Adenoid cystic ca. (palate)	Maxillary	44	V, VI	(–)	48	16
10	36/M	Adenoid cystic ca. (parotid)	Parasellar	60	II, III, VI, IX–XI	(–)	35	10
11	70/M	Adenoid cystic ca. (parotid)	Maxillary–nasal	127	(–)	(–)	36	12
12	67/M	Adenoid cystic ca. (maxilla)	Ethmoid	35	(–)	Yes	36	12
13	67/F	Adenoid cystic ca. (maxilla)	Maxillary	75	II	(–)	39	13
14	15/M	Adenoid cystic ca. (orbit)	Orbital	14	(–)	(–)	54	18
15	36/F	Adenoid cystic ca. (parotid)	Parasellar	13	VI	(–)	39	13
16	57/F	Epipharyngeal ca.	Epipharyngeal	39	V, VI	Yes	35	10
17	66/M	Epipharyngeal ca.	Epipharyngeal	94	(–)	Yes	45	18
18	60/M	Epipharyngeal ca.	Epipharyngeal	9	VI	Yes	30	15
19	59/M	Squamous cell ca. (nasal)	Ethmoid–frontal sinus	22	III, IV, VI	Yes	36	12
20	76/M	Squamous cell ca. (maxilla)	Maxillary	55	II	Yes	39	13
21	80/M	Squamous cell ca. (oral)	Maxillary	88	(–)	Yes	39	13
22	53/M	Tongue ca.	Middle fossa	55	(–)	(–)	35	10
23	43/M	Epithelioid hemangioendothelioma	Parasellar?	154	II	(–)	35	10
24	61/F	Esthesioneuroblastoma	Ethmoid	39	II	Yes	40	16

[a]ca.: carcinoma
[b]RTx: conventional external-beam radiation therapy covering the current tumor site

> 20% tumor diameter enlargement). From these values, the control rate can be calculated as [CR + PR + NC]/total. Further evaluation based on changes in neurological signs was made as well.

16.4 Results

Imaging and clinical follow-up was obtained in all 24 patients for 2–13 months after SRT (Tables 16.2 and 16.4).

In the metastasis group, seven of eight patients were alive at the end of the follow-up time of 2–12 months (median 9.5 months). One patient died from deterioration of primary hepatocellular carcinoma 9 months after the Novalis Radiosurgery SRT for skull base metastasis. The skull base tumor decreased in size and his clinical neurological symptoms of oculomotor palsy and facial dysesthesia had been improved after Novalis SRT. Seven patients of eight including this patient the tumors decreased in size until the end of the follow-up period or patient death. Only in one patient with cholangiocellular carcinoma, the lateral part of the tumor grew after the Novalis SRT. A second Novalis SRT (45 Gy in 15 fractions at 100% isodose) for the growing part was performed 5 months after the first SRT and the tumor was stable in size until 13 months after the first Novalis SRT. The neurological symptoms due to cranial nerve involvement were improved completely or partially in five patients out of eight.

Table 16.4 Results of Novalis stereotactic radiotherapy for skull base recurrence of malignant head and neck tumors

Case	Follow-up (months)	Local result	Cranial nerve signs	Survival	Remarks
9	12	CR	Unchanged	Alive	Lung metastasis was treated by Novalis SRT
10	3.5	PG	Worsened	Dead	Died from CSF dissemination
11	9	PR	None	Alive	
12	7	PR PG	None	Dead	Distant failure (2 months), died from lung metastasis
13	5	CR	Unchanged	Alive	
14	8	NC	None	Alive	
15	6	PR	Improved	Alive	Pain was relieved
16	9	PR	Worsened	Alive	
17	12	NC	None	Alive	Pain was relieved
18	2	PR	Improved	Alive	
19	9	CR	Unchanged	Alive	
20	6	PG	Unchanged	Alive	Repeat Novalis SRT was done for relapse
21	2	PG	None	Dead	Died from tumor progression
22	2	PG	None	Alive	Distant failure (2 months)
23	9	NC	Improved		
24	5	PR	Improved		

SRT stereotactic radiotherapy, *PR* partial remission, *NC* unchanged, *PG* progression

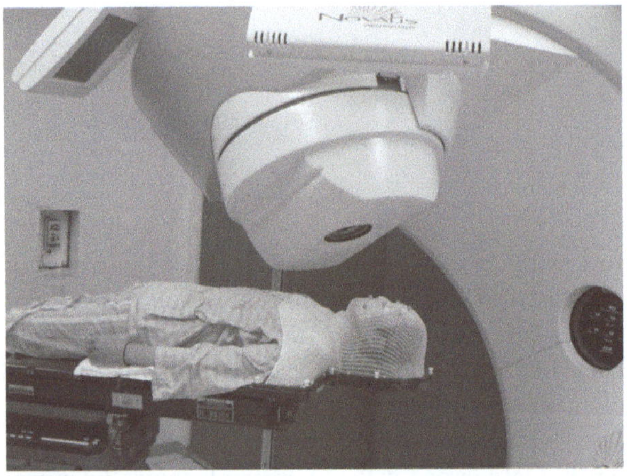

Fig. 16.1 Patient fixation using a head-neck-shoulder thermoplastic shell during Novalis stereotactic radiotherapy (SRT)

In recurrent head and neck tumor group, 13 patients were alive and 3 died during the follow-up period of 2–12 months (median 6.5 months). Two patients died from local tumor progression (squamous cell carcinoma) or cerebrospinal fluid space dissemination (adenoid cystic carcinoma, ACC). Another patient died from lung metastasis of ACC. The local tumor disappeared in three patients, decreased in size in five, was stable in three, and increased in size in five. In one patient Novalis SRT (39 Gy 13 fractions at 100% isodose) was performed again for the local tumor progression recently. In another patient lung metastatic tumor which had already existed at the time of SRT for skull base tumor was treated by Novalis. Cranial nerve symptoms which were due to local skull base tumors were improved in four out of ten patients and were stable in four. In two patients the neurological deficits deteriorated with or without tumor progression.

16.4.1 Illustrative Cases

Case 3: 38-year-old male, Fig. 16.2

The patient had nephrectomy for renal cell carcinoma of the right kidney. EBRT was done for iliac bone metastasis later. Radio-frequent ablation was done for lung metastasis 2 and 3 years later and it was also done for multiple bone metastases. Electron beam therapy was done for right occipital subcutaneous metastasis 1 year later. Then, 1 year later, the patient developed facial palsy on the left due to suboccipital skull base metastasis. Novalis SRT was performed for the skull base metastasis. A total dose of 40 Gy (at 100% isodose) in ten fractions was delivered. The tumor was covered by the 95% isodose area. The tumor decreased in size remarkably and right hemi-facial palsy was completely improved within 3 months after SRT.

Case 9: 36-year-old male, Fig. 16.3

The patient had 5-year history of ACC originating in the oral hard palate on the right side. The primary tumor was resected partially and EBRT followed. Then a recurrent tumor around the right optic canal developed and caused visual disturbance of the right eye. The right eye became completely blind after the surgical resection of the right orbital tumor. Then, the tumor recurred again in the right cavernous sinus extending to the right maxillary sinus and caused right abducens palsy and right facial dysesthesia. It was treated with

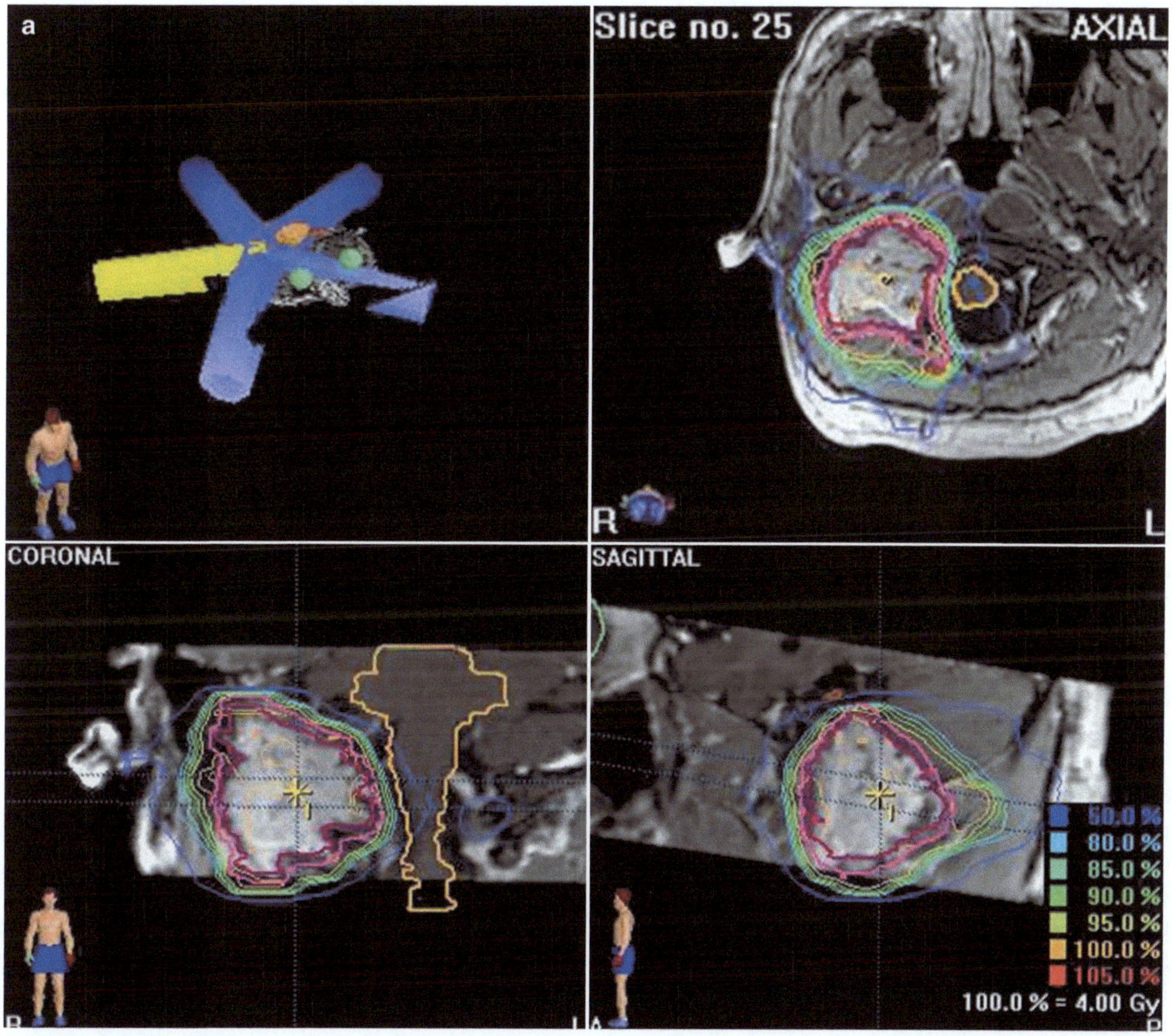

Fig. 16.2 Case 3: (**a**) Dose planning on BrainSCAN for skull base metastasis of renal cell carcinoma. (**b**) Axial magnetic resonance (MR) image with gadolinium (Gd) enhancement at Novalis SRT. (**c**) Axial MR image with Gd enhancement 4 months after SRT. Total dose of 40 Gy in ten fractions at 100% isodose was delivered by coplanar multi-beam intensity-modulated stereotactic radiotherapy. The right suboccipital skull base metastatic tumor was near complete disappearance within 4 months after SRT

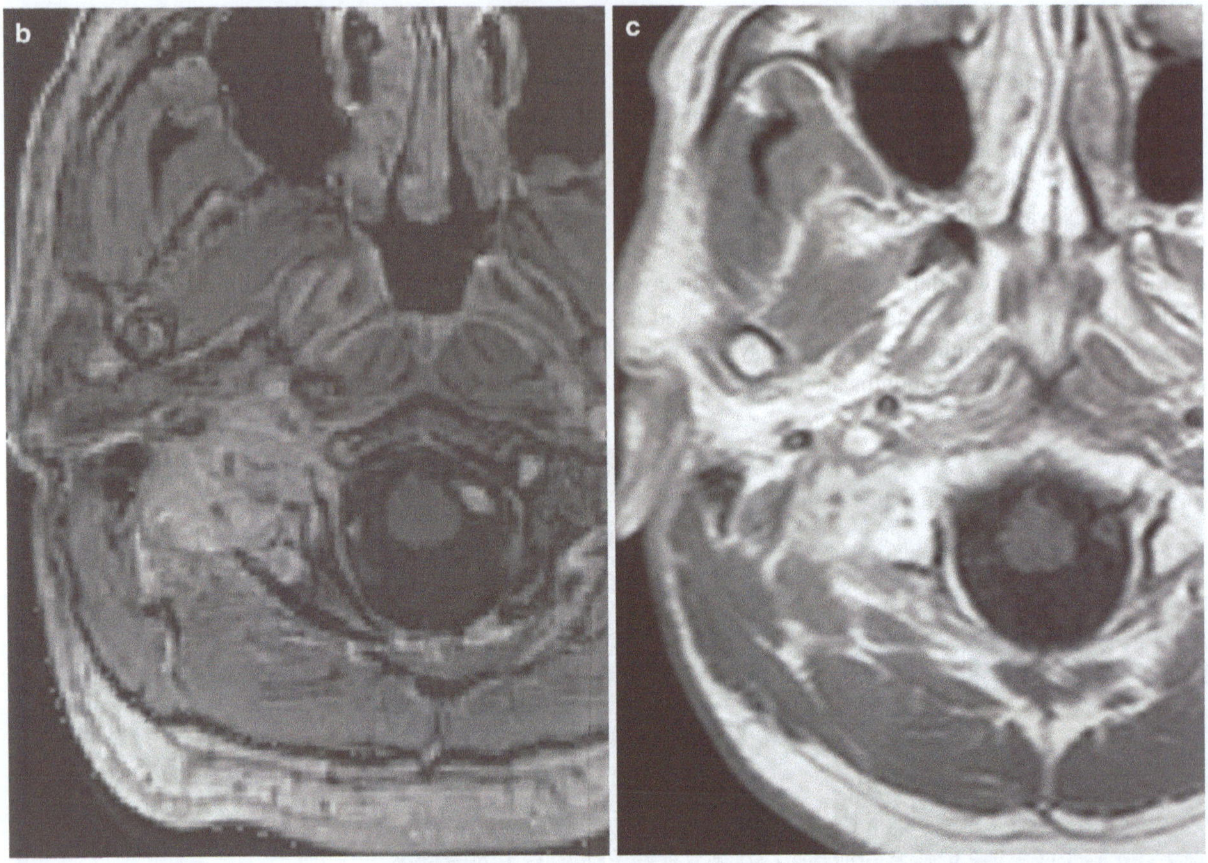

Fig. 16.2 (continued)

Novalis SRT with a total dose of 48 Gy in 16 fractions by coplanar intensity-modulated multi-beam. The tumor was remarkably decreased in size within 4 months after SRT.

Case 19: 59-year-old male, Fig. 16.4

The patient had suffered from squamous cell carcinoma originated in the left ethmoid sinus for 18 years. The primary tumor had been resected partially and EBRT was done. The tumor recurred in the left maxillary sinus 6 years later. Chemotherapy by intraarterial administration and EBRT with electron beam was done and maxillectomy followed. However, the tumor recurred in the left frontal sinus and maxillary sinus 6 years later again. Resection of the anterior skull base and conformal EBRT followed. In addition, reconstructive surgery of anterior skull base was performed. Then, relapse occurred in the right sphenoid sinus extending into the middle skull fossa 3 years later and EBRT was done. Recently, 2 years later, relapse in the frontal sinus and ethmoid sinus occurred and Novalis SRT was performed. This time, the area of radiation was overlapped partially with the areas of the first EBRT and the fourth EBRT. A total dose of 36 Gy at 100% isodose in 12 fractions was delivered by coplanar conformal multi-beam. The tumor disappeared within 6 months after Novalis SRT. The tumor had been of high uptake of 18 F-fluorodeoxyglucose–positron emission tomography (FDG-PET) before the SRT and the high-uptake area was gone on follow-up FDG-PET 6 months after SRT.

16.5 Discussion

Skull base metastases may invade critical structures including cranial nerves. Standard therapy of skull base metastases has been conventional EBRT to

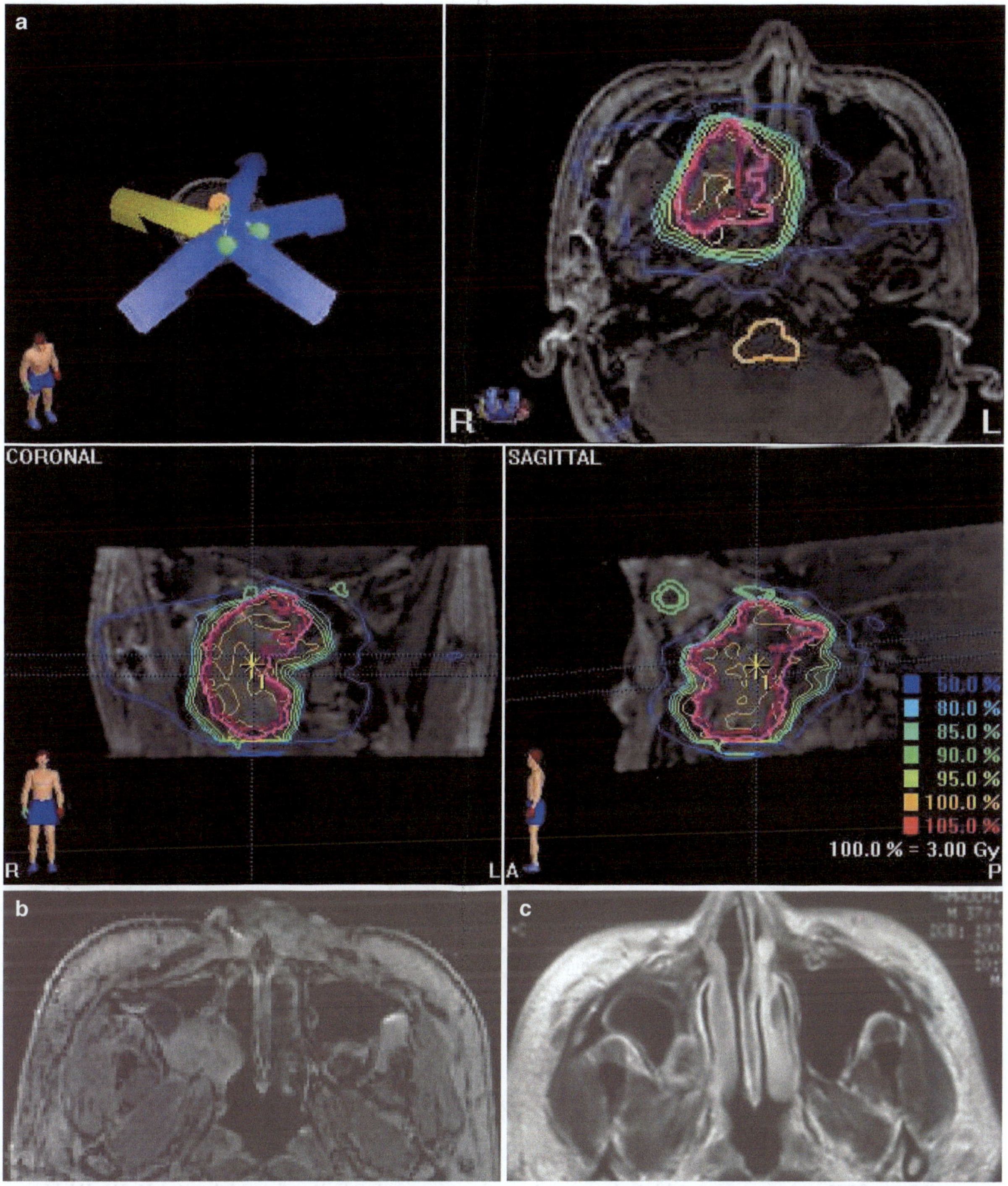

Fig. 16.3 Case 9: (**a**) Dose planning for maxillary relapse of adenoid cystic carcinoma. (**b**) Axial MR image with Gd enhancement at Novalis SRT. (**c**) Axial MR image with Gd enhancement 4 months after SRT. Total dose of 48 Gy in 16 fractions was delivered by coplanar multi-beam intensity-modulated stereotactic radiotherapy. The tumor was remarkably decreased in size within 4 months after SRT

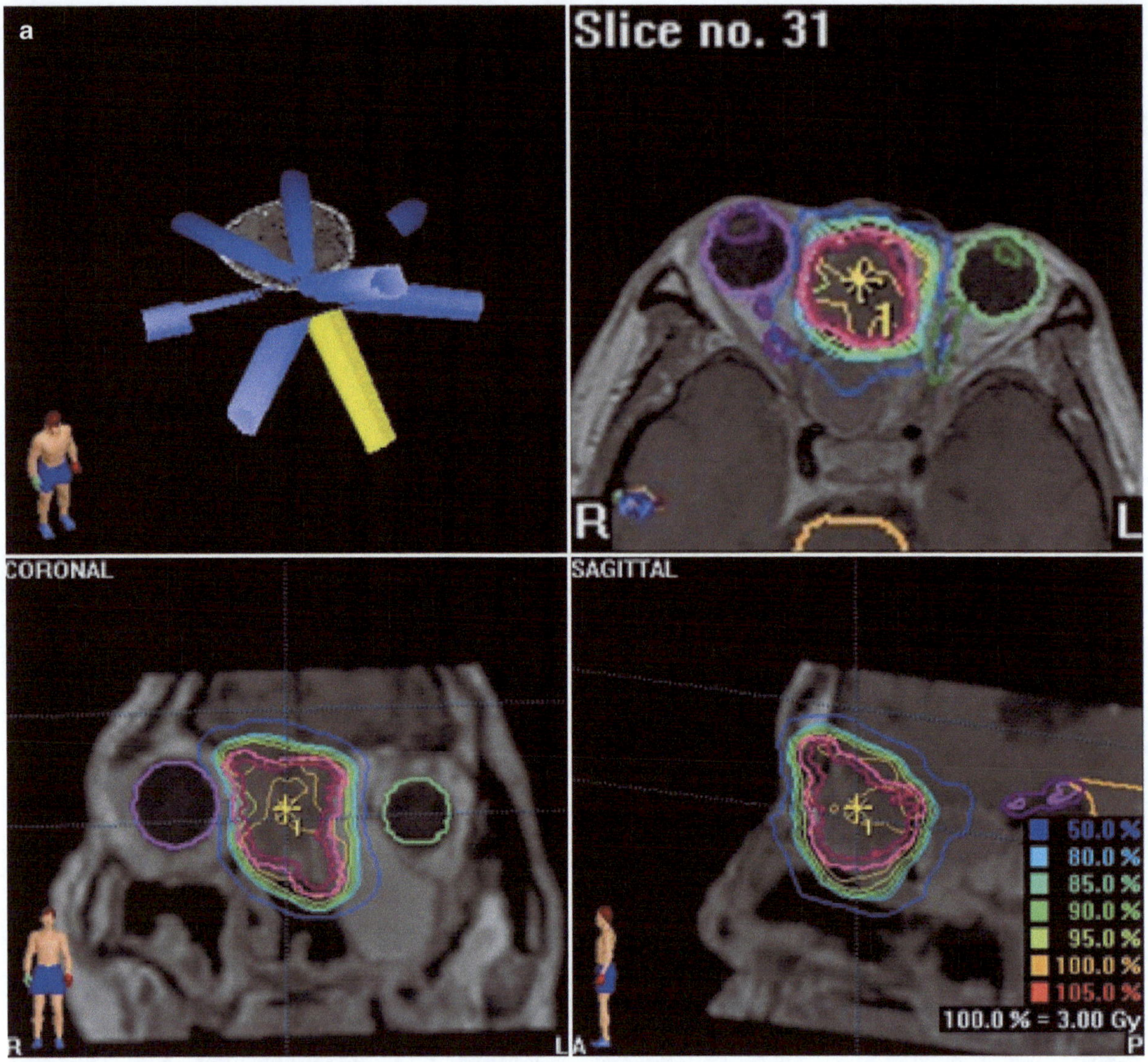

Fig. 16.4 Case 19: (**a**) Dose planning for relapse of squamous cell carcinoma in the frontal and ethmoid sinus. The recurrent tumor (**b**, axial MR image with Gd enhancement) was treated with Novalis SRT. A total dose of 36 Gy in 12 fractions was delivered by coplanar conformal multi-beam. The tumor disappeared within 6 months after SRT (**d**, axial MR image with Gd enhancement). The tumor presented high uptake of 18 F-fluorodeoxyglucose–positron emission tomography (FDG-PET) (**c**) and the high-uptake area was gone on follow-up FDG-PET 6 months after SRT (**e**)

relatively broad area including the tumor (Laigle-Donadey et al. 2005). However, stereotactic radiosurgery (SRS) or SRT can concentrate high dose on the target volume while sparing the critical structures adjacent the target. There have been few reports on SRS or SRT for skull base metastases. Formerly, Mori et al. reported successful treatment results of Gamma Knife® (Elekta, Stockholm, Sweden) single-session SRS for relatively small metastases (1.6–11.3 ml, median 3.1 ml) in sellar and/or cavernous sinus (Mori et al. 2006) causing pituitary dysfunction and deficits of cranial nerve II, III, IV, V, and VI in some of the cases. Three pituitary and/or cavernous tumors were stable in size and six tumors disappeared or decreased in size with median follow-up time of 4 months (range, 2–12 months). The control rate was 100% and cranial nerve symptoms were improved completely or partially in 67% (six cases

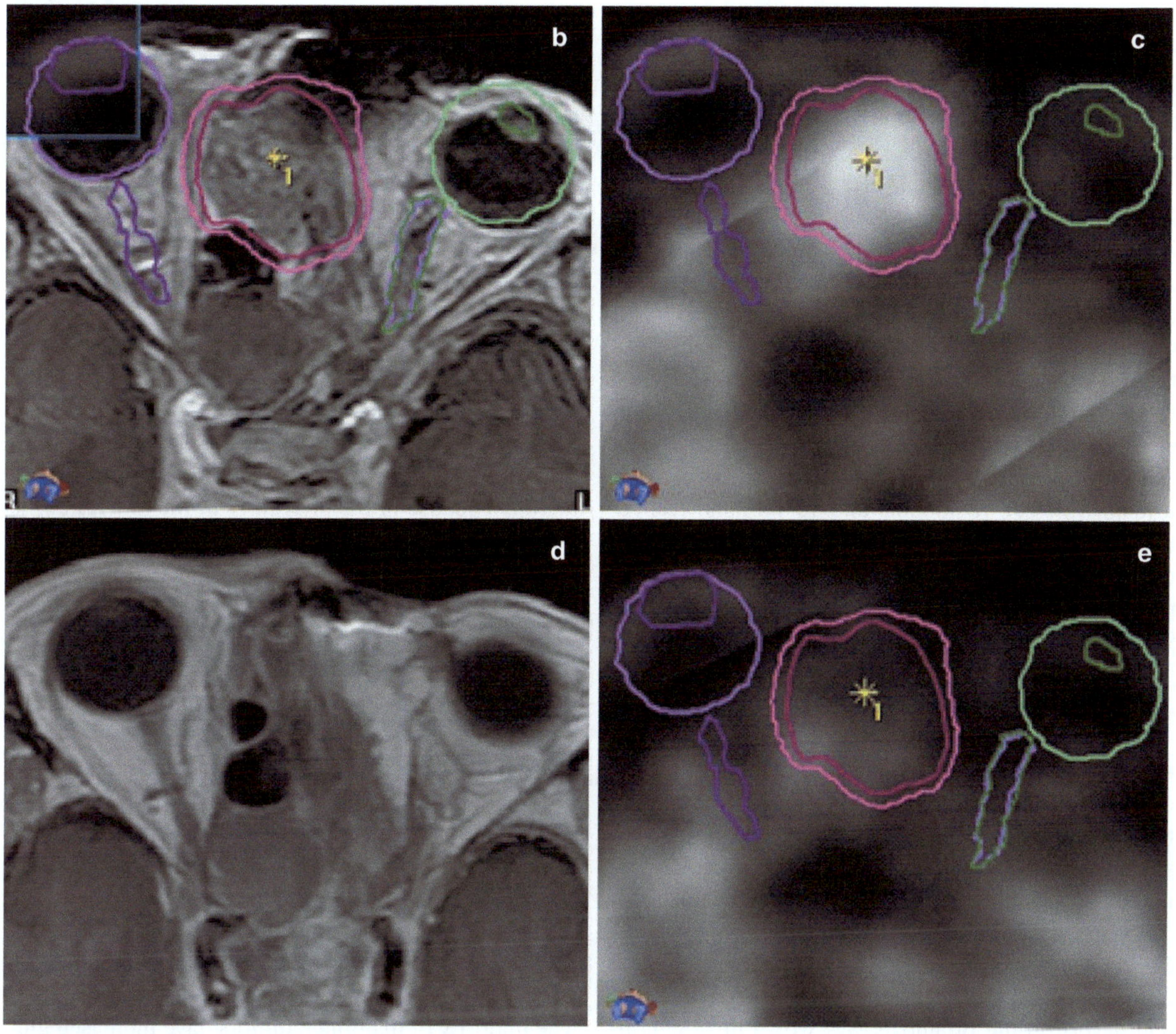

Fig. 16.4 (continued)

among nine). Two patients died during the follow-up time but the cause of death was systemic disease in both patients. No side effect due to SRS was observed. In this study, we reported successful results for palliation by Novalis SRT for large skull base metastases (45–112 ml, median 60 ml). All eight tumors were controlled until the end of the follow-up time or patient death, though retreatment was done in one patient. Cranial nerve symptoms improved fully or partially in five patients out of eight. SRT was thought to be safe and effective for skull base metastases, even if the tumor was relatively large.

For the initial treatment of head and neck cancers, conventional EBRT to the broad area including the adjacent lymph nodes with or without chemotherapy following surgical resection or biopsy is employed as primary standard therapy. However, head and neck cancers sometimes invade skull base area when they recur. Conventional re-irradiation is not adequate when relapse is inside or adjacent to the area of previous EBRT field. SRT can concentrate high dose on the target volume while sparing the critical structures adjacent the target. Furthermore, in certain cases SRT or intensity-modulated radiation therapy is valuable even in the initial radiotherapy, because of the proximity of the tumor to the orbits and optic pathways which are most valuable but most vulnerable structures to radiation injury.

There are some reports showing the effectiveness of SRS or SRT for head and neck cancers. Most study series describe the results of a small number of patients with various histologies (Ahn et al. 2000; Cmelak et al. 1997; Firlik et al. 1996; Kaplan et al. 1992; Kocher et al. 1998; Miller et al. 1997; Ryu et al. 2004), other than those on SRS or SRT for nasopharyngeal carcinoma (Chen et al. 2001; Dhanachai et al. 2007; Wu et al. 2007; Xiao et al. 2001). Formerly, Mori et al. reported successful treatment results of Gamma Knife SRS for relatively small skull base relapse of ACC (Mori et al. 2005). Oda et al. also reported results of Gamma Knife SRS for recurrent epipharyngeal carcinoma (EPC) (Oda et al. 2006). The control rate was 83% and 71% with median follow-up times of 18 months and 15 months, respectively. Wu et al. (2007) evaluated the results of SRT using LINAC-based system (Elekta) for locally persistent or recurrent nasopharyngeal carcinoma in 90 patients. The actuarial 3-year local-failure free survival rate at 3 years was 89% for persistent disease and 75% for recurrent disease.

The reported results of conventional EBRT for oronasal carcinomas have shown the difficulties to control the disease. Uchida et al. (2005) reported treatment results of conventional EBRT in 20 cases of squamous cell carcinoma and five cases of undifferentiated carcinoma of ethmoid sinus. Local control rate at 3 years and 5 years were 49% and 37% respectively. Survival rate at 3 years and 5 years were 34% and 24%. They reviewed reported series in the literature and described the prognosis was worse in squamous cell carcinoma and undifferentiated carcinoma than in adenocarcinoma and ACC. Recently, some results of SRS or SRT have been reported. Habermann et al. (2002) reported treatment results of surgical resection and Gamma Knife SRS in eight cases of nasal and paranasal carcinomas extending into the skull base. At 3 years after the treatment local relapse developed only in two cases. In four cases complete remission was obtained. One patient had distant relapse and one patient had lung metastasis. Voynov et al. (2006) reported treatment results of CyberKnife® (Accuray, Sunnyvale, CA, USA) SRS or SRT in 22 cases of recurrent head and neck squamous cell carcinoma after full dose conventional EBRT. They delivered 20–30 Gy in 1 to 8 fractions in recent cases. The local control rate at 2 years was 26% and the cause specific survival rate and the overall survival rate were 26% and 22% respectively. The median survival was 12 months. They concluded the prognosis of recurrent cases was not good but described a certain effect to improve the palliation of symptoms such as pain had obtained.

In this study, we showed preliminarily successful results of Novalis SRT for relapsed malignant skull base tumors of the head and neck. We treated 12 cases of recurrent tumors (five of ACC, three of EPC, and four of nasooral carcinomas) after prior treatments including EBRT, whether the field of which had included the current recurrent area or not. The results were favorable, though the follow-up time was not long. In addition, we treated two cases of ACC (Tables 16.3 and 16.4) by Novalis SRT as an initial radiotherapy because of the proximity of the tumors to the visual structures. In both cases the treated tumors were controlled until the end of the follow-up time.

Skull base epithelioid hemangioendothelioma (EH) is of histologically intermediate malignancy. It may be aggressive and extend to skull base invasively (Fernandes et al. 2006). Esthesioneuroblastoma may extend along the skull base (Bradley et al. 2003). It has invasive character and initial radiation treatment should be given to a broad area. We treated one case of EH as an initial radiation therapy because of proximity of the tumor to the optic pathways and treated one case of recurrent esthesioneuroblastoma after EBRT. The results were favorable in both cases.

FDG-PET is increasingly being used for detection of recurrent or residual disease in many tumor types. The majority of malignant tumors have increased glucose, amino acid and DNA metabolism. By using suitable tracers, malignant tumors can be differentiated from benign lesions. In head and neck cancers, FDG-PET is useful to detect relapse early because areas of tumor recurrence can be distinguished as high-uptake volume from radiation fibrosis, necrosis, and post-surgical changes. Gil et al. (2007) reported the findings of FDG-PET in skull base carcinomas. In all 12 cases of squamous cell carcinoma, sinusoidal undifferentiated carcinoma, clear cell carcinoma, EPC and adenocarcinoma, the tumors were of high uptake. Chan et al. (2006) also reported efficacy of FDG-PET to detect residual or recurrent EPC. O'Donnell et al. (2008) reported successful results of Gamma Knife SRS in two cases of locally recurrent EPC diagnosed early by FDG-PET scanning. In this study we demonstrated an illustrative case (Case 19) to show the usefulness of FDG-PET in identifying the target during the dose-planning and in following-up the tumor.

16.6 Conclusions

This study demonstrated the proof of principle and the potential of Novalis SRT for the treatment of skull base metastatic tumors and skull base relapse of head and neck malignant tumors, though the follow-up time was not long. Concerning skull base metastases from other visceral organ cancers, good local control was obtained by Novalis SRT and cranial nerve symptoms may be improved quickly. As for recurrence of malignant head and neck tumors, Novalis Radiosurgery SRT may be safe and effective as a salvage treatment. This study offers the potential to extend the use of Novalis SRT as an initial radiotherapy for certain selected head and neck malignant tumors, especially the tumors located adjacent to the orbits and optic pathways.

References

Ahn YC, Lee CK, Kin DY et al (2000) Fractionated stereotactic radiation therapy for extracranial head and neck tumors. Int J Radiat Oncol Biol Phys 48:501–505

Bradley PJ, Jones NS, Robertson I (2003) Diagnosis and management of esthesioneuroblastoma. Curr Opin Otolaryngol Head Neck Surg 11:112–118

Chan S-C, Ng S-H, Chang JT-C et al (2006) Advantage and pitfalls of 18 F-fluoro-2-deoxy-D-glucose positron emission tomography in detecting locally residual or recurrent nasopharyngeal carcinoma: comparison with magnetic resonance imaging. Eur J Nucl Med Mol Imaging 33:1032–1040

Chen H-J, Leung WL, Su C-Y (2001) Linear accelerator bases radiosurgery as a salvage treatment for skull base and intracranial invasion of recurrent nasopharyngeal carcinomas. Am J Clin Oncol CCT 24:255–258

Cmelak AJ, Cox RS, Afler JR et al (1997) Radiosurgery for skull base malignancies and nasopharyngeal carcinoma. Int J Radiat Oncol Biol Phys 37:997–1003

Dhanachai M, Kraiphibul P, Dangprasert S, Puatawpong P, Narkwong L, Laothamatas J, Kulaproditharom K, Sirachainan E, Yongvithisatid P (2007) Fractionated stereotactic radiotherapy in residual or recurrent nasopharyngeal carcinoma. Acta Oncol 46:828–833

Fernandes AL, Ratilal B, Mafra M, Magalhaes C (2006) Aggressive intracranial and extra-cranial epithelioid hemangioendothelioma: a case report and review of the literature. Neuropathology 26(3):201–205

Firlik KS, Kondziolka D, Lunsford LD et al (1996) Radiosurgery for recurrent cranial base cancer arising from the head and neck. Head Neck 18:160–166

Gil Z, Even-Sapir E, Margalit N et al (2007) Integrated PET/CT system for staging and surveillance of skull base tumors. Head Neck 29(6):537–545

Habermann W, Zanarotti U, Groell R et al (2002) Combination of surgery and Gamma Knife radiosurgery – A therapeutic option for patients with tumors of nasal cavity or paranasal sinuses infiltrating the skull base. Acta Otorhinolaryngol Ital 22:74–79

Kaplan ID, Adler JR, Jr H et al (1992) Radiosurgery for palliation of base of skull recurrences from head and neck cancers. Cancer 70:1980–1984

Kocher M, Voges J, Staar S et al (1998) Linear accelerator radiosurgery for recurrent malignant tumors of the skull base. Am J Clin Oncol CCT 21:18–22

Laigle-Donadey F, Taillibert S, Martin-Duverneuil N, Hildebrand J, Delattre JY (2005) Skull-base metastases. J Neurooncol 75:63–69

Miller RC, Foote RL, Coffy RJ et al (1997) The role of stereotactic radiosurgery in the treatment of malignant skull base tumors. Int J Radiat Oncol Biol Phys 39:977–981

Mori Y, Kobayashi T, Kida Y et al (2005) Stereotactic radiosurgery as a treatment for recurrent skull base adenoid cystic carcinoma. Stereotact Funct Neurosurg 83:202–207

Mori Y, Kobayashi T, Shibamoto Y (2006) Stereotactic radiosurgery for metastatic tumors in the pituitary gland and the cavernous sinus. J Neurosurg 105(Suppl):37–42

O'Donnell HE, Plowman PN, Khaira MK, Alusi G (2008) PET scanning and Gamma Knife radiosurgery in the early diagnosis and salvage "cure" of locally recurrent nasopharyngeal carcinoma. Br J Radiol 81:e26–e30

Oda K, Mori Y, Kobayashi T et al (2006) Stereotactic radiosurgery as a salvage treatment for recurrent epipharyngeal carcinoma. Stereotact Funct Neurosurg 84:103–108

Ryu S, Khan M, Yin F-F et al (2004) Image-guided radiosurgery of head and neck cancers. Otolaryngol Head Neck Surg 130:690–697

Uchida D, Shirato H, Onimaru R et al (2005) Long-term results of ethmoid squamous cell or undifferentiated carcinoma treated with radiotherapy with or without surgery. Cancer J 11:152–156

Voynov G, Heron DE, Burton S et al (2006) Frameless stereotactic radiosurgery for recurrent head and neck carcinoma. Technol Cancer Res Treat 5:529–535

Wu S-X, Chua DTT, Deng ML, Zhao C, Li F-Y, Sham JST, Wang H-Y, Bao Y, Gao Y-H, Zeng Z-F (2007) Outcome of fractionated stereotactic radiotherapy for 90 patients with locally persistent and recurrent nasopharyngeal carcinoma. Int J Radiat Oncol Biol Phys 69:761–769

Xiao J-P, Xu G-Z, Mial Y-J (2001) Fractionated stereotactic radiosurgery for 50 patients with recurrent or residual nasopharyngeal carcinoma. Int J Radiat Oncol Biol Phys 51:164–170

Part III

Functional Radiosurgery

Radiosurgery for Trigeminal Neuralgia: Indications, Results and Complications

17

Alessandra A. Gorgulho

17.1 Introduction

Trigeminal Neuralgia (TN) is a medical condition with one of the broadest therapeutic armamentarium varieties. This reflects the fact that none of current therapeutic options lead to definitive and long lasting pain relief in the absence of significant toxicity or assurance of no major post-operative complications. Anticonvulsants are recommended for those initially diagnosed with this condition. Medication side effects, despite classified as minor, significantly interfere with the quality of life of patients over time, as they need increased doses of medication to maintain pain control and/or they become more sensitive to the side effects with aging.

The annual incidence of Trigeminal Neuralgia is 4–5/100,000 people (Katusic et al. 1991). About a quarter of the patients diagnosed with TN will not respond to medication (Fields 1996), while another quarter will develop intolerance to medication (Farago 1987; Fromm et al. 1984). Despite the fact that half of the TN patients need surgical intervention, the exact criteria defining "medically refractory" TN has not yet been established (Broggi et al. 2008; Zakrzewska et al. 2005). Therefore, a common consensus regarding the optimal timing for surgery is still lacking. Studies evaluating quality of life in patients submitted to microvascular decompression showed that an absolute majority of the patients would have had surgery earlier (Zakrzewska et al. 2005; Zakrzewska and Patsalos 2002). The exact timing for recommendation of radiosurgery is even less standardized in comparison to other "traditional" surgical modalities. It is somewhat intuitive that patients and clinicians may consider surgical intervention earlier as the surgical techniques become less invasive. Still, the identification of specific subpopulations of TN patients who will better benefit from a particular treatment modality is heavily based on the neurosurgeon's level of comfort with each of the surgical alternatives.

17.2 Radiosurgery in the context of other surgical techniques for Trigeminal Neuralgia

Two systematic literature reviews (Cruccu et al. 2003; Tatli et al. 2008) rated microvascular decompression (MVD) as the surgical procedure leading to the highest long-lasting rate of pain control with the lowest rate of trigeminal sensory root dysfunction. MVD requires the patients to be eligible to receive general anesthesia and be submitted to a craniotomy. There is a small risk of more prominent complications as deafness, CSF leak, meningitis (aseptic and bacterial), stroke and even death (Barker et al. 1996; Broggi et al. 2000; Cruccu et al. 2003; Tatli et al. 2008; Zakrzewska et al. 2005). MVD is the single non-ablative surgical modality.

Radiofrequency rhizotomy (RFR) ranked as the second most effective surgical modality leading to pain control in a systematic literature review (Lopez et al. 2004b). Long term effectiveness of pain control is closely correlated with facial numbness occurrence (Broggi et al. 1990; Tatli et al. 2008). RFR is definitely the technique that leads to the highest incidence of complications among all ablative techniques. These complications include anesthesia dolorosa, bothersome

A.A. Gorgulho
Department of Neurosurgery, UCLA Medical Center, David Geffen School of Medicine at UCLA, 300 UCLA Medical Plaza, Suite B212, Los Angeles, CA 90095, USA
e-mail: a_gorgulho@yahoo.com

A.A.F. De Salles et al. (eds.), *Shaped Beam Radiosurgery*,
DOI: 10.1007/978-3-642-11151-8_17, © Springer-Verlag Berlin Heidelberg 2011

dysesthesias, keratitis, motor trigeminal root dysfunction and meningitis (Broggi et al. 1990, 2008; Lopez et al. 2004b). Only patients who are willing to accept facial numbness as a consequence of the intervention should be offered this option.

Fewer studies reporting on balloon compression (BC) meet the standards to be included in systematic literature reviews. Different systematic reviews (Lopez et al. 2004b; Tatli et al. 2008) placed BC as second or third most effective modality. Balloon compression leads to satisfactory pain relief at the cost of lower complications in comparison to RFR (Lopez et al. 2004b; Tatli et al. 2008) and the incidence of facial numbness is variable, subsiding over time (Mullan and Lichtor 1983; Skirving and Dan 2001). BC leads to the highest incidence of trigeminal motor root dysfunction (Tatli et al. 2008), while mild transient masticatory weakness is present in virtually all cases during the immediate post-operative period.

Glycerol injection leads to the lowest success rate of pain relief both at short term and mainly at long term. Recurrence rate is 62% at actuarial 5 years (Tatli et al. 2008). Anesthesia dolorosa and bothersome dysesthesia have been reported with this technique.

SRS emerges as the least invasive modality leading to good pain outcomes and low complication rates. Facial numbness is the most common complication with an incidence ranging from 2% to 54% depending on the treatment protocol followed. Anesthesia dolorosa has been reported by some authors (Pollock et al. 2002; Villavicencio et al. 2008), however the incidence is considerably lower compared to RFR. SRS is not the "definitive" surgical procedure for the TN condition; as none of the other procedures are either. Sustained pain relief rates with SRS are not the highest ones but the lack of invasiveness associated with low incidence of complications, in particular major complications, explain why radiosurgery has gained increased acceptability by the scientific community. The appeal of radiosurgery to patients shall become even stronger with the current possibility of frameless dedicated-Linac radiosurgery.

Rahimian et al. (2004) conducted a thorough evaluation of the geometrical accuracy and precision of a dedicated-Linac device equipped with robotic table (Novalis® Radiosurgery, Brainlab, Feldkirchen, Germany) using frameless radiosurgery on a phantom. The overall mean system deviation was 0.32 ± 0.42 mm considering inaccuracies in each step of the procedure including imaging, fusion, treatment planning, and treatment itself.

17.3 Radiosurgery Indications

Radiosurgery was initially indicated for patients who failed previous treatments or were not suitable to undergo anesthesia due to fragile medical condition. Nevertheless, the background provided by SRS literature data and the convenience of SRS treatment expanded its indication to patients not submitted to prior surgical procedures.

At UCLA, we use an algorithm previously discussed in one of our publications (Gorgulho and De Salles 2006) (Fig. 17.1). Elderly patients are offered radiosurgery as the initial surgical approach. Young patients and even older patients in good medical condition are recommended to have MVD, the gold-standard surgical procedure. Patients' candidates to MVD who refuse surgery are recommended to have radiosurgery. In our experience, it is relatively frequent to receive patients amenable to undergo MVD who prefer to try SRS procedure first. Patients are acknowledged about the shortcomings of SRS: latency time to accomplish pain control, more modest rates of sustained pain relief and higher rates of facial numbness in comparison to MVD. The intensity of facial numbness post-SRS is however subtle in the majority of the cases. Furthermore, MVD following prior SRS is not more difficult to perform (Shetter et al. 2005).

Patients under acute pain attack (i.e., not being able to eat or talk) receive intra-venous anticonvulsant infusion as the initial approach. They are not candidates to radiosurgery since the drawback of this technique is the time latency of on average 6–8 weeks to provide pain relief after radiation treatment (Adler et al. 2009; Chen et al. 2008; Herman et al. 2004; Matsuda et al. 2008; Pollock et al. 2002; Smith et al. 2003). If the pain is at V1, they are treated with BC; if the pain is at V2 or V3, they are treated with RFR. Our group does not recommend RFR for V1 pain, due to the possibility of corneal numbness and keratitis. In our practice we do not perform glycerol injection as a routine. A retrospective study comparing the effectiveness of radiosurgery and glycerol injection concluded that radiosurgery results are superior to glycerol in all aspects except in providing immediate pain control. These results suggest that radiosurgery is a better choice over glycerol injection for patients who are not under acute pain attacks (Henson et al. 2005).

As can be noticed in Fig. 17.1, patients have radiosurgery as the initial surgical procedure or at

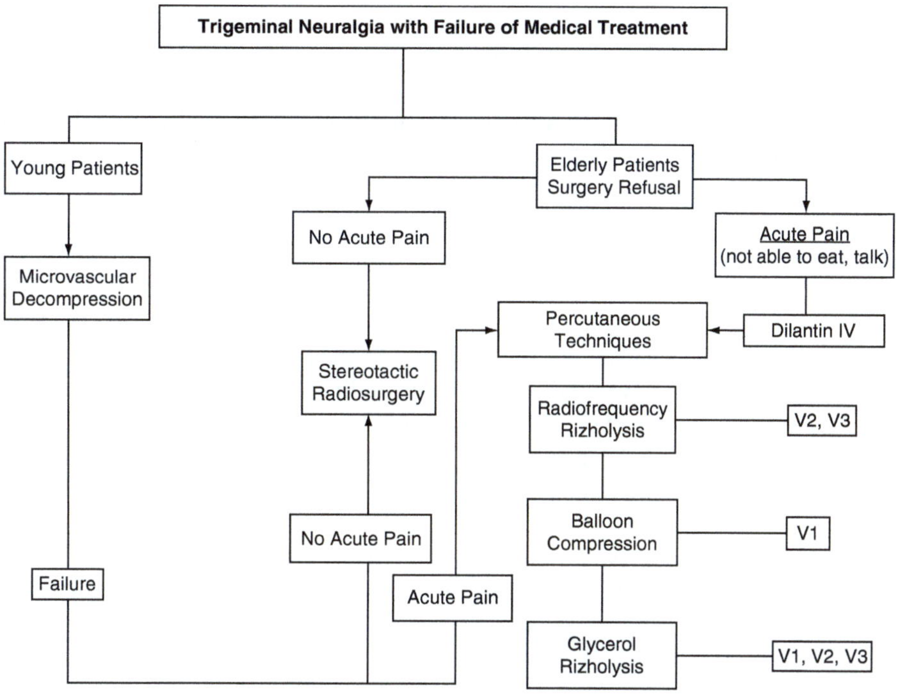

Fig. 17.1 Algorithm used for selection of the surgical modalities among patients with refractory trigeminal neuralgia. Young patients are offered micro-vascular decompression as first line surgical modality. Elderly patients are offered radiosurgery as the initial surgical approach. Patients experiencing acute pain attacks are offered balloon compression when V1 branch is involved or radiofrequency rhizotomy when pain does not involve V1. Radiosurgery is also offered at recurrence of MVD or any percutaneous technique

recurrence/failure of other surgical procedures. Our data (Smith et al. 2003) and that of others (Lopez et al. 2004a; Maesawa et al. 2001; Petit et al. 2003; Pollock et al. 2002) showed that patients receiving SRS as first surgical approach achieved better pain relief than those who had previous procedures. The explanation for this observation can go in two directions: either radiation works better in an intact nerve or patients having radiosurgery after a failure consist of a more "resistant" population to any treatment.

The current recommendations of other experts in surgical treatment of TN are summarized in the next couple paragraphs. Little et al. (2008a) described a similar approach to ours. They recommend SRS for elderly patients and for those refusing surgery since SRS offers a satisfactory rate of pain control and low rate of complication.

A retrospective study compared pain relief and post-treatment complications in 52 elderly patients (defined as ≥ 65 years) treated with MVD or SRS (Oh et al. 2008). Pain relief rates were higher with MVD than with SRS (63% vs. 55.5%, respectively), while recurrence rates were similar. Acute complications were higher in the MVD group with 6 out of 27 cases presenting with facial numbness, cerebral spinal fluid leakage, hearing impairment, herpes zoster infection and acute subdural hematoma. Chronic complications included 4 cases of bothersome facial and tongue numbness. For the SRS group, there were two cases of facial dysesthesia, mildly bothersome. The authors concluded that pain relief occurs sooner in patients treated with MVD but complications are more frequent in comparison to the SRS group and with surgical series including younger patients submitted to MVD. The authors concluded that SRS should be preferably recommended for this age group.

Broggi et al. (2008) suggest MVD as the initial approach for all the cases, not considering age a limiting factor per se. BC is offered as the second surgical option. For those who failed MVD or BC and accept to have facial numbness, they perform RFR.

In summary, different environments define different profiles of surgical experience. Besides, the surgical literature is extremely heterogeneous in terms of pain outcome definition, recurrence and complications, challenging the validity of the conclusions based on erratic reading of the series. This enhances the need for standardization of the reports (Zakrzewska and Lopez 2003) to allow future meta-analysis and prospective trials comparing the multiple techniques with long term follow-up.

17.4 Radiosurgery Indication for TN: A Historical Perspective

Stereotactic Radiosurgery was actually first used in humans to treat TN. The initial two patients treated by Lars Leksell experienced sustained pain relief for decades. However, when summarizing his life long experience with radiosurgery for TN in approximately 60 patients, Leksell wrote: "No definite conclusion should be drawn concerning the optimal dose of radiation or the exact mechanism and site of action in the root or the ganglion, or even the general applicability of the method". The interest on TN radiosurgery at the gasserian ganglia vanished due to poor pain relief rates observed in the initial series and also by the inadvertent discovery that glycerol (used to target the ganglia for radiosurgery) lead to pain improvement by itself. In the nineties, thin cuts MRI and the use of special sequences allowed the use of radiosurgery at the same site within the trigeminal pathway where modern microsurgery was performed (De Salles et al. 1997).

Recently, several authors reported their results of SRS for trigeminal neuralgia (Brisman 2004; Hasegawa et al. 2002; Herman et al. 2004; Kondziolka et al. 1996; Little et al. 2008a; Maesawa et al. 2001; Massager et al. 2004; Nicol et al. 2000; Petit et al. 2003; Pollock et al. 2001, 2005; Regis et al. 2006; Rogers et al. 2000; Smith et al. 2003; Urgosik et al. 2005; Young et al. 1998) (Table 17.1). There is however disagreement on the SRS approaches, centered mostly on the location of the target within the trigeminal complex and on the total radiation dose. There have been 249 patients treated with SRS for TN at UCLA from August/1995 to June/2008. As experience treating TN was accumulated, the treatment protocol was modified over time. A brief summary of our experience is provided in the next section.

Table 17.1 Summary of radiosurgery results for trigeminal neuralgia

Authors	Nb patients	Dose (Gy)	Initial pain relief (%)	Recurrence (%)	Numbness (%)	Follow-up (months)
Kondziolka et al. (1996)	50	60–90	94	6	6	18[d]
Young et al. (1998)	110	70–80	95.5	34	2.7	19.8[d]
Nicol et al. (2000)	42	90	95.2	4.8	16.7	14[e]
Pollock et al. (2001)	68	70 90	86 93	26 15	15 54	14.4[d]
Maesawa et al. (2001)	220	60–90	82.3	13.6	10.2	24[e]
Smith et al. (2003)	60	70–90	95.5[a] 79[b]	25.6	25	23[d]
Massager et al. (2004)	47	90	83	8	38.3	16[d]
Herman et al. (2004)	112 18[c]	75 70	78 93	22 NA	NA 11	37.5[e] 24.5[e]
Urgosik et al. (2005)	107	70–80	96	25	20	60[e]
Regis et al. (2006)	100	70–90	94	34	10	12[f]
Little et al. (2008a)	136	70–90	73.5	16.2	45	75[e]

[a]Patients not submitted to prior procedures
[b]Patients submitted to prior procedure
[c]Patients submitted to repeat SRS within the same series
[d]Mean follow-up
[e]Median follow-up
[f]Minimum follow-up
NA – information not available in the report

17.5 Isocenter Position and Radiation Dose Impacts on the Results of SRS for Trigeminal Neuralgia

17.5.1 UCLA Experience

Throughout the years, the isocenter position was brought closer to the root entry zone (REZ) and pons. Initially, patients were treated with the 20% isodose line of prescription tangential to the surface of the pons. Based on our own experience and reports of the literature, the isocenter was moved by bringing the 30% IDL tangential to the pons. And since March/2003, the isocenter was placed with the 50% IDL tangential to the pontine surface (Fig. 17.2).

The retrospective analysis of the 102 eligible patients evaluated the effect of isocenter position on the incidence of facial numbness. The strength of this study, in comparison to others in the literature, is the fact that only patients treated with the same maximal radiation dose (90 Gy) were included. Therefore, the groups analyzed differed exclusively in regards to maximal dose of radiation at the root entry zone (REZ) and brainstem and not to other portions of the trigeminal nerve. All the patients were treated with a dedicated-Linac radiosurgery device (Novalis Radiosurgery). The risk difference for facial numbness incidence between the group treated with the 30% IDL tangential to the pons and the group treated with the 50% IDL tangential to the pons was 19.7% (95% CI: 0.33–31.2%). No other variables significantly predict facial numbness occurrence in multivariate analysis. This is the first study to our knowledge, based on single center data analysis, showing increased occurrence of facial numbness according to pre-determined higher doses of radiation to the REZ/brainstem, while controlling for prescribed radiation dose (Gorgulho et al., unpublished).

Prior results published by UCLA group also showed a positive correlation between brainstem enhancement

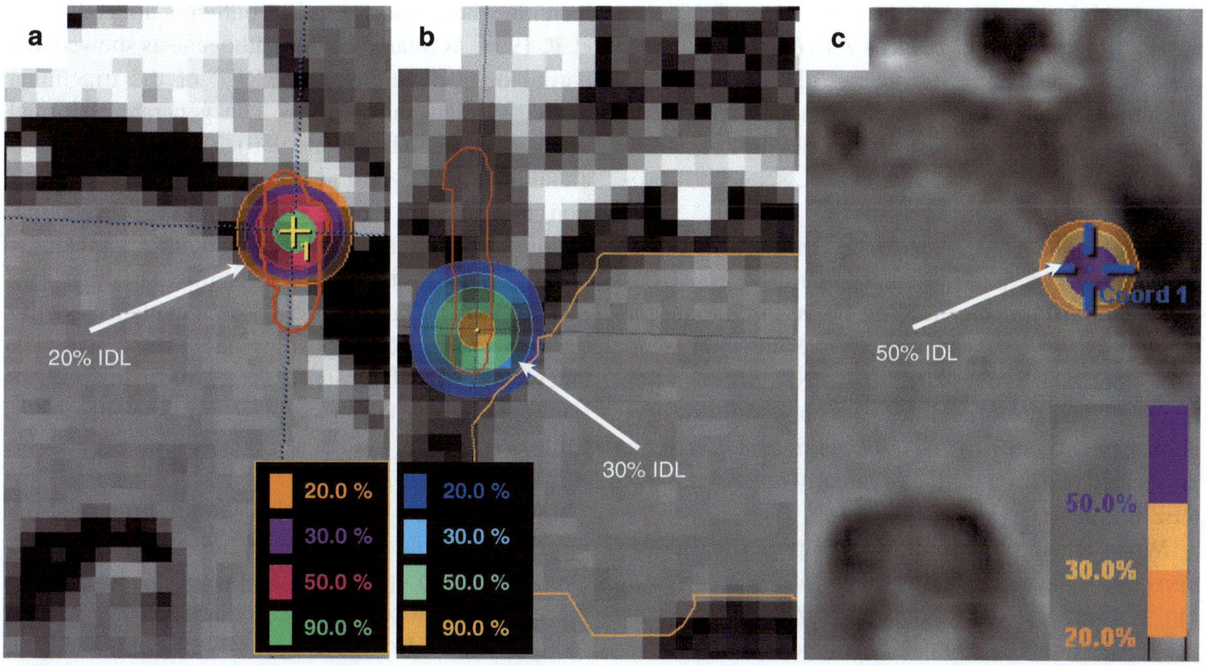

Fig. 17.2 The three protocols used at UCLA for radiosurgery treatment of Trigeminal Neuralgia. (**a**) Treatment plan showing the placement of the 20% isodoseline (IDL) tangential to the pontine surface (*orange circle* within the isodoseline distribution, *white arrow*). (**b**) The treatment protocol was modified bringing the isocenter closer to the brainstem surface. Notice the 30% isodoseline in *light blue*, indicated by the *arrow* in (b). The 20% IDL (*dark blue*) is encompassing a small amount of brainstem tissue. (**c**) Progressive move of the isocenter even closer to the root entry zone and brainstem. The 50% isodoseline is placed at the limit of the pontine surface. The *dark and light orange lines* represent the 20% and the 30% IDL, respectively, and were used for determination of the position of the isocenter throughout the initial years of radiosurgery experience at UCLA (a and b). The 50% IDL is shown by the *arrow* (*purple circle line*)

post-radiosurgery and excellent pain outcome (Gorgulho et al. 2006). This preliminary observation included 37 patients with post-operative MRI scans after SRS for classical and symptomatic trigeminal neuralgia. Among them, eight showed pons enhancement. A significantly better pain outcome was confirmed in a later analysis of 30 patients presenting with pons enhancement in the follow-up MRIs in comparison to the other patients of our series (Gorgulho et al. 2007). The radiological enhancement peaks around 12 months after radiation delivery. The enhancement time course follows the same time curve observed after radiosurgery for other indications, such as tumors and AVMs. The brainstem enhancement subsides over time and becomes inconspicuous at about 24 months post-radiosurgery but can still be noticed in a minority of cases after 28 months. In the context of TN, it is reassuring to observe such enhancement in the brainstem/REZ. Radiosurgery treatment of TN to the REZ target is challenging since either a 4 or a 5 mm collimator is used on a target measuring 3 mm in diameter (Chavez et al. 2005). The radiation dose is high, requiring a treatment time of at least 30–45 min, even for the devices with the highest monitor units available in the market. The accuracy of modern radiosurgery devices is comparable and can be improved in the context of TN SRS by the use of thin slice thickness MRI and specific sequences providing better visualization of the TN (i.e., CISS sequence). The TN lies suspended in the CSF of the pre-pontine cistern. Physicians should be conscious about minimal movement of the nerve throughout the respiratory cycle, especially considering total treatment time, which ranges from 30 to 90 min depending on the device. Therefore, the post-radiosurgery enhancement confirms that a substantial amount of the prescribed radiation dose was actually delivered to the REZ of the nerve (i.e., our target).

When treating TN with SRS, the prescribed radiation dose is the maximal dose, therefore when discussing delivered dose it means both maximal and prescribed doses. The ideal dose appears to be somewhere between 70 Gy and 90 Gy, since pain control was significantly poorer when less than 70 Gy was delivered to patients (Kondziolka et al. 1996), and 100 Gy caused nerve necrosis in baboons (Kondziolka et al. 2000).

Goss et al. (2003) described 25 patients with classical TN treated with a dedicated-Linac device (Novalis Radiosurgery) to the dose of 90 Gy. Dose volume histogram analysis disclosed a correlation between brainstem volume within the 50% IDL (≥ 0.008 cm^3) and occurrence of mild facial numbness.

17.6 Isocenter Position and Radiation Dose Impact on the Results of SRS for Trigeminal Neuralgia

17.6.1 Literature Analysis

The rational for placement of the isocenter in the root entry zone (REZ) is based on the accepted pathophysiological mechanism proposed for classical trigeminal neuralgia. The average distance of REZ from the TN emergence out of the brainstem in humans is 3 mm. It is known that the central myelin is more sensitive to injuries, including damage caused by radiation. Based on MVD surgical experience, this is the most common location where neurovascular conflict is noticed (Love et al. 1998). Research on TN pathogenesis showed that partial demyelination of the REZ of the trigeminal nerve, by mechanical injury, can generate abnormal action potentials (Burchiel 1980). These foci of demyelination would distort and augment sensory information transmission conveyed through the trigeminal circuitry. MVD reaches success in controlling pain by modifying trigeminal function in this particular segment of the trigeminal system. These evidences justify the choice of isocenter positioning with the 50% IDL tangential to the brainstem surface by many authors (Gorgulho et al. 2006; Gorgulho and De Salles 2006; Little et al. 2008b; Petit et al. 2003; Rogers et al. 2000) (Figs. 17.2c and 17.3).

Other authors, however, have the opinion that the increase in facial numbness is not worthy (Pollock et al. 2001) and optioned for a protocol with either a more distant isocenter positioning or a lower total radiation dose. Kondziolka et al. (1996) defined the isocenter position by the 30% isodoseline (IDL) touching the pons. Pollock et al. (2001) described the 20% as the median IDL at the brainstem surface when delivering 90 Gy and the 40% IDL when delivering 70 Gy. Nicol et al. (2000) and Hasegawa et al. (2002) also chose the 20% isodoseline tangential to the pons surface. Petit et al. (2003), Little et al.

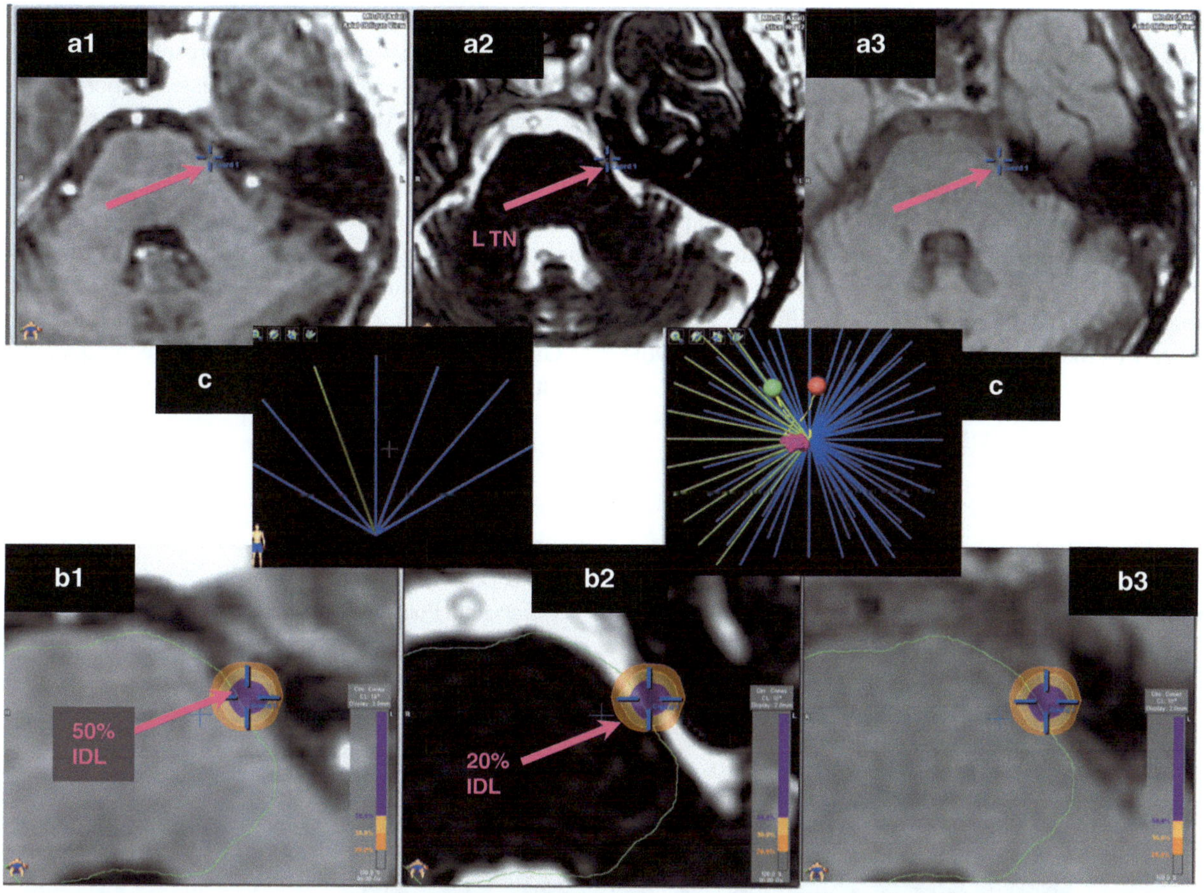

Fig. 17.3 MRI sequences used for targeting the trigeminal nerve. Figures A.1/A.2/A.3 shows the trigeminal nerve on axial cuts of T1 with contrast, *CISS* (constructive interference steady state) and T1 without contrast sequences, respectively. B.1/B.2/B.3 shows the dose distribution of the 20% (*dark orange circle*), 30% (*light orange*) and 50% (*purple*) radiation doses under magnified view. The C figures illustrate the 7 non coplanar dynamic arcs distribution as well as the automated segmentation of the brainstem (*structure in pink*) provided by the iPlan® RT Image software (Brainlab, Feldkirchen, Germany)

(2008a, b), and Rogers et al. (2000) are among those also using the 50% IDL tangential to the brainstem surface. Other groups propose to place the isocenter even further away the REZ, juxta-posterior to the gasserian ganglion.

Retrospective studies of Gamma unit series showed evidence for association between incidence of facial numbness and better pain outcomes (Massager et al. 2004; Pollock et al. 2002; Tawk et al. 2005). A meta-analysis performed by Pollock (2006) showed a positive correlation between excellent pain outcomes (pain free and medication free), occurrence of facial numbness, and radiation total dose. Pooled results of the series specifically analyzing the relationship between pain outcomes and facial numbness provided a higher statistical power to confirm this correlation.

A series of 100 patients enrolled in a prospective controlled trial showed excellent pain control (pain free and medication free) in 58% of the cases at minimum 1 year follow-up (Regis et al. 2006). These authors placed the isocenter just posterior to the gasserian ganglia. The analysis of predictive factors for SRS success was statistically significant for the length of the trigeminal nerve, the pre-pontine cistern surface and the distance between the shot emergence and the brainstem. The volume of trigeminal nerve per se submitted to a given dose of radiation did not correlate with pain control. Massager et al. also published a retrospective analysis of 47 patients treated with 90 Gy at the same target used by the Marseille group (Regis et al. 2006). A shorter distance between the target and the brainstem and higher radiation dose delivered to the brainstem was also predictive of successful pain control. The findings of a retrospective series published by Brisman and Mooij (2000), on 172 patients treated with 75 Gy, also corroborates these observations. The authors concluded: ".....that for a fixed radiosurgical dose the proximity to the radiosurgical target to brainstem is more important for pain relief than a more distal placement that would increase the nerve volume treated" (Fig. 17.4). In similarity, Massager et al. (2007) also concluded that "the radiobiological effect ....may be related to the energy delivered to the nerve root volume, rather than to the maximal dose delivered".

One group (Matsuda et al. 2008) recently published a retrospective analysis comparing results of patients treated at REZ vs. at the anterior cisternal portion of the trigeminal nerve. The conclusions were that the REZ target led to improved pain outcomes at short-term with a lower rate of bothersome sensory complications. There are important limitations in this analysis due to lack of control for radiation dose and significantly different length of follow-up available for both groups.

Given that radiosurgery is an ablative technique, the results presented in the literature are expected: good

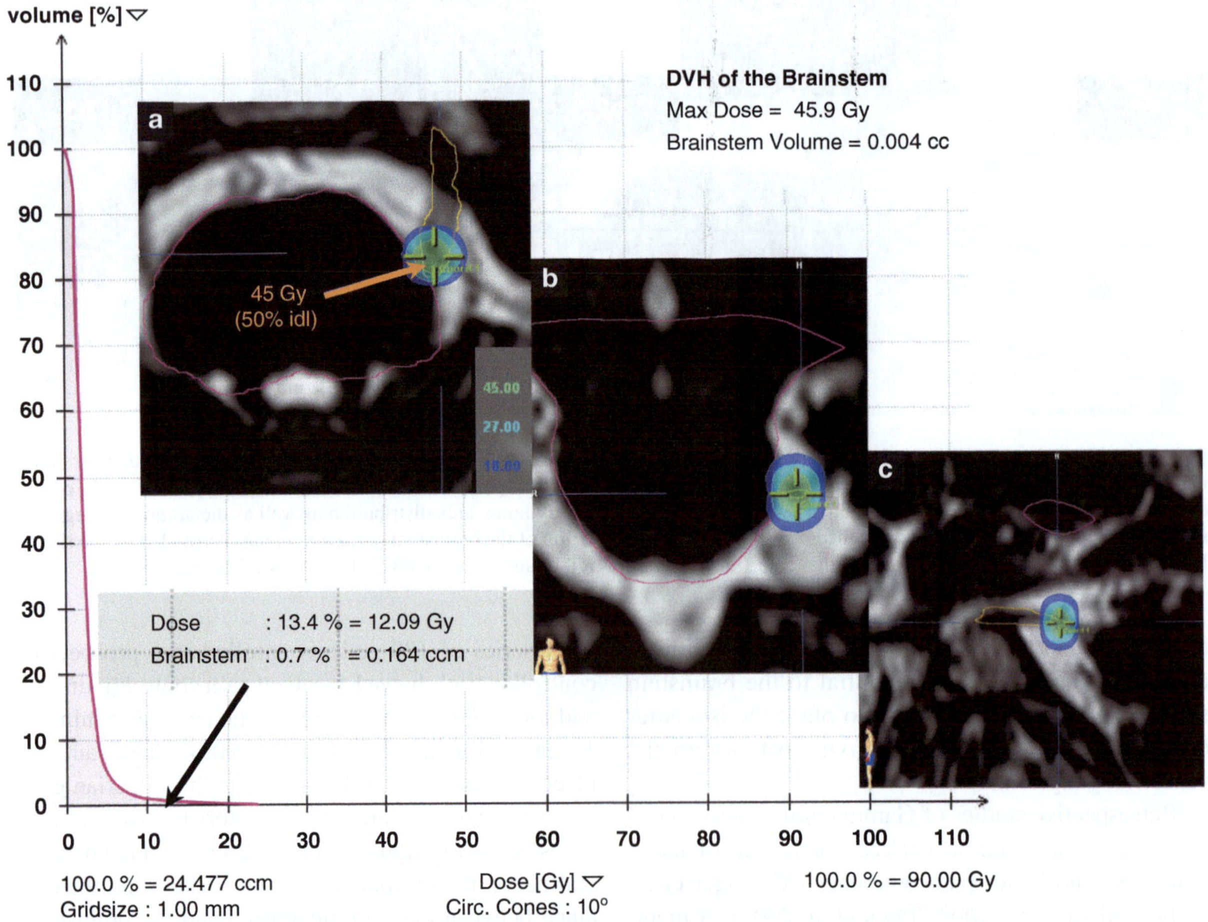

Fig. 17.4 Dose volume histogram of the brainstem showing that a volume of 0.164 cc receives 12 Gy. Some authors place the isocenter far anteriorly into the cisternal segment of the trigeminal nerve, aiming to spare any volume of brainstem from receiving 12 Gy. The radiosurgery dose distribution plan is shown in *axial, coronal and sagittal* (**a**, **b** and **c** figures) *views*. The 50% IDL corresponds to the dose of 45 Gy, displayed in *green*. The maximal dose of radiation to the brainstem is 45.9 Gy to a volume of 0.004 cc. This minimal volume of brainstem corresponds to 1 or 2 pixels of brainstem tissue visualized in the MRI image which is encroached within the 50% dose volume. This encroachment is a result of the positioning of the isocenter at the root entry zone of the trigeminal nerve by placing the 50% isodose line tangential to the pontine surface

results depend on the fine tuning between triggering pain relief vs. facial numbness. Bothersome dysesthesia and anesthesia dolorosa have been reported in radiosurgery series but its incidence has been low in the dedicated-Linac and Gamma-unit reports. The levels were significantly higher in the CyberKnife® (Accuray, Sunnyvale, CA, USA) series (Lim et al. 2005; Villavicencio et al. 2008).

Many authors observed a correlation between higher doses of radiation to the trigeminal nerve and more trigeminal nerve sensory deficits (Brisman 2004; Flickinger et al. 2001; Massager et al. 2007; Petit et al. 2003; Pollock 2006; Pollock et al. 2001). Their conclusions consubstantiate the concept discussed in the prior section (i.e., isocenter positioning), where the general trend was that as the radiation dose delivered to the REZ increases; better chances of pain relief and higher incidence of facial numbness are noticed.

In summary, the current evidence level is based on the comparison of the results among different series using either the lower or the higher radiation dose within the spectrum 70–90 Gy, acknowledging to the fact that treated populations, isocenter positioning, definition of outcome measures and follow-up protocols significantly differ. Moreover ad-hoc analyses on retrospective series elicit careful interpretation of the results derived from the data. Although the frequency of facial numbness post-SRS differs substantially among the series (Massager et al. 2004; Nicol et al. 2000; Smith et al. 2003), bothersome numbness is consistently observed in a minority of the cases (4–12%) (Petit et al. 2003; Pollock et al. 2002; Smith et al. 2003) and so far cannot be attributed to a minimal threshold dose of radiation. The precise dose to achieve better results and less recurrence within acceptable rates of sensory complications is still to be defined. The definition of where to place the isocenter also impacts in the final decision of the dose prescription.

The key question remains: where exactly lays the "sweet spot" triggering an optimal rate of pain relief without increasing sensory complications to unacceptable levels? Our experience and literature evidence points to the REZ. A double-blind randomized clinical trial comparing high and low radiation doses to the REZ/brainstem is required to provide definite evidence on pain outcome benefits at the cost of increased facial numbness incidence.

17.6.2 Relevance of the Dose Distribution at the Trigeminal Nerve

At UCLA, the routine is to use 7 arcs, equally distributed and weighted to achieve a circular dose distribution. Initially we attempted an oval dose distribution using dynamic arcs but felt that the circular dose distribution was preferable. Some Gamma unit protocols use selective channel blocking to limit the maximal radiation dose to the brainstem. It is not clear whether this technique significantly decreases the incidence of mild facial numbness while maintaining the same levels of pain control. This has been an explanation proposed by some authors (Massager et al. 2006) to justify different results obtained with the similar protocols but with different dosimetric and beam channel blocking protocols (Massager et al. 2004, 2007).

17.6.3 Relevance of the Trigeminal Nerve Length Submitted to Radiation

Irradiation of a longer portion of the nerve either with two isocenters or with non-isocentric technique resulted in increased incidence of sensory disturbance without benefits on pain control rates (Flickinger et al. 2001; Lim et al. 2005; Villavicencio et al. 2008). Non-isocentric radiosurgery series have varied the length of trigeminal nerve treated (3–12 mm) as well as the radiation dose. Pain outcomes have been similar to those reported by dedicated-Linac and Gamma-unit series but the incidence of anesthesia dolorosa, masticatory weakness, and extra-trigeminal nerve complications were significantly higher (Lim et al. 2005). Complications such as hearing loss, foot paresis, and diplopia have been described in non-isocentric series (Adler et al. 2009; Villavicencio et al. 2008). A recent publication (Adler et al. 2009) where the maximal nerve length was limited to 6 mm and the average maximal dose was 73.5 Gy showed lower incidence of complications with absence of the extra-trigeminal system ones. The length of follow-up was too short to establish whether or not this protocol will lead to the similar sustained pain response observed in the isocentric series. Short-term pain control was satisfactory.

17.7 Radiosurgery Treatment Protocol and Results

At UCLA our current treatment protocol consists of T1 and CISS (constructive interference steady state) MRI sequences with 1 mm and 2 mm slice thickness, respectively. These images are fused to 1.5 mm slice thickness CT scans. The CISS sequence offers an exquisite level of detailed anatomy of the trigeminal pathway from inside the Meckel's cave through the pre-pontine cistern until its entrance in the pons (Figs. 17.3 and 17.4). Accuracy remains an important aspect of the radiosurgery process. Consequently, every single detail counts to improve accuracy; imaging being an important step. Minimal inaccuracy can result in failure to reach a 3 mm target embedded in cerebral spinal fluid of the pre-pontine cistern with a 4 mm collimator. We have reported on the importance of special MRI sequencing (Chavez et al. 2005) to improve the stereotactic targeting (De Salles et al. 2003).

Since January/2008, the 4 mm collimator is used for TN radiosurgery at UCLA. Since the 4 mm collimator was not available until recently, radiosurgery was performed with the 5 mm collimator. Radiosurgery was performed with the 3 mm collimator in a few cases, requiring retreatment due to pain recurrence. The dosimetry of the 3 mm collimator is however challenging and the use of the 4 mm collimator, under this circumstance, is preferable.

Figure 17.3 illustrates the treatment plan protocol currently used at UCLA. In summary, 90 Gy is delivered with a 4 mm collimator to the REZ by positioning the isocenter with the 50% IDL tangential to the pons using a circular dose distribution, achieved with the use of 7 non-coplanar arcs equally distributed. The brainstem receives up to 45 Gy using this protocol but the volume of tissue submitted to this dose is very minimal (Fig. 17.4). The maximal dose of radiation delivered to the root entry zone and brainstem regions have been shown to be relevant for the clinical outcome after radiosurgery.

The results of our most recent series review on 179 patients treated at UCLA from August/1995 to January/2007 is presented in Fig. 17.5 (Smith et al. 2010) in print. The median age was 74 years (range: 32–90). One hundred thirty patients had essential TN while 39 had secondary TN. Radiation dose ranged from 75 to 90 Gy, the 5 mm collimator was used in 90% of the cases. The isocenter positioning was progressively brought closer to the brainstem during different periods of time as prior detailed in the text. Mean latency to pain relief was 1.92 months. At mean 28.8 months follow-up, 79.3% of the patients experienced excellent or good pain relief. The actuarial analysis (Fig. 17.5) shows that excellent pain relief (defined as pain free and medication free) for those diagnosed as essential TN is 85% at 1 year and 65% at 3 years. These results are among the best ones achieved with SRS technique. Facial numbness was observed in 49.7% of the cases; however, it was mild in the majority of the cases. A five grading scale was used to rate the intensity of numbness with 1 being very faint numbness and 5 complete anesthesia. The median numbness score was 2. No masticatory weaknesses, anesthesia dolorosa, hearing loss or keratitis were observed in our series.

Frameless radiosurgery for TN has been performed in 17 patients since July/2009 to March/2010 using a dedicated-Linac device (Novalis TX™, Brainlab, Feldkirchen, Germany) at UCLA. Our current protocol for frameless radiosurgery for TN includes Winston-Lutz test and ExacTrac® X-Ray (Brainlab, Feldkirchen, Germany) calibration tests performed at the day of the treatment, full ExacTrac performed for each treatment arc with table yaw rotations at planned angles and checking of each ExacTrac fusion by the medical physicist, neurosurgeon, and radiation oncologist. The correction tolerance for ExacTrac was established at 0.5 mm and 1.0°. After the initial ExacTrac and shifts correction, the validity of the ExacTrac positioning is verified, by redundancy, using Cone Beam CT at 0 table rotation.

17.7.1 Repeat Radiosurgery

There are few publications describing the use of different protocols in the retreatment of patients who failed or presented pain recurrence after initial SRS. It appears that recurrences after successful SRS respond well to retreatment while failures still do not significantly respond to a second radiosurgery (Herman et al. 2004). Some groups change the position of the isocenter to a more anterior target (Hasegawa et al. 2002), others decrease the radiation dose (Shetter et al., JNS 2002) and others use the same protocol for retreatment (Pollock et al. 2005). We repeat SRS using the same treatment protocol. So far, we have re-treated 16 patients. All the series uniformly describe the same findings: pain relief should be expected in about

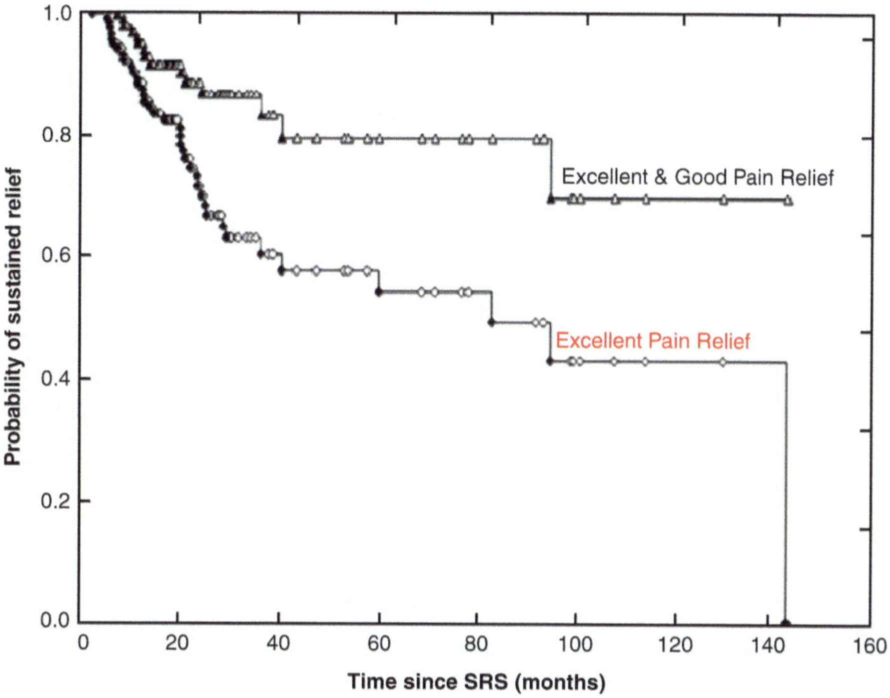

Fig. 17.5 *Kaplan Meier curve* of the 133 patients with classical trigeminal neuralgia in a retrospective series review of the 179 patients treated at UCLA with SRS for trigeminal pain during August/1995 to January/2007. The *triangle's curve* represents patients with excellent and good pain outcomes which includes those experiencing at least 50% of pain improvement up to those who are pain free with or without medication. The *diamond's curve* represents only patients who are pain free and medication free (excellent relief). The incidence of excellent pain control is 85% at 1 year and 65% at 3 years post-SRS. Satisfactory pain outcome (good and excellent relief) is 79.5% at 3 years

80% of the patients, "new" facial numbness incidence is higher and intensification of prior facial numbness is likely to occur. Therefore, patients should be carefully informed that they should expect more sensory complications when submitted to repeat SRS. The experience of the groups reporting repeated SRS is limited to few patients. Extended follow-ups are being acquired to establish the long-term effectiveness and safety of repeated SRS.

17.8 Conclusions

Radiosurgery is a good option in the surgical armamentarium available for TN. Despite the lack of consensus, it seems that SRS is considered the first surgical option for the elderly by the majority of the surgical community. An increasing percentage of younger patients have been treated initially with SRS due to the fact that this technique is the least invasive one, leading to satisfactory pain relief results and low complications rates. The major drawback of radiosurgery is the time latency between radiation delivery and pain relief.

Radiosurgery treatment protocols differ in regards to positioning of the isocenter within the trigeminal pathway and maximal radiation prescription dose. The concept of a higher dose of radiation specifically targeted to the root entry zone as a key factor to achieve better pain relief rates but at the cost of a higher incidence of facial numbness is suggested by our data as well as by the literature. However, longer follow-up is necessary to proof a long lasting effect of pain relief and rule out other sensory complications that may appear later on, such as deafferentation pain. A prospective double blind trial comparing different doses of radiation to the REZ is necessary to provide definition of the optimal radiosurgery treatment protocol. Also the standardization of pain relief scales, recurrence criteria and follow-up parameters should be kept as uniform as possible to allow for a closer comparison among radiosurgery reported results, including with other surgical modalities.

References

Adler JR Jr, Bower R, Gupta G et al (2009) Nonisocentric radiosurgical rhizotomy for trigeminal neuralgia. Neurosurgery 64:A84–A90

Barker FG 2nd, Jannetta PJ, Bissonette DJ et al (1996) The long-term outcome of microvascular decompression for trigeminal neuralgia. N Engl J Med 334:1077–1083

Brisman R (2004) Gamma knife surgery with a dose of 75 to 76.8 Gray for trigeminal neuralgia. J Neurosurg 100: 848–854

Brisman R, Mooij R (2000) Gamma knife radiosurgery for trigeminal neuralgia: dose-volume histograms of the brainstem and trigeminal nerve. J Neurosurg 93(Suppl 3): 155–158

Broggi G, Franzini A, Lasio G et al (1990) Long-term results of percutaneous retrogasserian thermorhizotomy for "essential" trigeminal neuralgia: considerations in 1000 consecutive patients. Neurosurgery 26:783–786, discussion 786–787

Broggi G, Ferroli P, Franzini A et al (2000) Microvascular decompression for trigeminal neuralgia: comments on a series of 250 cases, including 10 patients with multiple sclerosis. J Neurol Neurosurg Psychiatry 68:59–64

Broggi G, Ferroli P, Franzini A (2008) Treatment strategy for trigeminal neuralgia: a thirty years experience. Neurol Sci 29(Suppl 1):S79–S82

Burchiel KJ (1980) Abnormal impulse generation in focally demyelinated trigeminal roots. J Neurosurg 53:674–683

Chavez GD, De Salles AA, Solberg TD et al (2005) Three-dimensional fast imaging employing steady-state acquisition magnetic resonance imaging for stereotactic radiosurgery of trigeminal neuralgia. Neurosurgery 56:E628, Discussion E628

Chen JC, Greathouse HE, Girvigian MR et al (2008) Prognostic factors for radiosurgery treatment of trigeminal neuralgia. Neurosurgery 62:A53–A60

Cruccu G, Pennisi E, Truini A et al (2003) Unmyelinated trigeminal pathways as assessed by laser stimuli in humans. Brain 126:2246–2256

De Salles AAF, Solberg T, Medin P et al (1997) Linear accelerator radiosurgery for trigeminal neuralgia. In: Kondziolka D (ed) Radiosurgery, vol 2. Karger, Basel, pp 173–182

De Salles AAF, Frighetto L, Lacan G et al (2003) Radiosurgery can achieve precision needed for functional neurosurgery. Arch Neurol 60:1494–1496

Farago F (1987) Trigeminal neuralgia: its treatment with two new carbamazepine analogues. Eur Neurol 26:73–83

Fields HL (1996) Treatment of trigeminal neuralgia. N Engl J Med 334:1125–1126

Flickinger JC, Pollock BE, Kondziolka D et al (2001) Does increased nerve length within the treatment volume improve trigeminal neuralgia radiosurgery? A prospective double-blind, randomized study. Int J Radiat Oncol Biol Phys 51: 449–454

Fromm GH, Terrence CF, Maroon JC (1984) Trigeminal neuralgia. Current concepts regarding etiology and pathogenesis. Arch Neurol 41:1204–1207

Gorgulho AA, De Salles AA (2006) Impact of radiosurgery on the surgical treatment of trigeminal neuralgia. Surg Neurol 66:350–356

Gorgulho A, De Salles AA, McArthur D et al (2006) Brainstem and trigeminal nerve changes after radiosurgery for trigeminal pain. Surg Neurol 66:127–135, discussion 135

Gorgulho AS, Smith Z, Zrinzo L, Bezruky N, Moura AM, Agazaryan N, Selch M, De Salles AAF (2007) Results and complications of trigeminal neuralgia radiosurgery in patients presenting with pons enhancement in annual meeting of the American Association of Neurological Surgeons (AANS). Washington, DC. April 14–19, Oral Presentation 628, Scientific Program CD

Goss BW, Frighetto L, De Salles AA et al (2003) Linear accelerator radiosurgery using 90 gray for essential trigeminal neuralgia: results and dose volume histogram analysis. Neurosurgery 53:823–828, Discussion 828–830

Hasegawa T, Kondziolka D, Spiro R et al (2002) Repeat radiosurgery for refractory trigeminal neuralgia. Neurosurgery 50:494–500, Discussion 500–492

Henson CF, Goldman HW, Rosenwasser RH et al (2005) Glycerol rhizotomy versus gamma knife radiosurgery for the treatment of trigeminal neuralgia: an analysis of patients treated at one institution. Int J Radiat Oncol Biol Phys 63:82–90

Herman JM, Petit JH, Amin P et al (2004) Repeat gamma knife radiosurgery for refractory or recurrent trigeminal neuralgia: treatment outcomes and quality-oflife assessment. Int J Radiat Oncol Biol Phys 59:112–116

Katusic S, Williams DB, Beard CM et al (1991) Epidemiology and clinical features of idiopathic trigeminal neuralgia and glossopharyngeal neuralgia: similarities and differences, Rochester, Minnesota, 1945–1984. Neuroepidemiology 10:276–281

Kondziolka D, Lunsford LD, Flickinger JC et al (1996) Stereotactic radiosurgery for trigeminal neuralgia: a multiinstitutional study using the gamma unit. J Neurosurg 84:940–945

Kondziolka D, Lacomis D, Niranjan A et al (2000) Histological effects of trigeminal nerve radiosurgery in a primate model: implications for trigeminal neuralgia radiosurgery. Neurosurgery 46:971–976, Discussion 976–977

Lim M, Villavicencio AT, Burneikiene S et al (2005) CyberKnife radiosurgery for idiopathic trigeminal neuralgia. Neurosurg Focus 18:E9

Little AS, Shetter AG, Shetter ME et al (2008a) Long-term pain response and quality of life in patients with typical trigeminal neuralgia treated with gamma knife stereotactic radiosurgery. Neurosurgery 63:915–923, Discussion 923–914

Little AS, Shetter AG, Shetter ME et al (2008b) Salvage gamma knife stereotactic radiosurgery for surgically refractory trigeminal neuralgia. Int J Radiat Oncol Biol Phys 74(2): 522–527

Lopez BC, Hamlyn PJ, Zakrzewska JM (2004a) Stereotactic radiosurgery for primary trigeminal neuralgia: state of the evidence and recommendations for future reports. J Neurol Neurosurg Psychiatry 75:1019–1024

Lopez BC, Hamlyn PJ, Zakrzewska JM (2004b) Systematic review of ablative neurosurgical techniques for the treatment of trigeminal neuralgia. Neurosurgery 54:973–982, Discussion 982–973

Love S, Hilton DA, Coakham HB (1998) Central demyelination of the Vth nerve root in trigeminal neuralgia associated with vascular compression. Brain Pathol 8:1–11, Discussion 11–12

Maesawa S, Salame C, Flickinger JC et al (2001) Clinical outcomes after stereotactic radiosurgery for idiopathic trigeminal neuralgia. J Neurosurg 94:14–20

Massager N, Lorenzoni J, Devriendt D et al (2004) Gamma knife surgery for idiopathic trigeminal neuralgia performed using a far-anterior cisternal target and a high dose of radiation. J Neurosurg 100:597–605

Massager N, Nissim O, Murata N et al (2006) Effect of beam channel plugging on the outcome of gamma knife radiosurgery for trigeminal neuralgia. Int J Radiat Oncol Biol Phys 65:1200–1205

Massager N, Murata N, Tamura M et al (2007) Influence of nerve radiation dose in the incidence of trigeminal dysfunction

after trigeminal neuralgia radiosurgery. Neurosurgery 60: 681–687, Discussion 687–688
Matsuda S, Serizawa T, Nagano O et al (2008) Comparison of the results of 2 targeting methods in gamma knife surgery for trigeminal neuralgia. J Neurosurg 109(Suppl):185–189
Mullan S, Lichtor T (1983) Percutaneous microcompression of the trigeminal ganglion for trigeminal neuralgia. J Neurosurg 59:1007–1012
Nicol B, Regine WF, Courtney C et al (2000) Gamma knife radiosurgery using 90 Gy for trigeminal neuralgia. J Neurosurg 93(Suppl 3):152–154
Oh IH, Choi SK, Park BJ et al (2008) The treatment outcome of elderly patients with idiopathic trigeminal neuralgia: microvascular decompression versus Gamma Knife radiosurgery. J Korean Neurosurg Soc 44:199–204
Petit JH, Herman JM, Nagda S et al (2003) Radiosurgical treatment of trigeminal neuralgia: evaluating quality of life and treatment outcomes. Int J Radiat Oncol Biol Phys 56: 1147–1153
Pollock BE (2006) Radiosurgery for trigeminal neuralgia: is sensory disturbance required for pain relief? J Neurosurg 105(Suppl):103–106
Pollock BE, Phuong LK, Foote RL et al (2001) High-dose trigeminal neuralgia radiosurgery associated with increased risk of trigeminal nerve dysfunction. Neurosurgery 49: 58–62, Discussion 62–54
Pollock BE, Phuong LK, Gorman DA et al (2002) Stereotactic radiosurgery for idiopathic trigeminal neuralgia. J Neurosurg 97:347–353
Pollock BE, Foote RL, Link MJ et al (2005) Repeat radiosurgery for idiopathic trigeminal neuralgia. Int J Radiat Oncol Biol Phys 61:192–195
Rahimian J, Chen JC, Rao AA et al (2004) Geometrical accuracy of the Novalis stereotactic radiosurgery system for trigeminal neuralgia. J Neurosurg 101(Suppl 3):351–355
Regis JMP, Hayashi M, Roussel M, Donnett A, Bilet-Turc F (2006) Prospective controlled trial of gamma-knife surgery for essential trigeminal neuralgia. J Neurosurg 104: 913–924
Rogers CL, Shetter AG, Fiedler JA et al (2000) Gamma knife radiosurgery for trigeminal neuralgia: the initial experience of The Barrow Neurological Institute. Int J Radiat Oncol Biol Phys 47:1013–1019
Shetter AG, Rogers CL, Ponce F et al (2002) Gamma knife radiosurgery for recurrent trigeminal neuralgia. J Neurosurg 97:536–538
Shetter AG, Zabramski JM, Speiser BL (2005) Microvascular decompression after gamma knife surgery for trigeminal neuralgia: intraoperative findings and treatment outcomes. J Neurosurg 102(Suppl):259–261
Skirving DJ, Dan NG (2001) A 20-year review of percutaneous balloon compression of the trigeminal ganglion. J Neurosurg 94:913–917
Smith ZA, De Salles AA, Frighetto L et al (2003) Dedicated linear accelerator radiosurgery for the treatment of trigeminal neuralgia. J Neurosurg 99:511–516
Smith Z, Gorgulho A, MacArthur D et al (2010) Linear accelerator radiosurgery for trigeminal neuralgia: a single center experience in 179 patients with varied dose prescription and treatment plan, in Neurosurgery Department. University of California at Los Angeles, Los Angeles, p 29
Tatli M, Satici O, Kanpolat Y et al (2008) Various surgical modalities for trigeminal neuralgia: literature study of respective long-term outcomes. Acta Neurochir (Wien) 150: 243–255
Tawk RG, Duffy-Fronckowiak M, Scott BE et al (2005) Stereotactic gamma knife surgery for trigeminal neuralgia: detailed analysis of treatment response. J Neurosurg 102: 442–449
Urgosik D, Liscak R, Novotny J Jr et al (2005) Treatment of essential trigeminal neuralgia with gamma knife surgery. J Neurosurg 102(Suppl):29–33
Villavicencio AT, Lim M, Burneikiene S et al (2008) Cyberknife radiosurgery for trigeminal neuralgia treatment: a preliminary multicenter experience. Neurosurgery 62:647–655, Discussion 647–655
Young RF, Vermulen S, Posewitz A (1998) Gamma knife radiosurgery for the treatment of trigeminal neuralgia. Stereotact Funct Neurosurg 70:192–199
Zakrzewska JM, Lopez BC (2003) Quality of reporting in evaluations of surgical treatment of trigeminal neuralgia: recommendations for future reports. Neurosurgery 53:110–120, Discussion 120–112
Zakrzewska JM, Patsalos PN (2002) Long-term cohort study comparing medical (oxcarbazepine) and surgical management of intractable trigeminal neuralgia. Pain 95:259–266
Zakrzewska JL, Lopez BC, Kim SE et al (2005) Patient reports of satisfaction after microvascular decompression and partial sensory rhizotomy for trigeminal neuralgia. Neurosurgery 56:1304–1311

Stereotactic Radiosurgery for Movement Disorders

18

Leonardo Frighetto, Jorge Bizzi, and Paulo Oppitz

18.1 Introduction

Stereotactic radiosurgery (SRS) was developed with the aim of creating a minimally invasive technique capable of precisely generating a focal lesion in the brain. In his first procedure, Lars Leksell used an orthovoltage X-ray source adapted to his arc-centered stereotactic frame to treat a trigeminal neuralgia patient (Leksell 1951). At that point, his main goal was to develop a device to treat functional disorders of the brain, including intractable pain, movement disorders, and epilepsy. Although Leksell and his group described the utility of SRS in functional diseases (Leksell 1968; Steiner et al. 1980), the technique has advanced and proved its invaluable utility in the treatment of other major neurosurgical pathologies including brain arteriovenous malformations, metastases, malignant and benign tumors of the brain and skull base (De Salles et al. 2008; Friedman and Bova 1992; Kondziolka et al. 2008a; Sneed et al. 2002).

Almost 20 years after the development of the gamma unit, the interest for functional radiosurgery procedures returned in the beginning of the last decade (Lindquist et al. 1991; Rand et al. 1993). Probably encouraged by the advances in imaging and computerized software systems dedicated to radiosurgery planning, its applications to chronic pain syndromes, especially trigeminal neuralgia, as well as psychiatric and movement disorders have been used in many medical centers around the world (Bonnen et al. 1997; Duma et al. 1998, 1999; Friedman et al. 1996; Friehs et al. 1995; Kihlström et al. 1995; Ohye et al. 1996; Pan et al. 1996; Smith et al. 2003; Young et al. 1994). The application of SRS for movement disorders was also stimulated by the good results obtained with radiofrequency lesioning (Dogali et al. 1995; Goldman and Kelly 2000; Hariz and Bergenheim 2001; Jankovic et al. 1995; Laitinen et al. 1992; Linhares and Tasker 2000; Lozano et al. 1996; Tasker et al. 1997).

The literature related to SRS performed in order to treat movement disorders was developed using the gamma unit. In spite of the fact that there is no report of the utilization of the linear accelerator (Linac) based radiosurgery for the treatment of movement disorders, our group published three cases of thalamotomy using a dedicated 6 MV linac (Novalis® Radiosurgery, Brainlab, Feldkirchen, Germany) for treatment of chronic pain in the ventral medial/lateral posterior thalamus (Frighetto et al. 2004). The application of this dedicated Linac radiosurgery device (Novalis Radiosurgery) to perform lesions using a 3 mm collimator in the vervet monkey subthalamic nucleus and substantia nigra has also been reported and target accuracy was confirmed by histology (De Salles et al. 2001). Other reports have demonstrated the capability of dedicated Linacs to reach the necessary precision to treat small functional targets, including its clinical application for the treatment of trigeminal neuralgia. (Smith et al. 2003; Solberg et al. 1998).

This chapter represents a broad review of the usefulness of SRS for the treatment of movement disorders regarding its indications, techniques, applications and complications.

L. Frighetto (✉), J. Bizzi, and P. Oppitz
Department of Neurosurgery, Stereotactic Radiosurgery Section, Moinhos de Vento Hospital, Rua Tiradentes 333, 90560–030 Porto Alegre, RS, Brazil
e-mail: leonardo.frighetto@hmv.org.br; lfrighetto@hotmail.com

A.A.F. De Salles et al. (eds.), *Shaped Beam Radiosurgery*,
DOI: 10.1007/978-3-642-11151-8_18, © Springer-Verlag Berlin Heidelberg 2011

18.2 Indications and Patient Selection

The indications of SRS lesioning for movement disorders are essentially the same as the usual stereotactic open surgery. These include patients with tremor or rigid type Parkinson's disease (PD), essential tremor (ET) and tremor related to other medical conditions such as multiple sclerosis and trauma not controlled with the best medical therapy (Bonnen et al. 1997; Dogali et al. 1995; Duma et al. 1998; Friedman et al. 1996; Friehs et al. 1995; Goldman and Kelly 2000; Jankovic et al. 1995; Laitinen et al. 1992; Ohye et al. 1996; Pan et al. 1996; Rand et al. 1993; Young et al. 1996).

Since neurophysiology guided radiofrequency stereotactic surgery or deep brain stimulation (DBS) offers advantages over stereotactic radiosurgery, this procedure is reserved for a small subset of patients. These patients have conditions that may turn them into unacceptable candidates for invasive stereotactic neurosurgical intervention, including very elderly patients, high-risk surgical patients suffering from severe cardiac or pulmonary pathology and those using anticoagulants. In these cases, SRS can be the only available treatment option. There are also patients who may choose SRS to avoid an invasive surgical procedure (Duma et al. 1998; Friedman et al. 1999; Friehs et al. 1995; Ohye et al. 1996; Pan et al. 1996; Rand et al. 1993; Young et al. 1998a).

Invasive stereotactic surgery, including both radiofrequency lesioning and DBS may be associated with significant morbidity and possible mortality. These procedures carry an inherent risk of intracerebral hemorrhage, infection, seizures, brain displacement, tension pneumocephalus, and direct injury from probe placement, among others (Benabid et al. 1998; Starr et al. 1998; Tasker et al. 1997; Young et al. 1998a).

SRS is a less invasive procedure that does not involve opening of the cranium or incisions, with no risk of hemorrhage or meningitis from operative infection. The post-operative patient care is simpler and patients return earlier to their regular activities with a reduction in hospitalization time. The disadvantages of the technique include uncertain target determination due to the impossibility of confirming the lesion site intraoperatively with physiologic testing relying exclusively on anatomical targeting and a mean delay of 6 months for clinical improvement (Duma et al. 1998; Friedman et al. 1999; Friehs et al. 1995; Ohye et al. 1996; Pan et al. 1996; Rand et al. 1993; Young et al. 1998a).

18.3 Technical Aspects

18.3.1 Dose and Collimator Size

The safe and effective dose to be used for functional radiosurgery was not initially known. Previous reports by Leksell and his group disclosed that doses of 180–200 Gy were capable of creating a focal lesion in the brain for the treatment of chronic pain (Leksell 1968; Lindquist et al. 1992; Steiner et al. 1980).

The higher the maximum dose, the earlier the manifestations of a clinical effect can be perceived. On the other hand, a higher dose may induce more brain damage and introduce the possibility of severe delayed-onset complications. The initial high doses are currently being reduced with a tendency towards fewer complications. The currently accepted dose parameters vary between 120 and 160 Gy (Duma 2007; Kondziolka et al. 2008b; Ohye 2006).

Collimator size and number of isocenters have also been a matter of concern since the use of multiple isocenters and large size collimators were related to an increase in the complication rate (Duma 2007; Friehs et al. 1996; Ohye 2006; Young et al. 1998a).

18.3.2 Targeting

Target planning and choice of the real target are the most important factors in achieving better results in the treatment of movement-related disorders (Fig. 18.1). Ohye et al. (1996), initially described the displacement of the ideal target to perform a radiosurgical thalamotomy more medially and anteriorly, to avoid an unacceptably high dose to the internal capsule (IC) laterally and the sensory relay nucleus of thalamic ventralis caudalis nucleus caudally. This was achieved by preventing the 30% isodose line from extending into these structures. More recently, the same author placed the target in relation to a point that is a known percentage of that length behind the anterior thalamic pole. This new

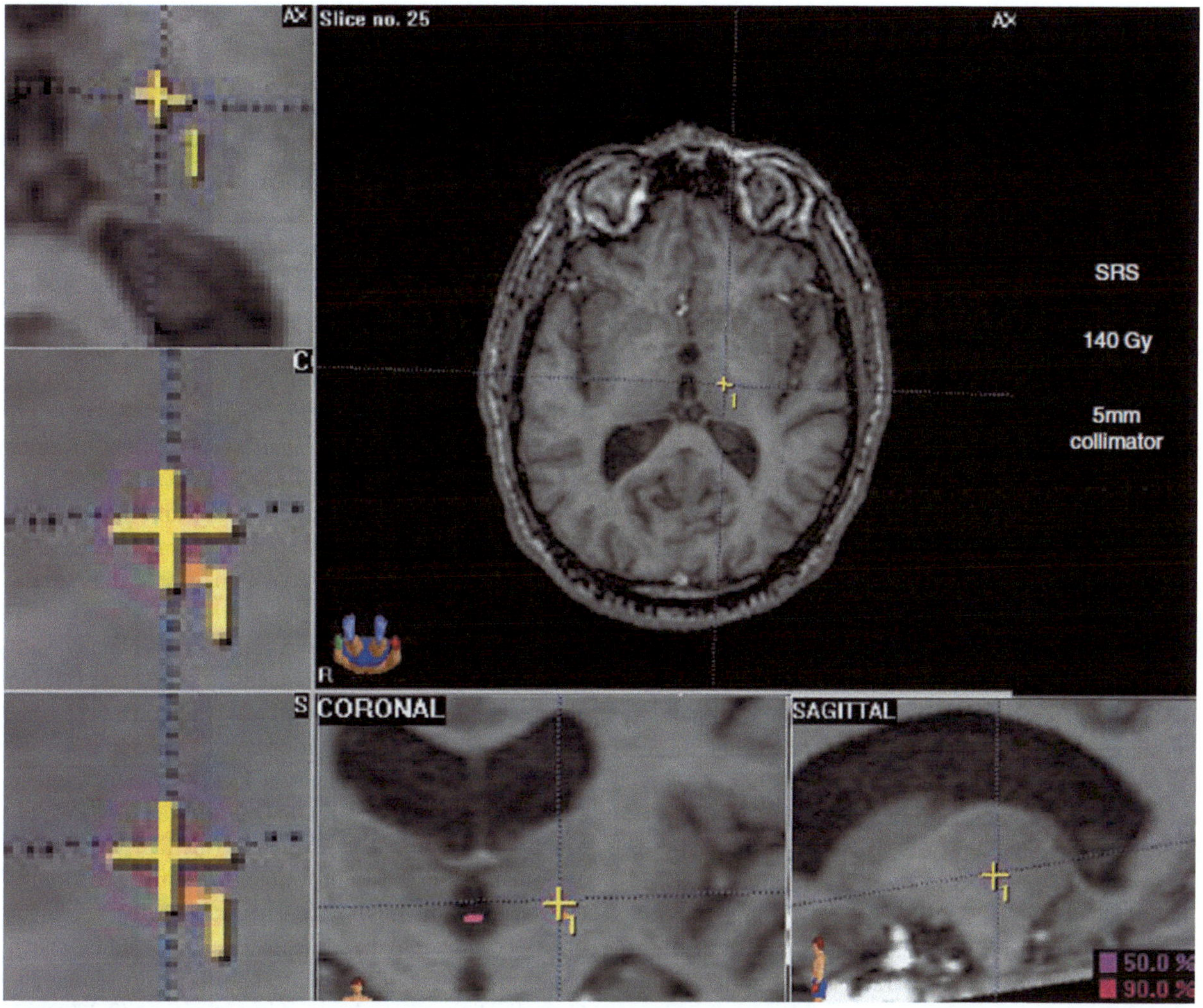

Fig. 18.1 Example of a radiosurgery thalamotomy performed at UCLA. The radiosurgery treatment consisted of 140 Gy delivered with a 5 mm collimator. Note the 50% (*purple*) and the 90% (*pink*) isodoselines in axial, coronal and sagittal views in the T1 MRI sequence (1 mm *slice thickness*). The patient was a 67 year-old gentleman with bilateral and debilitating essential tremor. He was not able to eat by himself nor write or use the keyboard of the computer. The patient had the following comor bidities: insulin-dependent diabetes mellitus, high blood pressure, prior cardiac bypass (2x), mild dementia and was on anti-coagulant therapy. He was considered not to be a good candidate for open surgery. At 5 months post-radiosurgery, his right hand tremor was almost completely controlled and the patient was able to perform daily living tasks on the right

method of calculating the desired target associated with the knowledge that the high signal zone surrounding a thalamic lesion is functionally almost intact, has encouraged the placement of the lesion closer to the real target point instead of shifting away to avoid capsular and sensory nucleus involvement (Ohye and Shibazaki 2002).

Kondziolka et al. (2008b), described the thalamotomy radiosurgery isocenter 2.5 mm superior to AC-PC (anterior commissure - posterior commissure) line, so that the inferior portion of the radiosurgery lesion would extend inferiorly to the AC-PC line. The 4 mm collimator was placed ¼ of the AC-PC line plus 1 mm anterior to PC and a point at half the width of the III ventricle plus 11 mm from the AC-PC line laterally. The 20% isodose line was kept medial to the IC (internal capsule).

There are still concerns related to MRI spatial inaccuracies, particularly for functional cases using this imaging modality alone without neurophysiological confirmation of the target. Modern protocols and high quality assurance MRI adjustments have corrected possible distortions of the MRI field, making this method sufficiently accurate for stereotactic targeting. Following such protocols, accuracy in the 1-mm range can be achieved (Lozano et al. 1996; Novotny et al. 2005; Sumanaweera et al. 1994; Young et al. 1998a).

Bednarz et al. (1999), studied the impact of geometrical distortions on the spatial accuracy of MRI-guided localization for functional radiosurgery comparing stereotactic coordinates of intracranial targets defined by MRI and CT. The average difference between the two modalities was only one pixel (or approximately 1 mm^3) along the X, Y, and Z axes. They concluded that the spatial accuracy of an MRI-based localization system can be comparable to that of CT with the added benefit of MRI resolution.

SRS is a closed skull procedure with no possibility of neurophysiological target verification. Therefore, the treatment success is dependent on anatomical target localization only.

The use of microelectrode stimulation and recording provides the surgeon the advantage to identify the intended target for lesioning electrophysiologically and is widely accepted in movement disorder surgery (Benabid et al. 1998; Burchiel et al. 1999; Jankovic et al. 1995; Linhares and Tasker 2000; Lozano et al. 1996). Although there are strong advocates for the microelectrode approach, there is in reality no documentation that such methods improve either the efficacy or safety of functional stereotactic procedures (Goldman and Kelly 2000; Tasker et al. 1997; Young et al. 1998a).

The necessity of electrophysiological target localization is probably higher in open skull procedures, in which loss of cerebrospinal fluid and brain shift may contribute to differences between the calculated anatomical target and the physiologically defined target. The closed brain technique in radiosurgery avoids these potential error-inducing mechanisms (Young et al. 1998a). Neurophysiological confirmation of the target is also important when it is defined using ventriculography or CT scanning (Alterman et al. 1995). The use of high definition MRI to calculate the target coordinates is another factor that makes the need for electrophysiological target localization questionable (Young et al. 1996). Dogali et al. (1995), reported that the electrophysiologically identified target for pallidotomy varied by a maximum of 1 mm from the anatomically determined target using MR imaging.

18.4 Thalamotomy

Radiosurgical thalamotomy for pain was one of the first performed functional radiosurgery procedures. Its application targeting the nucleus ventralis intermedius (VIM) has been performed by several authors in the treatment of tremor in patients with PD, ET, and tremor related to multiple sclerosis, trauma and or other causes. (Fig. 18.1) The reported results and complications with radiosurgery thalamotomy are comparable to those achieved using other methods (Duma et al. 1998; Friedman et al. 1999; Friehs et al. 1995; Ohye et al. 1996; Rand et al. 1993; Young et al. 1994).

Pan et al. (1996), described the treatment of eight patients with PD. Follow-up was available in six patients. Tremor disappeared in three and improved in the other three (Table 18.1). There was one case of contralateral limb weakness, which appeared 3 months after treatment.

Duma (2007), presented a series of 42 patients submitted to 46 lesions for the treatment of PD and ET. No change in tremor was observed in 4 patients (8.6%), mild improvement in 4 (8.6%), good improvement (more than 50%) in 13 (28%), excellent in 13 (28%) and complete elimination in 12 (26%). Clinical and radiological follow-up ranged from 6 to 90 months (median 30 months). The median time of improvements onset was 2 months (1 week to 8 months). Independent neurologist evaluations scoring of patient's response to treatment were obtained at regular clinical follow-up intervals. Complications were observed in one patient (2.3%) who was submitted to bilateral lesions and suffered a mild acute dysarthria 1 week after the treatment.

A comparison study was conducted between a subgroup of patients in whom "low-dose" lesions (mean 120 Gy) and those in whom "high-dose" lesions were made (mean 160 Gy) for purposes of dose–response information (Duma et al. 1998). There was better tremor reduction in the high-dose group (78% mean improvement) than in the low-dose group (56% mean improvement) ($p=0.04$). There were no neurological complications.

The largest series in the literature (Young et al. 2000) reported the results of 158 patients who underwent radiosurgery thalamotomy for the treatment of tremor. This group included 102 patients with PD, 52 with ET and four with other forms of tremor. After a median follow up, in patients with PD, of 47 months (range 11–93 months), 78 patients (76.5%)

Table 18.1 Literature review of radiosurgery thalamotomy series

Authors and year	Pathology	Patients	Lesions[a]	FU (months)	Excellent	Good	Mild	Failed	Complications
Li Pan et al. (1996)	PD	6	6	4.5 (2–9)	3 (50%)	3 (50%)	–	–	1 (16.6%)
Duma et al. (2007)	PD & ET	42	46	38 (NR)	25 (54%)	13 (28%)	4 (4.5%)	4 (8.6%)	1 (2.3%)
Duma et al. (1998)	PD	34	38	28 (6–58)	19 (50%)	11 (29%)	4 (10.5%)	4 (10.5%)	No
Niranjan et al. (2000)	ET	8	8	6 (2–11)	6 (75%)	2 (25%)	–	–	1 (12.5%)
Young et al. (2000)	PD	102	102	47 (11–93)	90 (88.2%)	–	–	12 (11.8%)	2 (1.9%)
Young et al. (2000)	ET	52	52	26 (NR)	48 (92.1%)	–	–	4 (7.8%)	1 (1.9%)
Ohye et al. (2002)	PD & ET	30	30	30 (24–96)	24 (80%)	–	–	6 (20%)	No

PD Parkinson's Disease, *ET* essential tremor, *NR* not reported, *FU* Median and range of follow-up
[a]Number of lesions

were completely tremor free, 12 patients (11.8%) were nearly free and 12 patients (11.8%) have failed the treatment. Blinded assessments of UPDRS tremor scores showed statistically significant improvements in overall tremor, action tremor, and tremor at rest. Statistically significant improvements were also seen in rigidity and maintained at 4-year follow-up evaluation.

The 52 patients with ET in this series were followed to a median time of 26 months. At 1-year follow-up, 92.1% of patients were completely or nearly tremor free, whereas in patients followed for 4 years, this percentage had decreased slightly to 88.2% (Table 18.1). The results in patients who presented other forms of tremor were not as good. Two patients showed modest improvements and the other two no improvement at all. One transient complication (0.66%) was reported in a patient who presented with balance disturbance, who improved just with observation. Two other permanent complications (1.3%) were reported between 6 and 12 months post-treatment. One patient experienced mild contralateral paresthesias in the face and upper extremity and another experienced mild weakness in both the contralateral arm and leg and very minimal dysphasia. In all three of these patients, the side effects were due to lesions, which became larger than expected, and not because of targeting errors.

The results of radiosurgery thalamotomy were considered as good as those published on radiofrequency thalamotomy or DBS. Essentially, 85–90% of patients showed significant improvements in tremor in short-term follow-up studies. These results have changed the use of the open lesioning technique in favor of radiosurgical thalamotomy in some centers (Duma et al. 1998; Kondziolka et al. 2008b; Ohye et al. 1996; Young et al. 1998a).

Ohye et al. (2002), presented a series of 53 patients submitted to radiosurgery thalamotomy. The reported results were based on 30 patients with at least 2 years of follow-up (median 30 months, range: 2–8 years) after the treatment. Clinical outcome was satisfactory in 24 patients (80%) with a reduction of the tremor to less than 25% of the preoperative state. Treatment failure was observed in six patients (20%), after one (two patients) or two (four patients) radiosurgery thalamotomies. There were no reported complications (Table 18.1).

Kondziolka et al. (2008b), reported a series of 31 patients harboring essential tremor submitted to radiosurgery thalamotomy with a mean follow-up of 36 months (4–96 months). Patients were treated with a single 4 mm collimator with a dose of 130–140 Gy. Of the 26 evaluable patients, 18 (69%) showed improvement in both action tremor and writing scores, 6 (23%) only in action tremor scores, and 3 (12%) in neither tremor nor writing. The authors used the Fahn-Tolosa-Marin clinical tremor rating scale (Fahn et al. 1993) to assess pre and postoperative tremor, showing that scores for both tremor and writing were found to be statistically significant. The typical response time was 1–4 months, although three patients had significant tremor improvement within 2 days. Two complications (7.7%) were reported in the study. One patient presented with transient mild right hemiparesis and dysphagia. Another patient suffered a mild right hemiparesis and speech impairment months after radiosurgery. In one case, a MRI follow-up study showed a larger than expected volume of contrast enhancement, which resolved over the next 18 months.

The Quality Standards Subcommittee of the American Academy of Neurology recently stated disadvantages of SRS, including dependence on anatomical imaging, delay of weeks to months for clinical results to occur, and risk of delayed progressive neurological deficits. Although the overwhelming majority of post-radiosurgery MRI studies depict a lesion in exactly the planned location with the expected appearance, they concluded that there is insufficient evidence to make recommendations regarding the use of SRS in the treatment of essential tremor. The advantage of SRS is that tremor relief can be provided to patients (particularly the elderly) who would not be good candidates to an open surgical procedure.

18.5 Imaging Changes

One of the major concerns about functional stereotactic procedures has been the matter of consistency and reproducibility of lesion size, given the variability in lesion volumes using identical radiosurgical parameters (Friehs et al. 1996; Kihlström et al. 1995; Lindquist et al. 1992; Young et al. 1998a). It is widely recognized in the literature that the volume of a thalamic lesion produced by SRS is so variable that it cannot be predicted beforehand (Duma et al. 1998; Friedman et al. 1996; Friehs et al. 1995; Ohye et al. 2002; Pan et al. 1996).

Usually, the initial MRI changes after radiosurgical thalamotomy reveal a circumscribed spherical lesion that enhanced with administration of gadolinium on T1-weighted images at a median of 1.5–3 months after radiosurgical lesioning (Duma et al. 1999; Kondziolka et al. 2008b; Young et al. 1998a). On T2-weighted images a mildly diffuse signal change is observed, representing what is believed to be edema, "radiation change", demyelination, or necrosis at a median of 4.5 months following treatment (Duma 2007; Duma et al. 1999). At 6–12 months after the procedure, the lesions enhanced intensely on T1-weighted images and the perilesional changes had diminished or disappeared (Young et al. 1998a). Usually, the peak lesion visualization and edema patterns become evident within 1 year of follow up (Duma et al. 1998). The T1 change represents necrosis and is approximately 4–5 mm and it maintained the same configuration in follow-up periods of up to 5 years (Duma 2007; Ohye et al. 2000; Young et al. 2000).

Another type of lesion was described in some cases with further increase in size up to 1 year. The extent of the size increase differs from case to case, from several hundred mm^3 to more than 4.0 cm^3. It may also differ from a round restricted to an irregularly expanding shape with or without streaking along the thalamocapsular border (Duma 2007; Friehs et al. 1996; Ohye et al. 2000). There was no correlation between the two types of lesion and the clinical effect on tremor, patient age at the time of SRS and the occurrence of clinical deficits (Ohye et al. 2000; Young et al. 1998a).

In a study comparing patients submitted to radiosurgery thalamotomy using "low" (120 Gy) and "high" dose (160 Gy), Duma et al. (1998), showed that the average T1 weighted gadolinium-enhanced lesion size was not different for either the low or high-dose groups. Although not statistically significant, there was a trend for the higher dose lesion to elicit a larger T2 signal change, or T2 "streaking". According to the author, it is unlikely that this represents necrosis because the presence of the streaking within the capsule or other thalamic nuclei never correlated with neurological impairment. The superior tremor control observed in the high-dose group may be a consequence of a "physiologically" larger lesion in this group, correcting for any target planning inaccuracies. In cases with surrounding enlarged reaction, cases of reoperation with microelectrode recording showed an almost normal neuronal activity in such a surrounding high signal zone and no related clinical side effect, proving that this area does not seem to be functionally damaged (Ohye et al. 2000).

18.6 Pallidotomy

The effectiveness of pallidotomy and pallidal stimulation in the control of the majority of the symptoms of PD, including rigidity, bradykinesia and levodopa-induced dyskinesias has already been demonstrated in the literature (Benabid et al. 1998; Burchiel et al. 1999; Dogali et al. 1995; Hariz and Bergenheim 2001; Laitinen et al. 1992; Lozano et al. 1996; Starr et al. 1998).

As in other functional stereotactic procedures precision is very important since inaccurate lesioning during the performance of pallidotomy may result in visual field defects, hemianopsia and sensory loss.

The feasibility and results demonstrated with radiosurgery thalamotomy induced many centers to bring SRS to other known functional targets. This evolution associated to the previously reported long term good results with radiofrequency pallidotomy (Hariz and Bergenheim 2001), made the globus pallidus internus (GPi) the natural next target to radiosurgery.

Radiosurgical pallidotomy was first reported by Rand (Rand et al. 1993), who used the technique in eight patients, four of whom had significant relief of contralateral rigidity. There were no reports of significant side effects.

Friedman et al. (1996) described four cases of PD who underwent unilateral pallidotomy using a 4 mm collimator and a dose of 180 Gy. No patient improved in a significant manner within the follow-up interval of 18 months. One patient developed a stroke related to radiation vasculopathy with severe radiation changes in the blood vessels adjacent to the radiosurgical lesion.

Bonnen et al. (1997), in a single case report, described a permanent contralateral homonymous hemianopsia and transient hemiparesis in a patient treated with radiosurgery pallidotomy. The resulting lesion was greater than expected.

A comparative study with 51 patients with PD who underwent pallidotomy was reported by Young et al. (1998b). Patients were divided in two groups, 29 were treated with radiosurgery and submitted to 34 lesions, while 22 were treated with radiofrequency and submitted to 25 lesions. The median follow-up in this series was 20.6 months (6–48 months). The evaluations of motor performance and postoperative assessments were obtained by blinded observers who had no role in or knowledge of the treatment course of these patients. The applied dose in the radiosurgery group was 120–140 Gy with the 4 mm collimator. In this study, complete or near complete relief of dyskinesias was observed in 13 out of 15 patients (86.6%) submitted to radiosurgery and in 10 of 12 (83.3%) in the radiofrequency group. The reduction in dyskinesias usually began 2–3 months after the radiosurgical procedure, with continued improvement noted over the next 3–6 months. The only complication was with one patient in the radiosurgery group (3.4%) who developed a lesion larger than expected (volume 950 mm^3) at 9 months postoperatively. This lesion was accompanied by a contralateral homonymous hemianopsia. Two other patients developed larger lesions than expected (520 mm^3 and 700 mm^3) but those were not associated with any clinical side effects. Thus, one of 29 patients (3.4%) and one of 34 lesions (2.9%) were associated with a clinical complication. According to the author, the results were equally as good as those obtained in the radiofrequency pallidotomies when electrophysiological localization was used. The results for patients submitted to simultaneous bilateral pallidotomies due to severe akinesia were not as good as to unilateral procedures.

As mentioned earlier for thalamotomies, the drawbacks of radiosurgical pallidotomy concern the latency between the procedure and the clinical benefit (2–3 months minimum) and the possibility that the lesion produced by radiosurgery will continue to enlarge on a delayed basis and involve adjacent normal structures.

Duma (2007) reported a series of 18 patients with PD who underwent stereotactic radiosurgical pallidotomy. Fifteen patients were treated using a single and three using two 4 mm collimator with a median maximum prescription dose of 160 Gy (range 90–165). Patients were submitted to independent neurologist evaluations and Unified Parkinson's Disease Rating Scale (UPDRS) (Martínez-Martín ct al. 1994) scoring of patient response to treatment at regular clinical follow-up intervals. The authors reported that the results were as not as good as expected. Over a median average follow-up of 8 months (range: 6–40 months), only six patients (33%) showed transient improvement in rigidity and dyskinesia. Three patients (17%) were unchanged and nine (50%) were worsened by the treatment. Of the six patients with improvement, two exhibited visual field deficits. Overall four (22%) had visual field deficit, three (16%) had speech or swallowing difficulties, 03 (16%) had worsening of their gait and one (5%) had numbness in the contralateral hemibody. Nine patients (50%) had one or more complications related to the treatment which were unresponsive to steroid treatment and considered to be permanent.

The explanation of the high complication rate in this series was related to the variability and unpredictability of the lesion size after radiosurgery targeting at the GPi. The differences in outcome comparing VIM and GPi targets led the authors to believe that there is a difference in sensitivity to radiation between these two nuclei. The increased susceptibility of the GPi is probably anatomical due to very small venous or arterial infarctions in the area, as a consequence of the tapering end supply provided by the lenticulostriate arteries (Friedman et al. 2002).

For the same dose at similar follow-up intervals (160 Gy maximum dose at 8 month follow-up) lesion sizes varied from 6 to 30 mm on T1-weighted MRI sequences with gadolinium enhancement. Immeasurable variability in edema patterns was visible at the same follow-up interval on T2-weighted MRI sequences. Follow-up MRI imaging at 1 year revealed accurately placed lesions but with variable and unpredicted sizes. Over time, lesions tended to decrease slightly, but in general were consistent throughout the course of follow-up (Duma et al. 1999).

The number of centers that have been performing radiosurgery pallidotomies compared to those performing thalamotomies, reflect the lack of reliability of the procedure and that other therapeutic options are superior to stereotactic radiosurgery targeting the GPi. The majority of the institutions have abandoned the procedure due to an unacceptable complication rate.

18.7 Conclusions

Advances in stereotactic techniques associated with improvements in MRI targeting, planning software and a better knowledge of SRS parameters brought the technique to a precision capable of performing focal and precise lesions in the basal ganglia for movement disorders.

Using modern functional SRS parameters, radiosurgery thalamotomy has become a safe and useful procedure for patients who are not suitable for an open surgical procedure. The reported results and complications of SRS are comparable to thalamic lesions generated by neurophysiologically guided radiofrequency procedures.

Complications were always related to the variability of lesion volumes using the same radiosurgical parameters, rather than related to stereotactic target precision. The factors related to this unpredictable thalamic reaction to high single dose radiation are still unknown.

Similar results and safety were not achieved with pallidal radiosurgery lesions. The results of radiosurgery pallidotomy are not homogeneous in the literature. Many reports disclosed an unacceptably high complication rate. Although just a few centers reported their results, the majority of them were not satisfactory, leading them to abandon the procedure.

Despite the fact that deep brain stimulation has supplanted lesioning as the first alternative in movement disorder surgery, stereotactic radiosurgery might still be the only treatment option for selected patients not eligible for conventional surgery targeting at the thalamus.

References

Alterman RL, Kall BA, Cohen H et al (1995) Stereotactic ventrolateral thalamotomy: is ventriculography necessary? Neurosurgery 37:717–722

Bednarz G, Downes MB, Corn BW, Curran WJ, Goldman HW (1999) Evaluation of the spatial accuracy of magnetic resonance imaging-based stereotactic target localization for gamma knife radio-surgery of functional disorders. Neurosurgery 45:1156–1161, Discussion 61–63

Benabid AL, Benazzouz A, Hoffmann D et al (1998) Long-term electrical inhibition of deep brain targets in movement disorders. Mov Disord 13(Suppl 3):119–125

Bonnen JG, Iacono RP, Lulu B, Mohamed AS, Gonzalez A, Schoonenberg T (1997) Gamma knife pallidotomy: case report. Acta Neurochir 139:442–445

Burchiel KJ, Anderson VC, Favre J, Hammerstad JP (1999) Comparison of pallidal and subthalamic nucleus deep brain stimulation for advanced Parkinson's disease: results of a randomized, blinded pilot study. Neurosurgery 6:1375–1382, Discussion 1382–1384

De Salles AA, Melega WP, Lacan G, Steele LJ, Solberg TD (2001) Radiosurgery performed with the aid of a 3-mm collimator in the subthalamic nucleus and substantia nigra of the vervet monkey. J Neurosurg 95:990–997

De Salles AA, Gorgulho AA, Selch M, De Marco J, Agazaryan N (2008) Radiosurgery from the brain to the spine: 20 years experience. Acta Neurochir Suppl 101:163–168

Dogali M, Fazzini E, Kolodny E et al (1995) Stereotactic ventral pallidotomy for Parkinson's disease. Neurology 45: 753–761

Duma CM (2007) Movement disorder radiosurgery—planning, physics and complication avoidance. Prog Neurol Surg 20: 249–266

Duma CM, Jacques DB, Kopyov OV et al (1998) Gamma knife radiosurgery for thalamotomy in parkinsonian tremor: a five-year experience. J Neurosurg 88:1044–1049

Duma CM, Jacques K, Kopyov OV (1999) Treatment of movement disorders using gamma knife stereotactic radiosurgery. Neurosurg Clin N Am 10:379–389

Fahn S, Tolosa E, Marin C (1993) Clinical rating scale for tremor. Parkinson's disease and movement disorders, 2nd edn. William & Wilkins, Baltimore, pp 271–280

Friedman WA, Bova FJ (1992) Linear accelerator radiosurgery for arteriovenous malformations. J Neurosurg 77(6):832–841

Friedman DP, Epstein M, Sanes JN et al (1996) Gamma knife pallidotomy in advanced Parkinson's disease. Ann Neurol 39:535–538

Friedman DP, Goldman HW, Flanders AE, Gollomp SM, Curran WJ Jr (1999) Stereotactic radiosurgical pallidotomy and thalamotomy with the gamma knife: MR imaging findings with clinical correlation – preliminary experience. Radiology 212:143–150

Friedman JH, Fernandez HH, Sikirica M, Stopa E, Friehs G (2002) Stroke induced by gamma knife pallidotomy: autopsy result. Neurology 58:1695–1697

Friehs GM, Ojakangas CL, Pachatz P et al (1995) Thalamotomy and caudatotomy with the gamma knife as a treatment for parkinsonism with a comment on lesion sizes. Stereotact Funct Neurosurg 64(Suppl 1):209–221

Friehs GM, Norén G, Ohye C et al (1996) Lesion size following gamma knife treatment for functional disorders. Stereotact Funct Neurosurg 66(Suppl 1):320–328

Frighetto L, De Salles A, Wallace R, Ford J, Selch M, Cabatan-Awang C, Solberg T (2004) Linear accelerator thalamotomy. Surg Neurol 62(2):106–113, Discussion 113–114

Goldman MS, Kelly PJ (2000) Stereotactic thalamotomy for medically intractable essential tremor. N Engl J Med 342: 461–468

Hariz MI, Bergenheim AT (2001) A 10-year follow-up review of patients who underwent Leksell's posteroventral pallidotomy for Parkinson disease. J Neurosurg 94(4): 552–558

Jankovic J, Cardoso F, Grossman RG et al (1995) Outcome after stereotactic thalamotomy for parkinsonian essential and other types of tremor. Neurosurgery 37:680–687

Kihlström L, Guo WY, Lindquist C et al (1995) Radiobiology of radiosurgery for refractory anxiety disorders. Neurosurgery 36:294–302

Kondziolka D, Mathieu D, Lunsford LD, Martin JJ, Madhok R, Niranjan A, Flickinger JC (2008a) Radiosurgery as definitive management of intracranial meningiomas. Neurosurgery 62(1):53–58, Discussion 58–60

Kondziolka D, Ong J, Lee J, Moore R, Flickinger J, Lunsford D (2008b) Gamma Knife thalamotomy for essential tremor. J Neurosurg 108(1):111–117

Laitinen LV, Bergenheim AT, Hariz MI (1992) Leksell's posteroventral pallidotomy in the treatment of Parkinson's disease. J Neurosurg 76:53–61

Leksell L (1951) The stereotaxic method and radiosurgery of the brain. Acta Chir Scand 102:316–319

Leksell L (1968) Cerebral radiosurgery. I. Gammathalanotomy in two cases of intractable pain. Acta Chir Scand 134: 585–595

Lindquist C, Kihlstrom L, Hellstrand E (1991) Functional neurosurgery – a future for the gamma knife? Stereotact Funct Neurosurg 57:72–81

Lindquist C, Steiner L, Hindmarsh T (1992) Gamma knife thalamotomy for tremor: report of two cases. In: Steiner L, Lindquist C, Forster D (eds) Radiosurgery: baseline and trends. Raven, New York, pp 237–243

Linhares MN, Tasker RR (2000) Microelectrode-guided thalamotomy for Parkinson's disease. Neurosurgery 46:390–395

Lozano A, Hutchison W, Kiss Z et al (1996) Methods for microelectrode-guided posteroventral pallidotomy. J Neurosurg 84:194–202

Martínez-Martín P, Gil-Nagel A, Gracia LM, Gómez JB, Martínez-Sarriés J, Bermejo F (1994) Unified Parkinson's disease rating scale characteristics and structure. The Cooperative Multicentric Group. Mov Disord 9(1):76–83

Novotny J Jr, Vymazal J, Novotny J, Tlachacova D, Schmitt M, Chuda P, Urgosik D, Liscak R (2005) Does new magnetic resonance imaging technology provide better geometrical accuracy during stereotactic imaging? J Neurosurg 102(Suppl):8–13

Ohye C (2006) From selective thalamotomy with microrecording to gamma thalamotomy for movement disorders. Stereotact Funct Neurosurg 84:155–161

Ohye C, Shibazaki T (2002) Location of the thalamic Vim nucleus. Its relation to the whole thalamic length. Funct Neurosurg 41:52–53

Ohye C, Shibazaki T, Hirato M, Inoue H, Andou Y (1996) Gamma thalamotomy for parkinsonian and other kinds of tremor. Stereotact Funct Neurosurg 66(1 Suppl):333–342

Ohye C, Shibazaki T, Ishihara J, Zhang J (2000) Evaluation of gamma thalamotomy for parkinsonian and other tremors: survival of neurons adjacent to the thalamic lesion after gamma thalamotomy. J Neurosurg 93(3 Suppl):120–127

Ohye C, Shibazaki T, Zhang J, Andou Y (2002) Thalamic lesions produced by gamma thalamotomy for movement disorders. J Neurosurg 97(5 Suppl):600–606

Ohye C, Shibazaki T, Sato S (2005) Gamma knife thalamotomy for movement disorders: evaluation of the thalamic lesion and clinical results. J Neurosurg 102(Suppl):234–240

Pan L, Dai J, Wang B et al (1996) Stereotactic gamma knife thalamotomy for the treatment of parkinsonism. Stereotact Funct Neurosurg 66(Suppl 1):329–332

Rand RW, Jacques DB, Melbye RW et al (1993) Gamma knife thalamotomy and pallidotomy in patients with movement disorders: preliminary results. Stereotact Funct Neurosurg 61(Suppl 1):65–92

Smith ZA, De Salles AA, Frighetto L, Goss B, Lee SP, Selch M et al (2003) Dedicated linear accelerator radiosurgery for the treatment of trigeminal neuralgia. J Neurosurg 99:511–516

Sneed PK, Suh JH, Goetsch SJ, Sanghavi SN, Chappell R, Buatti JM, Regine WF, Weltman E, King VJ, Breneman JC, Sperduto PW, Mehta MP (2002) A multi-institutional review of radiosurgery alone vs. radiosurgery with whole brain radiotherapy as the initial management of brain metastases. Int J Radiat Oncol Biol Phys 53(3):519–526

Solberg TD, DeSalles AAF, Medin PM, DeMarco JJ, Selch MT (1998) Technical aspects of LINAC radiosurgery for the treatment of small functional targets. J Radiosurg 1:115–127

Starr PA, Vitek JL, Bakay RA (1998) Ablative surgery and deep brain stimulation for Parkinson's disease. Neurosurgery 43: 989–1015

Steiner L, Forster D, Leksell L et al (1980) Gammathalamotomy in intractable pain. Acta Neurochir 52:173–184

Sumanaweera TS, Adler JR Jr, Napel S et al (1994) Characterization of spatial distortion in magnetic resonance imaging and its implications for stereotactic surgery. Neurosurgery 35:696–704

Tasker RR, Munz M, Junn FS et al (1997) Deep brain stimulation and thalamotomy for tremor compared. Acta Neurochir Suppl 68:49–53

Young RF, Jacques DS, Rand RW et al (1994) Medial thalamotomy with the Leksell gamma knife for treatment of chronic pain. Acta Neurochir Suppl 62:105–110

Young RF, Jacques DS, Rand RW et al (1995) Technique of stereotactic medial thalamotomy with the Leksell gamma knife for treatment of chronic pain. Neurol Res 17:59–65

Young RF, Vermeulen SS, Grim P et al (1996) Electrophysiological target localization is not required for the treatment of functional disorders. Stereotact Funct Neurosurg 66(Suppl 1): 309–319

Young RF, Shumway-Cook A, Vermeulen SS et al (1998a) Gamma knife radiosurgery as a lesioning technique in movement disorder surgery. J Neurosurg 89:183–193

Young RF, Vermeulen S, Posewitz A, Shumway-Cook A (1998b) Pallidotomy with the gamma knife: a positive experience. Stereotact Funct Neurosurg 70(1 Suppl):218–228

Young RF, Jacques S, Mark R, Kopyov O, Copcutt B, Posewitz A et al (2000) Gamma knife thalamotomy for treatment of tremor: long-term results. J Neurosurg 93(3 Suppl): 128–135

Stereotactic Radiosurgery for Epilepsy

19

Miguel Angel Celis, Olivia Amanda García Garduño,
and Sergio Moreno-Jiménez

19.1 Introduction

The original intention of Lars Leksell when he initiated stereotactic radiosurgery (SRS) in 1951 was to treat functional disorders such as Parkinson disease, chronic pain syndromes, and psychiatric conditions. Nowadays, SRS is also an emerging technology in the treatment of focal and non-focal epilepsy. Clinical cessation of seizures following SRS was observed in patients treated for arteriovenous malformations (Heikkinen et al. 1989) and cavernous malformations (Regis et al. 2000). Lindquist promoted the idea of a new approach for epilepsy surgery with Gamma Knife™ (Elekta, Stockholm, Sweden) radiosurgery (Lindquist et al. 1991).

Initial work on focused stereotactic irradiation for epilepsy was reported in 6 patients by Barcia-Salorio and then in 11 patients with long-term follow-up using an estimated dose range of 10–20 Gy (Barcia-Salorio et al. 1985; Barcia Salorio et al. 1994). In 1993, Régis and coworkers reported a selective amygdalohippocampal radiosurgery for mesial temporal lobe epilepsy (Régis et al. 1995). A recent publication of the Marseille group reported a total of 134 patients treated over 15 years, including 53 cases of MTLE, 61 cases of hypothalamic hamartomas, two cases of corpus callosotomy, and 12 of other causes (Régis et al. 2008). This report summarizes, to some extent, the patients and diseases that could be treated with radiosurgery.

M.A. Celis (✉)
Unidad de Radioneurocirugía,
Instituto Nacional de Neurología y Neurocirugía,
Insurgentes Sur 3877, Colonia La Fama,
C.P. 14269, México D.F.
e-mail: macelis@innn.edu.mx

O.A.G. Garduño
Laboratorio de Física Médica,
Instituto Nacional de Neurología y Neurocirugía,
Insurgentes Sur 3877, Colonia La Fama, C.P. 14269,
México D.F.
e-mail: oagarciag@innn.edu.mx

S. Moreno-Jiménez
Unidad de Radioneurocirugía,
Instituto Nacional de Neurología y Neurocirugía,
Insurgentes Sur 3877, Colonia La Fama,
C.P. 14269, México D.F.
e-mail: ser_radioneurocirugia@yahoo.com.mx

19.2 Mesial Temporal Lobe Epilepsy Radiosurgery (MTLE)

MTLE is considered the most frequent cause of drug resistant epilepsy in adults. The first treatment option for refractory cases is open surgery, which is safe and efficacious. However, radiosurgery is a less invasive method and does not carry the risk of peri-surgical complications such as bleeding, infection and post-operative pain (Rydenhag and Silander 2001). Moreover, there are reports on neuropsychological changes after temporal lobectomy. Thus, SRS may offer a non-invasive alternative to open surgery with the argument of less post-operative morbidity at less cost. The initial attempts to treat MTLE with SRS are from 1985. Barcia and co-workers treated six patients with a Co-60 unit using 10 mm circular collimators. The epileptic foci of these patients received an estimated dose of 10 Gy at periphery (Barcia-Salorio et al. 1985). In 1994, the same group reported the results on 11 patients treated for idiopathic focal epilepsy. From these patients, only four became seizure free. An additional five patients improved seizure frequency after 12 months follow-up (Barcia Salorio et al. 1994). In 1995, Régis and co-workers reported their pilot studies

A.A.F. De Salles et al. (eds.), *Shaped Beam Radiosurgery*,
DOI: 10.1007/978-3-642-11151-8_19, © Springer-Verlag Berlin Heidelberg 2011

showing a higher rate of seizure remission. The variability on the results reflects the difficulties for target definition and dose selection (Régis et al. 1995). The target volume used in SRS for MTLE involves: the amygdala, the head and anterior body of the hippocampus, and the parahippocampal gyrus with target volumes ranging from 4.3 to 9.0 cc. Regarding dose selection, reported doses used are between 10 and 25 Gy. The clinical results suggest that doses lower than 20 Gy are less effective than higher doses. However, higher doses increase the probability of radiation induced edema and neurological complications.

Dunoyer and coworkers, in 2002, reported four patients with medically uncontrolled seizures with localized seizure foci who were selected for stereotactic radiosurgery. Seizure foci were identified on the basis of ictal and interictal video-EEG recording. Magnetic resonance images (MRIs) were obtained before and after surgery. Ictal single-photon emission computed tomography (SPECT) was performed by using stabilized hexamethyl-propyleneamine oxime (HMPAO) with early injection after electrographic ictal onset (within 20 s). The favorable outcome obtained in three of our four cases indicated that in selected circumstances, stereotactic radiosurgery is a useful adjunct in the surgical management of pediatric epilepsy (Dunoyer et al. 2002).

In 2006, the Epilepsy Radiosurgery Study Group integrated by Universities of California at San Francisco and Charlottesville Virginia, conducted a multicenter prospective pilot study including eight US centers and 30 MTLE patients. Subjects were randomized to receive either low-dose (20 Gy) or high-dose (24 Gy) on mesial structures (amygdala, hippocampus and para-hippocampal gyrus). At 24-month follow-up the overall rate of seizure-free (from 18th to 24th month after radiosurgery) was 67%. However, in the high-dose group this study reported 85% seizure-free vs. 56% in the low-dose group (Barbaro et al. 2009).

Hippocampal sclerosis is defined by neuronal loss, mostly located in the granular layers of the dentate gyrus and the Ammon horn. This provokes a reactive synaptogenesis and progressive excitatory process able to initiate and propagate seizures. Antiepileptic drugs suppress seizure activity but don't stop synaptogenesis. Despite the combination of two or three antiepileptic drugs, 30% of patients remain refractory. Surgical extirpation of sclerotic hippocampus is curative. But a number of side-effects, depending on the type and extent of resection, are significant: transient or permanent hemiparesis, mild or major visual field defects, infection, transient anomia (only in surgery on the dominant temporal lobe) and permanent language difficulty (Behrens et al. 1997).

19.2.1 Patient Selection

In our center, patient selection criteria are the same as for refractory epilepsy surgery. Clinical epileptic symptoms, electrophysiological data (interictal EEG and ictal video-EEG recordings), imaging studies (high magnetic field MRI focused on mesial temporal lobe sclerosis), neuropsychological tests (Weschler memory tests, verbal dominance) and metabolic data (interictal hypometabolic area on affected temporal lobe) are collected. Specialists in each field analyze the information. Informed consent is obtained, and open surgery is also offered to patients and families. Neuroimaging follow-up is necessary; therefore, an MRI is taken at 4, 6, 8 and 12 months in order to detect early signs of brain edema or signs of temporal lobe herniation (Hoggard et al. 2008).

19.2.2 Imaging

The imaging protocol used for treatment planning at our center includes three sets of MRI T2-weighted sequences (axial, coronal and sagittal planes) acquired on a 3.0 T MRI scanner (Signa Excite, General Electric, USA) with the following parameters: 512×512 matrix image size, 1.5 mm slice thickness without gap and 0.5 mm in place image resolution. These images offer high spatial resolution and enhanced visualization of brain anatomy. A CT scan is used for stereotactic localization with 512×512 matrix image size, 1.0 mm slice thickness and 0.8 mm axial image resolution. The morphological information provided by the MRI images is co-registered with the CT stereotactic coordinate system using the image fusion tool of the planning software. We recommend the placement of the frame parallel to the hippocampus.

19.3 Corpus Callosotomy Radiosurgery

Van Wagenen's contribution, along with Wilder Penfield and others, exemplifies how developments in neurosurgery led directly to developments in neuroscience.

Though rarely recognized, primacy in performing corpus callosotomy for epilepsy should be ascribed to van Wagenen and primacy in describing the associated neuropsychological sequelae be attributed to Akelaitis, even if superseded by the later results of Gazzaniga and Sperry (Mathews et al. 2008).

Corpus Callosum (CC) resectioning may decrease the number and severity of seizures in patients with intractable epilepsy who are not candidates for focal resection. The CC can spread epileptic activity from one lobe to the contralateral hemisphere. Its surgical longitudinal section prevents epileptic discharges from spreading between the two hemispheres in severe generalized epilepsies. This procedure reduces generalized tonic and mainly atonic seizures accompanied with sudden falls (drop attacks) and consequent injury (Feichtinger et al. 2006). This procedure is offered to patients with severe medically intractable multifocal epilepsy. Open surgical CC section is usually well tolerated, but a number of risks and complications have been reported (Rydenhag and Silander 2001; Behrens et al. 1997). In a recent publication, seizure rate improvement of 77% was observed in a series of 95 patients with 11% of early postoperative morbidity, 4% transient neurological deficits and no mortality (Tanriverdi et al. 2009).

Some clinicians consider that surgical section of the CC plays a minor role in the overall context based on the fact that CC section provides only reduction on the frequency of the drop attacks and some generalized tonic seizures but does not promote complete suppression of epileptic activity (Feichtinger et al. 2006).

Corpus Callosotomy using SRS is a relative new way to treat epilepsy that presents primary generalized or secondary rapidly spread seizures in patients who are not good candidates to open microsurgical procedure. In 1999, Pendl et al. reported the use of Gamma Knife radiosurgery for a patient with Lennox-Gastaut syndrome and for another one prior submitted to an anterior third corpus callosotomy presenting with tonic-clonic seizures. After a mean follow-up of 38 months, the patients had improved their seizure frequency (Pendl et al. 1999). In 2007, Celis and co-workers reported a patient with Lennox-Gastaut syndrome treated with Novalis® Radiosurgery (Brainlab AG, Feldkirchen, Germany) using dynamic conformal arcs. After a follow up of 12 months, the patient presented a decrease of 83% in seizure frequency (Celis et al. 2007).

19.3.1 Patient Selection

Patients with Lennox-Gastaut syndrome are good candidates to undergo corpus callosotomy with SRS. Drop attacks are the best-controlled subtypes of seizures controlled with this procedure.

19.3.2 Imaging

The images used for all treatment planning were three sets of MRI T2-weigthed sequences (axial, coronal and sagittal planes) acquired on a 3.0 T MRI scanner (Signa Excite, General Electric, USA) with the following parameters: 512×512 matrix image size, 1.5 mm slice thickness without gap, and 0.5 mm in-place image resolution. These images offer high spatial resolution and enhanced visualization of brain anatomy. A CT scan was used for stereotactic localization with 512×512 matrix image size, 1.0 mm slice thickness, and 0.8 mm axial image resolution. The morphological information provided by the MRI images was co-registered with the CT stereotactic coordinate system using the image fusion tool of the treatment planning software.

19.4 Hypothalamic Hamartomas (HH)

Hypothalamic hamartomas (HH) are developmental malformations variably associated with central precocious puberty and gelastic (laughing) seizures (Arita et al. 1999). They can be classified as sessile or pedunculated lesions. Sessile hamartomas can be further divided into Type I (midline), II (lateral), III (intraventricular), and IV (giant) (Romanelli et al. 2008). A further classification proposed by Valdueza and colleagues is based on lesion size, width of attachment, distortion of the hypothalamus, and location of attachment. Valdueza Type II lesions, corresponding to medium/large sessile HHs broadly attached to the tuber cinereum or mammillary body with or without hypothalamic compression, are most commonly reported in clinical series focusing on the radiosurgical treatment of epileptogenic hypothalamic hamartomas (Romanelli et al. 2008).

In 1998, Arita et al. reported the first case of a patient with a HH suffering from gelastic and tonic-clonic seizures treated with SRS. The patient became seizure free at follow up of almost 2 years. The reported MRI findings indicated a complete disappearance of the hypothalamic mass. As a result of this report, a multicenter retrospective study was conducted including ten patients in seven centers worldwide. All patients improved with reduced seizure frequency, four being seizure-free after a follow-up period of 12–71 months. The authors advocated a prescription dose of 17 Gy to the periphery of the lesion. These findings have since been confirmed using linear accelerator based radiosurgery (Friehs et al. 2007).

19.4.1 Patient Selection

As reported by Regis and coworkers according to their own classification, type I hamartomas, defined as lesions deeply embedded in the hypothalamus, are safely and effectively treated with SRS. Type II hypothalamic hamartomas can be resected by either endoscopic or transcallosal approaches or be treated by radiosurgery depending on the parent's choice and severity of epilepsy. In small type III hamartomas, radiosurgery is a safer procedure, because of the very close relationship to the fornix and mammillary bodies. Types V (rarely epileptic) and IV are frequently operable by disconnection. Very large type VI (or mixed type) with a large component above the floor of the third ventricle must be disconnected, and then the upper remnant would be best treated by radiosurgery using a staged technique. Overall, when the lesion is sufficiently small, radiosurgery offers a rate of seizure control comparable to microsurgery with the advantage of carrying decreased risk of complications. The disadvantage of radiosurgery is the time delay between treatment delivery and achievement of seizure control (Regis et al. 2007).

19.4.2 Imaging

The images used for all treatment planning in our center were three sets of MRI T2-weigthed sequences (axial, coronal and sagittal planes) acquired on a 3.0 T MRI scanner (Signa Excite, General Electric, USA) with the following parameters: 512×512 matrix image size, 1.5 mm slice thickness without gap and 0.5 mm in-plane spatial resolution. These MRI sequences offer high spatial resolution and enhanced visualization of brain anatomy. A CT scan was used for stereotactic localization with 512×512 matrix image size, 1.0 mm slice thickness and 0.8 mm axial image resolution. MRI images were co-registered to the CT stereotactic coordinate system using the image fusion tool of the treatment planning system.

19.5 Cases Examples

19.5.1 Mesial Temporal Lobe Epilepsy

19.5.1.1 Case Description

A 68-year-old male presented with seizures at age 25. Seizure frequency included about 90 partial and 3 generalized seizures per day. The patient was treated with radiosurgery at age 64, with a mean dose of 20.0 Gy at the isocenter (18 Gy at the periphery of the target volume). The target volume was 6.24 cm^3.

19.5.1.2 Treatment Technique

Intensity modulated radiation surgery (IMRS) was used in order to protect the optical chiasm and pathways (using 9 Gy as the maximum dose constraint). A total of 13 fields were used with an unequal distribution weighted towards the target side (Fig. 19.1).

19.5.1.3 Outcome

At 20 months follow-up, the patient is seizure free and with significant (>50%) decrease in duration and number of auras (Fig. 19.2).

19.5.1.4 Center Experience Outlining the Target

Delineation of the target depends on the definition of the extent of the epileptogenic zone. The average target volume on 14 patients treated in our institution was 8.24 cm^3. An example of treatment planning is shown in Fig. 19.3.

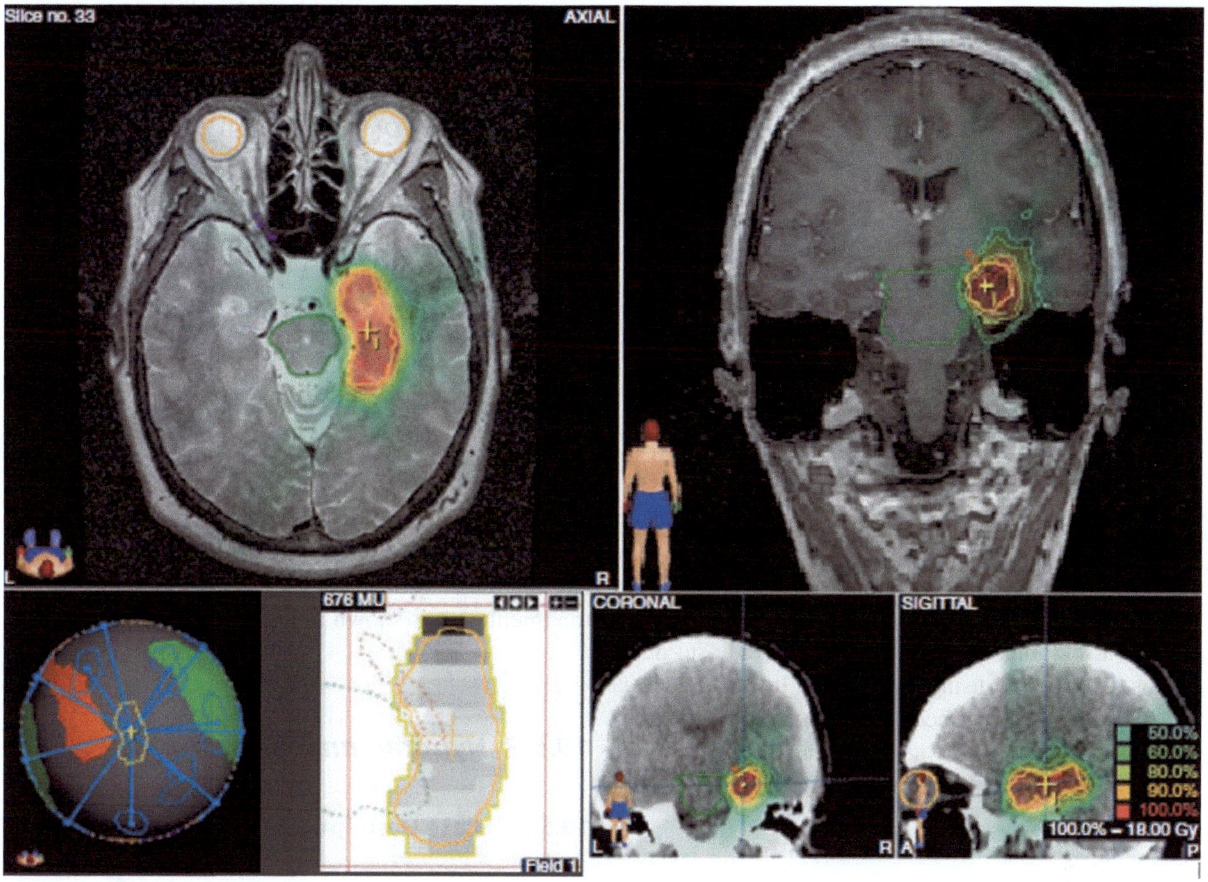

Fig. 19.1 Axial T2 and coronal T1 MRI images showing the dose distribution of a radiosurgery plan using 12 static fields for the treatment of a patient with MTLE. The dose prescribed at the periphery of the lesion was 18.0 Gy

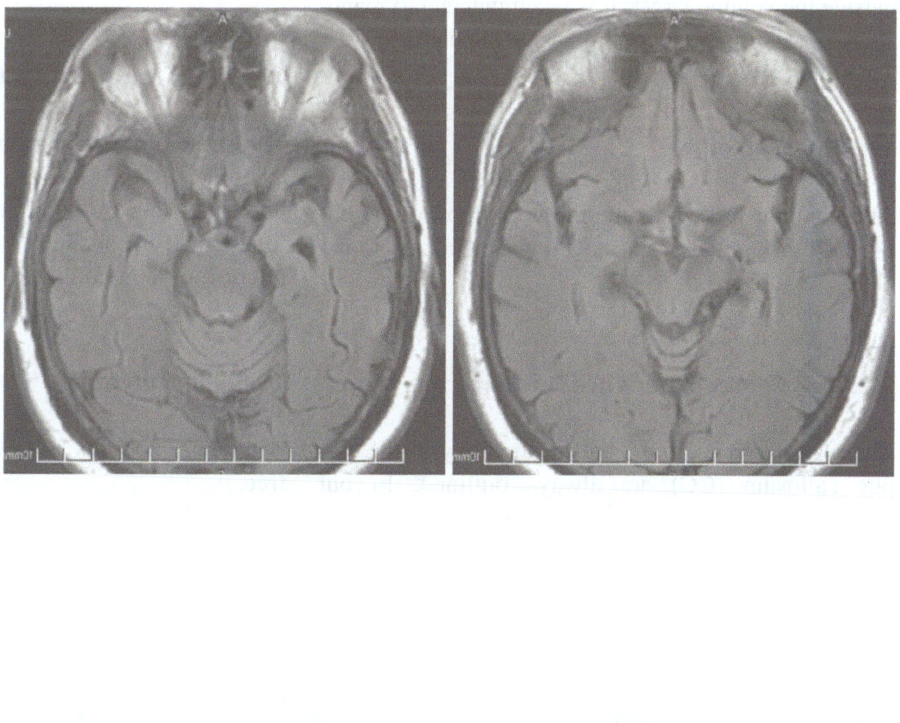

Fig. 19.2 Flair axial MRI images of the patients with MTLE at 2 years after radiosurgery treatment

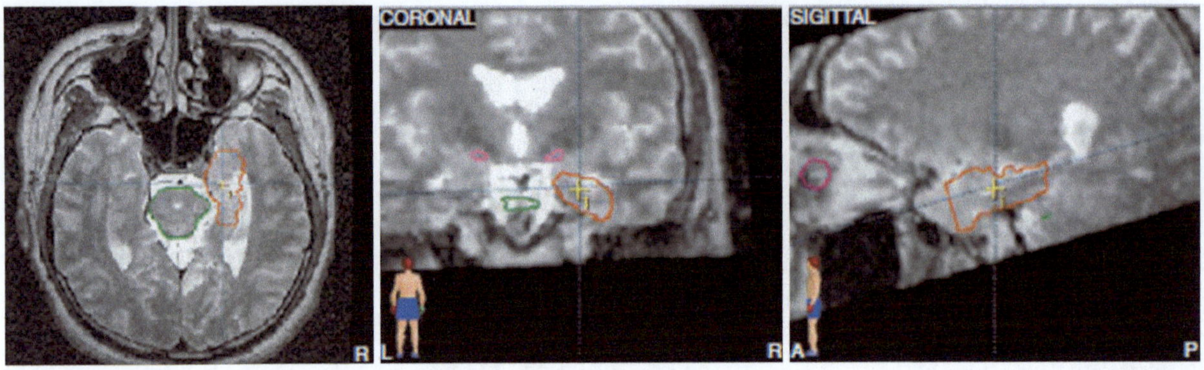

Fig. 19.3 T2 MRI images showing the mesial temporal lobe outlined on axial, sagittal and coronal views. The target volume depends on the definition of the extent of the epileptogenic zone

19.5.2 Corpus Callosotomy

19.5.2.1 Case Description

A 24-year-old male patient underwent a radiosurgical corpus callosotomy using a dedicated linear accelerator device. The prescribed dose was 36.0 Gy at the periphery of the rostrum, genu, and a half of the body of the corpus callosum.

19.5.2.2 Treatment Technique

A conformal dynamic arcs plan was achieved using a total of 11 arcs equally spaced. Due to the convex geometry of the CC, the isocenter was placed automatically outside the volume target. It is recommended to manually replace the isocenter point inside the outlined CC.

19.5.2.3 Outcome

At 32 months follow-up, there was an improvement of 84% on drop attacks and 65% on generalized tonic-clonic seizures.

19.5.2.4 Center Experience Outlining the Target

The rostrum, genu, and a half of the body of the corpus callosum (CC) are always outlined. In our experience with 13 patients treated, the average target volume was 0.70 cm^3, the average length was 5.5 cm and the mean width was 3.4 mm. An example of the treatment plan is shown in Fig. 19.4.

19.5.3 Hypothalamic Hamartoma

19.5.3.1 Case Description

An 18 year-old male presented with tonic seizures at age 2. At age 6, he experienced multiple types of seizures including gelastic and generalized tonic-clinic seizures. A hypothalamic hamartoma with a volume 1.32 cc was diagnosed.

19.5.3.2 Treatment Technique

The shape of the hamartoma dictates the choice of the technique used. If the lesion is small and round, it can be treated with arc-based treatments using circular collimation. If the shape is irregular, it can be done with micro-multileaf collimation (Fig. 19.5).

19.5.3.3 Outcome

After a 28 months follow-up, the patient is seizure free.

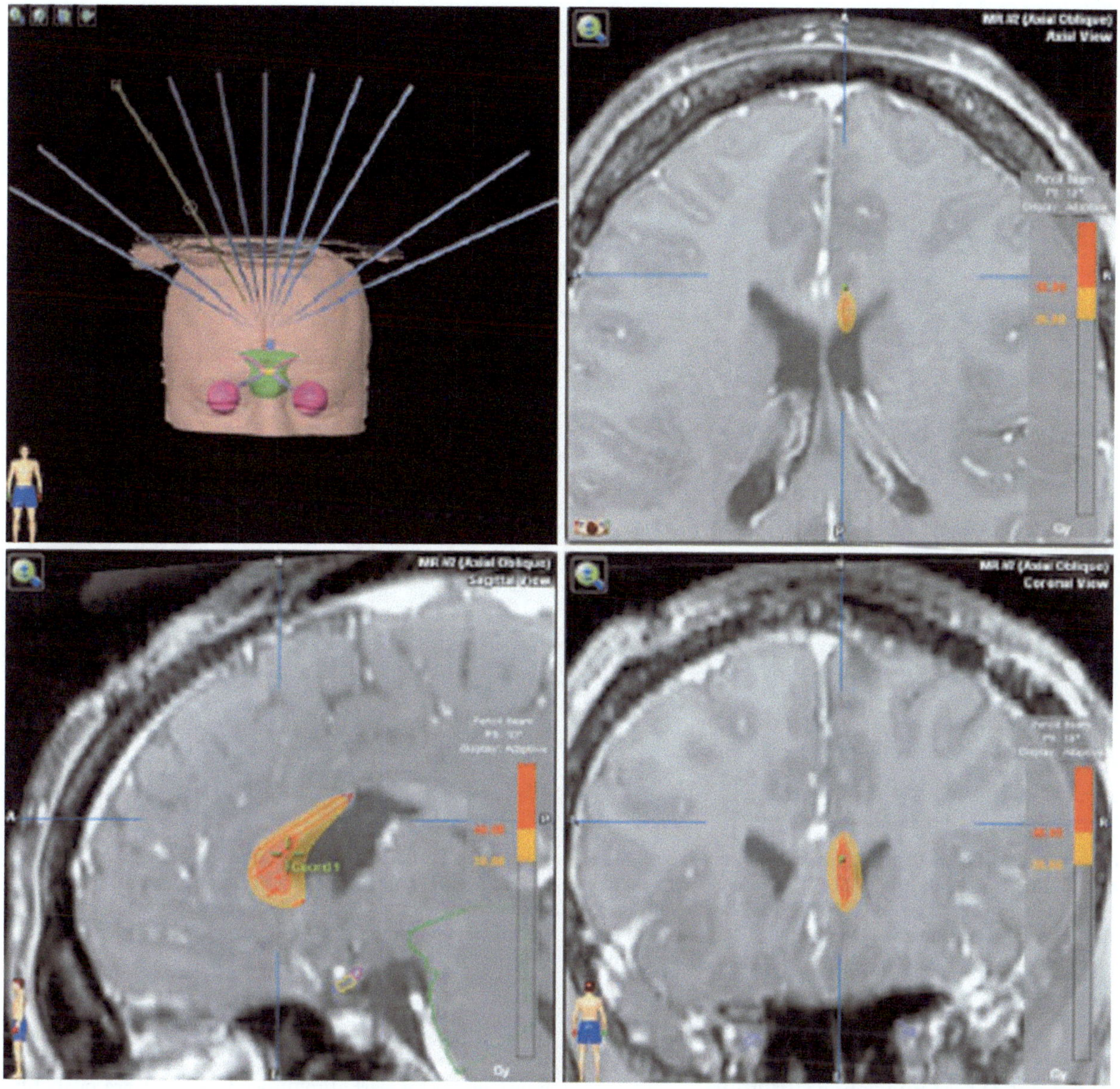

Fig. 19.4 Treatment planning MRI images showing the corpus callosum outlined in sagittal, axial and coronal views. The maximal dose was 40.0 Gy and the prescribed dose was 36.0 Gy. The plan was acquired using 11 non-coplanar dynamic arcs

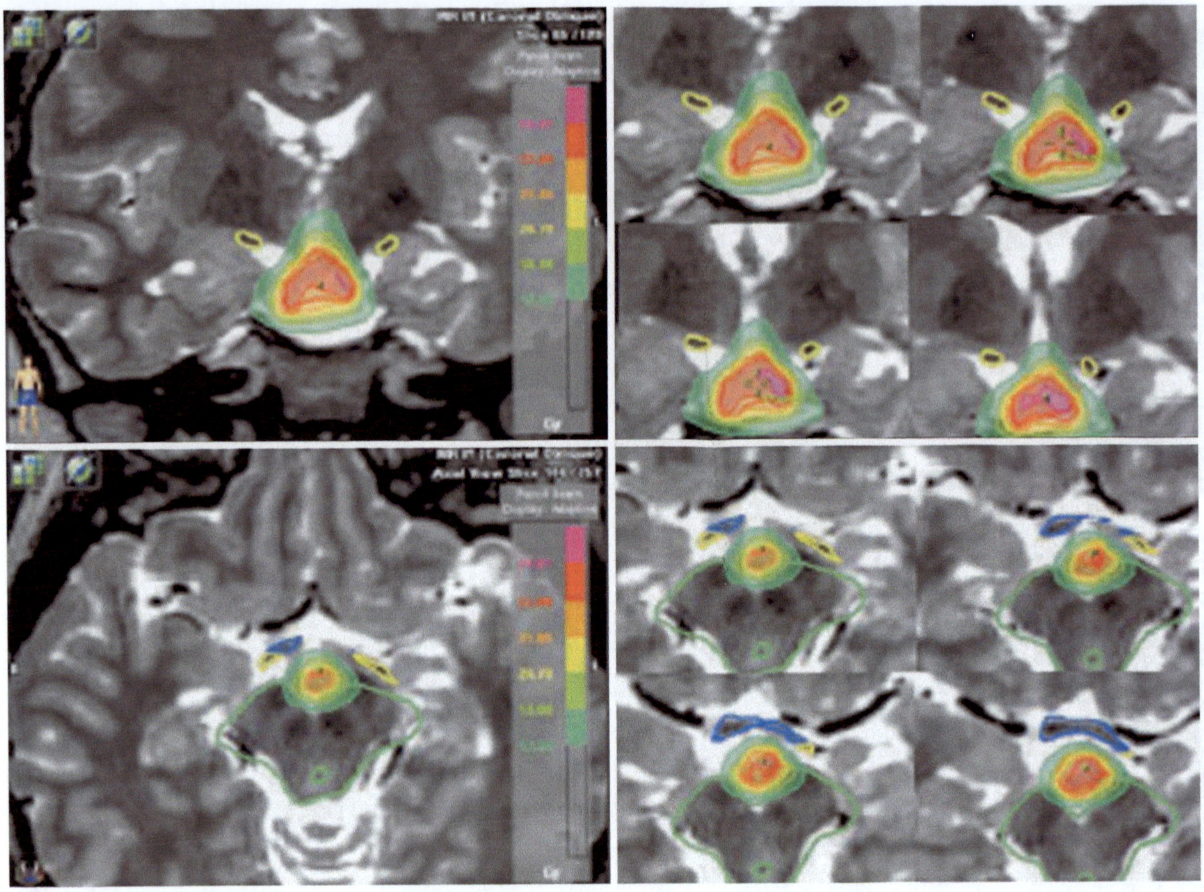

Fig. 19.5 (**a**) Hypothalamic hamartoma treatment using a 9 mm collimator. The dose was 22 Gy at isocenter and less than 9 Gy to the visual pathway and brainstem. Contiguous T2 coronal and axial slices show treatment volume and organs at risk: Optic pathway (yellow), optic apparatus (blue). (**b**) Treatment isocenter is at the cross-hair and gross target volume is shown in red. Dose-limiting critical structures identified: optic pathway (yellow), optic apparatus (blue) and brainstem (green) shown on contiguous T2 sagittal images and 3-D rendering

19.5.3.4 Center Experience Outlining the Target

The outlining includes the macroscopically seen tumor leaving a margin of 1 mm, taking extra caution with the optic pathway dose constraint.

19.6 Conclusions

Patients with MTLE at higher risk for open surgery due to the presence of the lesion in the dominant hemisphere for verbal/memory functions are probably the best candidates for radiosurgery treatment.

The efficacy of radiosurgery for the treatment of small hypothalamic hamartomas is comparable to microsurgery, with the advantage of decreased risk of post-operative complications inherent to the open procedure.

The analysis of our material, as well as other clinical and experimental data, suggests that the use of radiosurgery is beneficial on selected patients in whom a strict preoperative definition of the extent of the epileptogenic zone (or network) has been achieved and strict rules of dose planning are applied.

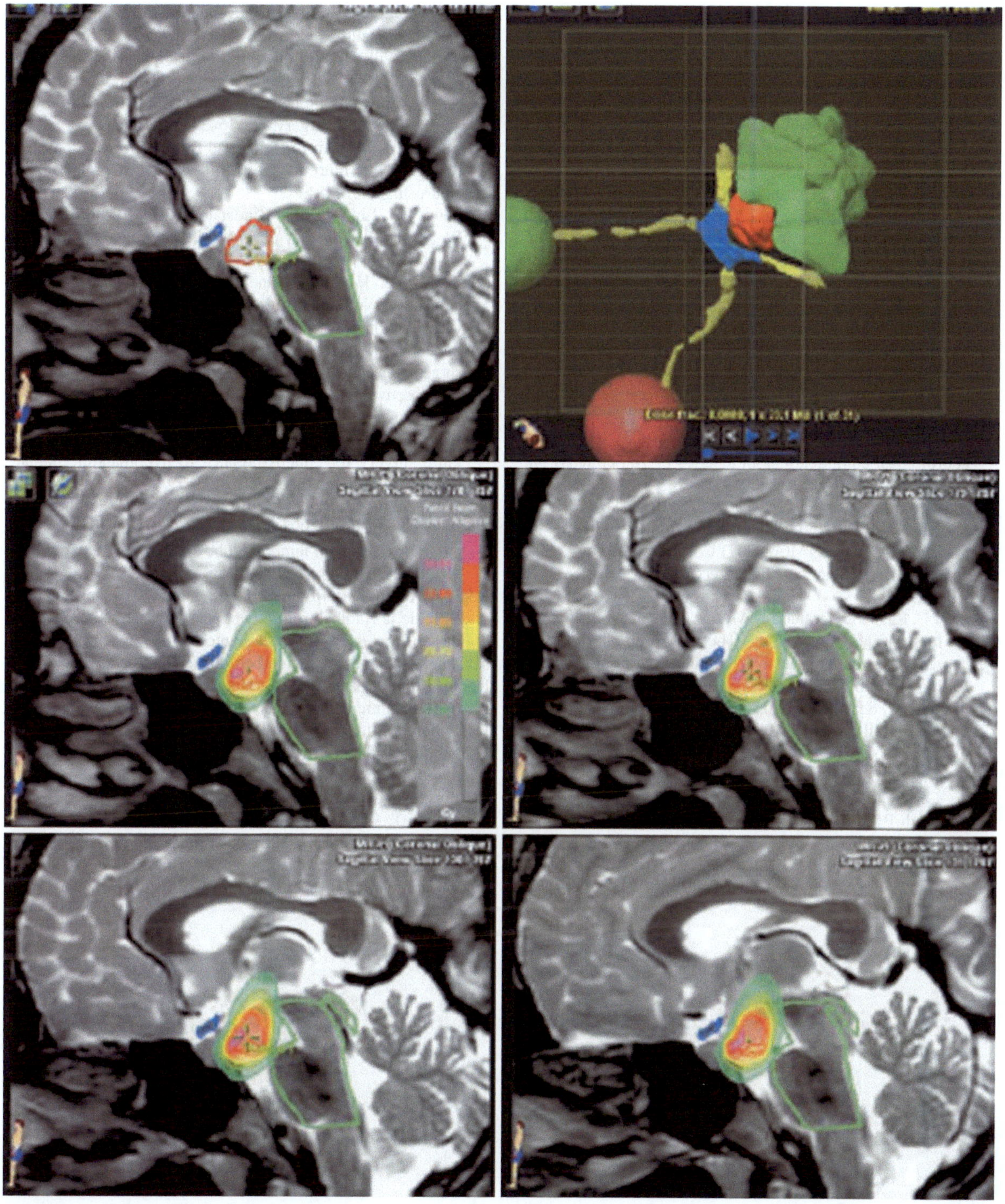

Fig. 19.5 (continued)

References

Arita K, Ikawa F, Kurisu K, Sumida M, Harada K, Uozumi T, Monden S, Yoshida J, Nishi Y (1999) The relationship between magnetic resonance imaging findings and clinical manifestations of hypothalamic hamartoma. J Neurosurg 91:212–220

Barbaro NM, Quigg M, Broshek DK, Ward MM, Lamborn KR, Laxer KD, Larson DA et al (2009) A multicenter, prospective pilot study of gamma knife radiosurgery for mesial temporal lobe epilepsy: seizure response, adverse events, and verbal memory. Ann Neurol 65:167–175

Barcia-Salorio JL, Roldan P, Hernandez G, Lopez Gomez L (1985) Radiosurgical treatment for epilepsy. Appl Neuro physiol 48:400–403

Barcia-Salorio JL, Barcia JA, Hernandez G, Lopez Gomez L (1994) Radiosurgery of epilepsy: long-term results. Acta Neurochir Suppl 62:111–113

Behrens E, Schramm J, Zentner J, König R (1997) Surgical and neurological complications in a series of 708 epilepsy surgery procedures. Neurosurgery 41:1–9

Celis MA, Moreno-Jiménez S, Lárraga-Gutiérrez JM, Alonso-Vanegas A, García-Garduño OA, Martínez-Juárez IE, Fernández-Gónzalez MC (2007) Corpus callosotomy using conformal stereotactic radiosurgery. Childs Nerv Syst 23: 917–920

Dunoyer C, Ragheb J, Resnick T, Alvarez L, Jayakar P, Altman N, Wolf A, Duchowny M (2002) The use of stereotactic radiosurgery to treat intractable childhood partial epilepsy. Epilepsia 43:292–300

Feichtinger M, Schröttner O, Eder H, Holthausen H, Pieper T, Unger F, Holl A, Gruber L, Kürner E, Trinka E, Fazekas F, Ott E (2006) Efficacy and safety of radiosurgical callosotomy: a retrospective analysis. Epilepsia 47:1184–1191

Friehs GM, Park MC, Goldman MA, Zerris VA, Noren G, Sampath P (2007) Stereotactic radiosurgery for functional disorders. Neurosurg Focus 23(6):E3

Heikkinen ER, Konnov B, Melnikov L, Yalynych N, Zubkov YN, Garmashov YA, Pak VA (1989) Relief of epilepsy by radiosurgery of cerebral arteriovenous malformations. Stereotact Funct Neurosurg 53:157–166

Hoggard N, Wilkinson ID, Griffiths PD, Vaughan P, Kemeny AA, Rowe JG (2008) The clinical course after stereotactic radiosurgical amygdalohippocampectomy with neuroradiological correlates. Neurosurgery 62:336–344

Lindquist C, Kihlström L, Hellstrand E (1991) Functional neurosurgery – a future for the gamma knife? Stereotact Funct Neurosurg 57:72–81

Mathews MS, Linskey ME, Binder DK (2008) William P. van Wegenen and the first corpus callosotomies for epilepsy. J Neurosurg 108:608–613

Pendl G, Eder HG, Schroettner O, Leber KA (1999) Corpus callosotomy with radiosurgery. Neurosurgery 45:303–307

Regis J, Bartolomei F, Kida Y, Kobayashi T, Vladyka V, Liscak R, Forster D, Kemeny A, Schröttner O, Pendl G (2000) Radiosurgery for epilepsy associated with cavernous malformation: retrospective study in 49 patients. Neurosurgery 47:1091–1097

Regis J, Scavarda D, Tamura M, Villeneuve N, Bartolomei F, Brue T, Morange I, Dafonseca D, Chauvel P (2007) Gamma knife surgery for epilepsy related to hypothalamic hamartomas. Semin Pediatr Neurol 14:73–79

Régis J, Peragut JC, Rey M, Samson Y, Levrier O, Porcheron D, Régis H, Sedan R (1995) First selective amygdalohippocampal radiosurgery for temporal lobe epilepsy. Stereotact Funct Neurosurg 64(suppl 1):193–201

Régis J, Arkha Y, Bartolomei F, Peragut JC, Chauvel P (2008) Rôle de la Radiochirurgie Gamma Knife dans le traitement des epilepsies pharmacorésistantes: situation actuelle, resultants et perspectives. Neurochirurgie 54:320–331

Romanelli P, Muacevic A, Striano S (2008) Radiosurgery for hypothalamic hamartomas. Neurosurg Focus 24:E9

Rydenhag B, Silander HC (2001) Complications of epilepsy surgery after 654 procedures in Sweden, September 1990–1995: a multicenter study based on the Swedish National Epilepsy Surgery Register. Neurosurgery 49:51–56

Tanriverdi T, Olivier A, Poulin N, Andermann F, Dubeau F (2009) Long-term seizure outcome after corpus callosotomy: a retrospective analysis of 95 patients. J Neurosurg 110:332–342

Spine Radiosurgery: Pain and Quality of Life Outcomes

20

Lilyana Angelov

20.1 Introduction

Spinal metastases are the most frequently occurring spine tumor and can arise in up to 30–50% of patients diagnosed with cancer (Wong et al. 1990; Heidecke et al. 2003; Ortiz Gomez 1995). The incidence and prevalence of bone metastases is expected to increase due to better detection and with the improvement of therapies for the primary malignancy that are prolonging patient survival. Early stages of spine metastases may be asymptomatic but delayed recognition of the problem and initiation of treatment can significantly impact a patient's quality of life (QOL) due to disabling pain, fractures or even paralysis from spinal cord compression (Ibrahim et al. 2008; Patchell et al. 2005).

Pain is the most common presentation of spine metastases affecting up to 90% of cancer patients (Helweg-Larsen and Sorensen 1994; Steinmetz et al. 2001). Spine pain can be mild to excruciating, debilitating, and difficult to manage and result in decreased QOL. Scoring tools such as the Brief Pain Inventory (BPI) and QOL assessment tools are useful during treatment to assess the impact of the disease at baseline and the overall effect of treatment. Further, QOL scores can predict survival in patients with cancer and have prognostic value independent of other factors (Coates et al. 1993, 1997). Using such assessment instruments to better understand the impact and role of stereotactic spine radiosurgery will serve to enhance our management of spine tumors and further help to guide our treatment strategies and improve our outcomes.

20.2 Radiation in the Treatment of Spine Metastases

The benefits of radiation therapy in the treatment of metastatic spine tumors are well established. It has been shown to reduce pain, control local disease progression and improve or retain neurological function (Wong et al. 1990; Cole and Patchell 2008; Loblaw et al. 2003; Helweg-Larsen 1996; Helweg-Larsen et al. 2000; Maranzano and Latini 1995; Maranzano et al. 2005a). While higher radiation dosages to the tumor result in greater tumor control (Maranzano et al. 2005b), the spine cord radiation tolerance limits the dose of conventional radiation that can be delivered (Wong et al. 1990; Maranzano et al. 2005b; Schultheiss 2008). As a result of these normal tissue tolerance constraints, there are often poor outcomes in terms of pain relief, tumor control and associated neurological deterioration, steroid use and decreased survival (Patchell et al. 2005; Price et al. 1986; Party 1999; Steenland et al. 1999).

In the past two decades, a number of technological advancements including improved patient immobilization (Lohr et al. 1999; Yenice et al. 2003; Wulf et al. 2000), precision radiation targeting and delivery using image-guided radiation therapy (IGRT) (Yenice et al. 2003; Ryu et al. 2003; Ryu et al. 2001; Murphy et al. 2001), and intensity modulated radiation therapy (IMRT) (Yu et al. 2008; Das et al. 2008) have begun to overcome some of the limitations of spine tumor radiation dosing.

L. Angelov
Head Section of Spine Tumors, Brain Tumor and Neuro-Oncology Center & Center for Spine Health, Neurological Institute, Cleveland Clinic, 9500 Euclid Avenue, S-73, Cleveland, OH 44195, USA
e-mail: angelol@ccf.org

A.A.F. De Salles et al. (eds.), *Shaped Beam Radiosurgery*,
DOI: 10.1007/978-3-642-11151-8_20, © Springer-Verlag Berlin Heidelberg 2011

Spine radiosurgery (SRS) is a novel treatment that stereotactically delivers high dose radiation in an accurate and conformal manner to the tumor in 1–5 fractions while its associated steep fall-off dose gradient protects adjacent normal structures. Hence, potentially tumor ablative doses of radiation can now be delivered to spinal tumors resulting in effective tumor control and substantial pain relief while simultaneously limiting the radiation to the adjacent normal structures minimizing both the acute and delayed morbidity and toxicity related to the treatment (Ryu et al. 2001, 2003; Gerszten et al. 2007; Bilsky et al. 2004; Benzil et al. 2004; De Salles et al. 2004; Medin et al. 2002). Many studies have reported local tumor control rates between 77% and 94% (Rock et al. 2004a, b; Gerszten et al. 1995, 2005a, b; Gerszten and Welch 2004) and included patients with tumors considered to be more radio-resistant such as colon or renal cell carcinoma (Gerszten et al. 2005b, 2007; Chang et al. 2007; Ryu et al. 2004; Rock et al. 2006; Sahgal et al. 2007; Yamada et al. 2005). As a result, enthusiasm for the role of spine radiosurgery in the management of spine tumors is rapidly growing.

Table 20.1 Key features of spine radiosurgery impacting outcomes

Effective and rapid pain palliation
High local tumor control rate
Non invasive
Outpatient treatment with no recovery time
Meaningfully improves QOL
Efficacy in radio-resistant histologies
Treatment option in patients previously irradiated with conventional external beam radiation therapy
Limited dose to adjacent normal tissue minimizing radiation impact (e.g.: spinal cord radio-toxicity, bone marrow reserve, post operative wound healing and infection rates)
Single fraction treatment advantageous to patients with limited life expectancy
Facilitated continuous/non-disrupted chemotherapy
May obviate the need for extensive spinal surgery
May decrease fusion/instrument failure when delivered after surgery compared to post-operative conventional radiation

20.3 Impact of Spine Radiosurgery

The most common indication for spine radiosurgery is pain and typically 70–90% of all patients treated present with tumor-related pain. Other indications for the procedure include: (1) initial tumor treatment often for radio-resistant histologies, (2) treatment after surgery for residual tumor and (3) local tumor progression after other treatment modalities such as surgery, conventional radiation and chemotherapy have failed. Table 20.1 lists several key features that impact and enhance the outcomes of patients with spine tumors when treated with stereotactic spine radiosurgery.

The impact of SRS on pain is significant both in the rapidity and degree of pain improvement as well as the proportion of patients that experience amelioration of this debilitating symptom. Several retrospective and prospective cohort studies have reported that SRS results in a high percentage of pain relief (either partial or complete) ranging 85–92% within a few days to weeks of treatment (Ryu et al. 2003, 2004; Gerszten et al. 2005b, 2007; Angelov 2009; Amdur et al. 2009). The largest single institution series is reported by Gerszten et al. (2007) reviewing 500 cases of spinal metastases treated by radiosurgery reporting 90% radiographic local tumor control for primary treated tumors. Long term pain improvement was noted to be 86%, and 85% of the patients presenting with neurological deficit, have improved. This clinical response is typically greater and more rapid than the results achieved with conventional radiation (Steenland et al. 1999). Efforts to prospectively evaluate the degree and timing of pain relief with SRS and its impact on QOL are in their early stages with this novel treatment paradigm and further studies are needed.

20.4 Measuring Pain Relief and QOL

The problem of pain in cancer is huge. Epidemiological surveys reviewing over 35,000 patients observed that 14–100% of cancer patients experience pain and patients with bone metastases reported cancer-related pain most frequently (Ahles et al. 1984; Goudas et al. 2005). In 2002, the NIH published a consensus statement on cancer symptom management where they noted the many cancer patients with pain, depression and fatigue receive inadequate treatment for their symptoms (NIH 2002). They strongly recommended that clinicians use a brief assessment tool to routinely evaluate their patients regarding their symptoms and initiate evidence-based treatments (NIH 2002; Ressel 2003). The problem with cancer pain however is that the pain is difficult to adequately assess and manage and physicians' assessment of patients' symptoms are often inaccurate (Dy et al. 2008; Holen et al. 2006).

Assessment tools need to be both reliable and validated and able to evaluate the relevant aspects of cancer pain including frequency, severity, and disruptiveness or interference. They have a role in initial patient screening, evaluating the impact of therapy and follow-up over time. Of particular value is the consistent reassessment of patients with the same pain scoring tools in order to understand the impact of pain management therapy in the short term as well as over time, adjust pain medication as appropriate and monitor for local or distal progression requiring further intervention. In this way, high quality objective care of patients with cancer pain can be provided.

However, pain relief is often affected by mood or insight and the impact of pain (or its relief through therapy) on QOL is a key component of a treatment evaluation. QOL is subjective and reflects a patient's perceptions of their physical, psychological and social well-being related to the cancer and its treatment. Yet, it is perhaps the most appropriate end-point that should be evaluated in the palliative setting, as such interventions are unlikely to lead to more traditionally measured end-points such as survival prolongation. Interventions should primarily aim at improving the QOL and limiting the impact of the disease as well as the toxicity of treatment.

Specifically related to spine metastases, advances in effective systemic treatment and more aggressive local interventions such as surgery in combination with radiation therapy (Patchell et al. 2005) have resulted in improved patient survival. Patients with prostate and breast cancer having bony metastases may have life expectancies in the 2–5 year range (Chow et al. 2009). In this setting, ameliorating pain as well as minimizing the skeletal and neurological complications to preserve mobility and function in these patients optimizes their QOL and should be aggressively pursued. In contrast, but also as essential to address, many advanced cancer or pre-terminal patients never complete radiation courses due to declining functional status, pain or the inconvenience of travel (Dy et al. 2008). In this context, single fraction radiation treatment as provided with SRS for spine metastases for example, may be more advantageous overall to the Quality Of Life of patients

To this end, as we manage patients with spine tumors who frequently present with significant pain and disability and a variable clinical course, the use of validated and appropriate pain assessment and QOL instruments should be promoted for use in both daily practice and clinical trials. Such longitudinal follow-up of patients provides information on specific disease symptoms and the effects of treatment on patients' lives. As well, it often helps to identify features of the patients' condition and the treatment that result in improved outcomes.

20.5 The Impact of SRS on Pain Relief and QOL Outcomes

While there are numerous pain assessment instruments, there has been no direct comparison between methods (Dy et al. 2008). However, in adult patients without cognitive impairment, a multidimensional pain assessment using the Brief Pain Inventory (BPI) (Cleeland and Ryan 1994; Daut et al. 1983) is often recommended (Holen et al. 2006; Caraceni et al. 2002). The BPI is a 17-item patient self–rating scale assessing demographic data, sensory and reactive pain components as well as use of medication. It has been deemed valid and reliable in patients with cancer (Daut et al. 1983; Jensen et al. 1999) and has been frequently employed in clinical trials. It was the key assessment tool in the Radiation Therapy Oncology Group study RTOG 97–14 to evaluate the impact of therapy on patients with bony metastases and is also the primary end-point measuring tool in the newly opened RTOG 06–31 study of image-guided radiosurgery/SBRT for localized spine metastases.

At our center, all patients are prospectively evaluated in terms of pain outcomes with BPIs prior to SRS. The questionnaire is administered for baseline pain assessment as well as at weeks 1, 2, 3 and 4 post treatment and then again every subsequent 3 months, while the patient continued to follow-up. In our series of 108 patients (154 treated targets), we found that pain scores were improved over baseline in 77% of patients ($p<0.001$) as early as 1 week post treatment and at 12 months post treatment 89% of the patients had continued pain improvement ($p<0.008$) over baseline as seen in Figure 20.1 This is

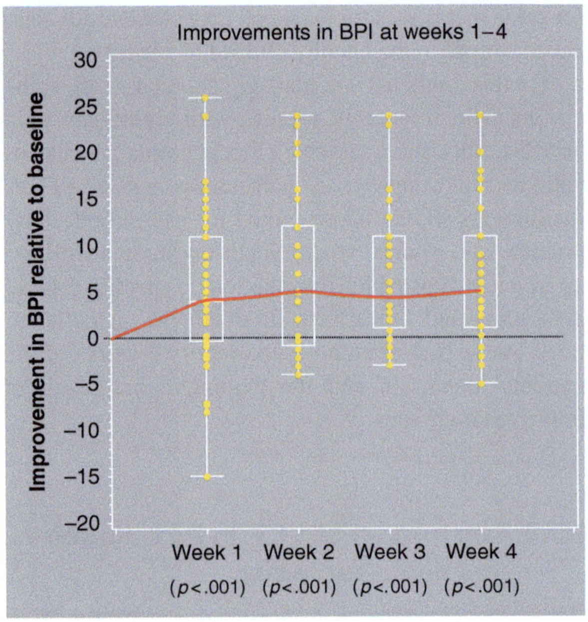

Fig. 20.1 Pain scores as assessed prospectively using the BPI assessment tool in a series 108 patients treated with single faction spine radiosurgery

consistent with other SRS studies including Ryu et al. (2008) where the overall pain control rate was 84% at 1 year and in the series of 200 patients with spine tumors published by Gagnon et al. (2009) where mean pain score decreased significantly ($p<0.001$) as assessed by the Visual Analog Scale, a decrease that persisted over the entire 4-year follow-up period ($p<0.05$).

In an encompassing review of the literature, Gerszten et al. (2009) identified 29 SRS studies and found that pain reduction was reported to be 85–100%, neurological recovery was 57–92% and local control rate was 75–100%. The authors compared these results to their review results of the literature regarding conventional radiation for spine metastases. They concluded that radiosurgery is superior in pain control, local control, and neurologic functional preservation.

In terms of the evaluation of QOL with SRS treatment, there are many cancer specific QOL questionnaires available. However, historically, bone metastases trials have employed the European Organization for Research and Treatment of Cancer Quality of Life group core questionnaire (EORTC QLQ-C30). Further, it is the most frequently used measure in cancer clinical trial research and well established as a QOL instrument for cancer patients in general and has been validated for use in palliative radiotherapy (Aaronson et al. 1993). Newer initiatives have created additional modules to supplement the EORTC QLQ-C30 and specifically address key disease or treatment related problems in patients with bone metastases such as the EORTC QLQ-BM2253, (Chow and Bottomley 2009), which is currently still being evaluated and validated. These will likely lead to a more profound understanding of the specific impact of bony metastases on QOL over time.

Since its inception, our SRS program has prospectively evaluated our patients with the EORTC QLQ-C30 that incorporates 9 multi-item scales; 5 functional scales (physical, role, cognitive, emotional and social), 3 symptom scales (fatigue, pain and nausea and vomiting) and a global QOL scale. Using this QOL tool, independent quality of life functional scores were significantly improved relative to baseline as early as 1 month post treatment in all patients with durable and statistically significant results seen over many months as demonstrated in Figure 20.2. Of note, this improvement in QOL was consistently seen even in those patients with more radio-resistant pathologies such as renal cell carcinoma (Angelov 2009) which is in stark contrast to the modest results seen with such cancers

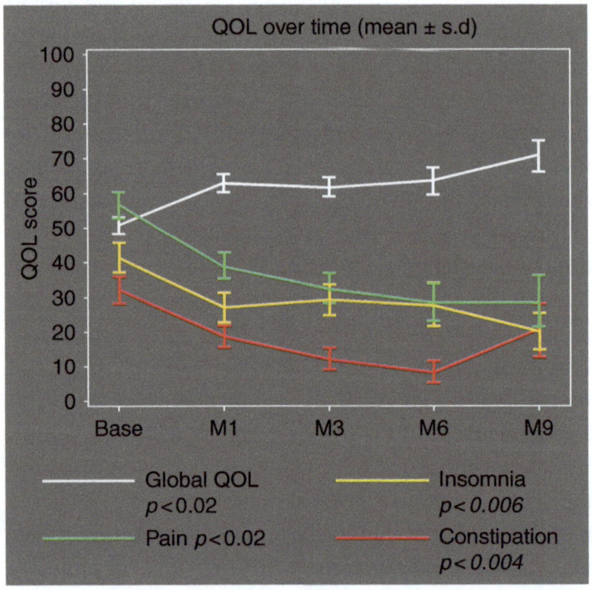

Fig. 20.2 EORTC QLQ-C30 assessment tool in patients treated with SRS ($n=108$ patients) demonstrates a significant improvement in pain, insomnia and constipation symptoms scale scores as well as the global QOL scores at months 1 (M1) through month 9 (M9) post treatment

when they metastasize to the spine and are treated with either surgery or conventional radiation.

20.6 Conclusion

Although a relatively new treatment modality, SRS is rapidly emerging as a promising major advancement in clinical medicine for the treatment and palliation of spine tumors. Its dose response/toxicity ratio is favorable both in terms of tumor control and rapid and durable pain relief and it is associated with limited post radiation spinal myelopathy (Gibbs et al. 2009). Patients are clearly experiencing the benefits of therapy.

However, as the long term survival of patients with cancer continues to dramatically increase, we need to remember to judiciously assess both the positive and negative effects of cancer and its treatment. To date there has been little systematic evaluation about the long term consequences of both standard and novel treatments in spine tumor patients and the impact on their QOL (Gotay 2003, 2004; Gotay et al. 2004; Gotay and Muraoka 1998; Gotay and Wilson 1998; Sankila and Coebergh 2004; Sankila et al. 1998). Multidisciplinary decision-making and a team approach to the very complex problem of spine metastases are essential to optimize patient outcomes and streamline care. Moving forward however, we also have a responsibility to understand and minimize treatment related sequelae. We will need to monitor the effects of long term symptoms or consequences of treatment toxicity. This should not only be a focus of research but also standard of care as our SRS and overall spine tumor management experience continues to grow (Harel and Angelov 2010).

References

Aaronson NK, Ahmedzai S, Bergman B et al (1993) The European Organization for Research and Treatment of Cancer QLQ-C30: a quality-of-life instrument for use in international clinical trials in oncology. J Natl Cancer Inst 85:365–376

Ahles TA, Ruckdeschel JC, Blanchard EB (1984) Cancer-related pain I. Prevalence in an outpatient setting as a function of stage of disease and type of cancer. J Psychosom Res 28:115–119

Amdur RJ, Bennett J, Olivier K et al (2009) A prospective, phase II study demonstrating the potential value and limitation of radiosurgery for spine metastases. Am J Clin Oncol 32(5):515–520

Angelov L (2009) Stereotactic Spine Radiosurgery (SRS) for pain and tumor control in patients with spinal metastases from renal cell carcinoma: a prospective study. Int J Radiat Oncol Biol Phys 75:s112–113

Benzil DL, Saboori M, Mogilner AY, Rocchio R, Moorthy CR (2004) Safety and efficacy of stereotactic radiosurgery for tumors of the spine. J Neurosurg 101(Suppl 3): 413–418

Bilsky MH, Yamada Y, Yenice KM et al (2004) Intensity-modulated stereotactic radiotherapy of paraspinal tumors: a preliminary report. Neurosurgery 54:823–830, Discussion 30–31

Caraceni A, Cherny N, Fainsinger R et al (2002) Pain measurement tools and methods in clinical research in palliative care: recommendations of an Expert Working Group of the European Association of Palliative Care. J Pain Symptom Manage 23:239–255

Chang EL, Shiu AS, Mendel E et al (2007) Phase I/II study of stereotactic body radiotherapy for spinal metastasis and its pattern of failure. J Neurosurg Spine 7:151–160

Chow E, Bottomley A (2009) Understanding the EORTC QLQ-BM22, the module for patients with bone metastases. Expert Rev Pharmacoecon Outcomes Res 9:461–465

Chow E, Hird A, Velikova G et al (2009) The European Organisation for Research and Treatment of Cancer Quality of Life Questionnaire for patients with bone metastases: the EORTC QLQ-BM22. Eur J Cancer 45:1146–1152

Cleeland CS, Ryan KM (1994) Pain assessment: global use of the Brief Pain Inventory. Ann Acad Med Singapore 23:129–138

Coates A, Thomson D, McLeod GR et al (1993) Prognostic value of quality of life scores in a trial of chemotherapy with or without interferon in patients with metastatic malignant melanoma. Eur J Cancer 29A:1731–1734

Coates A, Porzsolt F, Osoba D (1997) Quality of life in oncology practice: prognostic value of EORTC QLQ-C30 scores in patients with advanced malignancy. Eur J Cancer 33:1025–1030

Cole JS, Patchell RA (2008) Metastatic epidural spinal cord compression. Lancet Neurol 7:459–466

Das IJ, Cheng CW, Chopra KL, Mitra RK, Srivastava SP, Glatstein E (2008) Intensity-modulated radiation therapy dose prescription, recording, and delivery: patterns of variability among institutions and treatment planning systems. J Natl Cancer Inst 100:300–307

Daut RL, Cleeland CS, Flanery RC (1983) Development of the Wisconsin Brief Pain Questionnaire to assess pain in cancer and other diseases. Pain 17:197–210

De Salles AA, Pedroso AG, Medin P et al (2004) Spinal lesions treated with Novalis shaped beam intensity-modulated radiosurgery and stereotactic radiotherapy. J Neurosurg 101(Suppl 3):435–440

Dy SM, Asch SM, Naeim A, Sanati H, Walling A, Lorenz KA (2008) Evidence-based standards for cancer pain management. J Clin Oncol 26:3879–3885

Gagnon GJ, Nasr NM, Liao JJ et al (2009) Treatment of spinal tumors using cyberknife fractionated stereotactic radiosurgery: pain and quality-of-life assessment after treatment in 200 patients. Neurosurgery 64:297–306, Discussion 7

Gerszten PC, Welch WC (2004) Cyberknife radiosurgery for metastatic spine tumors. Neurosurg Clin N Am 15:491–501
Gerszten PC, Lunsford LD, Rutigliano MJ, Kondziolka D, Flickinger JC, Martinez AJ (1995) Single-stage stereotactic diagnosis and radiosurgery: feasibility and cost implications. J Image Guid Surg 1:141–150
Gerszten PC, Burton SA, Welch WC et al (2005a) Single-fraction radiosurgery for the treatment of spinal breast metastases. Cancer 104:2244–2254
Gerszten PC, Burton SA, Ozhasoglu C et al (2005b) Stereotactic radiosurgery for spinal metastases from renal cell carcinoma. J Neurosurg Spine 3:288–295
Gerszten PC, Burton SA, Ozhasoglu C, Welch WC (2007) Radiosurgery for spinal metastases: clinical experience in 500 cases from a single institution. Spine (Phila Pa 1976) 32:193–199
Gerszten PC, Mendel E, Yamada Y (2009) Radiotherapy and radiosurgery for metastatic spine disease: what are the options, indications, and outcomes? Spine (Phila Pa 1976) 34:S78–92
Gibbs IC, Patil C, Gerszten PC, Adler JR Jr, Burton SA (2009) Delayed radiation-induced myelopathy after spinal radiosurgery. Neurosurgery 64:A67–72
Gotay CC (2003) Quality of life assessment in cancer clinical research: current status and a look to the future. Expert Rev Pharmacoecon Outcomes Res 3:479–486
Gotay CC (2004) Assessing cancer-related quality of life across a spectrum of applications. J Natl Cancer Inst Monogr 33:126–133
Gotay CC, Muraoka MY (1998) Quality of life in long-term survivors of adult-onset cancers. J Natl Cancer Inst 90:656–667
Gotay CC, Wilson M (1998) Use of quality-of-life outcome assessments in current cancer clinical trials. Eval Health Prof 21:157–178
Gotay CC, Isaacs P, Pagano I (2004) Quality of life in patients who survive a dire prognosis compared to control cancer survivors. Psychooncology 13:882–892
Goudas LC, Bloch R, Gialeli-Goudas M, Lau J, Carr DB (2005) The epidemiology of cancer pain. Cancer Invest 23:182–190
Harel R, Angelov L (2010) Spine metastases: current treatments and future directions. Eur J Cancer 46(15):2696–2707
Heidecke V, Rainov NG, Burkert W (2003) Results and outcome of neurosurgical treatment for extradural metastases in the cervical spine. Acta Neurochir (Wien) 145:873–880, Discussion 80–81
Helweg-Larsen S (1996) Clinical outcome in metastatic spinal cord compression. A prospective study of 153 patients. Acta Neurol Scand 94:269–275
Helweg-Larsen S, Sorensen PS (1994) Symptoms and signs in metastatic spinal cord compression: a study of progression from first symptom until diagnosis in 153 patients. Eur J Cancer 30A:396–398
Helweg-Larsen S, Sorensen PS, Kreiner S (2000) Prognostic factors in metastatic spinal cord compression: a prospective study using multivariate analysis of variables influencing survival and gait function in 153 patients. Int J Radiat Oncol Biol Phys 46:1163–1169
Holen JC, Hjermstad MJ, Loge JH et al (2006) Pain assessment tools: is the content appropriate for use in palliative care? J Pain Symptom Manage 32:567–580
Ibrahim A, Crockard A, Antonietti P et al (2008) Does spinal surgery improve the quality of life for those with extradural (spinal) osseous metastases? An international multicenter prospective observational study of 223 patients. Invited submission from the Joint Section Meeting on Disorders of the Spine and Peripheral Nerves, March 2007. J Neurosurg Spine 8:271–278
Jensen MP, Turner JA, Romano JM, Fisher LD (1999) Comparative reliability and validity of chronic pain intensity measures. Pain 83:157–162
Loblaw DA, Laperriere NJ, Mackillop WJ (2003) A population-based study of malignant spinal cord compression in Ontario. Clin Oncol (R Coll Radiol) 15:211–217
Lohr F, Debus J, Frank C et al (1999) Noninvasive patient fixation for extracranial stereotactic radiotherapy. Int J Radiat Oncol Biol Phys 45:521–527
Maranzano E, Latini P (1995) Effectiveness of radiation therapy without surgery in metastatic spinal cord compression: final results from a prospective trial. Int J Radiat Oncol Biol Phys 32:959–967
Maranzano E, Bellavita R, Rossi R (2005a) Radiotherapy alone or surgery in spinal cord compression? The choice depends on accurate patient selection. J Clin Oncol 23:8270–8272, Author reply 2–4
Maranzano E, Bellavita R, Rossi R et al (2005b) Short-course versus split-course radiotherapy in metastatic spinal cord compression: results of a phase III, randomized, multicenter trial. J Clin Oncol 23:3358–3365
Medin PM, Solberg TD, De Salles AA et al (2002) Investigations of a minimally invasive method for treatment of spinal malignancies with LINAC stereotactic radiation therapy: accuracy and animal studies. Int J Radiat Oncol Biol Phys 52:1111–1122
Murphy MJ, Chang S, Gibbs I, Le QT, Martin D, Kim D (2001) Image-guided radiosurgery in the treatment of spinal metastases. Neurosurg Focus 11:e6
NIH (2002) State-of-the-science statement on symptom management in cancer: pain, depression, and fatigue. NIH Consens State Sci Statements 19:1–29
Ortiz Gomez JA (1995) The incidence of vertebral body metastases. Int Orthop 19:309–311
Party BPTW (1999) 8 Gy single fraction radiotherapy for the treatment of metastatic skeletal pain: randomised comparison with a multifraction schedule over 12 months of patient follow-up. Bone Pain Trial Working Party. Radiother Oncol 52:111–121
Patchell RA, Tibbs PA, Regine WF et al (2005) Direct decompressive surgical resection in the treatment of spinal cord compression caused by metastatic cancer: a randomised trial. Lancet 366:643–648
Price P, Hoskin PJ, Easton D, Austin D, Palmer SG, Yarnold JR (1986) Prospective randomised trial of single and multifraction radiotherapy schedules in the treatment of painful bony metastases. Radiother Oncol 6:247–255
Ressel GW (2003) NIH releases statement on managing pain, depression, and fatigue in cancer. Am Fam Physician 67:423–424
Rock JP, Ryu S, Yin FF, Schreiber F, Abdulhak M (2004a) The evolving role of stereotactic radiosurgery and stereotactic radiation therapy for patients with spine tumors. J Neurooncol 69:319–334

Rock JP, Ryu S, Yin FF (2004b) Novalis radiosurgery for metastatic spine tumors. Neurosurg Clin N Am 15: 503–509

Rock JP, Ryu S, Shukairy MS et al (2006) Postoperative radiosurgery for malignant spinal tumors. Neurosurgery 58:891–898, Discussion 8

Ryu SI, Chang SD, Kim DH et al (2001) Image-guided hypo-fractionated stereotactic radiosurgery to spinal lesions. Neurosurgery 49:838–846

Ryu S, Fang Yin F, Rock J et al (2003) Image-guided and intensity-modulated radiosurgery for patients with spinal metastasis. Cancer 97:2013–2018

Ryu S, Rock J, Rosenblum M, Kim JH (2004) Patterns of failure after single-dose radiosurgery for spinal metastasis. J Neurosurg 101(Suppl 3):402–405

Ryu S, Jin R, Jin JY et al (2008) Pain control by image-guided radiosurgery for solitary spinal metastasis. J Pain Symptom Manage 35:292–298

Sahgal A, Chou D, Ames C et al (2007) Image-guided robotic stereotactic body radiotherapy for benign spinal tumors: the University of California San Francisco preliminary experience. Technol Cancer Res Treat 6:595–604

Sankila R, Coebergh JW (2004) Cancer registries contribute to quality improvements in clinical care for all European cancer patients. Eur J Cancer 40:635–637

Sankila R, Olsen JH, Anderson H et al (1998) Risk of cancer among offspring of childhood-cancer survivors. Association of the Nordic Cancer Registries and the Nordic Society of Paediatric Haematology and Oncology. N Engl J Med 338:1339–1344

Schultheiss TE (2008) The radiation dose-response of the human spinal cord. Int J Radiat Oncol Biol Phys 71:1455–1459

Steenland E, Leer JW, van Houwelingen H et al (1999) The effect of a single fraction compared to multiple fractions on painful bone metastases: a global analysis of the Dutch Bone Metastasis Study. Radiother Oncol 52:101–109

Steinmetz MP, Mekhail A, Benzel EC (2001) Management of metastatic tumors of the spine: strategies and operative indications. Neurosurg Focus 11:e2

Wong DA, Fornasier VL, MacNab I (1990) Spinal metastases: the obvious, the occult, and the impostors. Spine (Phila Pa 1976) 15:1–4

Wulf J, Hadinger U, Oppitz U, Olshausen B, Flentje M (2000) Stereotactic radiotherapy of extracranial targets: CT-simulation and accuracy of treatment in the stereotactic body frame. Radiother Oncol 57:225–236

Yamada Y, Lovelock DM, Yenice KM et al (2005) Multifractionated image-guided and stereotactic intensity-modulated radiotherapy of paraspinal tumors: a preliminary report. Int J Radiat Oncol Biol Phys 62:53–61

Yenice KM, Lovelock DM, Hunt MA et al (2003) CT image-guided intensity-modulated therapy for paraspinal tumors using stereotactic immobilization. Int J Radiat Oncol Biol Phys 55:583–593

Yu CX, Amies CJ, Svatos M (2008) Planning and delivery of intensity-modulated radiation therapy. Med Phys 35:5233–5241

Part IV

Spinal and Other Extra-Cranial Applications

21 Spinal Cord Tolerance to Radiosurgery

Andrew Knight

21.1 Introduction

Stereotactic body radiotherapy (SBRT) is an emerging technology used for the treatment of spinal tumors. Its implementation allows effective dose escalation over conventional radiotherapy, which may improve tumor control. Additionally, it provides a treatment option for patients who are not candidates for conventional radiotherapy because of previous radiotherapy to the spinal cord. Finally, it has the potential to improve the quality of life for patients who may be spared a prolonged treatment course, and acute radiation toxicity. With potential advantages, come new challenges. Most critical among these challenges is to minimize the risk of spinal cord injury.

This chapter will serve as a review of the available evidence regarding the tolerance of the spinal cord to SBRT, and will include a brief discussion of the technical issues which must be addressed in order to amass useful clinical data on the subject.

21.2 Spinal Cord Tolerance to Conventional Radiation Therapy

Conventional radiotherapy to the spine results in a spinal cord dose which is equivalent to or higher than that of the target tumor (see Fig. 21.1.) In order to delivery clinically meaningful doses to the tumor without causing myelitis, radiotherapy is delivered in a protracted regimen, using relatively small daily doses. Case reports of myelitis after radiotherapy for head and neck tumors led to early recognition of the spinal cord as a structure sensitive to radiation (Ahlbom 1941). Later observations, including that of Wara et al. (1975) and (Lambert 1978), demonstrated a higher tolerance of the spinal cord than previously assumed in the setting of conventionally fractionated radiation, thus highlighting the importance of fraction size. The largest single-institution series of long-term survivors of radiotherapy to the spinal cord was presented by Marcus and Million in 1991, (Marcus and Million 1990) which confirmed that doses up to 50 Gy resulted in only rare cases of myelitis (<0.5% among long-term survivors.) These conclusions have been reaffirmed in review articles by Emami (Emami et al. 1991) and Schultheiss (Schultheiss et al. 1995; Schultheiss 2008).

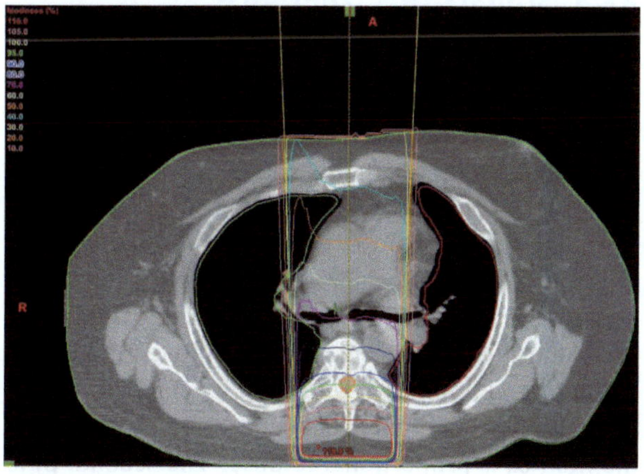

Fig. 21.1 Radiation dose-distribution from a typical posterior-anterior beam for treatment of metastatic tumor involving the vertebral body

A. Knight
Department of Radiation Oncology, David Geffen School of Medicine at UCLA, 200 UCLA Medical Plaza, Suite B265, Los Angeles, CA 90095, USA
e-mail: aknight@mednet.ucla.edu

A.A.F. De Salles et al. (eds.), *Shaped Beam Radiosurgery*,
DOI: 10.1007/978-3-642-11151-8_21, © Springer-Verlag Berlin Heidelberg 2011

Possible exacerbating factors for the development of radiation myelitis are neither well quantified nor elucidated. Caution has been advised in the setting of previous or planned treatment with chemotherapies known to be neurotoxic (Schultheiss et al. 1995). Also, there is some evidence that cord tolerance in the post-operative setting may also be impaired, given possible trauma or subclinical vascular injury (Linstadt et al. 1989).

21.3 Spinal Cord Tolerance to Hypofractionated Radiotherapy and Predictive Models

Radiation myelitis is thought to be a result of either glial or vascular injury (Schultheiss et al. 1995). While its precise biologic origin is controversial, significant work has been applied to modeling the likelihood of such injury. The linear-quadratic (LQ) model is the most widely accepted and employed model for predicting cell survival and toxicity. In this model, there are two components to cell killing by radiation: the first, α, is proportional to dose. The second, β, is proportional to the square of dose (Fowler 1989; Thames et al. 1982). The cell survival curve is modeled by the equation:

$$S = e(-\alpha D - \beta D2)$$

where S represents the fraction of cells surviving a dose D. The constants α and β are specific to the tissue irradiated.

Using the LQ model, one can calculate the biologically effective dose (BED), which is used to compare different fractionation regimens.

$$\text{BED} = (\text{nd}) \times (1 + \text{d}/\alpha/\beta),$$

where n is the number of fractions, d is the dose per fraction, and α/β (alpha-beta ratio) is the dose at which the α and β components contribute equally to cell killing. The alpha-beta ratio must be experimentally determined, but is often approximated as 10 Gy for malignant tumors, and 2–3 Gy for late responding normal tissues. Modeling of myelitis data has led to estimates of the alpha-beta ratio of the spinal cord to be approximately 2 Gy (Schultheiss et al. 1995; Schultheiss 2008). As such, when discussing spinal cord tolerance, doses are often presented as BED2, which refers to the BED assuming an alpha-beta ratio of 2 (see Table 21.1.)

It is important to recognize that the LQ model is not well validated for hypofractionated radiotherapy, and may incorrectly estimate the late toxicity of large doses per fraction. Similarly, its validity for predicting tumor control for radiosurgical doses has been questioned (Flickinger et al. 2002; Park et al. 2008). However, it is often employed as a starting point for comparing hypofractionated regimens.

Table 21.1 Column 1 lists various fractionation schemes used to treat spinal metastases. Column 2 gives the corresponding BED2. Column 3 gives the corresponding equivalent dose for treatment with 2 Gy per fraction, with respect to myelitis risk. Column 4 gives the corresponding equivalent dose, with respect to tumor control

Total dose/fraction number	BED2	Equivalent dose in 2 Gy fractions, for myelitis risk (α/β=2)	Equivalent dose in 2 Gy fractions, for tumor control (α/β=10)
8 Gy/1	40 Gy2	20.0 Gy	12.0 Gy
16 Gy/1	144 Gy2	72.0 Gy	34.7 Gy
20 Gy/1	220 Gy2	110 Gy	50.0 Gy
21 Gy/3	94.5 Gy2	47.3 Gy	29.8 Gy
24 Gy/3	120 Gy2	60.0 Gy	36.0 Gy
30 Gy/5	120 Gy2	60.0 Gy	40.0 Gy
35 Gy/5	158 Gy2	78.8 Gy	49.6 Gy
30 Gy/10	75 Gy2	37.5 Gy	32.5 Gy
50 Gy/25	100 Gy2	50.0 Gy	50.0 Gy

21.4 Spinal Cord Tolerance to Hypofractionated Radiation: Clinical Experience

The administration of large doses of radiation per treatment is thought to have a delayed deleterious effect on normal tissues, including the spinal cord, compared to a fractionated regimen of equivalent antitumor effect. Treatment with large single doses of radiation to the spinal cord has thus been generally restricted to the palliative setting. Because the interval for development of radiation-induced myelitis (often 1 year or more (Lambert 1978)) generally exceeds the life expectancy of these patients, limited useful data on single-dose spinal cord tolerance is available.

The most extensive clinical experience with hypofractionated radiotherapy to the spine is with 8 Gy in a single fraction for palliation of osseous metastases. RTOG 9714 randomized 898 patients with painful bone metastases to treatment with 8 Gy in a single fraction *versus* 30 Gy in 10 fractions (Hartsell et al. 2005). Approximately one half of these patients were treated to the spine. Although a late toxicity follow-up report of these patients has not been performed, no cases of myelitis have been observed (William Hartsell, personal communication.) Similarly, over 150 patients in the Dutch Bone Metastasis Study were treated for spine metastases with 8 Gy in a single fraction (Van der Linden et al. 2006; Van der Linden et al. 2005). No known myelitis cases were reported at the time of publication, and no cases of myelitis have been observed to date (Yvette van der Linden, personal communication).

Macbeth et al. published their experience with patients treated for small cell lung cancer, using a range of high-dose per fraction regimens (Macbeth et al. 1996). Among these patients, 114 were treated with a single fraction of 10 Gy, none of whom developed myelitis. An additional 524 patients were treated with 17 Gy, divided into two fractions given 1 week apart, three of whom developed myelitis. Of course, these data must be considered with caution, given the limited follow-up and survival of these patients.

Maranzano et al. have published several reports regarding treatment for metastatic spinal cord compression with 16 Gy in two 8 Gy fractions, separated by 1 week (Maranzano et al. 1997; Maranzano et al. 2001). In an initial report of 53 patients, no cases of myelitis were observed (Maranzano et al. 1997). In a subsequent long-term toxicity analysis, which included eight long-term survivors treated with this regimen, one had experienced myelitis (Maranzano et al. 2001).

While limited, the above data indicate that a single fraction dose of at least 8 Gy to the spinal cord is likely safe. The safety of other highly hypofractionated courses is not as well established. By extension, a maximum spinal cord dose of 8 Gy may be considered conservative for single fraction spine radiosurgery.

21.5 Reirradiation and Recovery of Occult Spinal Cord Injury

Symptomatic metastasis in a previously radiated field is a frequent indication for spine SBRT. In this setting, the accuracy and conformality of SBRT may provide an advantage over reirradiation by conventional radiotherapy. Nevertheless, the spinal cord will be exposed to some additional radiation dose. Recovery of the previous subclinical cord injury is an important consideration when deciding upon a reasonable cord dose limit for such treatment. Available data indicate that there is some recovery of spinal cord tolerance after radiotherapy, which increases with the time interval between radiation treatments.

Ang et al. conducted a series of reirradiation experiments on rhesus monkeys, in which animals were initially treated to 44 Gy in 2.2 Gy fractions (Ang et al. 2001). After an interval of 1–3 years, animals were retreated to a dose of either 57.2 or 66 Gy, also in 2.2 Gy fractions. Of the 45 animals that completed the treatment and extended observation, only 4 developed myelitis. Without some degree of repair of subclinical repair of radiation injury, nearly all of the animals would have been expected to develop myelitis. Of the several models the authors proposed to account for this repair, the most conservative suggests repair of more than 60% of the initial radiation injury during the 1–3 years between treatments.

Similarly, Nieder et al. reviewed published reports from 40 patients who were treated with reirradiation to the spinal cord (Nieder et al. 2005). While 11 patients developed myelopathy, no cases of myelopathy were seen in patients with an interval between treatments of greater than 2 months, and with no single course BED exceeding 102 Gy2 (equivalent to 51 Gy in 2 Gy fractions.) The authors concluded that the risk of myelopathy appears small for a cumulative BED of less than 135.5 Gy2, when the interval between treatments is at least 6 months, and no single treatment course BED exceeds 98 Gy2.

These limited data imply that the spinal cord has a significant ability to repair subclinical injury. Repair has been demonstrated most clearly in cases with initial treatment to a dose below spinal cord tolerance and a significant interval (1 year or more) between treatments.

21.6 Partial Volume Spinal Cord Tolerance

Despite the geometric advantages of SBRT over conventional radiotherapy, such treatment may still result in a significant radiation dose to a portion of the cord. This consideration is especially important when treating tumors that lie directly adjacent to the spinal cord. Respecting the tolerance of the spinal cord to single fraction or hypofractionated radiation may result in a "cold spot" in a portion of the tumor, creating a significant risk of recurrence. Alternatively, one may permit the maximum dose to the spinal cord to be high, while limiting this high-dose region to a small volume. The safety of the latter approach requires further investigation, although animal data and emerging clinical data are promising.

In order to understand the basis of partial volume spinal cord tolerance, it is helpful to consider the findings of Franklin et al. These investigators demonstrated that following a radiation-induced demyelinating injury to the rat spinal cord, oligodendrocyte progenitor cells (OPCs) migrate from the adjacent, undamaged spinal cord to remyelinate the injured region, thus preventing irreversible injury (Franklin et al. 1997). Their results demonstrated that demyelination injuries of lengths up to 2 mm were repaired. These findings indicate that a radiation-induced demyelination injury of a very short cord length may not result in clinical myelopathy.

Bijl et al. have conducted a series of experiments, also using a rat model, which further elucidate the partial volume effect of spinal cord radiation injury. These investigators found that the single fraction radiation dose required to cause myelopathy in 50% of subjects (ED50) was 20 Gy when treating a 20-mm length of spinal cord, 25 Gy for an 8-mm length, 54 Gy for a 4-mm length, and 88 Gy for a 2-mm length, lending support to the findings of Franklin et al. (Bijl et al. 2002).

In a subsequent experiment, these investigators applied a low-dose treatment to a large field ("bath"), followed by the same series of dose-escalated treatments to a short length of spinal cord in the middle of that field ("shower.") By doing so, they found that the tolerance advantage of the small field was greatly reduced (Bijl et al. 2006). For example, a "bath" dose of 4 Gy to 20 mm of cord, combined with a "shower" dose to the central 2 mm, was associated with an ED50 of 61 Gy for the combined dose (*versus* 88 Gy without the "bath" dose.) Such a finding is highly relevant to spine SBRT, since the dose gradient outside of the target volume results in a relatively large area of spinal cord receiving a lower, but significant radiation dose (see Fig. 21.2.) Notably, early results of hemicord radiosurgery using a porcine model also indicate a more modest partial volume dose tolerance advantage than indicated by the work of Franklin (Medin et al. 2008).

Also relevant to spine SBRT, Bijl et al. examined radiosensitivity of the rat spinal cord to radiation of different anatomic regions. In these experiments, the investigators treated either the central portion of the cord, with sparing of the lateral cord, or the lateral cord on one side (see Fig. 21.3.) (Bijl et al. 2005). All treatments involved a 20-mm length of cord. Treatment of

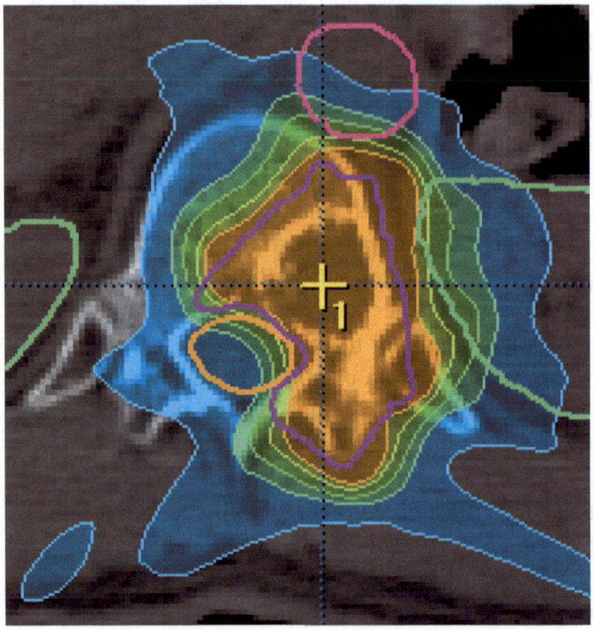

Fig. 21.2 Spine SBRT limits the high radiation dose to a very small volume of the spinal cord. However, a significant portion of the spinal cord is treated to a lower dose. This situation mimics the "bath and shower" experiment of Bijl et al. (2006)

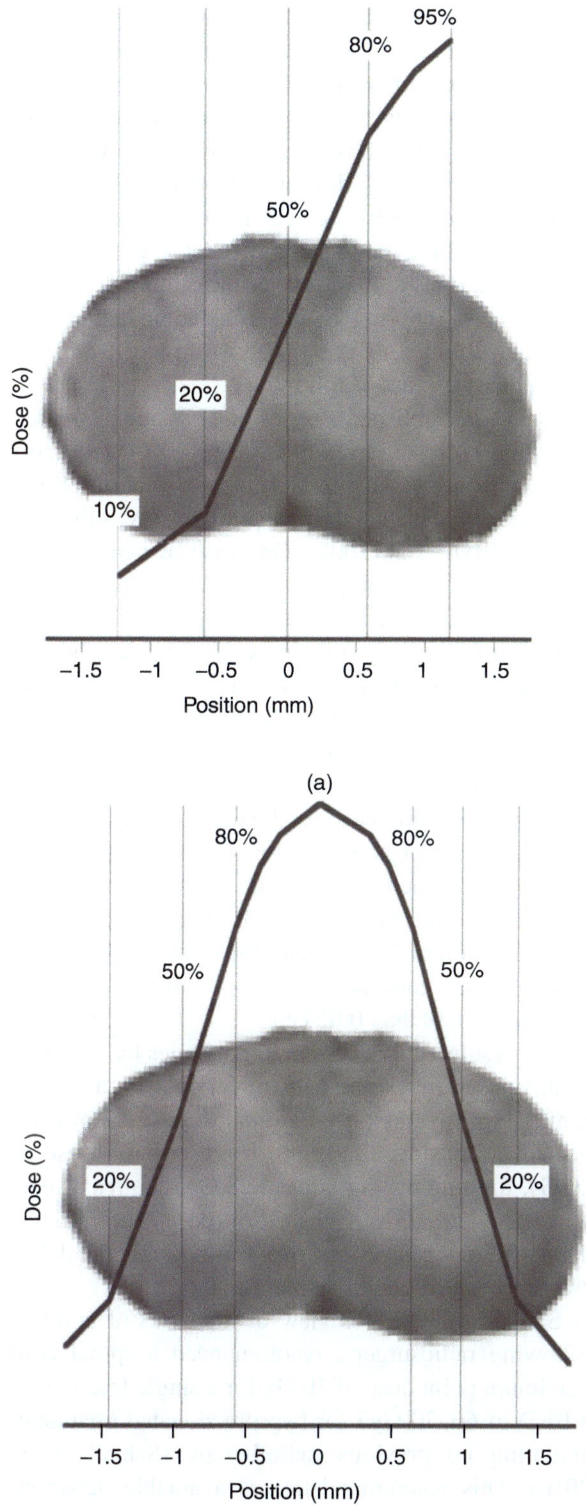

Fig. 21.3 Dose distribution profile used in experiments evaluating the impact of high doses of radiation across different areas of the cervical spinal cord of the rats. The different doses are projected over a transversal MRI slice of the cord. (From Bijl et al. 2005. Reprinted with permission)

the lateral cord was associated with an ED50 of approximately 30 Gy, which was significantly higher than the ED50 of 20 Gy observed with treatment of the entire cross-sectional area of the spinal cord. Treatment of the central cord was associated with an ED50 of 72 Gy, indicating a significantly higher radiation tolerance of the central than lateral cord. The authors considered regional differences in vascularity of the spinal cord a likely explanation for the findings. However, one must also consider the possibility that lateral cord injuries, which would affect the lateral corticospinal tract, would be more clinically evident than central cord injuries in this rat model.

While preliminary, this data raises the question of whether radiation dose to a small cross-sectional area of the spinal cord may be tolerated at relatively high doses. Further, it is possible that spinal tracts vary in radiosensitivity, with the lateral corticospinal tracts being relatively sensitive.

21.7 Treatment Accuracy: Implications for Interpreting Clinical SBRT Data

Data are accumulating regarding the safety of spine SBRT which may eventually confirm the preclinical evidence of partial volume tolerance of the spinal cord. However, this information must be interpreted in the context of the geometric uncertainty of SBRT.

The submillimeter tolerances of SBRT systems, as validated by manufacturers (www.varian.com, February 2009), are only a starting point for quantifying its overall accuracy. Uncertainty enters the system from a variety of sources which are not incorporated during validation of SBRT systems using a rigid anthropomorphic phantom (Jin et al. 2008; Ryu et al. 2003; Agazaryan et al. 2008a; Antypas and Pantellis 2008). These include CT to MRI fusion, physician contouring, patient position verification at the time of treatment, and intrafraction patient motion.

Methods of spinal cord contouring for SBRT planning have not been standardized, and have a significant impact on the reported spinal cord dose (Sahgal 2008). Further, MRI-guided contouring of the spinal cord requires high-quality MRI to CT fusion. This quality is impaired by changes in patient position during MRI *versus* CT planning, which often arises due to inconsistencies in patient immobilization between the two radiographic studies. Given concerns regarding CT to MRI fusion, as well as to add a margin of safety, some physicians use the bony spinal canal, as delineated by CT, as a surrogate for the spinal cord. The various methods of cord volume definition create variability of several millimeters, which has a significant impact on the reported spinal cord dose for an SBRT treatment.

While significant effort has been undertaken to validate the accuracy of image-guidance during SBRT (Jin et al. 2008), the largest source of treatment inaccuracy may be intrafraction patient motion. A series of CyberKnife treatments described by Hoogeman et al. demonstrated an unacceptable level of intrafraction motion among patients treated in the prone position, leading investigators to use the supine positioning for subsequent treatments. Among the 11 patients treated in the supine position from the same series, investigators noted a mean displacement of 1.2 mm from initial position at a time point of 15 min (Hoogeman et al. 2008). Alarmingly, one patient had a recorded displacement of 4.3 mm, observed 2 min after treatment started. Similar results have been observed in other CyberKnife® (Accuray, Sunnyvale, CA, USA) series (Murphy et al. 2003) as well as Novalis® Radiosurgery (Brainlab AG, Feldkirchen, Germany) series (Agazaryan et al. 2008b).

The dosimetric impact of inaccuracies in patient position has been examined. Guckenberger et al. created multiple treatment plans for nine patients with spinal tumors, each with simulated errors in translation and rotation (Guckenberger et al. 2007). This study demonstrated that in order to maintain a delivered spinal cord dose within 10% of the planned dose, translations must be limited to 2 mm in the transversal plane and 7 mm in the superior-inferior direction, and rotations errors must be limited to 5°. Similar findings have been observed by others (Wang et al. 2008). Notably, the impact of positioning inaccuracy on spinal cord dose is highly dependent on the radiation dose gradient adjacent to the cord. While a steep gradient is helpful for achieving treatment planning goals, it is also associated with increasing cord dose uncertainty in the setting of intrafraction patient motion.

21.8 Spinal Cord Tolerance to SBRT: Published Clinical Experience

Myelitis following SBRT has been rare to date, with a total of nine cases reported in the literature (Gwak et al. 2005; Gibbs et al. 2009; Gagnon et al. 2009; Ryu et al. 2007; Sahgal et al. 2010). Based on this experience, proposals of SBRT planning metrics have been set forth, none with universal acceptance.

In a relatively large series with significant follow-up, Gagnon et al. published their experience with 200 patients treated for 274 lesions with spine radiosurgery (Gagnon et al. 2009). Several fractionation schemes were used, with a median dose of 26 Gy administered in three fractions (21 Gy if prior radiation.) No myelitis has been reported to date, including among 82 patients with at least 1 year of follow-up and 40 patients with at least 2 years of follow-up.

Ryu et al. published a series of 177 patients treated with spine radiosurgery, without a history of prior radiation. Of these, 86 patients had at least 1 year of follow-up, and were included in a late toxicity subgroup analysis (Ryu et al. 2007). One case of myelitis was observed in this subgroup. Although the authors reported that dose of 10 Gy to no more than 10% of the defined spinal cord volume was safe, the case of observed myelitis would have met this dose constraint.

Gerszten et al. published a series of 73 patients with benign intradural extramedullary spine tumors treated with radiosurgery (Gerszten 2008). This series is particularly interesting because the nature of the patients' disease lends itself to longer follow-up than metastatic series. With a median follow-up of 37 months, three patients experienced myelitis, all of whom received a single fraction of 20 Gy. In all three cases, the volume of the spinal cord receiving more than 8 Gy was recorded as less than 0.02 cc.

The results of this benign tumor series by Gerszten et al. suggest that spine radiosurgery carries a significant risk of myelitis, even at modest doses. However, one must consider that, with a prescription dose of 20 Gy, limiting the cord dose to 8 Gy requires a steep dose gradient. Given the cord dose uncertainties described in the section above, it is possible the delivered dose was higher than planned.

Sahgal et al., in a review of the cases of myelitis following radiosurgery, recommended a spinal cord maximum point dose of 10 Gy for a single fraction, or a BED of 60–70 Gy2 for hypofractionated treatment, assuming no previous radiotherapy (Sahgal et al. 2010). This recommendation is a notable departure from practices which allow a higher dose to a limited volume of spinal cord. However, in light of the uncertainty regarding the dose actually delivered to the spinal cord during radiosurgery, it may be proven to be a reasonable approach.

Metrics for predicting myelitis in the setting of SBRT remain elusive. Reported series provide limited certainty regarding safety, as a relatively small numbers of patients have survival and follow-up beyond the time point (2 years or more (Lambert 1978)) at which myelitis may occur. Further, uncertainty regarding the actual delivered radiation dose to the spinal cord limits our ability to draw definite conclusions regarding partial volume tolerance.

21.9 Conclusions: Toward a Future of Certainty and Safety in Spine SBRT

Early experience with spine SBRT has been encouraging, with low rates of myelitis observed in both radiation naïve and previously radiated patients (Gibbs et al. 2009; Gagnon et al. 2009; Ryu et al. 2007; Gibbs et al. 2007; Yamada et al. 2008; Chang et al. 2007). The level of risk that is acceptable to patients and clinicians depends on clinical circumstances, and should be compared with that of conventionally fractionated radiotherapy when such treatment is feasible. Significant future research is necessary to better quantify this risk. This investigation may include animal experimentation to determine spinal cord tolerance to hypofractionated radiation, including outcomes in the setting of previous radiation, surgical intervention, and systemic therapy which may radiosensitize or impair post-radiation repair. Additionally, in order to maximally benefit from ongoing clinical research, it is vital that investigators develop methods which better quantify the dose actually delivered to the spinal cord during SBRT.

References

Agazaryan N, Tenn S, Selch M et al (2008a) Image-guided radiosurgery for spinal tumors: methods, accuracy, and patient intrafraction motion. Phys Med Biol 53:1715–1727

Agazaryan N et al (2008b) Image-guided radiosurgery for spinal tumors: methods, accuracy and patient intrafraction motion. Phys Med Biol 53:1715–27

Ahlbom H (1941) The results of radiotherapy of hypopharyngeal cancer at Radiumhemmut, Stockholm, 1930–1939. Acta Radiol 22:155–171

Ang K, Jiang G, Price R et al (2001) Extent and kinetics of recovery of occult spinal cord injury. Int J Radiat Oncol Biol Phys 50:1013–1020

Antypas C, Pantellis E (2008) Performance evaluation of a CyberKnife G4 image-guided robotic stereotactic radiosurgery system. Phys Med Biol 53:4697–4718

Bijl H et al (2002) Dose-volume effects in the rat cervical spinal cord after proton irradiation. Int J Radiat Oncol Biol Phys 52:205–211

Bijl H et al (2005) Regional differences in radiosensitivity across the rat cervical spinal cord. Int J Radiat Oncol Biol Phys 61:543–551

Bijl H, Van Luijk P, Van Der Kogel A et al (2006) Influence of adjacent low-dose fields on tolerance to high doses of protons in rat cervical spinal cord. Int J Radiat Oncol Biol Phys 64:1204–1210

Chang E et al (2007) Phase I/II study of stereotactic body radiotherapy for spinal metastases and its pattern of failure. J Neurosurg Spine 7:151–160

Emami B, Lyman J, Wesson M et al (1991) Tolerance of normal tissue to therapeutic irradiation. Int J Radiat Oncol Biol Phys 21:109–22

Flickinger J, Kondziolka D, Lunsford L et al (2002) An analysis of the dose response for arteriovenous malformation radiosurgery and other factors affecting obliteration. Radiother Oncol 63:347–54

Fowler JF (1989) The linear-quadratic formula and progress in fractionated radiotherapy. Br J Radiol 62:679–694

Franklin RJ et al (1997) Local recruitment of remyelinating cells in the repair of demyelination in the central nervous system. J Neurosci Res 50:337–344

Gagnon G, Nasr N, Henderson F et al (2009) Treatment of spinal tumors using CyberKnife fractionated stereotactic radiosurgery: pain and quality of life assessment after treatment in 200 patients. Neurosurgery 64:297–307

Gerszten P (2008) Radiosurgery for benign intradural spinal tumors. Neurosurgery 62:887–896

Gibbs I et al (2007) Image-guided robotic radiosurgery for spinal metastases. Radiother Oncol 85:185–190

Gibbs R, Patil C, Burton S et al (2009) Delayed radiation-induced myelopathy after spinal radiosurgery. Neurosurgery 64(Supplement):A67–A72

Guckenberger M et al (2007) Precision required for dose-escalated treatment of spinal metastases and implications for image-guided radiation therapy. Radiother Oncol 84:56–63

Gwak HS, Yoo HJ, Youn SM et al (2005) Hypofractionated stereotactic radiation therapy for skull base and upper cervical chordoma and chondrosarcoma: preliminary results. Stereotact Funct Neurosurg 83:233–243

Hartsell W, Scott C, DeSilvio M et al (2005) Randomized trial of short- versus long-course radiotherapy for palliation of painful bone metastases. J Natl Cancer Inst 97:798–804

Hoogeman M et al (2008) Time dependence of intrafraction patient motion assessed by repeat stereoscopic imaging. Int J Radiat Oncol Biol Phys 70:609–618

Jin J, Ryu S, Movasas B et al (2008) Evaluation of residual patient position variation for spinal radiosurgery using the Novalis image guided system. Med Phys 35:1087–1093

Lambert P (1978) Radiation myelopathy of the thoracic spinal cord in long term survivors treated with radical radiotherapy using conventional fractionation. Cancer 41:1751–1760

Linstadt D, Wara W, Sheline G et al (1989) Postoperative radiotherapy of primary spinal cord tumors. Int J Radiat Oncol Biol Phys 16:1397–1403

Macbeth F, Wheldon T, Reed N et al (1996) Radiation myelopathy: estimates of risk in 1048 patients in three randomized trials of palliative radiotherapy for non-small cell lung cancer. Clin Oncol 8:176–81

Maranzano E, Latini P, Corgna E et al (1997) Short-course radiotherapy (8 Gy x 2) in metastatic spinal cord compression: an effective and feasible treatment. Int J Radiat Oncol Biol Phys 38:1037–1044
Maranzano E, Bellavita R, Latini P et al (2001) Radiation-induced myelopathy in long-term surviving metastatic spinal cord compression patients after hypofractionated radiotherapy: a clinical and magnetic resonance imaging analysis. Radiother Oncol 60:281–288
Marcus R, Million R (1990) The incidence of myelitis after irradiation of the cervical spinal cord. Int J Radiat Oncol Biol Phys 19:3–8
Medin P et al (2008) Spinal cord tolerance to radiosurgical dose distributions: a swine model. Int J Radiat Oncol Biol Phys 72:S83
Murphy M et al (2003) Patterns of patient movement during frameless image-guided radiotherapy. Int J Radiat Oncol Biol Phys 55:1400–1408
Nieder C, Grosu A, Molls M et al (2005) Proposal of human spinal cord reirradiation dose based on collection of data from 40 patients. Int J Radiat Oncol Biol Phys 61:851–855
Park C, Papiez L, Timmerman R et al (2008) Universal survival curve and single fraction equivalent dose: useful tools in understanding potency of ablative radiotherapy. Int J Radiat Oncol Biol Phys 70:847–52
Ryu S et al (2003) Image-guided and intensity-modulated radiosurgery for patients with spinal metastasis. Cancer 97:2013–8
Ryu S et al (2007) Partial volume tolerance of the spinal cord and complications of single-dose radiotherapy. Cancer 109:628–36
Sahgal A (2008) Stereotactic body radiosurgery for spinal metastases: a critical review. Int J Radiat Oncol Biol Phys 71(3):652–65
Sahgal A et al (2010) Spinal cord tolerance for stereotactic body radiotherapy. Int J Radiat Oncol Biol Phys 77:548–553
Schultheiss TE (2008) The radiation dose-response of the human spinal cord. Int J Radiat Oncol Biol Phys 71:1455–1459
Schultheiss T, Kun L, Stephens L et al (1995) Radiation response of the central nervous system. Int J Radiat Oncol Biol Phys 31:1093–1112
Thames H, Withers H, Fletcher G et al (1982) Changes in early and late radiation responses with altered dose fractionation: implications for dose-survival relationships. Int J Radiat Oncol Biol Phys 8:219–226
Van der Linden Y, Dijkstra S, Leer J et al (2005) Prediction of survival in patients with metastases in the spinal column. Cancer 103:320–328
Van der Linden Y, Steenland E, Leer J et al (2006) Patients with a favourable prognosis are equally palliated with single and multiple fraction radiotherapy: results on survival in the Dutch Bone Metastasis Study. Radiother Oncol 78:245–253
Wang H et al (2008) Dosimetric effect of translational and rotational errors for patients undergoing image-guided stereotactic body radiotherapy for spinal metastases. Int J Radiat Oncol Biol Phys 71:1261–1271
Wara W, Phillips T, Schwade J et al (1975) Radiation tolerance of the spinal cord. Cancer 35:1558–1562
Yamada Y, Bilsky M, Fuks Z et al (2008) High-dose, single-fraction image-guided intensity-modulated radiotherapy for metastatic spinal lesions. Int J Radiat Oncol Biol Phys 71:484–490

Radiosurgery of the Malignant Spine Tumors

22

Samuel Ryu and Jack Rock

22.1 Introduction

Common malignant spine tumors are metastasis to the spine with or without epidural spinal cord compression, and less commonly, primary spine tumors to the bone, soft tissue or spinal cord. Treatment of these tumors may vary depending on the primary site, histology, and functional status of the patient. In this chapter, indication and the use of radiosurgery for malignant spine tumors will be discussed.

22.1.1 Spine Metastasis

Vertebral metastasis is a common oncological complication of many tumors. In the literature, spine metastases are usually included together with bone metastatic disease. Up to about 40% of patients presenting with bone metastasis will have spinal metastasis. Pain is the most common presenting symptom. It may be caused by intraosseous disease, spine instability, vertebral fracture, epidural compression, or nerve root impingement. Left untreated, the tumor may progress to cause neurological deficit. External beam radiation therapy has been used for palliation of pain. Overall pain response rate is about 50–60%, with complete response in about one third of the patients (Foro Arnalot et al. 2008; Chow et al. 2007; Falkmer et al. 2003). With the increasing survival of patients with metastatic disease, the need for durable sources of treatment to maintain the quality of life for these patients is imperative.

When spine metastasis involve a limited number of vertebrae, the prognosis and survival time are far longer than the diffusely widespread type metastasis. One-year survival rate was over 50%, and long-term survivors are more often seen (Ryu et al. 2007). The median time of prostate or breast cancers reach longer than 2 years in patients with solitary spine metastasis, whereas the survival time was shortest, about 6–8 months, in lung cancers. Thus, it is important to achieve rapid and durable pain control in patients with potentially long survival time. The improved tumor control of spine metastasis can be achieved by radiosurgery, which allows delivering high radiation doses for tumor control (as opposed to the palliative dose) and minimal radiation dose to the neighboring spinal cord.

Recent advances with patient immobilization and stereotactic localization as well as intensity-modulated beam planning and delivery made radiosurgery possible for spine lesions, which are usually irregular in shape and often associated with epidural or paraspinal mass. This process requires precise target definition, immobilization, and accurate image guidance. Presence of the spinal cord in immediate proximity to the target volume makes the radiosurgery challenging. The initial experience with spine radiosurgery required an invasive procedure that surgically anchored the stereotactic frame to the spinous process (Hamilton et al. 1996). With the use of more modern noninvasive

S. Ryu (✉)
Department of Radiation Oncology and Neurosurgery, Henry Ford Hospital, Detroit, MI, USA and
Department of Radiation Oncology, Henry Ford Hospital, 2799 West Grand Boulevard, Detroit, MI 48202, USA
e-mail: sryu1@hfhs.org

J. Rock
Department of Neurosurgery, Henry Ford Hospital, Detroit, MI, USA

A.A.F. De Salles et al. (eds.), *Shaped Beam Radiosurgery*,
DOI: 10.1007/978-3-642-11151-8_22, © Springer-Verlag Berlin Heidelberg 2011

technology, the targeting accuracy has been reported to be in the range of 1 mm (Ryu et al. 2003). The available pre-clinical and clinical studies have demonstrated the accuracy and precision of stereotactic targeting, rapid radiation dose fall off and clinical effectiveness of pain control from spinal metastasis. (Yin et al. 2002; Gerszten et al. 2007; Jin et al. 2008; Ryu et al. 2008).

Since the most common symptom of spine metastasis is pain, the prime goal of radiosurgery for spine metastasis should be pain control. The early reports of pain control by using single-dose radiosurgery are from a Henry Ford Hospital phase II study and the experience of the University of Pittsburgh. A Phase II trial at Henry Ford Hospital with radiosurgery dose escalation from 10 to 18 Gy demonstrated that consistent and durable pain control was achieved at doses over 14 Gy delivered in a single fraction. One-year actuarial pain control rate of the treated spine was 84% (Ryu et al. 2008). This was also consistent with the University of Pittsburgh experience that pain control was higher than 90% with single doses over 16 Gy with patients with breast cancer spine metastasis (Gerszten et al. 2005). There may be various factors affecting the pain outcomes including age, performance status, tumor histology, presence of neurological deficits or spinal lesions, and radiosurgery dose. However, none of these factors reached statistical significance in the study. There was a strong trend toward increased pain control with higher radiation dose. An experience from Memorial Sloan Kettering Cancer Center showed higher radiosurgery dose requirements (>20 Gy) for local control with higher incidences of vertebral compression fracture in up to 40% of the patients (Yamada et al. 2008; Rose et al. 2009). This experience has to be looked at more closely as to whether the compression fractures were directly related to the radiosurgery or if they were related to any other causes. Fractionated radiosurgery was also used with various fractionation schemes. The reported pain control by the fractionated radiosurgical schemes is reported to be in the 80–90% range, which is similar to the use of single-dose radiosurgery (Chang et al. 2007; Sahgal et al. 2008).

The target volume of spine radiosurgery varies depending on the tumor presentation and institutional preference. The most common type is vertebral body involvement and bone destruction. The involved segment of for vertebral body should be treated, preferably including both pedicles. When there is extensive posterior involvement invading the pedicle, more generous margin can be used including the involved vertebral body or both anterior and posterior elements. When only the posterior elements are involved the spinous process including both lamina can be treated. These are shown in Fig. 22.1, with examples of radiosurgery isodose distribution (Ryu et al. 2007). Some institutions use boost volumes to the grossly involved portion of the vertebral body.

The treatment algorithm of radiosurgery for spine metastasis is shown in Fig. 22.2. Radiosurgery is most frequently used to treat solitary spine metastasis and/or soft tissue extension causing epidural compression or paraspinal mass (Fig. 22.2a). Two contiguous spine segments can be treated with radiosurgery (Fig. 22.2b). In addition, radiosurgery may be used to treat separate multiple lesions that are not continuous to one another. At Henry Ford Hospital, up to three separate sites are treated with radiosurgery (Fig. 22.2c). When there is diffuse spine involvement with one or two levels of more clinical significance by either symptoms or epidural compression, radiosurgery can be used as a boost to those specific vertebrae spines concurrent with conventional external beam radiation therapy. In cases of more diffuse metastatic spine involvement, external beam radiation therapy or radionuclide therapy is indicated instead of radiosurgery. However, with more experience, we have found that patients with diffuse spine metastasis can also be treated successfully with radiosurgery to the symptomatic sites only, thus avoiding the protracted fractionated radiation therapy. This last practice is strictly for palliation purposes to avoid the number of hospital visits in critically ill and terminal patients.

Because of the radiation dose fall-off, it is inevitable to have higher dose reaching the spinal cord. We have reported the distance between 90% and 50% dose fall off at 5.26 mm in our early reports (Ryu et al. 2003). This led us to document all the radiosurgery cases with a dose-volume histogram. We have reported the partial volume spinal cord tolerance dose of 10 Gy to the 10% spinal cord volume, which is defined from 6 mm superior to the target volume to 6 mm inferior to the target volume (Ryu et al. 2007). This spinal cord volume was defined by image fusion of a simulation CT scan with contrast and MRI scans with T1 contrast and T2 images. Other institutions use a slightly different definition of spinal tolerance dose such as the maximum dose within the spinal cord or at the surface of the spinal cord. Whatever criteria are used, it is prudent to

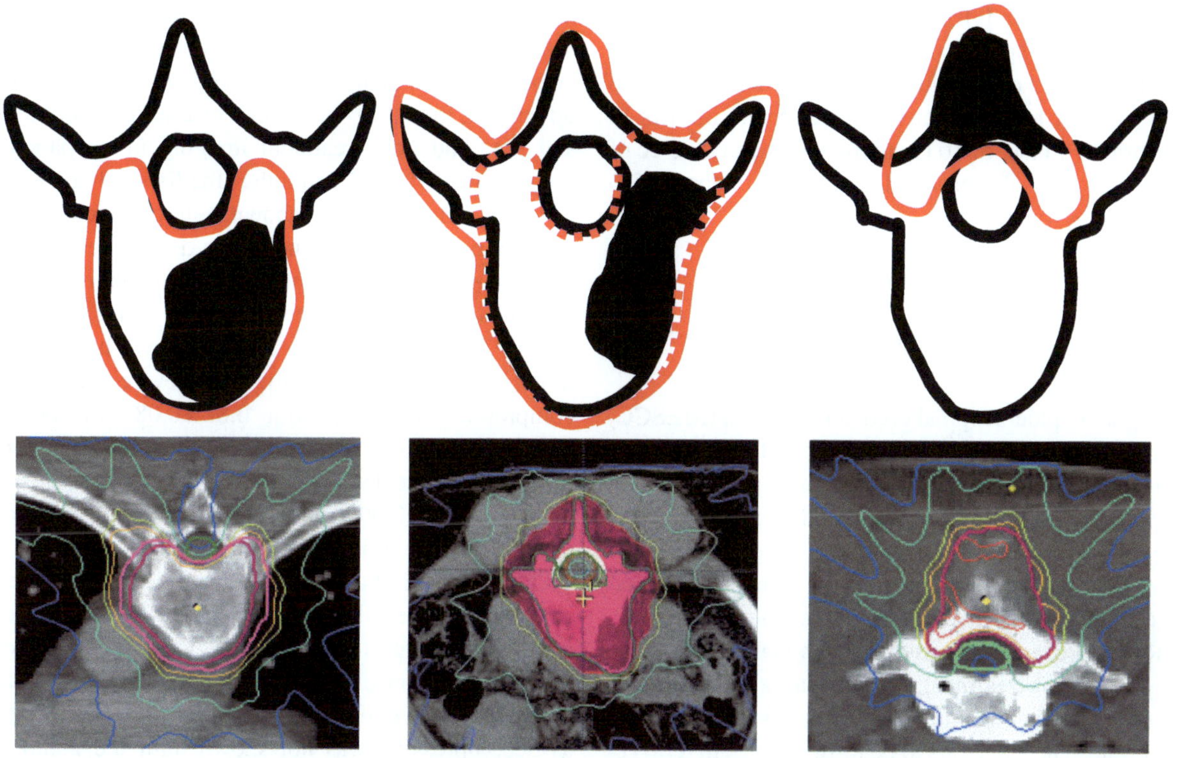

Fig. 22.1 Target volume of spine radiosurgery for spine metastasis. *Blackened* area represents metastatic tumor involvement. *Red lines* (*solid and dotted*) represent target volume. Example cases of radiosurgical isodose distribution are shown (Ryu et al. 2007)

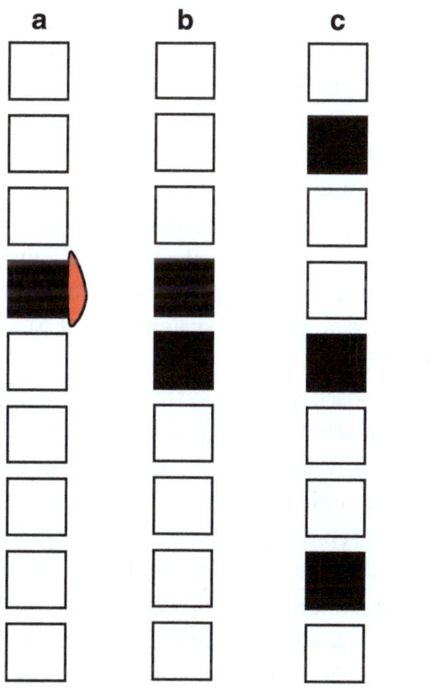

Fig. 22.2 Treatment algorithm of radiosurgery for spine metastasis. *Black squares* represent spines involved by metastasis. *Red ellipsoid* represents epidural extension

give special caution in image fusion, contouring the spinal cord, treatment planning, and interpreting the spinal cord dose distribution.

The experience of improved pain control by radiosurgery is being tested in Phase II/III study by the the RTOG trial 0631. In order to compile the radiosurgery experience and maintain quality control in the first 49 patients treated, there is an initial phase II component with a single dose of 16 Gy. When phase II study is over, there will be interim analysis for quality assurance. The trial will then continue with a Phase III study, randomized in 240 patients, between a single dose of 16 Gy (experimental arm) and external beam radiotherapy in a single dose of 8 Gy (control arm base on the previous RTOG 9714 trials of bone metastasis). The radiosurgical treatment method is the same as shown in Fig. 22.1, and the trial candidate patients are the same as shown in Fig. 22.2. The primary endpoint of this trial is pain control of the treated spine. Therefore, the patient should have a pain scale of ≥5 on a 1–10 visual scale to be registered for the trial. Secondary and tertiary endpoints are quality of life measurements and follow-up imaging studies. The partial volume spinal cord tolerance dose is 10 Gy to the 10% spinal cord volume, which is defined from 6 mm superior to the target volume to 6 mm inferior to the target volume, or 10 Gy to the volume of 0.35 cc of the spinal cord. The protocol is available on the RTOG Web site: www.rtog.org.

22.2 Epidural Spinal Cord Compression

Malignant epidural spinal cord compression (MESCC) is a common complication of cancer and has a substantial negative effect on quality of life and survival. It requires immediate diagnosis and treatment. It is important to pay attention to back pain, which is the most common presenting symptom. It is often associated with early or overt signs of neurological deficit. MRI has proven to be a useful tool in making the initial diagnosis. For treatment, various palliative care regimens of external beam radiotherapy have been used in the clinic. There appears to be no difference in terms of clinical outcome with the radiation dose or fractionation. A recent randomized study tested two radiation regiments of a short-course RT (8 Gy × 2 days) or a split-course RT (5 Gy × 3; 3 Gy × 5). There was no difference between these two arms; 56–59% back pain relief, 68–71% were able to walk, and 90% good bladder function (Maranzano et al. 2005). The role of aggressive surgical decompression has recently been demonstrated. Direct decompressive surgery combined with external beam radiotherapy can improve the ability to walk significantly compared to radiotherapy alone (Patchell et al. 2005). This indicates that the prime goal of treatment for spinal cord compression is to decompress the spinal cord and neuron elements. With this concept, another potential use of radiosurgery can be exploited for treatment of MESCC.

The use of radiosurgery for the purpose of epidural decompression has been tested at Henry Ford Hospital. A phase II trial was conducted examining the use of radiosurgery as the sole modality for spinal cord compression (Ryu et al. 2010). A total of 62 patients with 85 lesions of metastatic epidural compression were treated. The target volume encompassed the involved spine and epidural or paraspinal soft tumor component. The radiosurgery dose was 16–20 Gy in a single fraction. Steroids were tapered immediately after radiosurgery. The main criteria of inclusion into the trial were neurological status with muscle power of 4/5 or better. All patients had prospective clinical follow-up ranging from 1 to 48 months (median 11.5 months), and pre- and post treatment imaging in 36 patients ranging from 2 to 33 months (median 9.3 months). Primary endpoints were shown radiographically epidural tumor control and thecal sac decompression, on follow-up MRI scans. The results demonstrated that the mean epidural tumor volume reduction was 65 ± 14% at 2 months after radiosurgery. The epidural tumor area at the level of the most severe spinal cord compression reduced from 0.82 ± 0.08 cm^2 before radiosurgery to 0.41 ± 0.06 cm^2 after radiosurgery ($p < 0.001$). Thecal sac patency improved from 55 ± 4% to 76 ± 3% ($p < 0.001$). Overall, neurological function remained stable or improved in 81%.

The results indicate that radiosurgical decompression can be achieved, and thus radiosurgery can be used for the treatment of MESCC. Surgical decompression is effective because it removes the tumor immediately, whereas the effect of radiosurgery is not as immediate, as decompression was not shown until the 2 month post-treatment imaging study. Thus, an argument could be made that patients with minimal neurological signs (i.e., ambulatory patients) can be treated with radiosurgery, and surgery should be reserved for those who progress. Great caution is required for the use of radiosurgery for spinal cord compression as careful patient selection is required and the spinal cord is intimately located with the epidural tumor.

A future direction for the use of radiosurgery could be the development of a grading system for MESCC. It could be used to better select the patients who may benefit from radiosurgery for spinal cord compression. We proposed a grading system of MESCC and it is shown in Fig. 22.3.

The proposed grading system has two components: radiographic and neurological grades (Ryu et al. 2010). Radiographic grades (0–V) are Grade 0 – spine bone involvement only without spinal canal compromise; Grade I – the epidural tumor within the epidural fat with no thecal sac compression; Grade II – involvement of dura and arachnoid and mild compression of thecal sac; Grade III – when the tumor is impinging the spinal cord; Grade IV – spinal cord displacement with CSF still visible; and Grade V – frank spinal cord compression with CSF not visible between the tumor and the spinal cord. Neurological grading has five grades (A–E).

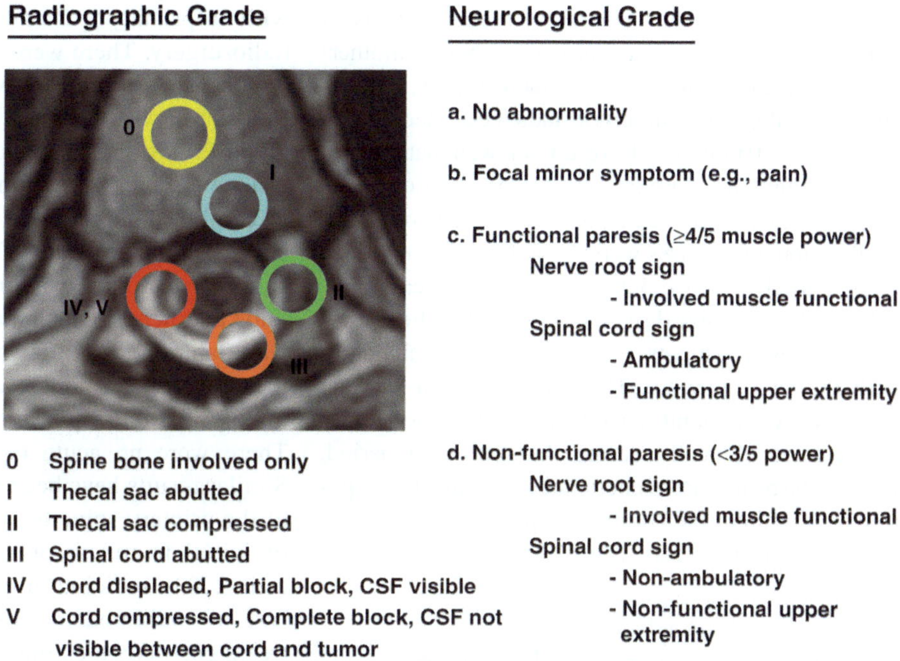

Fig. 22.3 Proposed grading system of spinal cord compression consisting of radiographic and neurological grades (Ryu et al. 2010)

In Grade A there are no symptoms. In Grade B, there is focal minor symptoms, such as pain or radiculopathy. Grade C is defined as functional paresis with muscle strength of 4/5. It may involve deficits from the nerve root or spinal cord. The involved muscle is functional and ambulatory. Grade D is defined as nonfunctional paresis with muscle strength of ≤3/5. It can be severe nerve root or spinal cord deficit with the involved muscle nonfunctional or nonambulatory. Grade E is plegic muscle strength, urinary or rectal incontinence.

We believe that combined radiographic and neurological grading is useful since the radiographic extent of epidural compression was not directly correlated with the neurological signs. Other clinical parameters such as rapidity of symptom development and subtle neurological changes are also important. The grading system is also useful for treatment decisions and response evaluation as well as outcome reporting. For example, Grade IIIc can be treated with radiosurgery, whereas Grades IIId and IVd are treated with surgical resection first. At our institution, the treatment options are reviewed at weekly multidisciplinary spine tumor board meetings. We currently use the muscle strength (≥4/5) as the most important indicator of patient selection for radiosurgery.

22.3 Intradural and Intramedullary (IDDM) Tumors

Intradural and intramedullary (IDIM) metastasis consists of leptomeningeal metastasis and intramedullary metastasis. Treatment of IDDM is more challenging and prognosis is dismal. Treatments are limited, but may help improve the clinical outcome (Waki et al. 2009; Dam-Hieu et al. 2009). The use of radiosurgery for IDDM is not known.

A retrospective review of the Henry Ford Hospital experience suggests that radiosurgery can be used in selective patients (Shin et al. 2009). Nine patients with 11 IDIM metastases were treated; 4 intradural extramedullary and 7 intramedullary lesions. The average target volume was 3.4 cm^3 (range 0.4–12.0). The mean radiosurgery dose was 13.8 Gy with a range of 10–16 Gy, in single session, prescribed to the 90% isodose line. The spinal cord dose exceeds our published guideline of 10 Gy to the 10% volume, which was used for the treatment of epidural compression (Ryu et al. 2007). Instead, we allowed higher radiation dose to the spinal cord in immediate vicinity to the target tumor. The decision was made on an individual basis by balancing the neurological status and general oncological status of tumor spread with estimated prognosis. No chemotherapy was given concurrently with radiosurgery, but was continued after radiosurgery as indicated. Median follow-up was 10 months. The results showed that the presenting symptoms were improved in eight cases (80%, 8/10), unchanged in one case and worsened in one case. Radiographic responses were: complete response 22% (2/9), partial response 33% (3/9), stable disease 33% (3/9), and progressive disease in 11% (1/9). After radiosurgery, seven patients (78%) remained ambulatory until the last follow-up. The overall median survival after SRS was 8 months. There was no radiation toxicity detected clinically during the follow-up period. Indeed, the results are encouraging. Although the experience is limited, radiosurgery appears to be effective and safe to treat patients with IDIM metastases.

22.4 Primary Tumors of the Spine and Spinal Cord

Primary spine or spinal cord tumors are not common. The usual initial treatment is surgical resection and multimodality treatment with radiation and/or chemotherapy. While many primary cord tumors are relatively radioresponsive, most of the primary spine tumors tend to be radioresistant, such as chondrosarcomas, chordomas, and osteogenic or soft tissue sarcomas. Radiosurgery can be used as part of combined modality treatment in the initial or recurrent setting. However, the experience with radiosurgery for the treatment of primary malignant tumors of the spine or the spinal cord is limited; therefore, the role of radiosurgery can be exploited. Radiosurgery seems to be a reasonable primary and or adjuvant therapeutic modality that might improve the local tumor control by increasing the total radiation dose compared to the standard fractionated external beam radiation therapy. Radiosurgery can also be delivered as an adjuvant therapy to the surgical cavity. Most of the primary malignant tumors of the spine have high rates of local recurrence and most are relatively radio resistant. Therefore, higher radiation doses should be delivered to the surgical cavity and to the gross tumor volume.

The interim clinical experience at Henry Ford Hospital was analyzed with a total of 26 patients with 36 primary spine and cord tumors treated with radiosurgery. There were 7 patients with spinal cord tumors, and 19 patients with primary spine tumors. Radiosurgery doses were a single session of 12–18 Gy in 29 lesions, and fractionated in 6 lesions. Ten lesions were recurrent tumors after the initial therapy of combined surgery and radiation. Median follow-up was 12 months (range 2–42 months) with imaging studies and clinical examination. The patients' symptoms and neurological status improved in 56%, and was stable in 28% after radiosurgery. The one-year local tumor control rate was 94%; complete response in 26%, partial response in 26%, and stable in 42%. There were no acute or long-term complications. Similar results have been reported after radiosurgery of the primary spine or spinal cord tumors as a part of initial treatment or recurrent setting (Gerszten et al. 2003). Judicious use of radiosurgery in the context of multimodality treatment can improve the treatment outcome. Further experience, preferably clinical trials, is needed.

References

Chang EL et al (2007) Phase I/II study of stereotactic body radiotherapy for spinal metastasis and its pattern of failure. J Neurosurg Spine 7(2):151–160
Chow E et al (2007) Palliative radiotherapy trials for bone metastases: a systematic review. J Clin Oncol 25(11): 1423–1436
Dam-Hieu P et al (2009) Retrospective study of 19 patients with intramedullary spinal cord metastasis. Clin Neurol Neurosurg 111(1):10–17
Falkmer U et al (2003) A systematic overview of radiation therapy effects in skeletal metastases. Acta Oncol 42(5–6): 620–633
Foro Arnalot P et al (2008) Randomized clinical trial with two palliative radiotherapy regimens in painful bone metastases: 30 Gy in 10 fractions compared with 8 Gy in single fraction. Radiother Oncol 89(2):150–155
Gerszten PC et al (2003) CyberKnife frameless single-fraction stereotactic radiosurgery for benign tumors of the spine. Neurosurg Focus 14(5):e16
Gerszten PC et al (2005) Single-fraction radiosurgery for the treatment of spinal breast metastases. Cancer 104(10): 2244–2254
Gerszten PC et al (2007) Radiosurgery for spinal metastases: clinical experience in 500 cases from a single institution. Spine 32(2):193–199

Hamilton AJ et al (1996) LINAC-based spinal stereotactic radiosurgery. Stereotact Funct Neurosurg 66(1–3):1–9

Jin JY et al (2008) Evaluation of residual patient position variation for spinal radiosurgery using the Novalis image guided system. Med Phys 35(3):1087–1093

Maranzano E et al (2005) Short-course versus split-course radiotherapy in metastatic spinal cord compression: results of a phase III, randomized, multicenter trial. J Clin Oncol 23(15): 3358–3365

Patchell RA et al (2005) Direct decompressive surgical resection in the treatment of spinal cord compression caused by metastatic cancer: a randomised trial. Lancet 366(9486):643–648

Rose PS et al (2009) Risk of fracture after single fraction image-guided intensity-modulated radiation therapy to spinal metastases. J Clin Oncol 27(30):5075–5079

Ryu S et al (2003) Image-guided and intensity-modulated radiosurgery for patients with spinal metastasis. Cancer 97(8): 2013–2018

Ryu S et al (2007) Partial volume tolerance of the spinal cord and complications of single-dose radiosurgery. Cancer 109(3):628–636

Ryu S et al (2008) Pain control by image-guided radiosurgery for solitary spinal metastasis. J Pain Symptom Manage 35(3):292–298

Ryu S, Rock J, Jain R, Lu M, Anderson A, Jin JY, Rosenblum M, Movsas M, Kim JH (2010) Radiosurgical decompression of epidural spine metastasis. Cancer 116(9):2250–2257

Sahgal A, Larson DA, Chang EL (2008) Stereotactic body radiosurgery for spinal metastases: a critical review. Int J Radiat Oncol Biol Phys 71(3):652–665

Shin DA, Huh R, Chung SS, Rock J, Ryu S (2009) Stereotactic spine radiosurgery for intradural and intramedullary metastasis. Neurosurg Focus 27(6):E10–E16

Waki F et al (2009) Prognostic factors and clinical outcomes in patients with leptomeningeal metastasis from solid tumors. J Neurooncol 93(2):205–212

Yamada Y et al (2008) High-dose, single-fraction image-guided intensity-modulated radiotherapy for metastatic spinal lesions. Int J Radiat Oncol Biol Phys 71(2):484–490

Yin FF et al (2002) A technique of intensity-modulated radiosurgery (IMRS) for spinal tumors. Med Phys 29(12): 2815–2822

Benign Spinal Tumors

23

Michael Selch

23.1 Introduction

Benign neoplasms account for approximately one third of all spinal tumors (Conti et al. 2004). Their frequency is increased in patients with neurofibromatosis Type 1 or 2. These lesions may be restricted to the thecal sac, the extra-thecal portions of the nerve sheath, or some combination of these locations (Celli et al. 2005). Benign spinal tumors typically present with a constellation of weakness, pain and/or sensory disturbance (Cherqui et al. 2007; Conti et al. 2004). Gross total resection is the standard of care for benign spinal tumors and complete removal rates are in excess of 95% in most neurosurgical experiences (Conti et al. 2004; Lot and Bernard 1997; Seppala et al. 1995a, b). Surgical cure, however, may require sacrifice of one or more nerve roots (Celli 2002; Celli et al. 2005; Kim et al. 1989; Safavi-Abbasi et al. 2008; Seppala et al. 1995a). Surgical intervention, moreover, may exacerbate underlying neurological symptoms or produce new, permanent deficits (Conti et al. 2004; Levy et al. 1986; Lot and Bernard 1997; Safavi-Abbasi et al. 2008; Seppala et al. 1995a, b). Subtotal tumor removal in an attempt to avoid neurological morbidity may result in tumor regrowth (Levy et al. 1986; Lot and Bernard 1997; Seppala et al. 1995b; Chang 1998). Stereotactic radiosurgery (SRS) has been demonstrated safe and effective for a variety of benign intracranial tumors. By extension, a similar radiotherapeutic approach should prove efficacious for spinal tumors of similar histology.

M. Selch
Department of Radiation Oncology, David Geffen School of Medicine at UCLA, 200 UCLA Medical Plaza, Suite B265, Los Angeles, CA 90095, USA
e-mail: mselch@mednet.ucla.edu

23.2 Technique of Image-Guided Spinal Radiosurgery at UCLA

Accuracy of intracranial SRS is traditionally assured by application of a minimally invasive head frame providing fiducial markers for determining three-dimensional target coordinates and a system for precise patient immobilization. Spinal radiosurgery approaches utilizing transcutaneously implanted bony fiducial markers or rigid external body frames have been reported (Blomgren et al. 1995; Chang et al. 2003; Hamilton et al. 1995; Lohr et al. 1999; Takacs et al. 1999).

Frameless, image-guided spinal radiosurgery is a technique for delivering accurate, conformal irradiation free of the requirement for fixed fiducials or cumbersome immobilization devices (Teh et al. 2007). The system in use at UCLA has been described elsewhere and will be reviewed in this chapter (Agazaryan et al. 2008; Yin et al. 2002a). Patients eligible for spinal radiosurgery are those who are deemed unresectable, refuse surgery, or for whom surgery is contraindicated due to comorbid conditions.

Patients undergoing image-guided spinal radiosurgery at UCLA are immobilized with a noninvasive device (BodyFIX®, Medical Intelligence, Schwabmunchen, Germany). This system utilizes a fiberglass base plate and a patient cushion compatible with CT and MRI (Total Body BlueBAG®, Medical Intelligence, Schwabmunchen, Germany). The cushion is custom-molded to the individual patient contour for comfort and ease of repositioning for imaging and treatment

A.A.F. De Salles et al. (eds.), *Shaped Beam Radiosurgery*,
DOI: 10.1007/978-3-642-11151-8_23,

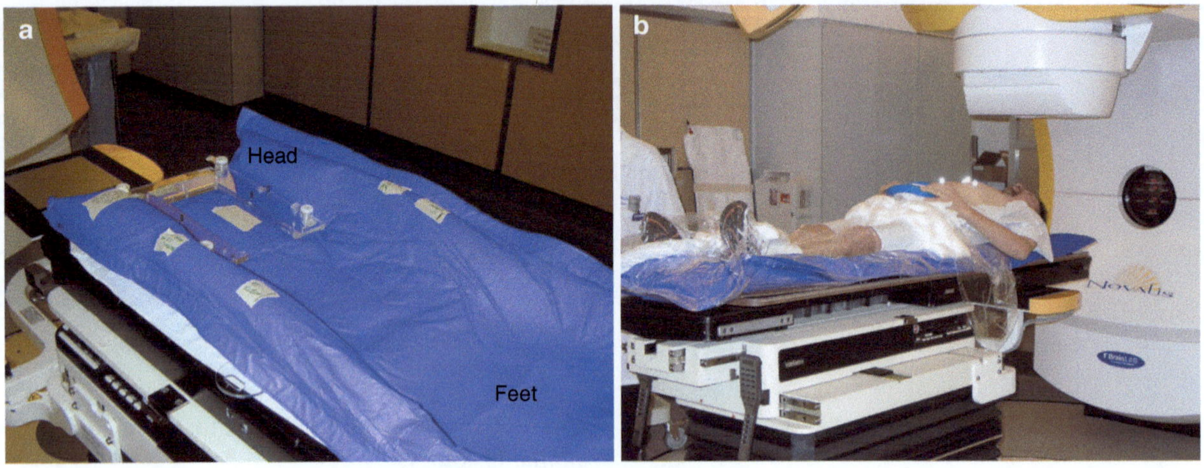

Fig. 23.1 (**a**) "Blue Bag" custom-molded immobilization device for spinal radiosurgery at UCLA. (**b**) Patient positioning using "Blue Bag" system

(Fig. 23.1). Additional immobilization can be accomplished with a separate clear plastic cover sheet extending from hips to feet that adheres to the patient via a vacuum system (Fig. 23.2). Patients with cervical spine lesions are further immobilized with a CT/MRI compatible custom-molded face mask (Fig. 23.3). In order to minimize spine motion during respiration, patients are immobilized in the supine position. Under fluoroscopic imaging, Yin et al. noted spine motion of less than 1 mm in the supine position (Yin et al. 2002a).

Treatment planning for spinal radiosurgery requires both CT and MRI scanning. A large bore CT simulator (Sensation® Open, Siemens Medical Solutions,

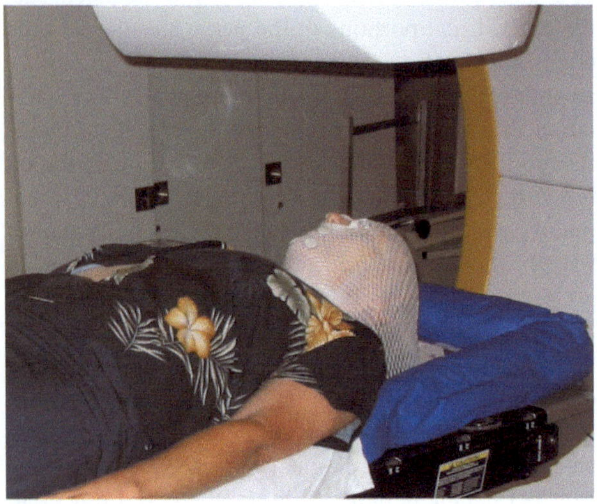

Fig. 23.3 Additional face mask immobilization for cervical spine radiosurgery

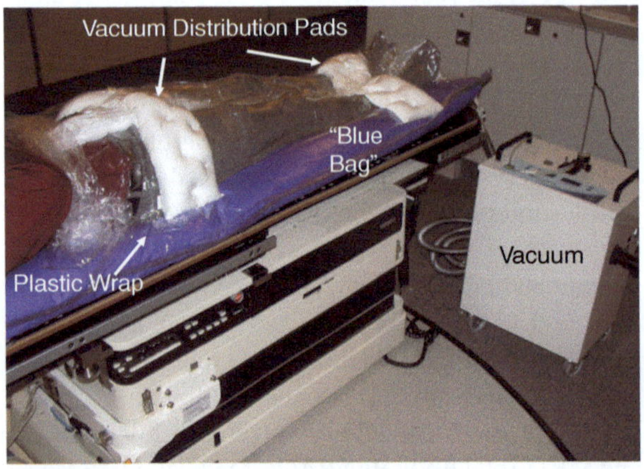

Fig. 23.2 Plastic wrap/vacuum system for additional patient immobilization during spinal radiosurgery

Malvern, PA) is used with spiral acquisition and 1.5-mm axial slice thickness without spacing. Multiple surface infrared reflecting skin markers are placed prior to CT imaging (Fig. 23.4). These markers are used for localization during treatment planning. The planning system used for image-guided spinal radiosurgery at UCLA establishes the relative location of the surface markers with respect to the target isocenter. Contrast-enhanced MRI with 2-mm axial slice thickness through the region of interest is obtained for

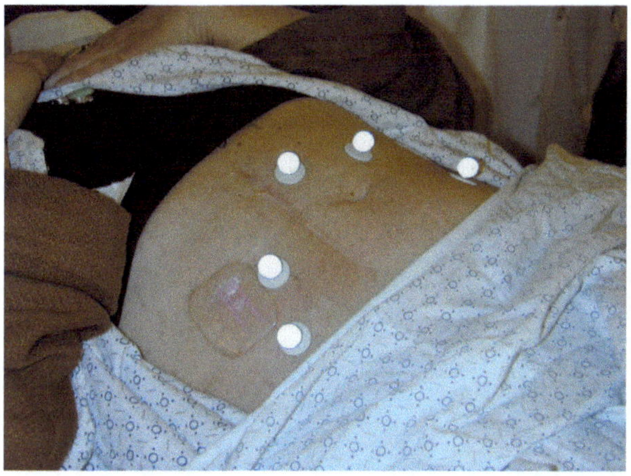

Fig. 23.4 Image displays five infrared reflectors on patient's abdomen

superior anatomic delineation and eventual image fusion during treatment planning.

Treatment plans are generated using a dedicated, commercially available system (first iPlan RT image 3.0 / BrainSCAN 5.31 and now iPlan image 4.0 and iPlan dose 4.0), Brainlab AG, Feldkirchen, Germany). CT and MRI images are fused for all patients. Target GTV (gross target volume) and objects at risk (OARs) are contoured by the radiation oncologist and neurosurgeon using the contrast-enhanced axial, coronal, and sagittal MRI. For benign tumors, no additional margin for CTV (clinical target volume) is added. An additional margin for the PTV (planning target volume) of 1–3 mm is added to account for errors in imaging, patient positioning, and intrafractional motion (Fig. 23.5). This added margin may be reduced near OARs such as the spinal cord at the discretion of the responsible physicians. The volume of spinal cord or cauda equina contoured during treatment planning typically extends 6 mm above and below the target according to the recommendation of Ryu et al. (Ryu et al. 2007). The imaging definition of the "spinal cord" is controversial in the setting of radiosurgery. Some investigators contour the entire bony canal as depicted on CT images as the spinal cord OAR. Other investigators utilize the soft tissue volume of the cord as depicted on T2-weighted MRI with or without a 1–2 mm additional margin. The approach at UCLA has been to contour the cord on the T2-weighted MRI without additional margin. It is recognized that this approach may result in a small geometric discrepancy

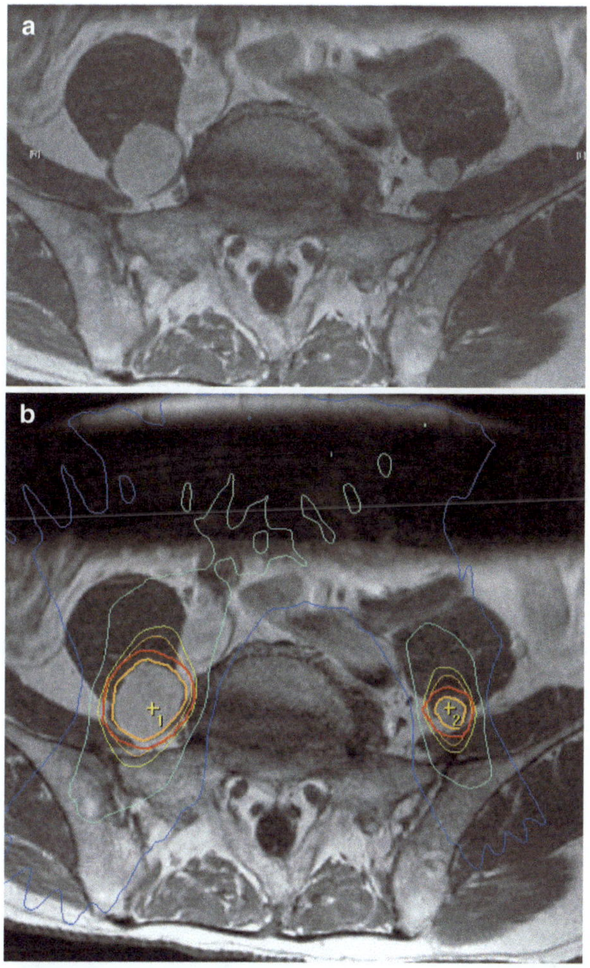

Fig. 23.5 (**a**) Axial MRI demonstrating bilateral L4 neurofibromas in a patient with neurofibromatosis. (**b**) Axial MRI demonstrates isodose lines for spinal radiosurgery. Each target was irradiated with three dynamic arcs. Isodose lines displayed: 90% (*yellow*); 80% (*light green*); 50% (*teal*); 30% (*blue*). The targets (*thick yellow*) received 12 Gy prescribed at the 90% isodose line encompassing the target plus a 2-mm margin (*thick orange*)

due to possible distortions in the CT-MRI fusion protocol. Treatment plans for benign tumors use either 6–8 intensity-modulated beams or 2–5 dynamic shaped conformal arcs (Figs. 23.6–23.8). Intensity-modulated treatment plans are generated using an inverse planning algorithm based on the dynamically penalized likelihood method and a pencil beam dose calculation algorithm. Dosimetric characteristics of the Novalis® Radiosurgery system (Brainlab AG, Feldkirchen, Germany) have been described elsewhere (Cosgrove

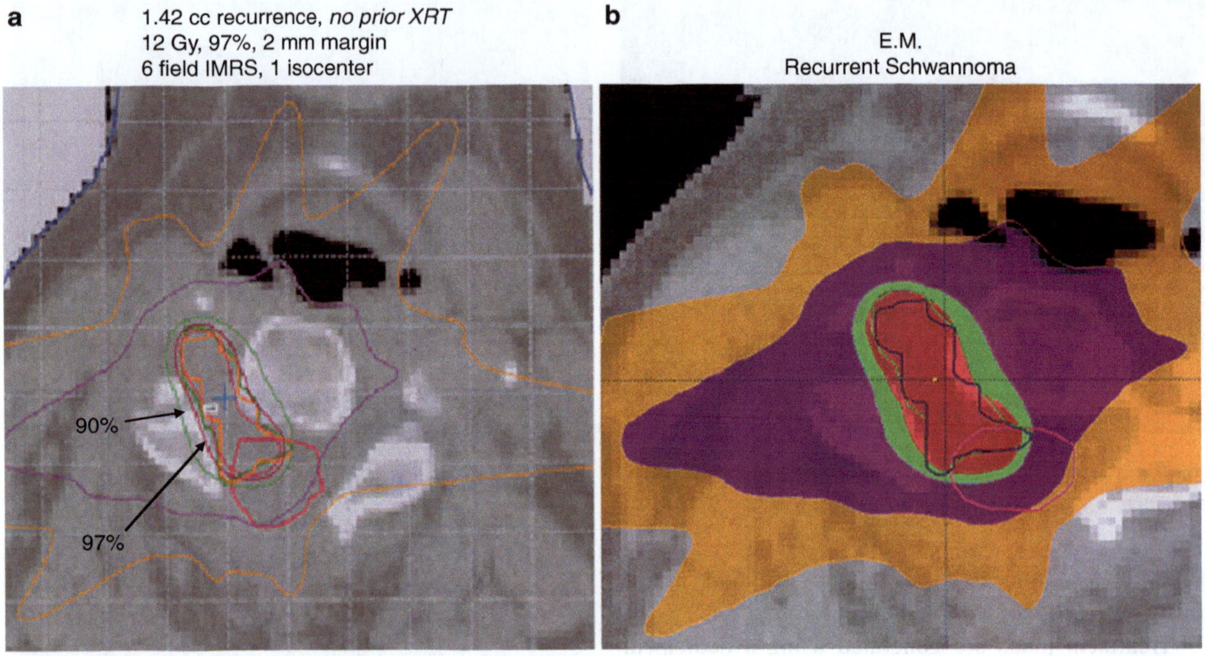

Fig. 23.6 (**a**) Intensity-modulated isodose distribution for a recurrent cervical spine schwannoma. The target received 12 Gy prescribed at the 97% isodose line, which encompassed the tumor (*dark orange line*) plus a 2-mm margin. The target was irradiated with six coplanar beams. (**b**) Dose wash distribution of the plan demonstrated in (**a**)

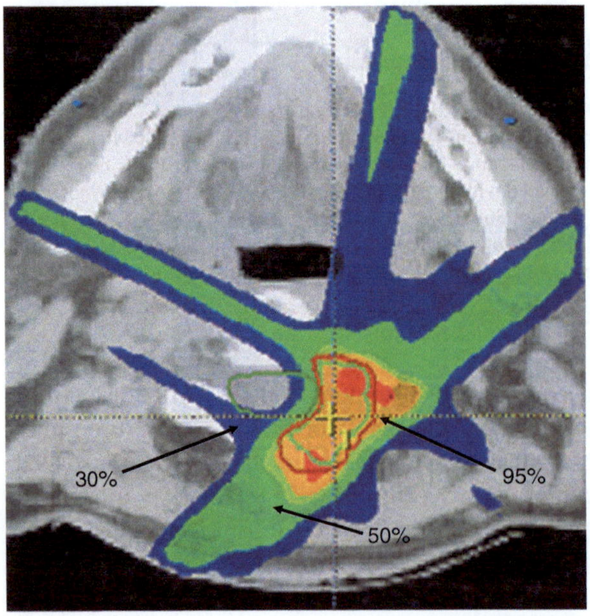

Fig. 23.7 Intensity-modulated plan for a cervical spine hemangioblastoma. The target (*green line*) plus a 2-mm margin (*red line*) was treated to a dose of 12 Gy prescribed at the 95% isodose line

et al. 1999; Yin et al. 2002b). Treatment planning information is exported to the image guidance system for eventual patient positioning.

Accurate target localization for spinal radiosurgery at UCLA involves both automated patient positioning and integrated image-guided devices (ExacTrac® X-Ray, Brainlab AG, Feldkirchen, Germany). The treatment planning process establishes and stores a unique geometric relationship between the surface infrared reflectors and the target isocenter. The ExacTrac device consists of two infrared cameras capable of generating and detecting infrared signals from the surface reflectors and a computerized control system. Prior to treatment, the patient is positioned on the accelerator couch using the previously fashioned immobilization device and the reflectors are reattached in their original surface position. Infrared signals are analyzed real time and the current position of the surface markers is compared to the stored position established from the planning CT. The system instructs the treatment couch to automatically position the patient and planned target isocenter near to the accelerator isocenter. A separate video camera system is coupled to the infrared

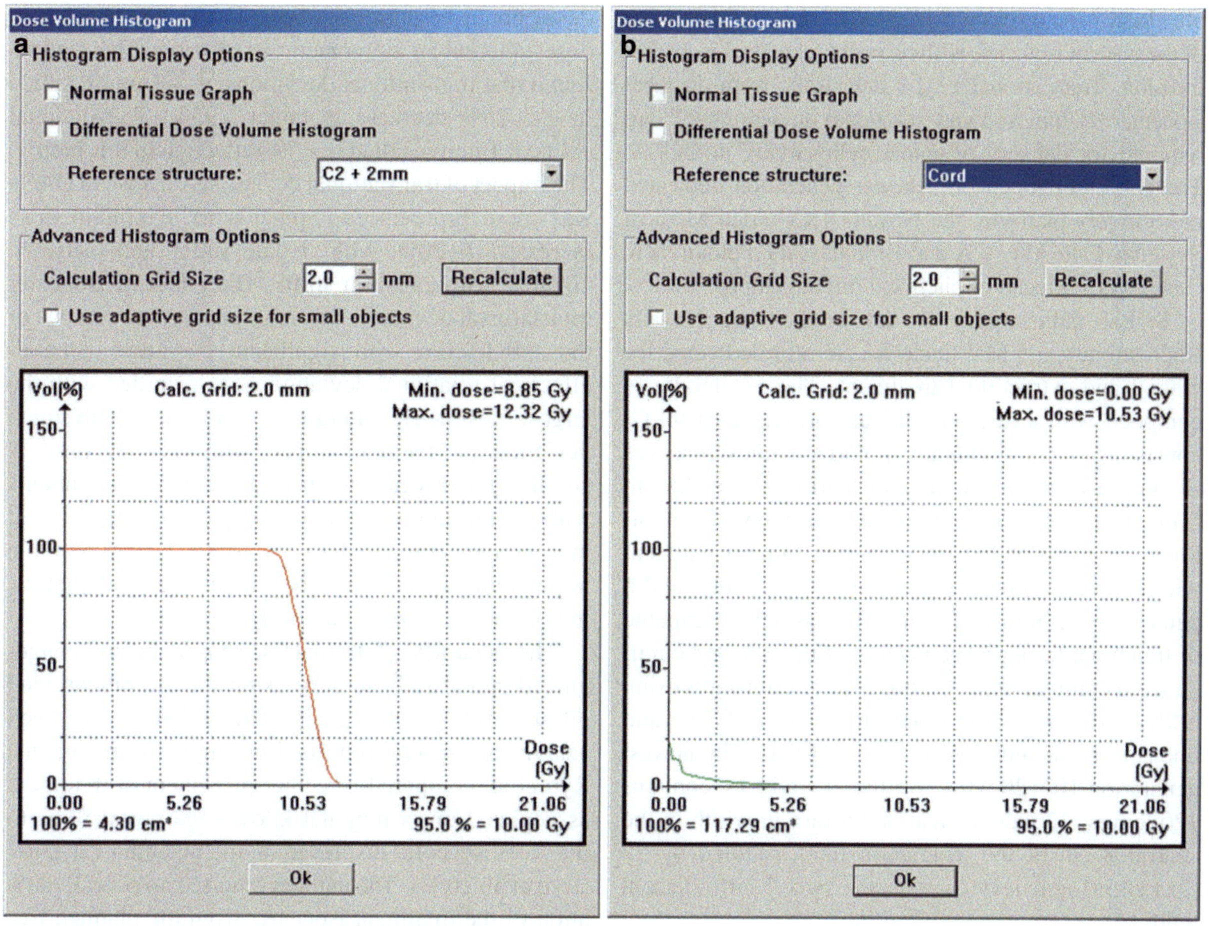

Fig. 23.8 (**a**) Dose-volume histogram for the target lesion displayed in Fig. 23.7. (**b**) Dose-volume histogram for the spinal cord from the same patient

system to provide visual confirmation of patient positioning. The real-time coordinates of the target isocenter are calculated after automated positioning and the system reports the positioning error of the actual isocenter compared to the preplanned ideal isocenter. Given the vagaries of reflector placement and patient respiration, slight discrepancies between ideal and actual isocenter placement can be expected.

Final patient positioning is achieved using radiographic image guidance based upon kV images of vertebral anatomy generated by ExacTrac. The radiographic image guidance system consists of a pair of ceiling-mounted flat panel amorphous silicon detectors and a pair of floor-mounted kV X-ray sources. The X-ray sources project obliquely onto the detectors from medial to lateral, superior to inferior, and posterior to anterior. A pair of oblique digital radiographs is obtained after initial infrared-based patient positioning. Vertebral anatomy in these images is compared to a pair of digitally reconstructed radiographs (DRRs) from the original planning CT generated in the same orientations as the in-room kV images. The system automatically compares the internal bony anatomy of the kV images with the DRRs to determine the current position of the spinal column relative to the preplanned or ideal position. The kV-DRR comparison is a 2D–3D registration process termed 6D fusion (Jin et al. 2006). A system described by Chang et al. replaces the kV oblique images with real-time CT scans and the process is termed 3D–3D registration (Chang et al. 2007). The system determines isocenter translational and yaw rotational deviations between the kV images and the DRRs for the patient positioning based on initial infrared positioning. These deviations are evaluated by the radiation oncologist and any required corrections in patient position are automatically performed by ExacTrac. The 2D–3D registration process is repeated after automatic position correction to confirm placement of the current isocenter with respect to the ideal isocenter location. Translational *x*, *y*, *z* deviations from an ideal isocenter <1 mm and yaw rotational deviations <2° are required for delivery of spinal radiosurgery at UCLA. The robot 6D couch on a newer generation dedicated radiosurgery platform, the Novalis Tx (Varian Medical Systems, Palo Alto, CA and Brainlab AG, Feldkirchen, Germany), corrects for pitch and roll deviations.

Spinal radiosurgery is delivered using Novalis Radiosurgery, a 6 MV linear accelerator dedicated for cranial and extracranial treatment. The accelerator is equipped with a micro-multileaf collimator (mMLC) consisting of 52 individually motorized tungsten leaves shaping a maximum treatment field of 9.8 × 9.8 cm (m3®, Brainlab AG, Feldkirchen, Germany). The collimator consists of 26 pairs of leaves: 14 pairs with leaf width 3.0 mm, 6 pairs with 4.5-mm-leaf width, and 6 pairs with 5.5-mm-leaf width. The system is capable of treatment through beams/arcs using attached circular fixed collimators, conformal static beams/arcs using mMLC, dynamic conformal arcs using mMLC, and intensity-modulated beams using mMLC. The newest generation HD120 MLC on the Novalis Tx contains 120 leaves: 32 pairs of leaves 2.5 mm in width in the central 8 cm of the irradiation field, saddled by 28 (2x14) 5.0 mm leaf pairs in the two 7 cm adjacent fields.

23.3 Accuracy of Image-Guided Spinal Radiosurgery

Small deviations of isocenter placement at the time of spinal radiosurgery compared to the ideal isocenter determined during image-based planning could have profound effects on dose distribution both for the target lesion and for adjacent critical normal tissue. Wang and associates examined the potential dosimetric effects of isocenter translational shifts and rotational deviations. The investigators initially planned radiosurgery for 20 patients with metastatic spinal lesions (Wang et al. 2008). Multiple additional plans were then generated for each isocenter that included various translational and rotational deviations simulating possible patient positioning errors. In this model system, the distance from the metastatic tumor GTV to the crucial OAR was small so substantial changes in delivered doses could be anticipated due to the steep falloff in dose inherent in stereotactic irradiation. The authors found that translational deviations of 2–3 mm resulted in a 5–25% decrease in target V95%. Translational shifts of 1 mm resulted in <5% reduction in this metric. The impact of translational deviations on dose to OARs was more pronounced. Spinal cord maximum dose increased 5–20% with 1-mm shifts and between 10–80% with 2–3-mm shifts. The effect of isocenter translational deviation was most apparent in regions of the spinal cord with significant curvature. Smaller effects of rotational deviation were recorded with the largest dosimetric alterations associated with pitch deviation and the least impact with yaw deviation. A similar analysis has not been performed for patients with benign tumors which are typically of a different morphology compared to metastatic lesions but the implications of isocenter deviations are, nonetheless, important in all spinal radiosurgery cases.

The accuracy of frameless, shaped beam, image-guided spinal radiosurgery using the aforementioned infrared/radiographic positioning technique has been analyzed in several reports. In a study of ten patients, Ryu et al. compared isocenter placement at treatment as depicted on orthogonal kilovoltage portal films to the ideal isocenter displayed on the planning CT DRR (Ryu et al. 2003). The authors reported an overall deviation of the treatment isocenter from the planned isocenter of 1.36 ± 0.11 mm. In a second report from this group using portal film comparison, average lateral, longitudinal, and vertical deviations of a planned isocenter were 0.8 ± 0.9 mm, 0.7 ± 0.7 mm, and 0.9 ± 0.5 mm, respectively, in 25 patients (Yin et al. 2002a). The overall root-mean-square deviation was 1.6 ± 0.9 mm. The authors noted no significant difference in deviation of isocenter placement between cervical, thoracic, or lumbar targets. The average deviation in phantom-measured isodose distribution compared to calculated distribution was 2% with a maximum difference of 4%. In a phantom study using both implanted fiducial and bony anatomy fusion techniques, this same group analyzed the overall positioning accuracy of a planned isocenter with the actual isocenter placement in the treatment room (Yan et al. 2003). They reported average lateral, longitudinal, and vertical deviations of 0.6 ± 0.3 mm, 0.5 ± 0.2 mm, and 0.7 ± 0.2 mm, respectively. There were no significant differences in deviation magnitude between implanted fiducial and bony anatomy positioning techniques. The impact of planning CT slice thickness varying from 2 to 8 mm on accuracy of isocenter placement was also evaluated. Isocenter deviation from ideal was least with 2-mm imaging thickness and was significantly worse with thicknesses >5 mm.

Although initial positioning of the target isocenter at the linear accelerator isocenter is highly accurate as the foregoing has demonstrated, patient movement during the time of multi-beam or multi-arc treatment delivery (i.e., intrafractional movement) is a potential source of additional dosimetric error (Wang 2008). Agazaryan and associates monitored intrafractional motion in 15 patients with 20 treatment sites using repeat 2D–3D fusion prior to each beam or arc subsequent to the initial isocenter placement (Agazaryan et al. 2008). Vertebral anatomy movement along all three axes of translation up to 3 mm was recorded between sequential measurements. These translational shifts could occur within 5 min of initial isocenter confirmation. Depending upon the axis of interest, translational offsets for the cervical spine varied from −3 mm to 1 mm, for the thoracic spine from −1 mm to 2.5 mm, and for the lumbar spine from −2 mm to 1.5 mm. Average mean yaw rotational offset was 0.1° (standard deviation 0.9°). As a result of this study, intrafraction monitoring of patient position during spinal radiosurgery has become routine at UCLA.

Patient movement during spinal radiosurgery can be minimized by the supine position. Hoogeman et al. analyzed patient movement during CyberKnife® (Accuray, Sunnyvale, CA, USA) spinal radiosurgery using repeated stereoscopic radiographs during treatment (Hoogeman et al. 2008). The total displacement vector was minimal for supine patients. Observed displacements were <2.8 mm in 95% of cases over a 15-min interval. The systematic error for supine patients increased linearly an average of 0.7 mm for all three components of translation over 15 min. The mean displacement, however, was only 0.1 mm and the overall three-dimensional systematic error was 1.2 mm at 15 min. Greater displacements were recorded for patients treated in the prone position. Even after 1 min, 95% of observed displacements were <3.1 mm and reached a maximum of 12 mm by 15 min. The overall three-dimensional systematic error for prone patients was 2.2 mm at 15 min. The largest component of systematic error for the prone patients was in the anterior direction, implying progressive ventral spine "sag" as treatment progressed. Random displacement errors were, on average, 1 mm larger for prone compared to supine patients.

23.4 Dose Selection for Benign Tumors

Dose selection for the treatment of benign spinal tumors has been influenced by the results of SRS for intracranial lesions of similar histology as well as current concepts regarding tolerance of the spinal cord to large single doses of irradiation. Flickinger et al. demonstrated 98% local control following single fraction doses of 11–18 Gy (median 13 Gy) for acoustic neuromas (Flickinger et al. 2001). The authors found no significant difference in local control rate between patients receiving <13 Gy compared to >14 Gy. According to Kollova et al., the rate of volume reduction following >12 Gy SRS for meningiomas was significantly higher than after <12 Gy ($p=0.012$) (Kollova et al. 2007). Dose necessary to control hemangioblastoma is controversial. In a multi-institutional series of 38 intracranial hemangioblastomas, Patrice and associates reported that lesions recurring after cranial SRS received a median peripheral dose of 14 Gy compared to a median of 16 Gy for locally controlled tumors ($p=0.023$) (Patrice et al. 1996). In a retrospective review of 93 intracranial hemangioblastomas, Wang et al. reported that the mean marginal SRS dose was 14.2 Gy for tumors progressing after treatment compared to 18 Gy for tumors that responded or remained stable ($p<0.01$) (Wang et al. 2005). Centers delivering >18 Gy to all patients report local control rates of 97% for hemangioblastomas (Bijl et al. 2005; Tago et al. 2005) Niemela et al., by contrast, advocated 10–15 Gy for small-medium sized tumors (Niemela et al. 1996).

The threshold tolerance of the spinal cord for myelopathy following radiosurgery remains undefined. Assuming the tolerance of the human spinal cord is 50 Gy delivered in standard 1.8–2 Gy fractions, the linear-quadratic model (alpha/beta value for cord =2 Gy) would predict an isoeffective single-dose tolerance of 13 Gy. There is considerable experience with single fraction palliative spinal cord radiotherapy in humans. Rades et al. reported no myelopathy in a group of 199 patients receiving 8 Gy in a single fraction for vertebral metastases (Rades et al. 2005a). Follow-up was >12 months in 65 patients in this experience. These investigators subsequently reported a randomized trial of five palliative schedules including 261 patients receiving 8 Gy single fraction (Rades et al. 2005b). Follow-up >12 months was available for 33% of this group and no cases of myelopathy were recorded. McBeth and associates reported a randomized trial of three regimens for inoperable lung cancer including 114 patients receiving 10 Gy single fraction and 524 patients receiving 17 Gy in two fractions (McBeth et al. 1996). No myelopathy was encountered in the single fraction patients although three patients developed cord injury after the two-fraction scheme.

In vivo animal experiments confirm the tolerance of the spinal cord to single fraction irradiation. Lo et al. delivered 12–75 Gy to T9-L4 in mouse spinal cord. After 18–24 months follow-up, there was little or no detectable functional injury associated with doses <16 Gy (Lo et al. 1991). Above this threshold, the incidence of detectable cord injury was dose dependent. The ED50 for mild, moderate, and severe cord injury was 19, 21, and 24 Gy, respectively. Hopewell and colleagues irradiated various lengths of rat cervical cord to 18–70 Gy (Hopewell et al. 1987). The ED50 for white matter injury following exposure of 16 mm of cord was 21.5 Gy.

These human and animal experiences represent homogeneous irradiation (i.e., entire width) of a long length of spinal cord. Spinal radiosurgery, however, delivers inhomogeneous irradiation to a restricted length of cord so the concept of partial volume tolerance becomes crucial for understanding the threshold doses for myleopathy. There are several lines of evidence suggesting that as the volume of the irradiated cord decreases the threshold dose for white matter injury increases substantially. In the mouse model used by Lo et al., the ED50 for myelopathy increased from 21 Gy following irradiation of a 2.2-cm length of cord to 31 Gy for a 1.5-cm length and 70 Gy for a 1-cm length (Lo et al. 1991). In the rat model of Hopewell et al., the ED50 for white matter injury increased from 20 Gy for a 1.6-cm length of cord irradiated to 22 Gy for a 0.8-cm length and 25 Gy for a 0.4-cm length (Hopewell et al. 1987). Bijl and associates irradiated variable lengths (2–20 mm) of the rat spinal cord with the plateau region of a proton beam (Bijl et al. 2002). In all animals, the entire width of spinal cord was irradiated. The ED50 for 20-mm length exposure was 20.4 Gy and for 8 mm 24.9 Gy. As the length of irradiated cord decreased further, the tolerance of the cord increased markedly. The ED50 for a 4-mm and 2-mm length of irradiation was 54 and 88 Gy, respectively. An explanation for partial cord tolerance is provided by the experiments of Franklin et al. (Franklin et al. 1997) This group demonstrated migration from unirradiated spinal cord of myelin-producing oligodendrogliocytes into a region of cord previously injured chemically and then exposed to 40 Gy single dose through a window of varying width. These recruited oligodendrogliocytes were capable of re-myelinating damaged cord. The authors documented that the effective distance over which this recruitment and migration occurs was limited to 1–2 mm. It must be emphasized that the experimental design of (Biji et al. 2002) and (Franklin et al. 1997) involved irradiation of the cord without beam penumbra. Bijl et al. subsequently demonstrated that a low dose of priming irradiation (4–18 Gy) could abrogate recruitment/migration of "uninjured" oligodendrogliocytes, resulting in a decrease in the ED50 (Bijl et al. 2003). This finding implies that the volume of spinal cord within the low-dose region must be respected in dosimetry planning for spinal radiosurgery.

Partial volume tolerance of the human spinal cord to radiosurgery was analyzed by Ryu and colleagues in a series of 177 patients with 230 metastatic lesions (Ryu et al. 2007). The treatment planning spinal cord constraint used by this group was <10 Gy to 10% of the cord volume. The investigators arbitrarily defined the cord volume as 6 mm above and below the target GTV. The average dose to the 10% cord volume in this experience was 9 Gy. Average dose to this specific cord volume was significantly related to prescribed dose but unrelated to target volume or cord level. Among the 86 patients surviving at least 1 year, the average dose to the 30%, 20%, 10%, 5%, and 1% cord volumes was 6, 7, 8.6, 9.8, and 10.7 Gy, respectively. The maximum spinal cord point doses for these specific partial volumes were 10.9, 12.4, 13, 14.9, and 15.8 Gy, respectively. The authors reported a single case of myelopathy occurring in a patient receiving 9.6 Gy to the 10% partial volume and a point maximum of 14.4 Gy. The authors concluded that an acceptable estimate of partial cord tolerance is 10 Gy to the 10% volume.

The topographic distribution of radiosurgery dose may also be important in determining partial volume tolerance of the spinal cord. Bijl and associates demonstrated regional sensitivity differences in the mouse cord. Using the plateau proton beam technique, a 20-mm length of either the lateral or the central cord was irradiated (Bijl et al. 2005). The ED50 for the lateral cord varied from 29 to 33 Gy compared to 72 Gy for the central cord. Histologic analysis demonstrated only white matter changes without accompanying gray matter injury. The results imply that the lateral corticospinal tract in humans may be less tolerant of spinal radiosurgery than the anterior tract or other ventral cord structures.

Single-dose tolerance of the cauda equine is unknown. This portion of the nervous system is tolerant of conventionally fractionated radiotherapy. According to Pieters and associates, the estimated TD5/5 and TD 50/5 were 55 and 72 Gy for males and 67 and 84 Gy for females (Pieters et al. 2006).

23.5 Results of Spinal Radiosurgery for Benign Tumors

Since January 2002, 29 patients with 43 benign tumors have undergone image-guided spinal radiosurgery at UCLA. Patient age ranged from 17 to 78 years (median 61 years). Nine patients had neurofibromatosis type 1 or 2. There were 26 nerve sheath tumors, 13 hemangioblastomas, 3 choroid plexus papillomas, and 1 meningioma. Tumor volume ranged from 0.05 to 14.7 cc (median 1.9 cc). The largest tumor dimension ranged from 0.9 to 4.1 cm (median 2.1 cm). Seventeen tumors were located on the surface of the cord, 11 were "dumbbell" lesions extending from the intraspinal nerve sheath to the extra-foraminal nerve sheath, 7 involved only the intraspinal nerve sheath, 6 were extra-foraminal, and 2 were confined to the nerve sheath within the spinal nerve foramen. Seventeen tumors were located in the cervical spine, 14 in the thoracic spine, 11 in the lumbar spine, and 1 was sacral. Fourteen tumors caused sensory disturbance, 12 caused pain, 10 caused weakness, and 11 lesions were asymptomatic. Histopathology was available on nine patients following subtotal removal. These patients were treated for imaging evidence of tumor regrowth or persistent symptoms. Presumptive histopathology in the remaining patients was established after removal of nerve sheath tumors elsewhere (neurofibromatosis patients), history of intracranial hemangioblastoma/choroid plexus tumors elsewhere or by clinico-radiologic findings compatible with a benign tumor.

All tumors were treated with a single isocenter. Forward planned dynamic arcs were used for 35 tumors and 8 were treated with intensity-modulated beams. Prescribed dose ranged from 12 to 15 Gy (median 12 Gy). Dose was prescribed at the 90–97% isodose line (median 90%). The maximum spinal cord dose was <12 Gy. Patients have been followed a median of 18 months (range 7–60 months). Local failure was defined as >2 mm increase in any linear tumor dimension persisting on two or more consecutive studies. Tumor response was defined as decrease in mean tumor dimension >2 mm persisting on two or more consecutive studies. Stable tumor was defined as no change in size or change <2 mm.

The actuarial local control rate following spinal radiosurgery for benign tumors was 95%. One hemangioblastoma recurred 12 months after treatment. Tumor responded in 32% and the remainder were stable (Fig. 23.9). Central tumor hypodensity was noted in two neurofibromas treated in the same patient (Fig. 23.10). Symptomatic improvement has been uncommon. Sensory disturbance improved in 2/14 sites, pain reduction in 1/13 sites, and decreased motor weakness in 1/10 sites. None of the patients developed new neurologic symptoms. Delayed transient worsening of preexisting symptoms occurred in two patients. There has been no clinical or radiographic evidence for spinal cord injury or major organ toxicity.

Larger experiences with spinal radiosurgery for benign tumors have been reported by investigators using CyberKnife technology. Dodd et al. reported a series of 55 pathologically proven or presumed lesions followed at least 6 months after treatment (median 23 months) at Stanford University (Dodd et al. 2006). Eligible patients had well-circumscribed tumors, no evidence of spinal instability, and minimal compromise of spinal cord function. There were 30 schwannomas, 16 meningiomas, and 9 neurofibromas. Overall tumor volume ranged from 0.136 to 24.6 cc (median 2.18 cc). The authors aimed for a single fraction dose of 16–30 Gy prescribed at the 80% isodose line. The spinal cord dose constraint was <10 Gy to <0.2 cc cord volume defined as 1 cm above and below the lesion. If this constraint could not be satisfied due to tumor proximity to the cord, the patient received multi-fraction radiosurgery with a constraint of <8 Gy to <0.4 cc of spinal cord. Overall, 37% of patients were treated with a single fraction and 42% with two fractions. Fiducial markers were placed percutaneously into vertebral segments above and below the target for the purpose of image guidance during irradiation. CT/MRI fusion for treatment planning was not routinely employed.

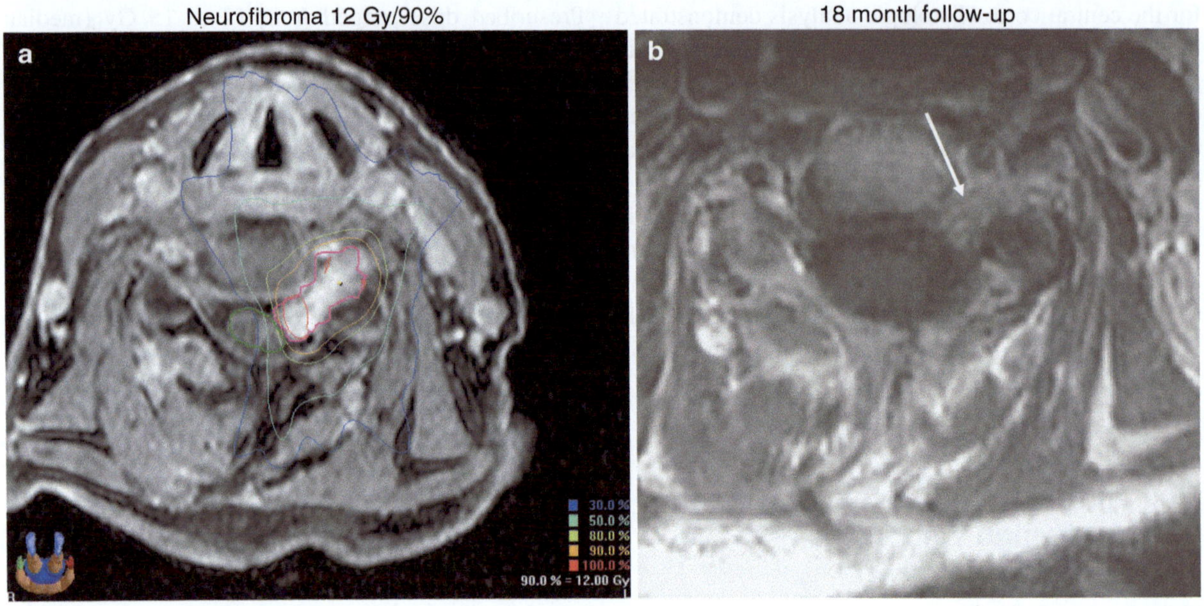

Fig. 23.9 (**a**) Isodose plan for a C6 nerve sheath tumor. The target (*thick pink*) received 12 Gy prescribed at the 90% isodose line. Isodose lines displayed: 100% (*thin red*); 90% (*yellow*); 80% (*light green*); 50% (*teal*); 30% (*blue*). (**b**) Axial contrast-enhanced MRI 18 months after spinal radiosurgery shows disease stability

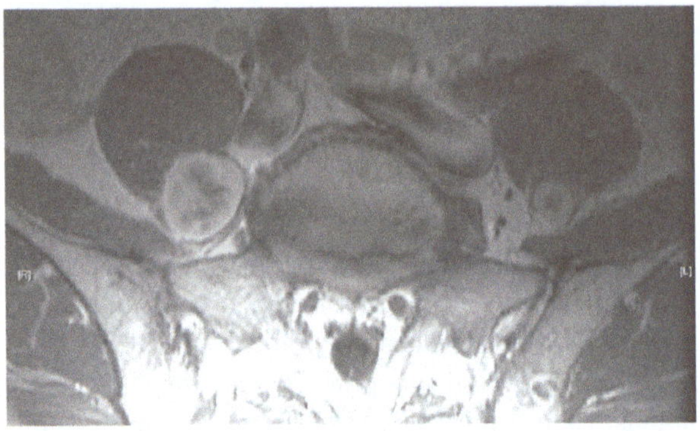

Fig. 23.10 Axial contrast-enhanced MRI 6 months after spinal radiosurgery of the patient displayed in Fig. 23.5. The image demonstrates bilateral loss of central tumor contrast enhancement without increase in tumor size

Local control was reported in 29 of 30 schwannomas. Tumor was stable in size in 56% and reduced in 40%. One tumor was removed due to slight increase in size. In this group, one third described improvement in pain, weakness, or sensory disturbance but 18% were clinically worse. There were no local relapses in the 15 meningiomas available for follow-up. Tumor remained stable in 67% and responded in 33%. Minor worsening of pretreatment symptoms was reported in 30% of cases. All nine neurofibromas were controlled although one was resected due to persistence of symptoms. One patient developed evidence of posterior column deficit 8 months after receiving 24 Gy in 3 fractions for a 7.56 cc C7/T1 meningioma recurrent after prior surgery. Dose-volume histogram analysis revealed 1.7 cc of the cord received >8 Gy per fraction.

Gerzsten et al. reported a series of 73 proven or presumed lesions followed a median of 37 months at the University of Pittsburgh (Gerszten et al. 2008). There were 35 schwannomas, 25 neurofibromas, and 13 meningiomas. Selection criteria mirrored those of the Stanford group. Tumors that occupied more than 50% of the epidural space within the cervical or thoracic spine were not considered radiosurgery candidates. Overall tumor volume ranged from 0.3 to 93 cc (median 4 cc). The authors aimed for a single fraction dose of 17 Gy prescribed at the 80% isodose line with at least 80% of the target within the prescription line. The maximum point dose constraint for the spinal cord dose was 8 Gy and for the cauda equina 10 Gy. If the constraint could not be satisfied due to tumor proximity, target coverage was sacrificed. CT/MRI fusion was not routine.

All 35 schwannomas were controlled although two unchanged tumors were eventually resected after developing new numbness. Pain was significantly reduced in 14 of the 17 schwannomas symptomatic before radiosurgery. All 25 neurofibromas were controlled and pain responded in 8/13. All 13 meningiomas were locally controlled. Three patients developed spinal cord toxicity compatible with a Brown-Sequard syndrome 5–13 months after radiosurgery. All three targets were located in the cervical spine and received a prescribed dose of 20 Gy. The volume of spinal cord receiving >8 Gy was less than 0.02 cc in all cases. MRI disclosed T2-weighted changes in the ipsilateral dorsal column in all cases. Strength returned to normal in two of the patients. Two of the patients had undergone prior surgery for their benign tumor. Prior surgery has been reported to increase the rate of cranial neuropathy after SRS for acoustic neuroma (Liscak et al. 1999).

In conclusion, image-guided spinal radiosurgery using a dedicated linear accelerator is an emerging technology that has been safely and effectively applied to benign tumors. The accuracy of this approach rivals that of the CyberKnife. It is free of the requirement for transcutaneous placement of bony fiducial markers. Finally Shaped Beam Radiosurgery, which can shape or modulate the beam on the target from any angular position by using a micro MLC (Micro Multileaf or HD120) is substantially more efficient than cone based treatments which must fill-in-the-dose by repeated cone-based repositioning.

The relatively low rate of symptomatic improvement associated with the absence of spinal cord injury following 12 Gy as used in our experience implies that there may be a role for dose escalation. Further clinical experience is required to conclusively establish the single-dose tolerance of the human spinal cord to large single-dose irradiation.

References

Agazaryan N, Tenn SE, DeSalles AAF et al (2008) Image-guided radiosurgery for spinal tumors: methods, accuracy and patient intrafraction motion. Phys Med Biol 53: 1715–1727

Bijl HP, van Luijk P, Coppes RP et al (2002) Dose-volume effects in the rat cervical spinal cord after proton irradiation. Int J Radiat Oncol Biol Phys 52:205–211

Bijl HP, van Luijk P, Coppes RP et al (2003) Unexpected changes of rat cervical spinal cord tolerance caused by inhomogeneous dose distributions. Int J Radiat Oncol Biol Phys 57:274–281

Bijl HP, van Luijk P, Coppes RP et al (2005) Regional differences in radiosensitivity across the rat cervical spinal cord. Int J Radiat Oncol Biol Phys 61:543–551

Blomgren H, Lax I, Naslund I et al (1995) Stereotactic high dose fraction radiation therapy of extracranial tumors using an accelerator. Acta Onco 34:861–870

Celli P (2002) Treatment of relevant nerve roots in nerve sheath tumors: removal or preservation. Neurosurgery 51:684–692

Celli P, Trillo G, Ferrante L (2005) Extrathecal intraradicular nerve sheath tumor. J Neurosurg Spine 3:1–11

Chang SD, Meisel JA, Hancock SL et al (1998) Treatment of hemangioblastomas in von Hippel-Lindau disease with linear accelerator-based radiosurgery. Neurosurgery 43:28–35

Chang S, Main W, Martin D et al (2003) An analysis of the accuracy of the CyberKnife: a robotic frameless stereotactic radiosurgical system. Neurosurgery 52:140–147

Chang EL, Shiu AS, Mendel E et al (2007) Phase I/II study of stereotactic body radiotherapy for spinal metastasis and its pattern of failure. J Neurosurg Spine 7:151–160

Cherqui A, Kim DH, Se-Hook K et al (2007) Surgical approaches to paraspinal nerve sheath tumors. Neurosurg Focus 22: 1–10

Conti P, Pansini G, Mouchaty H et al (2004) Spinal neurinomas: retrospective analysis and long-term outcome of 179 consecutively operated cases and review of the literature. Neoplasm 61:35–44

Cosgrove VP, Jahn U, Pfaender M et al (1999) Commissioning of a micro-multileaf collimator and planning system for stereotactic radiosurgery. Radiother Oncol 50:325–336

Dodd RL, Ryu MR, Kamnerdsupsphon P et al (2006) CyberKnife radiosurgery for benign intradural extramedullary spinal tumors. Neurosurgery 58:674–685

Flickinger JC, Kondziolka D, Niranjan A et al (2001) Results of acoustic neuroma radiosurgery: an analysis of 5 years' experience using current methods. J Neurosurg 94:1–6

Franklin RJM, Gilson JM, Blakemore WF (1997) Local recruitment of remyelinating cells in the repair of demyelination in the central nervous system. J Neurosci Res 50:337–344

Gerszten PC, Burton S, Ozhasoglu C et al (2008) Radiosurgery for benign intradural spinal tumors. Neurosurgery 62: 887–896

Hamilton AJ, Lulu BA, Fosmire H et al (1995) Preliminary clinical experience with linear accelerator-based spinal stereotactic radiosurgery. Neurosurgery 36:311–319

Hoogeman MS, Nuyttens JJ, Levendag PC et al (2008) Time dependence of intrafraction patient monitoring assessed by repeat stereoscopic imaging. Int J Radiat Oncol Biol Phys 70:609–618

Hopewell JW, Morris AD, Dixon-Brown A (1987) The influence of field size on the late tolerance of the rat spinal cord to single doses of X-rays. Br J Radiol 60:1099–1108

Jin JY, Ryu S, Faber K et al (2006) 2D/3D image fusion for accurate target localization and evaluation of a mask based system in fractionated stereotactic radiotherapy of cranial lesions. Med Phys 33:4557–4566

Kim P, Ebersold MJ, Onofrio BM et al (1989) Surgery of spinal nerve Schwannoma. Risk of neurological deficit after resection of involved root. J Neurosurg 71:810–814

Kollova A, Liscak R, Novotny J et al (2007) Gamma knife surgery for benign tumors. J Neurosurg 107:325–336

Levy WJ, Latcharo J, Hahn JF et al (1986) Spinal neurofibroma: a report of 66 cases and a comparison with meningiomas. Neurosurgery 18:331–334

Liscak R, Vladyka V, Urgosik D et al (1999) Acoustic neurinoma and its treatment using the Leksell γ-knife as a primary or secondary treatment. J Radiosurg 2:13–22

Lo YC, McBride WH, Withers HR (1991) The effect of single doses of radiation on mouse spinal cord. Int J Radiat Oncol Biol Phys 22:57–63

Lohr F, Debus J, Frank C et al (1999) Noninvasive patient fixation for extracranial stereotactic radiotherapy. Int J Radiat Oncol Biol Phys 45:521–527

Lot G, Bernard G (1997) Cervical neuromas with extradural components: surgical management in a series of 57 patients. Neurosurgery 41:813–822

McBeth Fr, Wheldon TE, Girling DJ et al (1996) Radiation myelopathy: estimates of risk in 1048 patients in three randomized trials of palliative radiotherapy for non-small cell lung cancer. Clin Oncol 8:176–181

Niemela M, Lim YJ, Soderman M et al (1996) Gamma knife radiosurgery in 11 hemangioblastomas. J Neurosurg 85: 591–596

Patrice SJ, Sneed PK, Flickinger JC et al (1996) Radiosurgery for hemangioblastoma: results of a multiinstitutional experience. Int J Radiat Oncol Biol Phys 35:493–499

Pieters RS, Niemierko A, Fullerton BC et al (2006) Cauda equine tolerance to high-dose fractionated irradiation. Int J Radiat Oncol Biol Phys 64:251–257

Rades D, Stalpers LJ, Hulshof MC et al (2005a) Effectiveness and toxicity of single-fraction radiotherapy with 1 × 8 Gy for metastatic spinal cord compression. Radiother Oncol 75: 70–73

Rades D, Stalpers LJ, Veninga T et al (2005b) Evaluation of five radiation schedules and prognostic factors for metastatic spinal cord compression. J Clin Oncol 23:3366–3375

Ryu S, Yin FF, Rock J et al (2003) Image-guided and intensity-modulated radiosurgery for patients with spinal metastases. Cancer 97:2013–2118

Ryu S, Jin JY, Jin R et al (2007) Partial volume tolerance of the spinal cord and complications of single-dose radiosurgery. Cancer 109:628–636

Safavi-Abbasi S, Senoglu M, Theodore N et al (2008) Microsurgical management of spinal schwannomas: evaluation of 128 cases. J Neurosurg Spine 9:40–47

Seppala MT, Haltia MJJ, Sankila RJ et al (1995a) Long-term outcome after removal of spinal neurofibromas. J Neurosurg 82:572–577

Seppala MT, Haltia MJJ, Sankila RJ et al (1995b) Long-term outcome after removal of spinal Schwannomas: a clinicopathologic study of 187 cases. J Neurosurg 83:621–626

Tago M, Terahara A, Shin M et al (2005) Gamma knife surgery for hemangioblastomas. J Neurosurg 102(suppl):171–174

Takacs II, Hamilton AJ, Lulu BA et al (1999) Frame based stereotactic spinal radiosurgery: experience from the first 19 patients treated. Stereotact Funct Neurosurg 73:69

Teh BS, Paulino AC, Lu HH et al (2007) Versatility of the Novalis system to deliver image-guided stereotactic body radiation therapy (SBRT) for various anatomical sites. Technol Cancer Res Treat 6:347–354

Wang EM, Pan L, Wang BJ et al (2005) The long-term results of gamma knife radiosurgery for hemangioblastomas of the brain. J Neurosurg 102(Suppl):225–229

Wang H, Shiu A, Wang C et al (2008) Dosimetric effect of translational and rotational errors for patients undergoing image-guided stereotactic body radiotherapy for spinal metastases. Int J Radiat Oncol Biol Phys 71:1261–1271

Yan H, Yin FF, Kim JH (2003) A phantom study on the positioning accuracy of the Novalis Body system. Med Phys 30: 3052–3060

Yin FF, Ryu S, Ajlouni M et al (2002a) A technique of intensity-modulated radiosurgery (IMRS) for spinal tumors. Med Phys 29:2815–2822

Yin FF, Zhu J, Yan H et al (2002b) Dosimetric characteristics of Novalis shaped beam surgery unit. Med Phys 29: 1729–1764

Stereotactic Body Radiotherapy for the Lung

24

Yukinori Matsuo, Keiko Shibuya, Masaru Narabayashi, and Masahiro Hiraoka

24.1 Introduction

Lung cancer is the leading cause of cancer-related deaths both in the US (Jemal et al. 2008) and in Japan (Center for Cancer Control and Information Services, National Cancer Center 2007). Approximately 62,000 patients died of lung cancer during 2005 in Japan. Surgery is accepted as the standard care for stage I non-small cell lung cancer (NSCLC), and application of radiotherapy is limited to medically inoperable patients. Clinical outcomes of conventional radiotherapy for stage I NSCLC were inferior to those of surgery. The overall survival rate of conventional radiotherapy for medically inoperable patients with stage I NSCLC is approximately 15% (Sibley 1998).

Stereotactic body radiotherapy (SBRT) is a newly emerging radiotherapy treatment method to deliver a high dose of radiation to the target, utilizing either a single dose or a small number of fractions with a high degree of precision within the body, according to the American Society for Therapeutic Radiology and Oncology and American College of Radiology practice guidelines (Potters et al. 2004). Lax et al. developed the first stereotactic body frame with vacuum pillow stabilization for SBRT (Lax et al. 1994).

Blomgren et al. published the first report on SBRT using the stereotactic body frame in 1995 (Blomgren et al. 1995). They treated 42 tumors in the lung and liver of 31 patients. The local rate of no progressive disease was 80%. Uematsu et al. developed a frameless system (FOCAL unit) that consisted of a linear accelerator, an X-ray simulator, computed tomography (CT), and a table (Uematsu et al. 1998). They performed SBRT for 66 lung tumors in 45 patients using this system. Local progression was observed only in 2 of the 66 tumors (3%). Several researchers studied SBRT for lung tumors after these reports, and their results were also promising (see next section).

These promising results encouraged multi-institutional oncology groups to conduct trials of SBRT for the lung. The Radiation Therapy Oncology Group (RTOG) and Japan Clinical Oncology Group (JCOG) started the RTOG 0236 protocol and JCOG 0403 protocol (Hiraoka and Ishikura 2007), respectively. RTOG 0236 is a phase II trial of SBRT for medically inoperable stage I/II NSCLC. JCOG 0403 is a phase II trial of SBRT for T1N0M0 NSCLC in both operable and inoperable patients. Patient accrual was closed for both RTOG 0236 and JCOG 0403. The clinical outcomes of these trials are awaited.

SBRT has been one of the important options for the treatment of lung cancer. Since this treatment was covered by the governmental health insurance in Japan in 2004, the number of patients who have received SBRT has been increasing. SBRT for lung cancer was performed in 2,104 cases at 53 institutions by November 2004 in Japan according to a report by Nagata et al. (2006).

Y. Matsuo, K. Shibuya, M. Narabayashi, and M. Hiraoka (✉)
Department of Radiation Oncology and Image-applied Therapy, Graduate School of Medicine, Kyoto University, 54 Kawara-cho, Shogoin, Sakyo-ku, 6068507 Kyoto, Japan
e-mail: hiraok@kuhp.kyoto-u.ac.jp

A.A.F. De Salles et al. (eds.), *Shaped Beam Radiosurgery*,
DOI: 10.1007/978-3-642-11151-8_24,

24.2 Brief Summary of the Current Literature Results

24.2.1 Primary Non-small Cell Lung Cancer (NSCLC)

Table 24.1 summarizes reports on SBRT outcomes for NSCLC. Although there are some variations in dose-fractionation and patient characteristics (e.g. operability), SBRT outcomes are much better than those of conventional radiotherapy.

There are two large series of multi-institutional studies that retrospectively surveyed clinical outcomes of SBRT for NSCLC. Onishi et al. reviewed 257 patients who received SBRT for stage I NSCLC during 1995–2004 at 14 institutions in Japan (Onishi et al. 2007). Local progression occurred in 14.0% of patients. The overall 3-year and 5-year survival rates were 56.8% and 47.2%, respectively. The local recurrence rates were 8.4% in patients who received a biological effective dose (BED) of 100 Gy or more at the isocenter, and 42.9% in patients receiving less than 100 Gy in BED. The difference was significant ($p<0.001$). Baumann et al. retrospectively reviewed results of SBRT for 138 patients with medically inoperable stage I NSCLC treated during 1996–2003 at five centers in Sweden and Denmark (Baumann et al. 2006). Local failure was observed in 12% of patients. The overall 3-year and 5-year survival rates were 52% and 26%, respectively. Local failure was associated with tumor size, target definition and central or pleura proximity. There was a significant advantage in survival for the group receiving a dose above 55.6 Gy in equivalent dose in 2 Gy fractions (EQD2). According to Baumann, 55.6 Gy in EQD2 at the PTV periphery corresponds to BED 100 Gy at the isocenter as in Onishi's study.

24.2.2 Metastatic Lung Cancer

There are several reports on SBRT for metastatic lung cancer (Table 24.2). Up to two lesions were simultaneously treated in most of these reports, except for that by Okunieff (up to five lesions). The local control rate was more than 60% and the overall survival rate was more than 30% at 2 years. These outcomes were thought to be comparable to surgical metastatectomy (The International Registry of Lung Metastases Writing Committee 1997).

24.2.3 Toxicity

Onishi et al. reported that pulmonary complications above grade 2 were observed in 5.4%, grade 3 esophagitis in 0.8%, and grade 3–4 dermatitis in 1.2% in the retrospective study of 257 SBRT patients (Onishi et al. 2007). In Baumann's retrospective study, grade 3–4 toxicity was observed in 10.1% (Baumann et al. 2006).

Table 24.1 SBRT for primary lung cancer

Author	No. of patients	Dose	Local control	Overall survival
Nagata (2005)	45	48 Gy/4 fr at IC	95% (T1)	83% (T1, 3 yr)
			100% (T2)	72% (T2, 3 yr)
Timmerman et al. (2006)	70	60–66 Gy/3 fr at PTV periphery	95% (2 yr)	54.7% (2 yr)
Hoyer et al. (2006)	45	45 Gy/3 fr at IC	85% (2 yr)	48% (2 yr)
Zimmermann et al. (2006)	68	24–40 Gy/3–5 fr at PTV periphery	88% (3 yr)	51% (3 yr)
Hof et al. (2007a)	42	19–30 Gy/1 fr at IC	67.9% (3 yr)	37.4% (3 yr)
Koto et al. (2007)	31	45 Gy/3 fr, or 60 Gy/8 fr at IC	77.9% (T1, 3 yr)	71.7% (3 yr)
			40.0% (T2, 3 yr)	

Abbreviations: *IC* isocenter, *fr* = fraction, *yr* = year

Table 24.2 SBRT for pulmonary metastasis

Author	No. of patients	Dose	Local control	Overall survival
Wulf et al. (2004)	51	26 Gy/1 fr, or 30–37.5 Gy/3 fr at PTV periphery	80%	33% (2 yr)
Okunieff et al. (2006)	50	50–55 Gy/ 10–11 fr at IC	83%	25% (3 yr)
Hof et al. (2007b)	61	12–30 Gy/ 1 fr at IC	63.1% (3 yr)	47.8% (3 yr)
Norihisa et al. (2008)	34	48–60 Gy/ 4–5 fr at IC	90% (2 yr)	84.3% (2 yr)

Abbreviations: *IC* isocenter, *fr* = fraction, *yr* = year

Baumann et al. reported on toxicity in a multi-institutional phase II study of SBRT for medically inoperable stage I NSCLC, which was performed at seven different centers in Sweden, Norway and Denmark (Baumann et al. 2008). Grade 3 toxicity was seen in 21% of the patients, and no grade 4 or 5 toxicity was reported.

One of the most striking data on toxicity after SBRT for the lung is the article published in 2006 by Timmerman et al. (2006). They reported that grade 5 toxicity was observed in 6 patients (8.6%), and grade 3–4 was in another 8 patients (11.4%) of 70 patients who underwent SBRT for NSCLC with a prescription dose of 60–66 Gy in 3 fractions. Such severe toxicities were associated with tumor location. Patients treated for tumors in the peripheral lung demonstrated a 2-year freedom from severe toxicity in 83% compared with 54% for patients with central tumors. Based on this study, central tumor was excluded from the RTOG trial 0236. Early toxicity report of RTOG 0236 showed grade 3–4 pulmonary toxicity in 15% (Timmerman and Paulus 2007).

24.3 Targeting Issues

This section and the following sections described our SBRT practice for the lung in Kyoto University (Takayama et al. 2005). We performed SBRT for one or two tumors in the lung less than 5 cm in diameter. Two kinds of body frame, Stereotactic Body Frame (Elekta, Stockholm, Sweden) and BodyFIX (Medical Intelligence, Schwabmünchen, Germany), are used to attain accurate and precise patient positioning and immobilization. The former has built-in reference indicators which provide accurate determination of target co-ordinates. In our experience, daily setup errors with Stereotactic Body Frame were within 5 mm in 90%, 100%, and 93% of all verifications in mediolateral, anteroposterior, and craniocaudal directions, respectively (Negoro et al. 2001). BodyFIX is composed of relatively radiolucent materials which allow image guidance with X-ray. Since we started to use the Novalis® Radiosurgery system (Brainlab AG, Feldkirchen, Germany) for lung SBRT in April 2008, the BodyFIX system is used for most cases of SBRT in Kyoto University.

X-ray fluoroscopy is performed to measure tumor movement before CT scan. When the tumor moves more than 8–10 mm in the craniocaudal direction, we use a small abdominal pressing plate called a "diaphragm control" which suppresses the movement of the diaphragm and reduces respiratory motion of the tumor. After fluoroscopy, the patient is moved to the CT room. CT scan is performed under free-breathing with a slow scan or "long-scan-time" technique which can visualize a major part of the trajectory of the tumor by scanning each slice for a time longer than the respiratory cycle.

24.4 Outlining the Lesion

Delineation policy depends on the management of respiratory motion in SBRT for the lung. Internal target volume (ITV) which encompasses the whole trajectory of the tumor motion should be delineated when irradiation is performed under free-breathing. When you use a kind of gating technique, you should delineate gross tumor volume (GTV) or clinical target volume (CTV) during appropriate phases of respiration. In Kyoto University, SBRT for the lung is performed under free-breathing; therefore the ITV method is used.

The ITV is first delineated using CT, and then the ITV is extended to reflect the fluoroscopic evaluation of tumor movement, if necessary. We delineate both the solid area (tumor itself), which could be seen even using a mediastinal window setting (window width of 350 Hounsfield units (HU) and window level 40 HU, typically), and the surrounding obscure area, which could be seen only under a lung CT window setting (window width of 2,000 HU and window level of –700 HU). The obscure area is considered to indicate either microscopic tumor invasion or respiratory tumor motion. Neither GTV nor CTV is defined because the delineated ITV includes both of these. We do not extend the target to include whole area of spiculation or pleural indentation around the tumor. After contouring on CT, we compare the ITV on CT with the tumor motion evaluated on fluoroscopy. If the delineated ITV is insufficient to encompass respiratory motion, we appropriately extend the ITV. Planning target volume (PTV) is defined by adding a 5-mm margin of setup error to the ITV.

The planning organ-at-risk volumes (PRVs) are defined for lung, spinal cord, esophagus, stomach, intestine, trachea, bronchus, pulmonary artery and other organs at risk (OARs). The margin between PRV and OAR is 5 mm, except for the spinal cord and lung. The PRV for the spinal cord is defined as a 3-mm margin with the spinal canal delineated on CT images. The PRV for the lung is the bilateral pulmonary parenchyma outside the PTV.

24.5 Dose Decision

In dose prescription of SBRT for the lung, prescription point (isocenter or PTV periphery) and inhomogeneity correction (no correction, simplistic 1-D correction, or superposition/convolution) are important. These issues are discussed below.

We prescribe 48 Gy in 12-Gy fractions at the isocenter for primary lung cancer and 56 Gy in 14-Gy fractions for metastatic lung cancer, respectively. The Batho power law method is used as an inhomogeneity correction algorithm. Calculated BEDs at the isocenter are 105.6 Gy and 134.4 Gy for primary lung cancer and lung metastasis (under $\alpha/\beta = 10$ Gy), respectively.

Non-coplanar static beams (5–8 ports) with 6-MV X-rays are used. The margin between the PTV and the field edge is 5 mm, as a rule.

Dose constraints for OARs are the same as those of JCOG 0403 (Table 24.3).

Table 24.3 Dose constraints of organs at risk (OARs) for the Japan Clinical Oncology Trial 0403 protocol (as of September 2008)

PRV	Constraints
Lung	Mean dose ≤ 18 Gy
	40-Gy irradiated volume ≤ 100 cc
	V15 ≤ 25%
	V20 ≤ 20%
Spinal cord	Maximal dose ≤ 25 Gy
Esophagus and pulmonary artery	40-Gy irradiated volume ≤ 1 cc
	35-Gy irradiated volume ≤ 10 cc
Stomach and intestine	36-Gy irradiated volume ≤ 10 cc
	40-Gy irradiated volume ≤ 100 cc
Trachea and main bronchi	40-Gy irradiated volume ≤ 10 cc
Other organs	48-Gy irradiated volume ≤ 1 cc
	40-Gy irradiated volume ≤ 10 cc

24.6 Representative Case

24.6.1 Patient History

The patient was a 75-year-old male. He was receiving medication for asthma and emphysema. A coin lesion was detected on follow-up chest X-ray. CT scan was performed subsequently, and it demonstrated an 18-mm solitary tumor in the upper lobe of the left lung. CT-guided biopsy was performed to confirm histology of the lung tumor, and squamous cell carcinoma was detected. There was no evidence of metastasis either in regional lymph nodes or in distant organs. Clinical stage of lung cancer was determined as T1N0M0 stage IA. Pulmonary function test showed borderline operability and the patient chose SBRT rather than surgery for the treatment of lung cancer.

24.6.2 Simulation

Stereotactic Body Frame (Elekta) was used for fixation of the patient body. Fluoroscopic evaluation showed that the tumor motion was 2, 4, and 3 mm in the craniocaudal, mediolateral and anteroposterior directions, respectively. The motion was too small to use a diaphragm control. CT images were acquired under free breath using a slow scan technique.

24.6.3 Treatment Planning

Eclipse® (Varian Medical Systems, Palo Alto, CA) was used in SBRT planning for the patient. The ITV was delineated on the CT images including the obscure area that surrounded the solid tumor (Fig. 24.1). Since the ITV based on CT was thought to be sufficient to encompass the motion evaluated with fluoroscopy, extension of the ITV to compensate for tumor motion was not considered necessary. The PTV was made by adding a 5-mm margin to the ITV. The lung, spinal cord and aorta were defined as OARs in this case. PRV was set for each OAR.

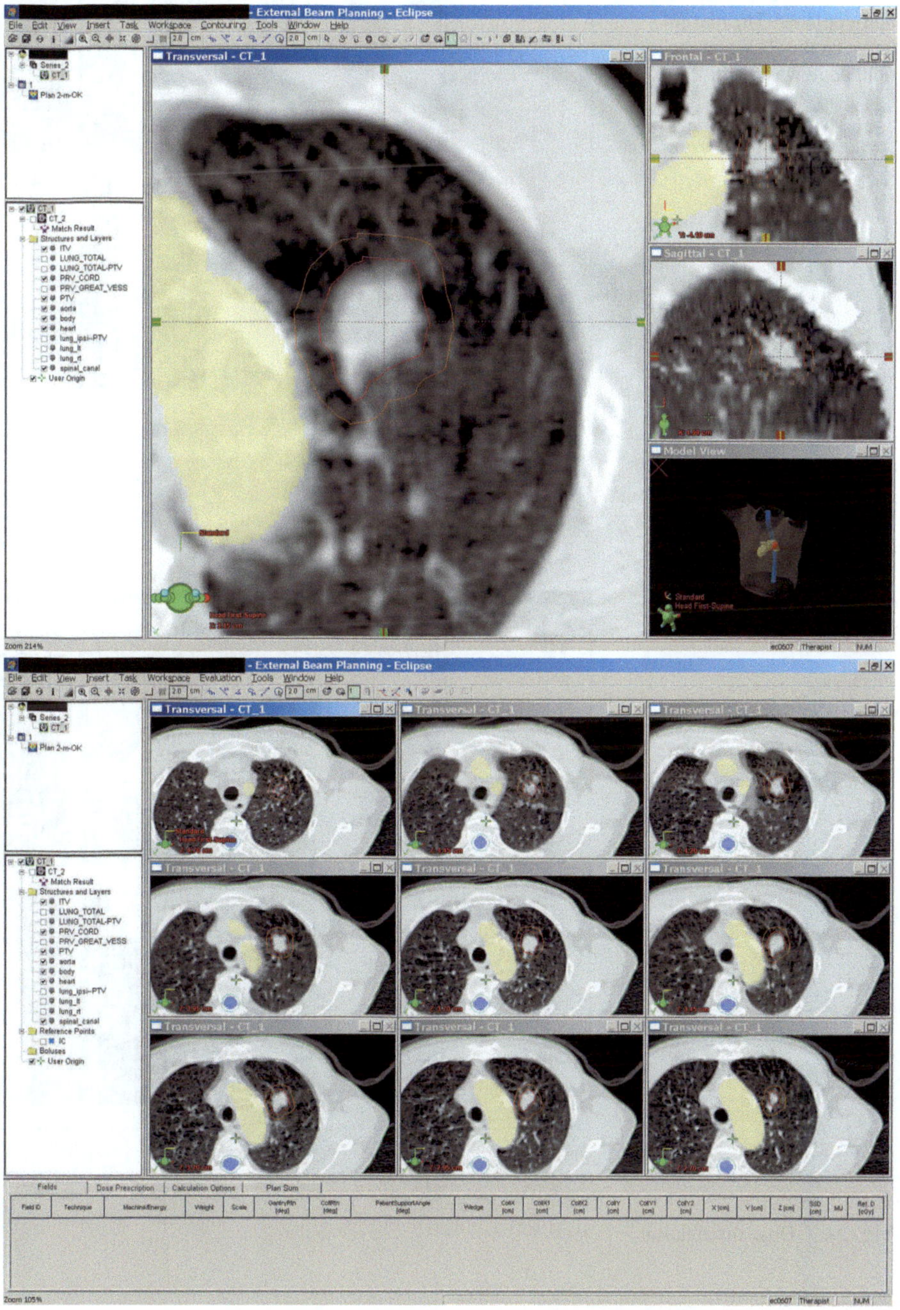

Fig. 24.1 Target delineation. The red line and the orange line indicate the ITV and the PTV, respectively. The margin between the ITV and the PTV was 5 mm

Six beams (two coplanar beams and four non-coplanar beams) were arranged for the PTV (Fig. 24.2). Prescription dose was 48 Gy at the isocenter in 12-Gy fractions. Dose distribution was calculated using the Batho power law correction (Fig. 24.3).

Dose coverage for the PTV was satisfactory. Minimal dose, maximal dose and D95 for the PTV were 43.7, 49.0, and 45.7 Gy, respectively. OAR doses were acceptable according to the dose constraints (Table 24.3). Mean dose and V20 in the lung

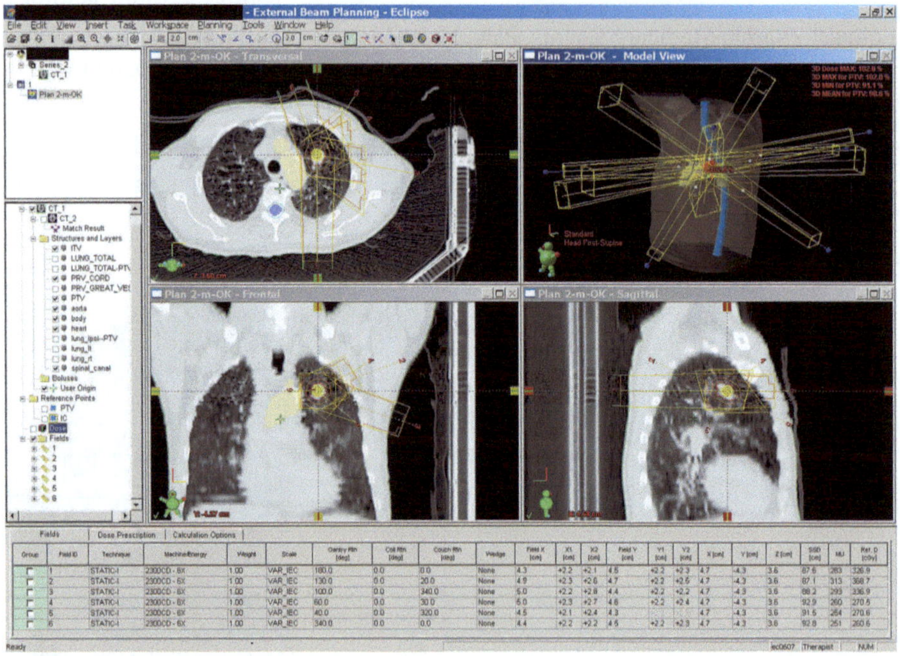

Fig. 24.2 Beam arrangement. Six beams were arranged for the PTV. Two of the six beams were coplanar, and the remaining four beams were non-coplanar. The margin between the PTV and the field edge was 5 mm

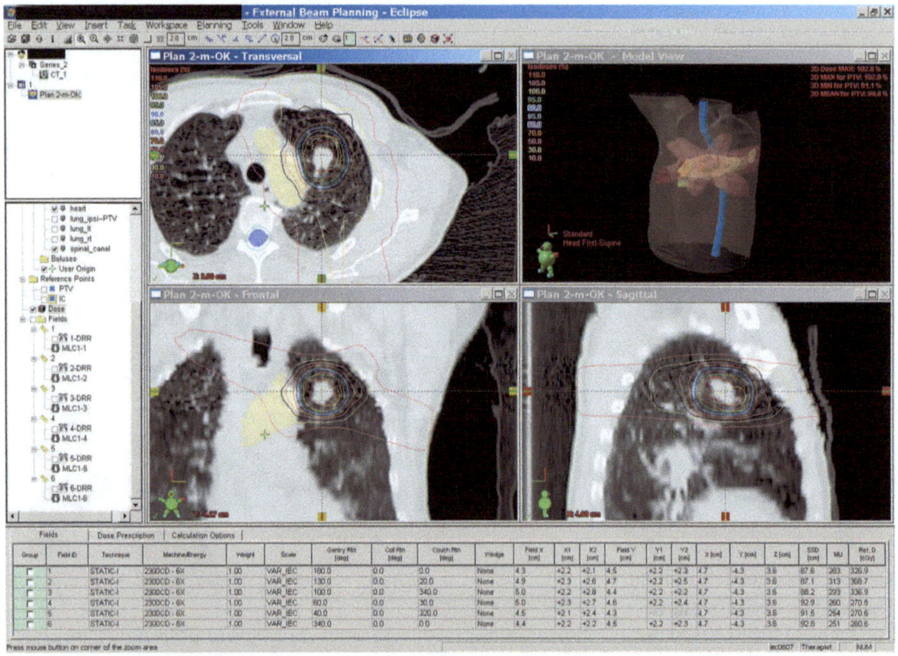

Fig. 24.3 Dose distribution

were 2.5 Gy and 3.3%, respectively. Maximal dose in the PRV for the cord was 7.2 Gy. V40 Gy and V48 Gy in the PRV for the aorta were 0 and 2.6 cc, respectively.

24.6.4 Clinical Outcome

Four fractions of SBRT were delivered in 8 days. There was no acute adverse effect during the treatment session (Fig. 24.4).

The tumor shrank to 12 mm in diameter 6 weeks after SBRT. Asymptomatic radiation pneumonitis was observed on CT images at 3 months. The lung injury changed to a scar at 10 months. There was no sign of local recurrence on CT 3 years after SBRT. There has not been any evidence of disease progression to date. There is no adverse effect during the follow-up, except asymptomatic pneumonitis findings on CT.

24.7 Discussions

24.7.1 Prescription Point and Inhomogeneity Correction

Prescription point should be considered in planning of SBRT. Most of the Japanese studies (including JCOG 0403) are based on isocenter prescription. On the other hand, the US studies (including RTOG 0236) prescribed dose at the PTV periphery.

Inhomogeneity correction is also important in radiotherapy planning for the lung. A dry run study to

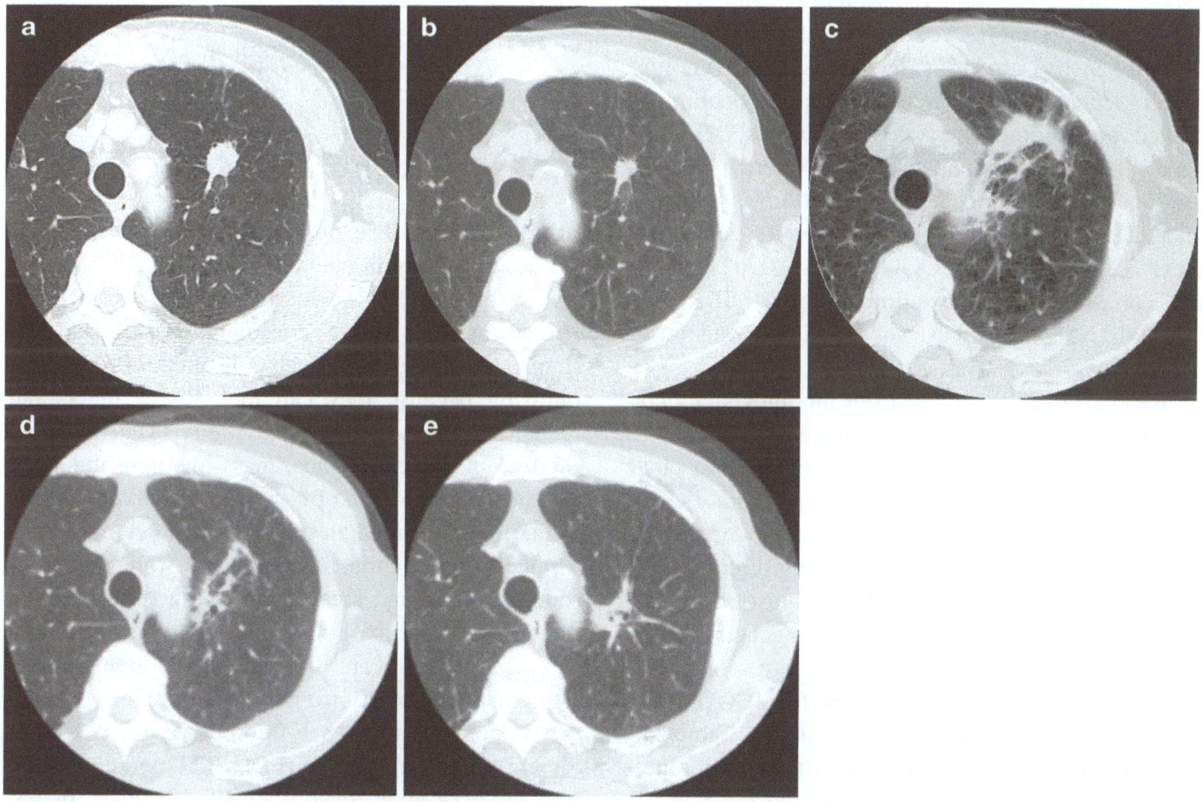

Fig. 24.4 CT changes after SBRT: (**a**) before SBRT – an 18-mm solitary tumor was in the upper lobe of the left lung; (**b**) 6 weeks after SBRT – the tumor shrank to 12 mm in diameter; (**c**) 3 months after SBRT – asymptomatic radiation pneumonitis was observed; (**d**) 10 months after SBRT; (**e**) 3 years after SBRT – local recurrence was not observed

assess interinstitutional variations in SBRT planning before the start of JCOG 0403 showed that dose calculation algorithm was a significant factor in the interinstitutional variations (Matsuo et al. 2007a).

Task Group No. 65 of the Radiation Therapy Committee of the American Association of Physicists in Medicine classified inhomogeneity correction algorithms into four categories according to the level of anatomy sampled for scatter calculation and the inclusion or exclusion of electron transport (Task Group No. 65 of the Radiation Therapy Committee of the American Association of Physicists in Medicine 2004). The task group recommends that the superposition/convolution algorithm be considered in order to ascertain dosage at tumor/lung interfaces in radiation planning for the lung, and that simplistic 1-dimensional equivalent path corrections are reasonable only for point dose estimations for lung tumors. It is generally accepted that dose distributions with superposition/convolution algorithms or Monte Carlo algorithms (classified as category four algorithms) are more accurate than those with older inhomogeneity correction algorithms. However, most SBRT reports were based on older algorithms or lacked an inhomogeneity correction. JCOG 0403 used simplistic 1-dimensional equivalent path corrections as inhomogeneity correction algorithms, and RTOG 0236 used no inhomogeneity correction. Next SBRT trial of JCOG (protocol 0702), which is a phase I dose escalation study of SBRT for T2N0M0 NSCLC, will use superposition/convolution algorithms.

We evaluated the influences of inhomogeneity corrections for comparison between protocols of JCOG 0403, JCOG 0702 and RTOG 0236 (Matsuo et al. 2008). SBRT plans were recalculated with Eclipse (Varian) under the same monitor units under the following three conditions of heterogeneity correction: Batho power law correction (BPL), anisotropic analytical algorithm (AAA), and no heterogeneity correction (NC). BPL, AAA and NC are considered inhomogeneity correction settings for JCOG 0403, JCOG 0702, and RTOG 0236, respectively. Table 24.4 is a summary of the results. Significant differences were observed except between BPL and AAA in isocenter dose or between AAA and NC in minimal dose of PTV.

Table 24.4 Differences in dose-volumetric data between heterogeneity correction algorithms

		BPL	AAA	NC	Differences
IC		48.0	48.4	44.7	BPL, AAA>NC
ITV	D95	46.4	44.4	42.5	BPL>AAA>NC
	Min.	45.4	42.5	41.5	BPL>AAA>NC
	Mean	47.8	46.8	44.4	BPL>AAA>NC
PTV	D95	45.3	42.3	41.3	BPL>AAA>NC
	Min.	42.5	39.0	38.9	BPL>AAA, NC
	Mean	47.4	45.7	44.1	BPL>AAA>NC

Data are shown in Gy. Inequality signs (>) mean significant differences by Tukey HSD test.

Abbreviations: *IC* isocenter, *BPL* Batho power law, *AAA* anisotropic analytical algorithm, *NC* no correction of inhomogeneity, *ITV* internal target volume, *PTV* planning target volume

Inhomogeneity correction algorithms make rapid progress. Monte Carlo based algorithms are now available in clinical practice. Figure 24.5 shows an example case using a new Monte Carlo algorithm in iPlan® RT Dose 4.0 (Brainlab AG, Feldkirchen, Germany).

24.7.2 Detection of Local Recurrence

Early detection of local recurrence after SBRT is desired, especially in operable cases that can undergo salvage surgery. However, early detection is sometimes difficult because dense consolidations overlap the tumor on follow-up CT. Such consolidations could be confusing because they can look like a mass, and are called "mass-like consolidations (Matsuo et al. 2007b)." In our experience, mass-like consolidations were observed in 68% of cases that underwent SBRT for the lung at a median of 5 months after treatment. Although most of the consolidations were radiation-induced lung injury, local recurrence was observed in about 10% of the mass-like consolidations. We could not find any significant differences on CT findings to distinguish lung injury from local recurrence.

It is possible that 18 F-fluorodeoxyglucose positron emission tomography (FDG-PET) would help to interpret mass-like consolidations. However, in our experience, maximal standardized uptake values (SUVmax) after SBRT tend to remain high even in

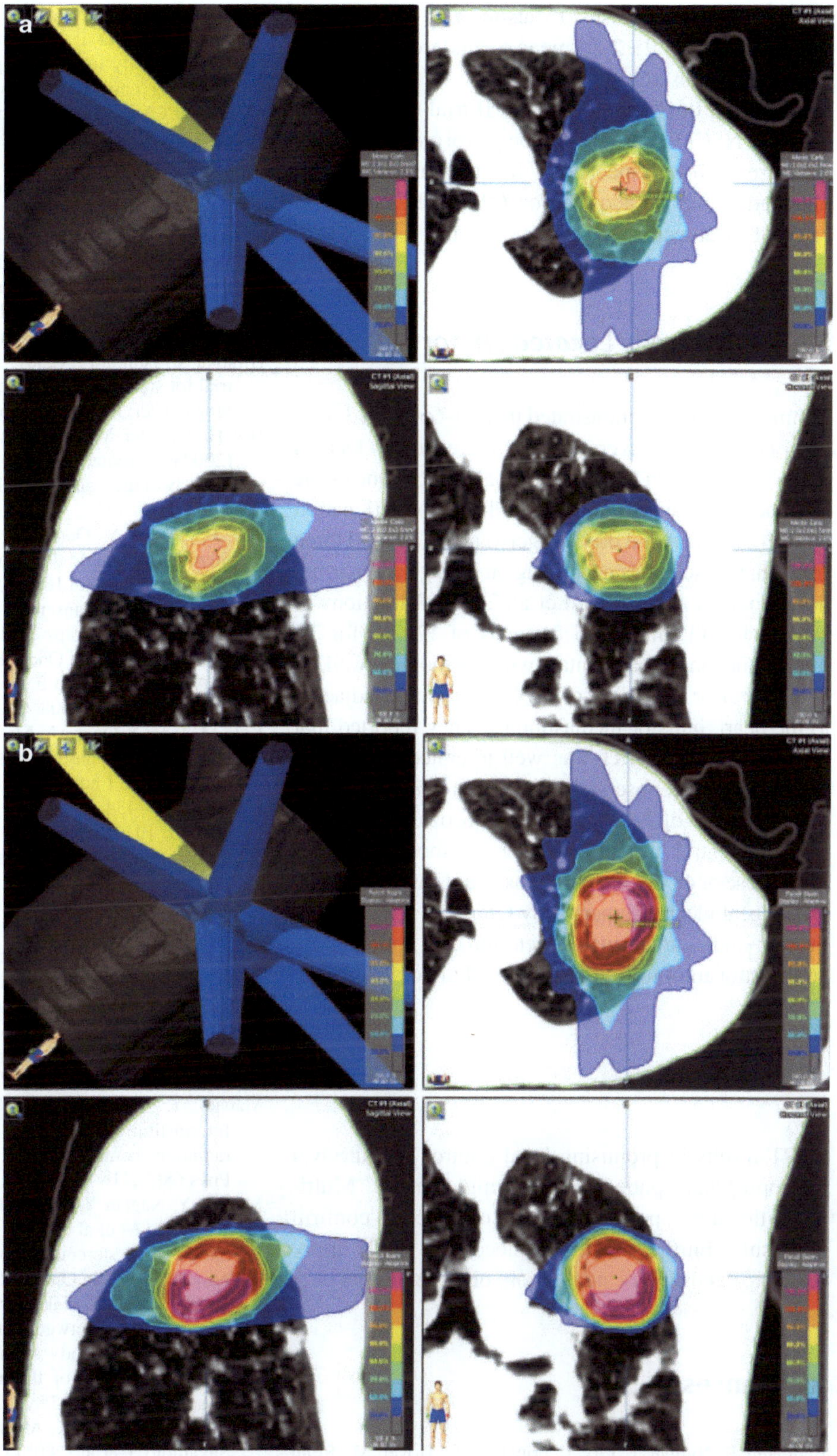

Fig. 24.5 Comparison of dose distributions between algorithms. (**a**) Dose distributions calculated with Monte Carlo algorithm. The isocenter dose was 48.0 Gy. D95 for the PTV was 36.2 Gy. (**b**) Dose distributions calculated with path length correction method under the same monitor units as in Fig. 24.5a. The isocenter dose was 49.3 Gy. D95 for the PTV was 49.4 Gy. Doses for the PTV in path length correction might be overestimated compared with Monte Carlo algorithm

locally controlled cases (Matsuo Y et al. 2010). SUVmax was 4.9±2.2 (mean±standard deviation) within 6 months after the treatment.

In RTOG 0618 that is a phase II trial of SBRT for operable NSCLC, surgery will be performed in patients who are highly suspected of local recurrence. New knowledge may be acquired on CT and FDG-PET in cases of local recurrence from this trial.

24.7.3 Centrally Located Tumor

Timmerman et al. demonstrated that 60–66 Gy in 3 fractions could cause severe toxicity for centrally located tumors in the lung (Timmerman et al. 2006). One of the approaches to central tumor is mild hypofractionation with a mild fractional dose. Lagerwaard et al. used three fractionation schemes depending on T stage and normal tissue toxicity (Lagerwaard et al. 2008); 3 fractions of 20 Gy (for T1 tumors), 5 fractions of 12 Gy (for T1 tumors showing broad contact with the thoracic wall, or T2 tumors), or 8 fractions of 7.5 Gy (for tumors adjacent to the heart, hilus or mediastinum). They reported that this risk-adapted SBRT was well tolerated and severe late toxicity was observed in less than 3% of patients. Eight fractions of 7.5 Gy may be a reasonable approach for most central tumors. However, we should note that lower dose of 48 Gy in 8 fractions could cause a grade 5 esophageal ulcer as reported by Onimaru et al. (2003). Further studies are needed to determine an optimal dose and fractionation for centrally located tumors.

24.8 Conclusions

SBRT results in promising local control and survival in appropriate patients with lung tumors. Multi-institutional prospective trials are expected to confirm the results. Further studies are needed to safely apply SBRT to centrally located tumors or large tumors.

References

Baumann P, Nyman J, Lax I, Friesland S, Hoyer M, Rehn Ericsson S et al (2006) Factors important for efficacy of stereotactic body radiotherapy of medically inoperable stage I lung cancer. A retrospective analysis of patients treated in the Nordic countries. Acta Oncol 45(7):787–795

Baumann P, Nyman J, Hoyer M, Gagliardi G, Lax I, Wennberg B et al (2008) Stereotactic body radiotherapy for medically inoperable patients with stage I non-small cell lung cancer – a first report of toxicity related to COPD/CVD in a non-randomized prospective phase II study. Radiother Oncol 88(3):359–367

Blomgren H, Lax I, Näslund I, Svanström R (1995) Stereotactic high dose fraction radiation therapy of extracranial tumors using an accelerator. Clinical experience of the first thirty-one patients. Acta Oncol 34(6):861–870

Center for Cancer Control and Information Services, National Cancer Center (2007) Cancer Statistics in Japan 2007. [Online]. Available from HYPERLINK. http://ganjoho.ncc.go.jp/public/statistics/backnumber/2007_en.html

Hiraoka M, Ishikura S (2007) A Japan clinical oncology group trial for stereotactic body radiation therapy of non-small cell lung cancer. J Thorac Oncol 2(7 Suppl 3):S115–S117

Hof H, Muenter M, Oetzel D, Hoess A, Debus J, Herfarth K (2007a) Stereotactic single-dose radiotherapy (radiosurgery) of early stage nonsmall-cell lung cancer (NSCLC). Cancer 110(1):148–155

Hof H, Hoess A, Oetzel D, Debus J, Herfarth K (2007b) Stereotactic single-dose radiotherapy of lung metastases. Strahlenther Onkol 183(12):673–678

Hoyer M, Roed H, Hansen AT (2006) Prospective study on stereotactic radiotherapy of limited-stage non–small-cell lung cancer. Int J Radiat Oncol Biol Phys 66(4):S128–S135

Jemal A, Siegel R, Ward E, Hao Y, Xu J, Murray T et al (2008) Cancer statistics, 2008. CA Cancer J Clin 58(2):71–96

Koto M, Takai Y, Ogawa Y, Matsushita H, Takeda K, Takahashi C et al (2007) A phase II study on stereotactic body radiotherapy for stage I non-small cell lung cancer. Radiother Oncol 85(3):429–434

Lagerwaard FJ, Haasbeek CJ, Smit EF, Slotman BJ, Senan S (2008) Outcomes of risk-adapted fractionated stereotactic radiotherapy for stage I non-small-cell lung cancer. Int J Radiat Oncol Biol Phys 70(3):685–692

Lax I, Blomgren H, Näslund I, Svanström R (1994) Stereotactic radiotherapy of malignancies in the abdomen. Methodological aspects. Acta Oncol 33(6):677–683

Matsuo Y, Nakamoto Y, Nagata Y, Shibuya K, Takayama K, Norihisa Y et al (2010) Characterization of FDG-PET images after stereotactic body radiation therapy for lung cancer. Radiother Oncol 97(2):200–204

Matsuo Y, Takayama K, Nagata Y, Kunieda E (2007a) Interinstitutional variations in planning for stereotactic body radiation therapy for lung cancer. Int J Radiat Oncol Biol Phys 68(2):416–425

Matsuo Y, Nagata Y, Mizowaki T, Takayama K, Sakamoto T, Sakamoto M et al (2007b) Evaluation of mass-like consolidation after stereotactic body radiation therapy for lung tumors. Int J Clin Oncol 12(5):356–362

Matsuo Y, Nagata Y, Nakamura M (2008) Differences in dose-volumetric data between heterogeneity correction algorithms for stereotactic body radiation therapy for lung cancer: is there any impact of the algorithms on local control? Int J Radiat Oncol Biol Phys 72(1):S638–S639

Nagata Y, Takayama K, Matsuo Y, Norihisa Y, Mizowaki T, Sakamoto T et al (2005) Clinical outcomes of a phase I/II study of 48 Gy of stereotactic body radiotherapy in 4 fractions for primary lung cancer using a stereotactic body frame. Int J Radiat Oncol Biol Phys 63(5):1427–1431

Nagata Y, Matsuo Y, Takayama K (2006) Survey of stereotactic body radiotherapy in Japan. Int J Radiat Oncol Biol Phys 66(3):S150–S151

Negoro Y, Nagata Y, Aoki T, Mizowaki T, Araki N, Takayama K et al (2001) The effectiveness of an immobilization device in conformal radiotherapy for lung tumor: reduction of respiratory tumor movement and evaluation of the daily setup accuracy. Int J Radiat Oncol Biol Phys 50(4):889–898

Norihisa Y, Nagata Y, Takayama K, Matsuo Y, Sakamoto T, Sakamoto M et al (2008) Stereotactic body radiotherapy for oligometastatic lung tumors. Int J Radiat Oncol Biol Phys 72(2):398–403

Okunieff P, Petersen AL, Philip A, Milano MT, Katz AW, Boros L et al (2006) Stereotactic Body Radiation Therapy (SBRT) for lung metastases. Acta Oncol 45(7):808–817

Onimaru R, Shirato H, Shimizu S, Kitamura K, Xu B, Fukumoto S-i et al (2003) Tolerance of organs at risk in small-volume, hypofractionated, image-guided radiotherapy for primary and metastatic lung cancers. Int J Radiat Oncol Biol Phys 56(1):126–135

Onishi H, Shirato H, Nagata Y, Hiraoka M, Fujino M, Gomi K et al (2007) Hypofractionated stereotactic radiotherapy (HypoFXSRT) for stage I non-small cell lung cancer: updated results of 257 patients in a Japanese multi-institutional study. J Thorac Oncol 2(7 Suppl 3):S94–S100

Potters L, Steinberg M, Rose C, Timmerman R, Ryu S, Hevezi JM et al (2004) American Society for Therapeutic Radiology and Oncology and American College of Radiology practice guideline for the performance of stereotactic body radiation therapy. Int J Radiat Oncol Biol Phys 60(4):1026–1032

Sibley GS (1998) Radiotherapy for patients with medically inoperable Stage I nonsmall cell lung carcinoma: smaller volumes and higher doses – a review. Cancer 82(3): 433–438

Takayama K, Nagata Y, Negoro Y, Mizowaki T, Sakamoto T, Sakamoto M et al (2005) Treatment planning of stereotactic radiotherapy for solitary lung tumor. Int J Radiat Oncol Biol Phys 61(5):1565–1571

Task Group No. 65 of the Radiation Therapy Committee of the American Association of Physicists in Medicine (2004) AAPM Report No. 85: Tissue inhomogeneity corrections for megavoltage photon beams. Medical Physics Publishing

The International Registry of Lung Metastases Writing Committee (1997) Long-term results of lung metastasectomy: prognostic analyses based on 5206 cases. J Thorac Cardiovasc Surg 113(1):37–49

Timmerman RD, Paulus R (2007) Toxicity analysis of RTOG 0236 using stereotactic body radiation therapy to treat medically inoperable early stage lung cancer patients. Int J Rad Biol Phys 69(3):S86

Timmerman R, McGarry R, Yiannoutsos C, Papiez L, Tudor K, DeLuca J et al (2006) Excessive toxicity when treating central tumors in a phase II study of stereotactic body radiation therapy for medically inoperable early-stage lung cancer. J Clin Oncol 24(30):4833–4839

Uematsu M, Shioda A, Tahara K, Fukui T, Yamamoto F, Tsumatori G et al (1998) Focal, high dose, and fractionated modified stereotactic radiation therapy for lung carcinoma patients: a preliminary experience. Cancer 82(6): 1062–1070

Wulf J, Haedinger U, Oppitz U, Thiele W, Mueller G, Flentje M (2004) Stereotactic radiotherapy for primary lung cancer and pulmonary metastases: a noninvasive treatment approach in medically inoperable patients. Int J Radiat Oncol Biol Phys 60(1):186–196

Zimmermann FB, Geinitz H, Schill S, Thamm R, Nieder C, Schratzenstaller U et al (2006) Stereotactic hypofractionated radiotherapy in stage I (T1–2 N0 M0) non-small-cell lung cancer (NSCLC). Acta Oncol 45(7):796–801

Stereotactic Body Radiation Therapy for Tumors of the Pancreas

25

Percy Lee and Brian Yeh

25.1 Introduction

More than 42,000 new cases of pancreatic cancer are diagnosed each year in the United States. Pancreatic cancer is the fourth leading cause of cancer-related deaths, and is the second leading cause of digestive cancer-related deaths. Even with the most aggressive combined modality therapy, the overall 5 year survival currently remains less than 5% (Jemal et al. 2009).

25.1.1 Surgery

Surgery with R0 resection (> 1 mm surgical margins) is the only treatment currently available with curative potential for patients with locally advanced pancreatic cancer (Verbeke 2008). However, local control and survival for patients, even after surgery, remain poor. Furthermore, because pancreatic cancer frequently presents at a late stage, only 15–20% of pancreatic cancer patients are candidates for resection (Varadhachary et al. 2006). Approximately 52% of patients present with metastatic disease, and another 26% present with locally advanced unresectable tumors (Jemal et al. 2009).

Recently, a distinct subset of "borderline resectable" patients has been described for which there is no standard of care (Verbeke 2008). These patients have tumors that about the superior mesenteric artery (SMA) or celiac artery, encase a short segment of the common hepatic artery, or occlude the superior mesenteric vein (SMV), portal vein (PV) or SMV-PV confluence over a short segment. Many of these patients who undergo surgery do not achieve a gross total resection, with an estimated R0 rate of approximately 30% (Verbeke et al. 2006). Their outcomes are similar to patients that have unresectable disease (Verbeke 2008). More innovative treatment options are needed in order to improve the overall survival in this group of patients.

25.1.2 Chemotherapy

First-line chemotherapy for locally advanced and metastatic pancreatic cancer is gemcitabine, a nucleoside analog. In the pivotal trial for which the FDA approved this drug, patients treated with gemcitabine had a modest improvement in survival compared to patients treated with 5FU from 4.41 to 5.56 months (Burris et al. 1997). In addition, nearly 25% of patients receiving gemcitabine were noted to have a clinical benefit compared to 5% of patients receiving 5FU. To date, no randomized phase III study adding a second agent to gemcitabine chemotherapy has been shown to result in a meaningful improvement in overall survival compared to gemcitabine alone.

25.1.3 Radiation Therapy

Radiation therapy is a widely accepted treatment modality for pancreatic cancer. The Gastrointestinal Tumor Study Group (GITSG) carried out a series of

P. Lee (✉) and B. Yeh
Department of Radiation Oncology, David Geffen School of Medicine at UCLA, 200 UCLA Medical Plaza, Suite B265, Los Angeles, CA 90095, USA
e-mail: percylee@mednet.ucla.edu

A.A.F. De Salles et al. (eds.), *Shaped Beam Radiosurgery*,
DOI: 10.1007/978-3-642-11151-8_25, © Springer-Verlag Berlin Heidelberg 2011

landmark studies that demonstrated the effectiveness of radiation therapy as both adjuvant and definitive treatment in pancreatic cancer (Kalser and Ellenberg 1985; Moertel et al. 1981). Modern radiation treatments have increasingly used conformal fields and dose escalation to enhance tumor control. Efforts to increase radiation dose to the pancreatic tumor without risking normal tissue injury have generally required relatively invasive techniques such as interstitial implantation of radioactive isotopes or intraoperative radiotherapy (IORT). Historically, the local control rates for conventional fractionated radiotherapy have ranged from 25% to 50% (Willett et al. 2005). Local progression from tumor leads to significant morbidity, including gastric outlet obstruction and pain.

The development of stereotactic body radiation therapy (SBRT) was led by a need to dose-escalate radiation therapy and improve tumor control of deep-seated tumors. Defining features include: (1) rigorous immobilization due to the longer treatment times; (2) image guidance for accurate set-up of patient from simulation to treatment; (3) use of multiple fields, or large-angle arcs of small aperture fields to reduce dose to surrounding normal tissue; (4) use of internal surrogates such as gold fiducial markers rather than relying on external tattoos for patient positioning; (5) strategy to account for organ and tumor motion; and (6) use of highly ablative doses of radiation therapy in few sessions (typically 1–5) in order to achieve higher rates of local control (Potters et al. 2004; Papiez et al. 2003).

25.2 Radiobiology

Classical radiobiology describes the relationship between radiation dose and cell survival using fractionated small doses of radiation. The most widely accepted model is the linear-quadratic formula (Fowler 1989). However, many have doubted whether this model is applicable for SBRT where much higher doses per fraction of radiation is delivered in a few fractions (Guerrero and Li 2004). Namely, some have argued that the linear-quadratic model might over predict the treatment effect (Park et al. 2008). However, much higher doses per fraction, as in SBRT, may have additional cellular cytotoxicities not accounted for by models developed for conventional fractionated radiation therapy. At doses per fraction above 7 Gy, microvascular endothelial apoptosis is thought to contribute to increased tumor control (Garcia-Barros et al. 2003). More research is needed to understand the cell survival characteristics of high dose per fraction radiation therapy in order to develop better predictive models for outcomes in SBRT.

The pancreas presents challenges in regards to being able to safely deliver SBRT. The head of the pancreas, where majority of tumors reside, is in close proximity to the C-loop of the duodenum, which is exquisitely sensitive to radiation therapy. For example, delivery of conventionally fractionated radiation (1.8–2 Gy/day) to more than 50 Gy results in damage to the small bowel such as ulcerations, stenosis, bleeding, and perforation. Furthermore, the pancreas move with respiration, as well as with peristalsis that is not easily predictable.

25.2.1 Single Dose

Stereotactic body radiotherapy delivering a single dose of 25 Gy prescribed to the isodose surface covering 95% or greater of the PTV is feasible and safe to administer in patients with locally advanced unresectable pancreatic cancer (Koong et al. 2004). The 50% isodose line was only allowed to cover the proximal duodenal wall. This dose resulted in greater than 90% local control and effectively palliated symptoms related to local tumor growth. Based on these results, a subsequent phase II study was completed which assessed the efficacy of combining a standard 5 week course of chemoradiotherapy with 45 Gy and either concurrent 5-FU or concurrent capecitabine, followed by a stereotactic radiotherapy boost with 25 Gy to the primary tumor in patients with locally advanced unresectable pancreatic cancer (Koong et al. 2005). In this cohort of 19 patients, a local control rate of 94% was achieved. However, all of the patients eventually developed metastases with a median time to progression of 17.5 weeks.

More recently, another phase II study integrating 25 Gy single-dose stereotactic body radiotherapy with gemcitabine chemotherapy in patients with unresectable pancreatic cancer was completed (Schellenberg et al. 2008). This study, involving 16 patients, confirmed the excellent local control rate observed in previous studies. The median overall survival was

11.4 months, the median time to progression was 9.7 months, and the 1 year survival was 50%. There were no significant acute GI toxicities. However, they did observe seven cases (44%) of grade 2 or greater late toxicity, and one case of grade 4 late toxicity (duodenal perforation).

In a retrospective review of 77 patients treated with 25 Gy single-dose stereotactic body radiotherapy for unresected pancreatic cancer, a 1 year local control rate of 84% was observed (Chang et al. 2009). Distant metastasis was the most common site of failure, and the 1 year progression-free survival was 9%, with a 1 year overall survival rate of 21%. No grade 4 acute toxicities were observed. However, four cases (5%) of grade 2 or 3 acute toxicity were reported. One of these four patients had also received external-beam radiotherapy with 45 Gy. Ten patients experienced grade 2 or greater late toxicity. Of these ten patients, three had also received external-beam radiotherapy. The 12 month actuarial rate of grade 2 or greater late toxicity was 28%. The authors concluded that SBRT for pancreatic adenocarcinoma was effective for local control, but is associated with risk of toxicity. They recommended additional strategies to reduce complications and that SBRT should be done with special attention to quality assurance.

25.2.2 Fractionated Stereotactic Body Radiotherapy

Fractionated stereotactic body radiotherapy for unresectable pancreatic cancer has been studied in a phase II trial from Denmark (Hoyer et al. 2005). 45 Gy in three fractions was prescribed to the center of the tumor, with the 95% isodose surface covering the CTV (tumor and surrounding edema) and the 67% isodose surface covering the PTV. The CTV was expanded 5 mm transversely and 10 mm longitudinally to form the PTV. Of the 22 patients in the study, six (27%) developed local progression; however, five of these six also had tumor progression outside the irradiated volume at the same time. The median progression-free survival was 4.8 months, and the 1 year progression-free survival rate was 9%. Acute toxicity was substantial. At baseline, 14 patients (64%) were observed to have grade 2 or greater toxicity. Five patients (22%) experienced significant GI toxicity (severe mucositis, gastric or duodenal ulceration, perforated gastric ulcer). In all five cases, part of the stomach or duodenum received at least 30 Gy. Of note, the volume treated to the prescription dose in this study was much larger than those in the Stanford study due to differences in margins and target delineation.

Other studies include a series of nine patients who had positive margins after resection from the University of Pittsburgh. They received a single fraction of 16–24 Gy (Parikh et al. 2008). All were alive at a mean follow-up of 5 months with 100% local control. They reported no acute toxicity. Georgetown University reported a retrospective series of 20 patients with local recurrence after definitive chemoradiation therapy, and eight with recurrence after surgery and adjuvant therapy (Lominska et al. 2008). All of the patients had received a prior dose of 50.4 Gy of conventional fractionated radiation therapy with concurrent chemotherapy. They were treated with 20–30 Gy delivered in 3–5 fractions. The median survival was 5.3 months, with 25% of the patients alive 8 months after treatment. One patient developed a bowel obstruction and another patient developed per-pancreatic abscess, both occurring in patients receiving three fractions. 85.7% of the patients were locally controlled. Tables 25.1 and 25.2 summarize the published studies showing outcome and toxicity of SBRT for pancreatic cancer.

25.3 U.C.L.A. Approach

At U.C.L.A., we utilize Novalis TX™ Radiosurgery (Brainlab AG, Feldkirchen, Germany) to deliver SBRT for pancreatic tumors. The Novalis TX is a commercially available linear accelerator specifically designed for image-guided radiation therapy (IGRT) and stereotactic body radiotherapy (SBRT). This machine combines a conventional high-energy linear accelerator with a kV imager, cone beam CT, and respiratory gating. Because of these innovations, it is possible to deliver highly accurate, stereotactic radiation treatments. This machine eliminates the uncertainties of tumor location and is able to correct for real time changes in tumor motion as a result of respiration during treatment.

The successes with SBRT in achieving a high local control rate with acceptable toxicity in unresectable pancreatic cancer patients led us to hypothesize that

Table 25.1 Results of stereotactic body radiation therapy (SBRT) for pancreatic cancer

Group	Patients	Previous RT	SBRT dose	Local control	Distant control	Median survival (months)	One-year survival
Stanford Phase I (Koong et al. 2004)	15 LA	2/15	15–25 Gy × 1	100% (25 Gy)	0% (25 Gy)	11	NR
Stanford Boost (Koong et al. 2005)	16 LA	16/16; 45 Gy with 5-FU	25 Gy × 1	94%	0%	8.3	15%
Stanford gemcitabine (Schellenberg et al. 2008)	16 LA	No	25 Gy × 1	81%	0%	11.4	50%
Danish phase II (Hoyer et al. 2005)	19 LA; 3 LR	No	10 Gy × 3	57%; 2 PR	13%	5.7	5%
Beth Israel Deaconess (Mahadevan et al. 2007)	21 LA; 3 LR	No; 3/3	8–12 Gy × 3	79% at 8 months	55% at 8 months	NR	75% at 8 months
Beth Israel Deaconess (Mahadevan et al. 2007)	8 PM	No	10 Gy × 1	100% at 8.8 months	75% at 8.8 months	NR	75% at 8.8 months
University of Pittsburgh (Parikh et al. 2008)	9 PM	2/9	16–24 Gy × 1	100% at 5 months	89% at 5 months	NR	NR
Georgetown University (Lominska et al. 2008)	28 LR	28/28; Median dose 50.4 Gy with chemo	20–30 Gy total; 3–5 fractions	86% (12/14)	43%	5.3	25% at 8 months

LA locally advanced, *LR* locally recurrent, *PM* positive margins, *PR* partial response, *NR* not reported
Adapted from Chang and Saif (2008)

Table 25.2 Toxicity of stereotactic body radiation therapy (SBRT) for pancreatic cancer

Group	Acute toxicity	Late toxicity	Notes
Stanford Phase I (Koong et al. 2004)	33% grade 1–2 GI	NR	
Stanford Boost (Koong et al. 2005)	69% grade 1–2 GI 12.5% grade 3 GI	12.5% grade 2 duodenal ulcers	
Stanford gemcitabine (Schellenberg et al. 2008)	12.5% grade 2 GI 6.3% grade 3 GI	31.3% grade 2 GI 6.3% grade 3 GI 6.3% grade 4 GI	47% had late toxicities 4–10 months after SBRT
Danish phase II (Hoyer et al. 2005)	79% grade 2+ at 14 days	18% "severe" GI mucositis/ ulceration 4.5% grade 4 gastric perforation	Increased pain, nausea, and decreased performance status seen at 14 days vs. baseline
Beth Israel Deaconess (Mahadevan et al. 2007 Nov 1)	25% grade 2 GI	4% grade 3 GI 4% grade 3 vascular	Toxicities reported for locally advanced and Local recurrence patients only
University of Pittsburgh (Parikh et al. 2008)	0%	NR	Limited follow-up
Georgetown University (Lominska et al. 2008)	NR	7% GI (1 abscess, 1 bowel obstruction)	

NR not reported
Adapted from Chang and Saif (2008)

pre-operative SBRT can improve the gross total resection rates in patients with borderline resectable pancreatic cancer. We currently use a three fraction regimen (12 Gy×3 over 5–7 days) for a total dose of 36 Gy of SBRT preoperatively in patients with borderline or marginally resectable disease as well as locally advanced unresectable tumors (Figs. 25.1 and 25.2). This fractionation scheme has a similar tumoricidal effect, but has potentially less normal tissue effect compared to 25 Gy in a single fraction based on BED calculations. The goal is to improve outcomes in this subset of patients. Given the relatively high rate of leaving microscopic or gross disease behind at the time of surgery, additional local therapy is warranted. Pancreatic cancer patients who undergo pancreatectomy whose disease is not completely resected fare as poorly as patients with unresectable disease to begin with. Conversely, patients who are able to undergo an R0 resection have improved survival compared to those who only achieve an R1 (gross or microscopic residual disease) (Raut et al. 2007). Therefore, achieving an R0 resection may result in improved overall survival. Neoadjuvant conventional fractionated radiotherapy in combination with chemotherapy has been used to achieve an acceptable R0 resection rate of approximately 40% (Katz et al. 2008; Massucco et al. 2006). Pre-operative radiation has the potential advantage of enhanced radiosensitivity from improved oxygenation of a pre-surgical field, reduced tumor seeding by surgical handling, and reduced toxicities due to a smaller radiation field. Furthermore, SBRT has been demonstrated to produce excellent local control and response

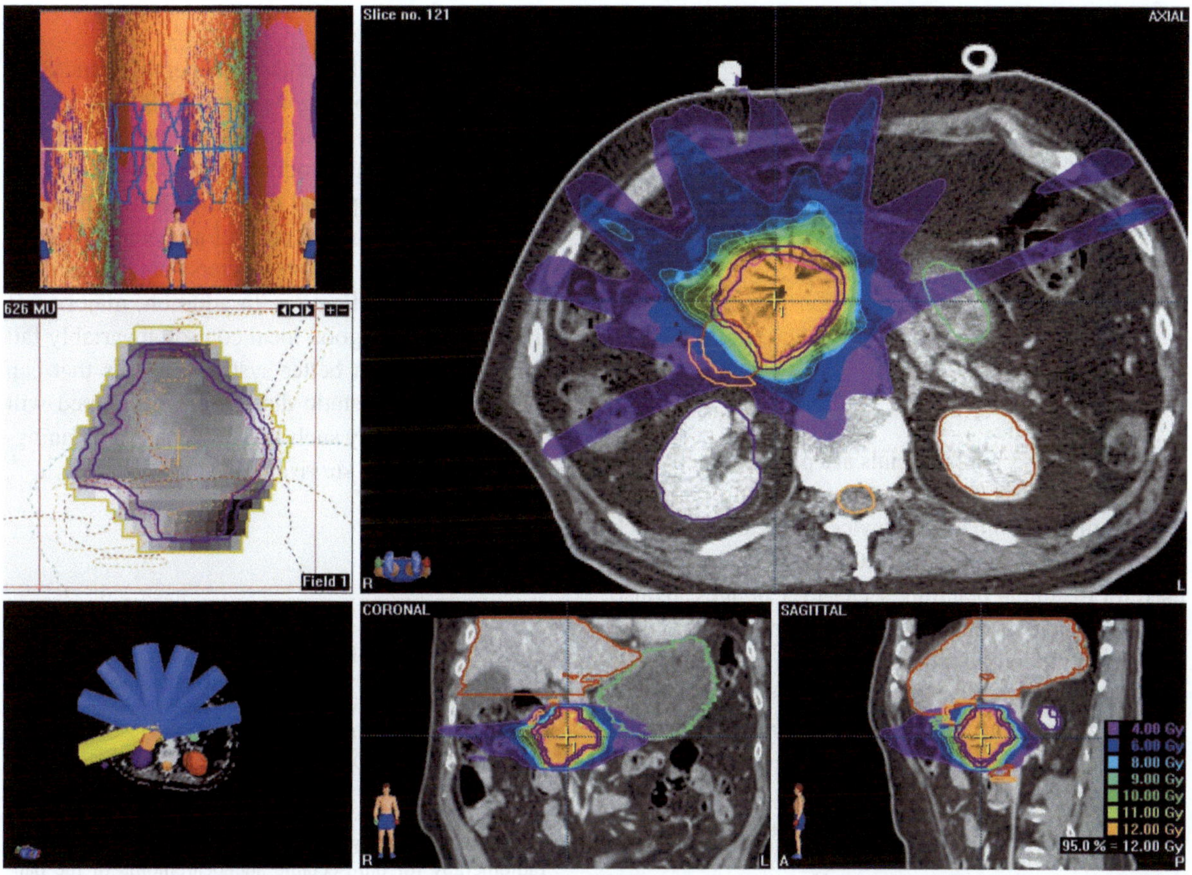

Fig. 25.1 Intensity modulated stereotactic radiosurgery treatment plan for a patient with locally advanced pancreatic adenocarcinoma treated at UCLA to a dose of 36 Gy in 3 fractions with the Novalis TX. 95% of the PTV (0–3 mm expansion of the ITV) is encompassed by the 100% prescription line. No more than 5% of the contoured duodenum risk object (1 cm above and below the GTV) receives more than 30 Gy, and no more than 50% of the contoured duodenum risk object receives more than 21 Gy. The contralateral duodenal wall closest to the GTV is limited to 18 Gy

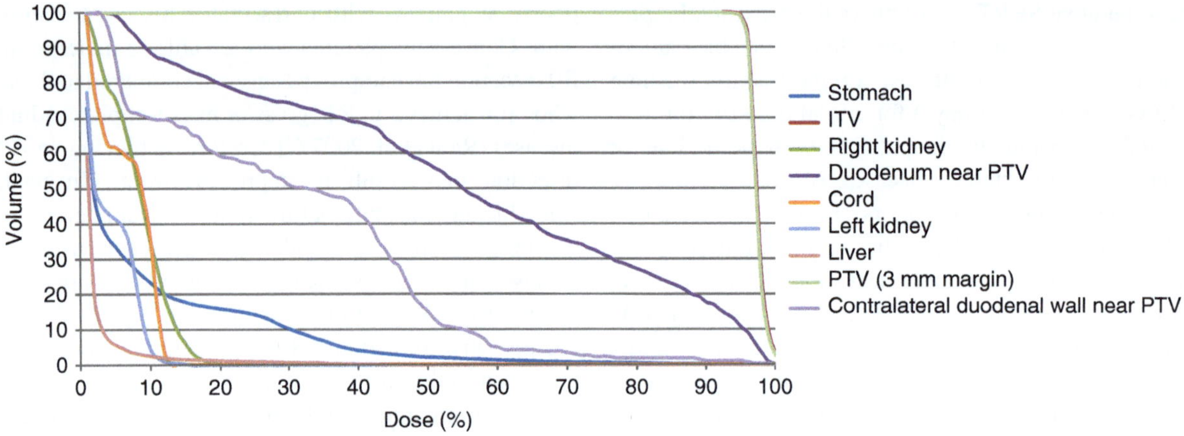

Fig. 25.2 Dose volume histogram (DVH) of the above treatment plan showing GTV, ITV, and PTV coverage as well as the DVH for the organs at risk: duodenum, small bowel, stomach, kidneys, liver, and spinal cord

in patients with unresectable disease. SBRT compared to fractionated conventional radiation has the additional benefits of a potentially higher biological effect, greater accuracy and precision, and a significantly shorter treatment course allowing patients to proceed to surgery sooner. We hypothesize that pre-operative SBRT alone can achieve as good if not improved R0 resection rate in borderline or marginally resectable pancreatic cancer patients with acceptable toxicity profiles.

25.3.1 Technique

Logistically, 2–3 gold fiducials are placed directly into the tumor under CT guidance for targeting purposes. A custom immobilization device is created for each patient, and four-dimensional CT (4D-CT) images are used for treatment planning. FDG-PET images are also used for treatment planning. An internal target volume (ITV) is contoured based on the 4D-CT, and the ITV is expanded by 0–3 mm (except for expansion into the duodenum or stomach) to form the PTV. 36 Gy in three fractions is prescribed to the isodose surface which covers the 95% of the PTV. No more than 5% of the contoured duodenum risk object (1 cm above and below the GTV) receives more than 30 Gy, and no more than 50% of the contoured duodenum risk object receives more than 21 Gy. For pancreatic head lesions, the dose to the contralateral duodenal wall closest to the GTV is limited to a total dose of 18 Gy. A Whipple procedure will be attempted within 4 weeks after SBRT.

25.4 Conclusions

Surgery is still the gold standard in operable pancreatic cancer. Recently publications using SBRT for locally advanced pancreatic cancer have shown promising local control, but can produce substantial acute and late toxicities. The optimal dose and fractionation for SBRT for pancreas tumor as well as potential use of radiosensitizer and radioprotectors are areas that require further investigation. In addition, majority of the patients, despite good local control, invariably fail distantly. Only when better systemic agents that can eradicate micrometastatic disease are developed will effective local therapy such as SBRT make a meaningful impact on patient survival.

References

Burris HA 3rd, Moore MJ, Andersen J et al (1997) Improvements in survival and clinical benefit with gemcitabine as first-line therapy for patients with advanced pancreas cancer: a randomized trial. J Clin Oncol 15(6):2403–2413

Chang BW, Saif MW (2008) Stereotactic body radiation therapy (SBRT) in pancreatic cancer: is it ready for prime time? JOP 9(6):676–682

Chang DT, Schellenberg D, Shen J et al (2009) Stereotactic radiotherapy for unresectable adenocarcinoma of the pancreas. Cancer 115(3):665–672

Fowler JF (1989) The linear-quadratic formula and progress in fractionated radiotherapy. Br J Radiol 62(740):679–694

Garcia-Barros M, Paris F, Cordon-Cardo C et al (2003) Tumor response to radiotherapy regulated by endothelial cell apoptosis. Science 300(5622):1155–1159

Guerrero M, Li XA (2004) Extending the linear-quadratic model for large fraction doses pertinent to stereotactic radiotherapy. Phys Med Biol 49(20):4825–4835

Hoyer M, Roed H, Sengelov L et al (2005) Phase-II study on stereotactic radiotherapy of locally advanced pancreatic carcinoma. Radiother Oncol 76(1):48–53

Jemal A, Siegel R, Ward E et al (2009) Cancer statistics, 2009. CA Cancer J Clin 59(4):225–249

Kalser MH, Ellenberg SS (1985) Pancreatic cancer. Adjuvant combined radiation and chemotherapy following curative resection. Arch Surg 120(8):899–903, Erratum in: Arch Surg 1986 Sep;121(9):1045

Katz MH, Pisters PW, Evans DB et al (2008) Borderline resectable pancreatic cancer: the importance of this emerging stage of disease. J Am Coll Surg 206(5):833–846

Koong AC, Le QT, Ho A et al (2004) Phase I study of stereotactic radiosurgery in patients with locally advanced pancreatic cancer. Int J Radiat Oncol Biol Phys 58(4):1017–1021

Koong AC, Christofferson E, Le QT et al (2005) Phase II study to assess the efficacy of conventionally fractionated radiotherapy followed by a stereotactic radiosurgery boost in patients with locally advanced pancreatic cancer. Int J Radiat Oncol Biol Phys 63(2):320–323

Lominska CE, Nasr NM, Silver NL, Gagnon GJ (2008) Salvage stereotactic radiosurgery for locally recurrent previously irradiated pancreatic cancer. Int J Radiat Oncol Biol Phys 72(1):S276–S277

Mahadevan A, Shanmugam L, Kaplan I et al (2007) Fractionated radiosurgery for pancreas cancer. Int J Radiat Oncol Biol Phys 69(3):S307

Massucco P, Capussotti L, Magnino A et al (2006) Pancreatic resections after chemoradiotherapy for locally advanced ductal adenocarcinoma: analysis of perioperative outcome and survival. Ann Surg Oncol 13(9):1201–1208

Moertel CG, Frytak S, Hahn RG et al (1981) Therapy of locally unresectable pancreatic carcinoma: a randomized comparison of high dose (6000 rads) radiation alone, moderate dose radiation (4000 rads + 5-fluorouracil), and high dose radiation + 5-fluorouracil: The Gastrointestinal Tumor Study Group. Cancer 48(8):1705–1710

Papiez L, Timmerman R, DesRosiers C, Randall M (2003) Extracranial stereotactic radioablation: physical principles. Acta Oncol 42(8):882–894

Parikh SD, Burton SA, Heron DE et al (2008) Stereotactic radiosurgery in patients with resected pancreatic carcinomas with positive margins. Int J Radiat Oncol Biol Phys 72(1): S272–S273

Park C, Papiez L, Zhang S et al (2008) Universal survival curve and single fraction equivalent dose: useful tools in understanding potency of ablative radiotherapy. Int J Radiat Oncol Biol Phys 70(3):847–852

Potters L, Steinberg M, Rose C et al (2004) American Society for Therapeutic Radiology and Oncology and American College of Radiology practice guideline for the performance of stereotactic body radiation therapy. Int J Radiat Oncol Biol Phys 60(4):1026–1032

Raut CP, Tseng JF, Sun CC et al (2007) Impact of resection status on pattern of failure and survival after pancreaticoduodenectomy for pancreatic adenocarcinoma. Ann Surg 246(1): 52–60

Schellenberg D, Goodman KA, Lee F et al (2008) Gemcitabine chemotherapy and single-fraction stereotactic body radiotherapy for locally advanced pancreatic cancer. Int J Radiat Oncol Biol Phys 72(3):678–686

Varadhachary GR, Tamm EP, Abbruzzese JL et al (2006) Borderline resectable pancreatic cancer: definitions, management, and role of preoperative therapy. Ann Surg Oncol 13(8):1035–1046

Verbeke CS (2008) Resection margins and R1 rates in pancreatic cancer–are we there yet? Histopathology 52(7):787–796

Verbeke CS, Leitch D, Menon KV et al (2006) Redefining the R1 resection in pancreatic cancer. Br J Surg 93(10):1232–1237

Willett CG, Czito BG, Bendell JC, Ryan DP (2005) Locally advanced pancreatic cancer. J Clin Oncol 23(20):4538–4544

Prostate SBRT

26

Guy Soete

26.1 Clinical Aspects

Prostate cancer (PC) is currently the most common male cancer in most western countries, representing 30% of malignant tumors in men (Jemal et al. 2006). The major prognostic factors in localized prostate cancer are Gleason score, initial prostate-specific antigen (iPSA) and T stage. The terms "organ confined" and "locally advanced" disease refer to T1-T2 and T3-T4 respectively. These three prognostic factors are combined in nomograms that predict the risk of microscopic extracapsular extension, seminal vesicle (SV), and nodal involvement (D'Amico et al. 1999; Partin et al. 1997). They provide a scientific basis for treatment choice (local, locoregional and/or hormonal), allow radiation oncologists to choose the clinical target volume (CTV: prostate ± SV ± iliac lymph nodes), and ultimately predict patient outcome (Kattan et al. 1998; Kattan et al. 2001; Kattan et al. 2000). Men with indolent tumors and limited life expectancy have least to gain from submitting them to the hazards of curative treatment (Albertsen et al. 2005) and are managed by watchful waiting. "Active surveillance" (AS) refers to the strict follow-up of indolent PC in young men, leaving the possibility of a curative treatment in case of evolution to an aggressive cancer. The only active treatment that has been compared to watchful waiting in a contemporary randomized trial is radical prostatectomy (RP). RP showed a significant survival benefit and is therefore considered the gold standard for the treatment of young men with organ confined PC (Bill-Axelson et al. 2005). Whether this holds true with current high dose - high precision radiotherapy (RT) techniques remains controversial. Freedom from biochemical failure (FFBF) after RP, brachytherapy (BT) and high-dose contemporary RT are comparable (Kupelian et al. 2004).

The different treatment modalities cause different amounts of chronic bladder, bowel, and sexual dysfunction (Merrick et al. 2005; Miller et al. 2005; Potosky et al. 2004; Talcott et al. 1998). Urinary continence is mainly impaired after RP with 10–30% of patients requiring pads after treatment compared to 5–10% after RT or BT. Obstructive and irritative urinary complaints are mainly reported after BT and RT. Bowel dysfunction with cramps, bleeding, diarrhea and bowel urgency is reported by 10–20% of patients after RT. Erectile dysfunction is reported in 60–90% of the patients after RP compared to 50–60% after RT and BT.

26.2 General Aspects of Prostate Cancer Radiotherapy

26.2.1 Dose Escalation

When PSA was introduced in the late 1980s, it became apparent that the majority of patients treated with the low radiation doses (≤70 Gy) used at that time experienced a rising post-treatment PSA, indicating subsequent clinical failure. This prompted radiotherapists to stepwise escalate the dose. Four large reports on dose escalation in the PSA era (Hanks et al. 2000; Lyons et al. 2000; Pollack et al. 2000; Zelefsky et al. 1998) and five randomized trials (Dearnaley et al. 2005; Peeters et al. 2006; Pollack et al. 2002; Shipley et al. 1995; Zietman et al. 2005) have since then been

G. Soete
UZ Brussels, Laarbeeklaan 101, B-1090 Jette, Belgium
e-mail: guy.soete@uzbrussel.be

A.A.F. De Salles et al. (eds.), *Shaped Beam Radiosurgery*,
DOI: 10.1007/978-3-642-11151-8_26, © Springer-Verlag Berlin Heidelberg 2011

Table 26.1 Risk group definition and results from non-randomized and randomized dose-escalation trials

Non-randomized comparisons (Hanks et al. 2000; Lyons et al. 2000; Pollack et al. 2000; Zelefsky et al. 1998)		Data from phase III trials (Peeters et al. 2006; Zietman et al. 2005)	
Risk group definition	Benefit for high dose?	Benefit for high dose?	Risk group definition
Low: T1–2 and Gleason 2–6 and PSA < 10	No	Conflicting	Low: T1–2 and Gleason 2–6 and PSA < 10
Intermediate: all other	Yes	Yes	Intermediate: all other
High: presence of >1 adverse factors (T3–4, Gleason 7–10 or PSA > 10) or PSA > 20 combined with at least one other adverse factor	No	Yes	High: T3–4 and/or Gleason 8–10 and/or PSA >20 ng/ml

published. Of notice, different risk group definitions were used. As a consequence, the "high risk" patients in the randomized trials are different from the "high risk" from the non-randomized data (Table 26.1). The latter can in fact be considered "very high risk", which might explain the different findings in the non-randomized reports compared to the randomized trials.

The non-randomized comparisons of doses of 76–78 Gy to ~70 Gy consistently showed a benefit in terms of FFBF for intermediate risk patients. No significant gain was observed for low risk and results were conflicting for high risk patients.

The two most recent phase III trials provided data according to risk group (Table 26.1). The Massachusetts General Hospital (MGH) trial (393 patients, 70.2 Gy vs. 79.2 Gy) showed a significant gain in 5 year-FFBF from 61% to 80% as well as a gain in local control from 47% to 67%. Overall survival was identical in both arms. On subgroup analysis, the difference remained significant for the low and intermediate risk group. No conclusions could be drawn for the high risk group which consisted of only 33 patients (Zietman et al. 2005). The Dutch trial (664 patients, 68 Gy vs. 78 Gy) demonstrated a significant benefit of 5 year-FFBF from 54% to 64%. No other endpoints were reported. On subgroup analysis, the gain in the intermediate and high risk group remained significant. In contrast to the MGH trial, no benefit was observed for low risk patients (Peeters et al. 2006).

It can be concluded that dose escalation to doses ~78 Gy compared to ≤ 70 Gy favors the intermediate and high risk subgroups. Its role remains unclear for low risk patients. Delivering doses in the order of 78 Gy by means of old RT techniques resulted in a high rate of severe side effects, especially radiation rectitis. Two recent technical developments have dramatically increased the precision of radiation dose delivery and permit safe delivery of high radiation doses: conformal RT techniques (CRT) and image guided radiotherapy (IGRT).

26.2.2 Conformal and Image Guide Radiotherapy

The goal of external beam RT is to induce clonogenic cell death to the tumor cells with minimal collateral damage to the surrounding healthy tissues (bladder, rectum, penile bulb). CRT and IGRT contribute to achieve this goal in two distinct ways. CRT provides dose distributions accurately shaped to the planning target volume (PTV). Intensity modulated RT (IMRT) can be considered a sophisticated type of CRT. IMRT allows for "dose painting" (the on purpose delivery of different doses to different regions in the PTV) and creating steep dose gradients and concave dose distributions. This is of particular importance in PC where the posterior border of the PTV may be concave and touches the rectal wall.

At least equally important as conformality is the accurate spatial delivery of the conformal dose distribution to the PTV. IGRT refers to the use of imaging (e.g. X-rays, CT or ultrasound) instead of skin drawings and lasers for more accurate patient positioning. These technologies bear in common that they intend to reduce setup errors. Setup errors are by convention reported as 1 standard deviation (SD) for the patient population (Kutcher et al. 1995). So-called "margin-recipes" mathematically relate the SD of organ motion and patient setup errors to margins required for adequate target coverage (Bel et al. 1996; van Herk et al. 2000). Ultimately IGRT should allow for narrowing the safety margins around the CTV, less normal tissue irradiation, and a reduction of side-effects. IGRT techniques are even more important in hypofractionated RT for PC. Such schedules are increasingly being used and the risk of impaired cure due to geographical miss is statistically larger compared to classical fractionation (Song et al. 2006).

26.2.3 Hypofractionation

Normal tissues and tumors show different sensitivities to changes in fractionation due to their varying ability to repair sublethal radiation damage (SLD). This sensitivity can be quantified through the α/β ratio in the linear-quadratic model (Thames et al. 1982). Early responding normal tissues (~acute toxicity) and most tumors inefficiently repair SLD. They are therefore relatively insensible to fractionation (~high α/β ratio) and cell kill is mainly the function of the total dose and treatment time. Late responding normal tissues efficiently repair SLD between fractions (~low α/β ratio). Therefore, fractionating will preferentially spare late responding normal tissues compared to most tumors (and early responding normal tissues). This has been the basis for "conventional fractionation" that uses fractions in the order of 2 Gy.

Combined analysis of patient outcome after RT and BT has recently led to the assumption that the α/β ratio of PC is lower than for most other tumors. Values between 1.2 and 4 Gy have been proposed (Brenner and Hall 1999; Brenner et al. 2002; Chappell et al. 2004; Fowler et al. 2001; Kal and Van Gellekom 2003; King and Mayo 2000; Wang et al. 2003). The low α/β ratio of prostate cancer could allow for radiation schedules that are more convenient (fewer fractions and shorter overall treatment time).

Some clinical data on hypofractionation have been reported (Kupelian et al. 2005; Livsey et al. 2003; Lloyd-Davies et al. 1990; Mahadevan et al. 2005; Ritter et al. 2005; Tsuji et al. 2005). Acute toxicity rates after hypofractionated RT vary with the specific fraction size, total dose, and overall treatment time that are being used, but the different groups agree that it is higher than for conventional fractionation. In addition, three randomized trials comparing hypofractionation to conventional fractionation have been published (Lukka et al. 2005; Pollack et al. 2006; Yeoh et al. 2006). Severe (grade 3–4) toxicity occurred in ~3% of the patients in both arms. The dose levels used in the Canadian (Lukka et al. 2005) and Australian (Yeoh et al. 2006) trials (~65 Gy) would be considered inappropriately low today. In the most recent trial, Pollack et al. used doses ~80 Gy but long-term results from this trial are not available yet (Pollack et al. 2006). In conclusion, hypofractionated RT for PC at present must be considered an experimental treatment.

26.3 Novalis® Radiosurgery-Conformal Image-Guided Radiotherapy: The UZ Brussels Experience

26.3.1 Introduction

The Novalis® Radiosurgery system (Brainlab AG, Feldkirchen, Germany) was one of the first commercially available CRT/IGRT systems. For a detailed description of the different positioning and treatment delivery options we refer to the physics chapter (part III). Since its first use in the treatment of PC at the UZ Brussels (UZB) in 2000, over 600 PC patients have been treated. The system has been the subject of several studies regarding patient positioning, treatment delivery, and clinical patient outcome (Arcangeli et al. 2009; Engels et al. 2009; Linthout et al. 2007; Soete et al. 2002a, 2002b, 2006a, b, c, 2007; Verellen et al. 2002; Verellen et al. 2003), which will be summarized in the following paragraphs.

26.3.2 Procedure

Patients treated with Novalis Radiosurgery at UZB are a selected group of men with either a low (<10%) risk of microscopic nodal involvement or proven pathologically node negative after laparoscopic lymphadenectomy. For other cases we consider whole pelvic irradiation indicated (Roach et al. 2003) which is not compatible with Novalis Radiosurgery (maximum field size at isocenter distance 9.8×9.8 cm).

Implanted markers for prostate visualization were rarely used till 2006. At present 50% of the patients receive marker implantation. Three gold seeds are placed under transrectal ultrasound guidance (GoldlockTM,

Beampoint, Kista, Sweden). The classical simulation has not been abandoned. Its purpose is to have skin drawings available at the moment of planning CT in order to avoid systematic rotational errors between the planning CT and the treatment. One could argue that this has become redundant since the introduction of the Robotics Tilt Module. The ability of the latter system to correct for rotational errors is however limited (to 2.5°, 3° and 10° for tilt, roll and yaw respectively). Patients are scanned with the infrared (IR) markers in place and with filled bladder.

The first steps in the planning procedure are the automatic marker localization and delineation of CTV, bladder and rectum. For patients with a low risk (<10%) of SV involvement, the CTV consists of the prostate only. Else it is limited to the proximal half of the SV (Kestin et al. 2002). CTV to PTV margins in anteroposterior (AP), craniocaudal (CC) and left-right (LR) directions are 10–10–6 mm for patients without implanted markers and 5–5–3 mm for those with markers. The prescribed isocenter dose is 78 Gy for intermediate risk patients and 70 Gy for low and high risk, defined as in the retrospective reports available at that time (Table 26.1).

Late rectal toxicity appears to be the limiting factor in dose escalation and the significant rectal dose-volume thresholds that have been reported are fairly consistent. The following dose-volume thresholds for the rectum are applied: Rvol 75 Gy, Rvol 70 Gy, Rvol 60 Gy and Rvol 50 Gy (i.e. the rectal volume receiving 75, 70, 60, and 50 Gy) should be <10%, <25%, <50% and <60% of the rectal volume. Late G2–3 rectal toxicity is observed in 5–10% and >25% of patients respectively, below and above these thresholds (Boersma et al. 1998; Fiorino et al. 2003; Kuban et al. 2003; Zapatero et al. 2004). Dose-volume constraints for (partial) bladder irradiation are far less established and not taken into account during planning.

Patients are treated in supine position with conventional head, knee and ankle support. Positioning involves either daily co-registration of X-rays with digitally reconstructed radiographs (DRR) from the planning CT or - if available - marker fusion. In 2005 the Robotics Tilt Module was installed under the treatment couch, allowing for full 6° of freedom-setup correction.

Based on clinical findings (cf. paragraph 3.5), some changes in the procedure were implemented over the last few years. At present, all patients receive rectal enema for the planning CT, in case of markers, isotropic margins of 6 mm are used and all patients are treated with 78 Gy.

26.3.3 ExacTrac® X-Ray Positioning

The setup accuracy of ExacTrac X-ray was first assessed by phantom measurements (Verellen et al. 2003). Various combinations of known translational and rotational deviations were introduced and compared to the translational and rotational deviations that were actually detected by the system. Residual errors (i.e. after accepting the proposed shifts and repositioning of the phantom) were measured by the hidden target test. The overall 3-D displacement vector for the co-registration of X-rays with DRR was 0.6 ± 0.9 mm. For marker fusion, an even smaller value of 0.3 ± 0.4 mm was obtained. The residual errors (95% confidence interval) were 2–4 mm for DRR co-registration and 1–2 mm for markers. The next logical step was to investigate setup-accuracy in a clinical setting. Data were acquired from a total of 984 treatment fractions in 58 patients. Setup errors were determined by measuring the distance from the beam isocenter to the anterior, superior, and midline aspect of the pubic bone on orthogonal Megavolt images.

The following positioning procedures were compared:

1. Conventional positioning with skin drawings and lasers
2. ExacTrac positioning using IR markers
3. ExacTrac X-ray co-registration of X-rays with DRRs without correction for rotations
4. ExacTrac X-ray co-registration of X-rays with DRRs with correction for rotations (Robotics Tilt Module).
5. ExacTrac X-ray marker fusion without correction for rotations

Figure 26.1 represents the pooled data from the various published studies (Soete et al. 2002a, b, 2006b, 2007). The stepwise implementation of the different positioning procedures gradually reduced setup uncertainty. Ultimately in step 4, the setup errors became comparable to the accuracy of the measurement itself. Since that time the use of Megavolt images to verify setup has been abandoned at the UZB. It has been suggested that couch corrections prior to treatment might cause secondary counteract patient motion (Lauve et al. 2006). In the experience of UZB, secondary patient motion is below 2 mm and 2° for translations and rotations rsp. in over 90% of cases (Linthout et al. 2007). The setup accuracy in case of implanted marker is comparable to step 4 but obviously offers the additional advantage of direct prostate targeting and overcomes the problem of interfraction prostate motion. ExacTrac X-ray marker

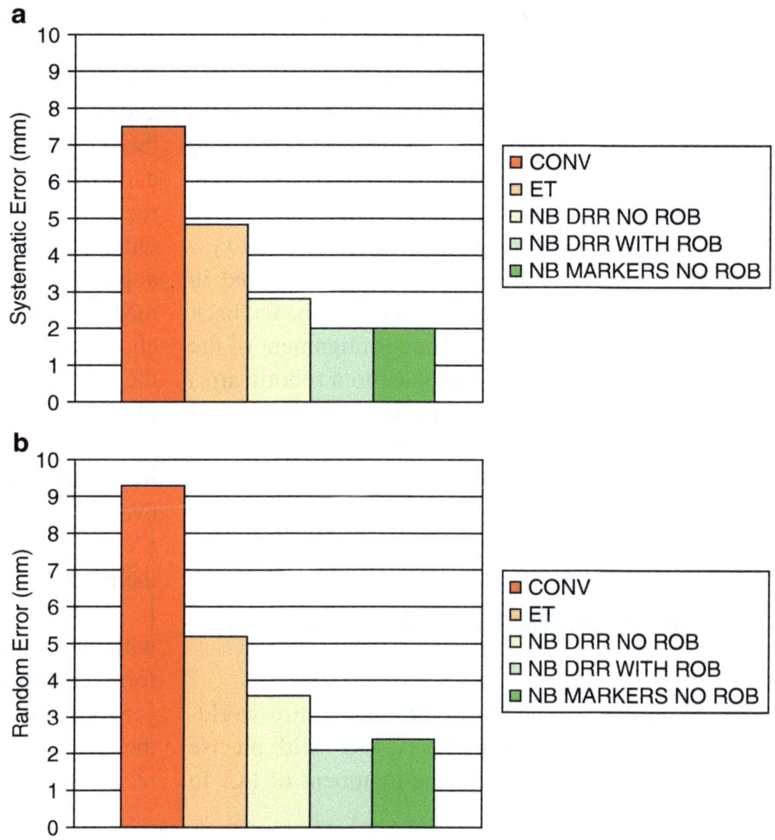

Fig. 26.1 Systematic (**a**) and random (**b**) setup errors represented as the overall 3-D displacement vector for different positioning methods: *1* Conventional positioning with skin drawings and lasers (*CONV*), *2* ExacTrac positioning (*ET*), *3* ExacTrac X-ray co-registration of X-rays with DRRs without correction for rotations by Robotics Tilt Module (*NB BRR NO ROB*), *4* ExacTrac X-ray co-registration of X-rays with DRRs with Robotics (*NB BRR WITH ROB*) and *5* ExacTrac X-ray marker fusion without Robotics (*NB MARKERS NO ROB*)

fusion with correction for rotations (Robotics Tilt Module) is currently under investigation.

The ideal IGRT system would allow for daily prostate imaging without possible introduction of errors due to image-acquisition itself, do so within a reasonable time frame, without the necessity for implanted markers and preferentially without exposing the patient to radiation. A solution that combines all these features does not exist so far.

The technical tools that are currently most frequently used for PC IGRT are Electronic Portal Imaging (EPI), X-ray positioning, ultrasound and CT based positioning. EPI was the first widely used IGRT modality (Hanks et al. 2000). The main difference between EPI and the Novalis Body X-ray positioning procedure is that EPI is a time consuming procedure that verifies positioning whereas ExacTrac X-ray is a positioning procedure. The linac time including X-ray positioning and irradiation is short (around 10') which is a prerequisite for daily use. The images are kV and therefore of better quality compared to EPI. The radiation exposure to the patient for a 78 Gy treatment is estimated 40 mSv which is at least 10x less compared to EPI or IGRT using daily CT images (Verellen et al. 2003). A disadvantage, which this system has in common with EPI, is that prostate visualization requires implantation of radio-opaque markers.

More recently, ultrasound and CT (kV or MV, cone beam or fan beam) for daily prostate positioning have been introduced in clinical practice (Court et al. 2003; Huang et al. 2002; Jaffray et al. 2002; Lattanzi et al. 1999; Mackie et al. 2003; Pouliot et al. 2006). Daily ultrasound positioning is an attractive method because no radiation is involved and the prostate itself is positioned without the need for implanted markers. However, with ultrasound positioning, there are concerns about the possible introduction of errors during image acquisition by pressure to the patient's lower abdomen (Langen et al. 2003; Vvan den Heuvel and Powell 2003). Positioning systems based on CT imaging allow for volumetric prostate imaging without the need for markers. Because of time requirements and radiation exposure to the patient they are generally used in off-line setup correction instead of daily use.

Intrafraction prostate motion remains one of the limiting factors for reducing the PTV to CTV safety margins. Tools to deal with intrafraction prostate motion should combine tumor tracking, provide motion feedback to the multileaf collimator or linac and finally target tracking by dynamic MLC or dynamic movement of the linac itself. The only system combining these features that has reached clinical implementation so far is the CyberKnife™ (Accuray, Sunnyvale, USA). It uses X-ray information as the ExacTrac X-ray system. The position of the target can be monitored in fluoroscopy mode and this information can be fed back to the robot, allowing for continuous alignment of the beam (generated by a linac mounted to a robotic arm) with the target. Drawbacks of this system are the need for implanted markers and fluoroscopy and the long (30–40') treatment time (Gibbs 2006).

26.4 Novalis Conformal Arc and Intensity Modulated Radiotherapy

The UZ Brussels is currently the only centre worldwide that uses conformal arc RT (CART) with precise beam shaping by mMLC for the treatment of PC. In daily routine, a CART plan is first calculated aiming at coverage of the CTV by the 100% isodose (78 Gy) and the PTV by the ≥90% isodose (70.2 Gy). Gantry start and stop angles are 200° and 160° (the posterior 40° "wedge" is not used in order to avoid the stabilizing carbon bars underneath the treatment couch). If the rectal dose-volume criteria are met, the plan is accepted. Otherwise an IMRT plan is calculated (five static fields at gantry angles 0°, 75°, 135°, 225° and 285°, with the mMLC in dynamic MLC mode). To some extent the choice is a coincidental one, since it depends upon the specific "snapshot" anatomical situation on the planning CT.

The shape of the PTV was shown to be of crucial importance for the choice of treatment delivery (Verellen et al. 2002). For a concave PTV (prostate + SV), IMRT is clearly superior to conformal arc therapy in achieving rectal sparing. A clinical example is given in Fig. 26.2. For a convex PTV (prostate without SV), IMRT does not perform better than conformal arc therapy. Both are able to create an inhomogeneous dose distribution (i.e. PTV underdosage) in the overlap zone with the rectum. For CART, the rectum is blocked from the lateral angles (90 ± 10°

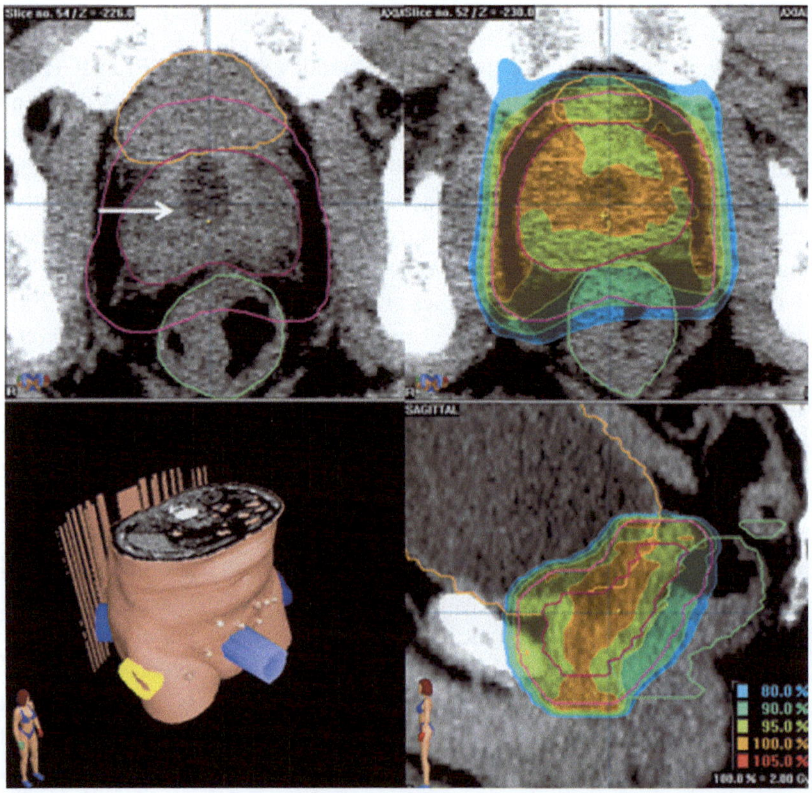

Fig. 26.2 PC treatment planning with Novalis IMRT. This 64-year old man underwent a TUR for urinary obstruction (TUR-defect indicated by arrow). A PC stage T1a was discovered, Gleason 7, iPSA 10 ng/ml. The risk of SV involvement was estimated 20% and the base of the SV was included in the CTV. This patient was under anticoagulant treatment which he was afraid to interrupt. Therefore no markers were implanted and margins around the CTV were set as 10–10–6 mm AP-CC-LR. Because of the concave shape of the PTV, rectal sparing could not be adequately obtained with CART. The high-dose region in the IMRT plan coincides with the concavity in the PTV

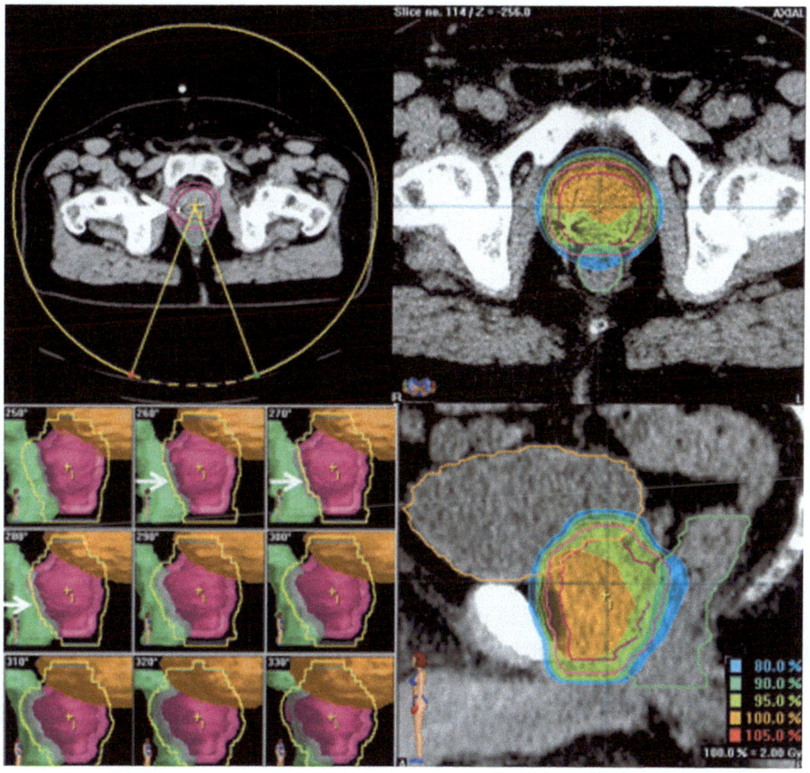

Fig. 26.3 PC treatment planning with Novalis CART. This asymptomatic 75-year-old man underwent random prostate biopsies because of an elevated PSA of 7 ng/ml. A T1c PC was found, Gleason 6. The risk of SV involvement was <10% and CTV consisted of prostate only. Markers were implanted and isotropic margins of 6 mm around the CTV were used. Because of the convex shape of the PTV, adequate target coverage and rectal sparing could be obtained with CART by blocking the rectum from the lateral angles of the arc (*arrow*)

and 270 ± 10°) resulting in a posterior blurred dose distribution in order to meet rectal dose-volume constraints and at the same time provide adequate dose coverage of the PTV. A clinical illustration is given in Fig. 26.3.

In case of a convex target, conformal arc therapy is the treatment of choice because of several advantages compared to IMRT. Planning and treatment are faster by a factor of about 5. CART is equally faster compared to other conformal non-IMRT techniques with multiple static beams because for each treatment fraction the parameters for irradiation need to be entered only once instead of for each separate field. Apart from the advantage in terms of economics, shorter treatment time is more convenient to patients and intrafraction movements will be less important as compared to IMRT. Finally, total body radiation exposure is directly related to the beam-on time which is much higher with IMRT (more "wasted photons"). At UZB 8 out of 10 patients are treated with CART. We must however emphasize that this situation is related to the selection of patients with mainly organ confined disease in which the SV were either not or only partially treated.

26.4.1 Clinical Results

Data on the clinical outcome of patients treated with Novalis conformal IGRT are available for both conventional fractionation (Engels et al. 2009; Soete et al. 2006c) and hypofractionation (Arcangeli et al. 2009; Soete et al. 2006a). Toxicity was scored according to RTOG/EORTC criteria (Cox et al. 1995). For FFBF the Phoenix-definition ("nadir + 2") was used (Roach et al. 2006).

The first group consists of 238 men treated between 2000 and 2004 with a median follow-up of 60 months (25–93 m). Patient characteristics are given in Table 26.2. Patients in the intermediate risk group were treated with 78 Gy; the others with 70 Gy. HT was prescribed in one-third of them. At that time the margins around the PTV were 10–10–6 mm and 5–5–3 mm in the AP, CC and LR direction for patients without ($n = 213$) and with implanted markers ($n = 25$) respectively. Treatment was mainly delivered by conformal arc RT (230 patients); IMRT was used in the remaining eight patients.

The early toxicity profile was excellent given the absence of grade 3–4 and the low rate of RTOG grade 2 (i.e. requiring medication) side effects: GI 6% and GU

Table 26.2 Disease characteristics of 238 patients treated with Novalis image guided CART (number of patients)

T stage		Gleason score		Initial PSA		UZB risk group	
1	(124)	2–6	(171)	0–4	(14)	low	(105)
2	(92)	7	(55)	>4–10	(128)	intermediate	(120)
3	(22)	8–10	(12)	>10–20	(74)	high-very high	(13)
				>20	(22)		

16%. Five-year freedom from severe grade 3–4 late side effects was 100% for GI and 99.4% for GU. Five-year FFBF is excellent with rates of 93%, 86% and 77% for the low, intermediate and high risk group respectively (Fig. 26.4). As expected, on multivariate analysis, higher risk group and lower dose were associated with impaired FFBF ($p<0.001$ and $p=0.027$ rsp.). The same was true for the presence of a distended rectum on the planning CT ($p=0.023$). To our surprise, the use of markers for patient positioning resulted in a trend for worse FFBF ($p=0.047$).

The experience with hypofractionation is more limited and follow-up for this group is insufficient to draw definitive conclusions regarding late side effects and FFBF. This group consists of 33 men treated between 2004 and 2006 with a median follow-up of 14 months (2–34 m). These patients were treated in a prospective phase II trial investigating a RT schedule consisting of 56 Gy delivered in 16 fractions of 3.5 Gy over a 4 week treatment time. For an α/β estimation between 1.5 and 4 Gy this corresponds to a dose of 70–80 Gy in conventional 2 Gy fractions. HT was prescribed in 17 of these 33 patients. The same margins were used as for the patients treated with conventional RT. Markers were used in six patients. Treatment was delivered by conformal arc RT in 27 patients and by IMRT in six patients.

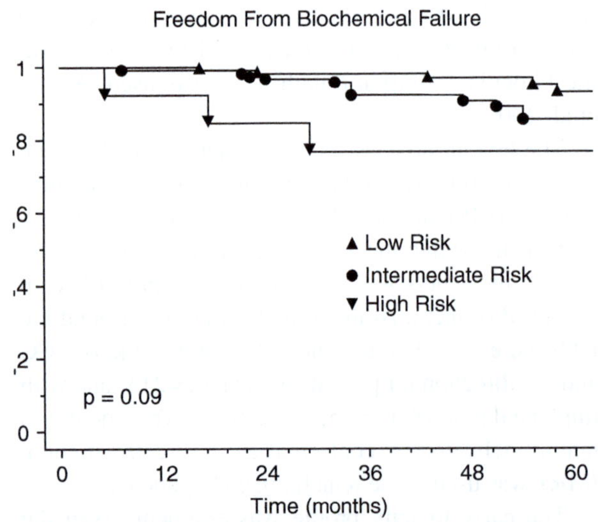

Fig. 26.4 Kaplan-Meier graph representing FFBF of 238 patients treated with Novalis image guided CART

Only one severe early side effect occurred (grade 3 GU)… The percentages of "minor to moderate" (grade 1 or more) and "moderate" (grade 2 or more) GI and GU side effects was significantly higher compared to the control group of patients treated with conventional fractionation (Table 26.3). However all side effects had disappeared 2 months after treatment. So far only one patient experienced severe late toxicity (grade 3 GU). Two-year FFBF appears equally favorable with rates of 100%, 86%, and 80% for the low, intermediate, and high risk group respectively. Further follow-up is needed to confirm these data.

Recently, several groups have demonstrated the negative impact on FFBF of a distended rectum on the planning CT (de Crevoisier et al. 2005; Heemsbergen et al. 2007). We were able to confirm this and at present all patients receive rectal enema for the planning CT (Soete et al. 2006a). In the 25 patients in whom implanted markers were used for positioning, arbitrary chosen non-uniform margins of 3 mm LR and 5 mm in the AP and CC were applied to compensate for intrafraction prostate motion. The very narrow LR margin may lead to an underdosage of the lateral portion of the

Table 26.3 Percentage acute GI and GU toxicity for conventional ($n=238$) and hypofractionated ($n=33$) prostate treatments with Novalis

	GI		GU	
	≥grade 1	≥grade 2	≥grade 1	≥grade 2
Conventional	25	6	53	16
Hypofractionation	56	16	84	38

peripheral zone where most tumors arise. Second, in retrospect it turned out that the planning system is unable to handle CC margins that are not a multiple from the planning CT slice-thickness (2 mm). Therefore, the real CC margin was not the requested 5 mm but 4 mm instead. Third, the beam penumbra for a conformal arc plan is usually smaller than for static beams, rendering target coverage even more challenging if inadequate margins are used. Based upon data concerning intrafraction prostate motion that have been published since then and the margin recipe by Van Herk et al. (Aubry et al. 2004; van Herk et al. 2000) isotropic margins of 6 mm are considered appropriate for marker positioning. Based on the favorable toxicity profile, all patients are treated with 78 Gy since 2006.

The implementation of the Novalis system for PC treatment was not an isolated event. Several other factors have undoubtedly contributed to the favorable results. Patients treated with Novalis are selected for a low risk of nodal involvement and are not exposed to the hazards of whole pelvic irradiation. In contrast to the situation prior to Novalis, the SV are not or only partially included in the CTV. For rectal sparing evidence-based dose-volume constraints are used. At present, we systematically combine RT with long-term HT in all patients with locally advanced disease (Bolla et al. 2002; Pilepich et al. 2005). Short term HT is prescribed for T1-T2 disease in the presence of a Gleason score 7–10 or an iPSA > 10 ng/ml (D'Amico et al. 2004).

26.5 Conclusion and Future Directions

The Novalis Radiosurgery system offers PC patients the opportunity for precise high-dose CRT and IMRT. Because the different components are fully integrated it is a fast procedure suitable for routine clinical use. ExacTrac X-ray was shown to perform accurately both on phantom measurements and in a clinical setting. From a clinical point of view severe side effects are a rare event and biochemical control appears favorable. These results are equally affected by patient selection and changes in clinical practice over time.

A weak point of ExacTrac X-ray is the need for implanted markers to compensate for interfraction prostate motion. It has in common with most other IGRT systems that continuous monitoring intrafraction organ motion with dynamic correction is not feasible. Intrafraction motion has been mentioned earlier as a limiting factor for reduction of margins around the CTV. A second limiting factor is the delineation uncertainty of the prostate on planning CT, mainly in the apical region. Magnetic resonance imaging and recently available CT-MRI co-registration software allow for more precise prostate delineation. Other advantages of MRI are the possibility to visualize the gross tumor volume, the ability to detect extracapsular extension or SV invasion not detected by transrectal ultrasound and the visualization of the penile bulb (Wallner et al. 2002; Wang et al. 2006). Avoiding penile bulb irradiation is believed to be beneficial with regard to erectile function (Mangar et al. 2006; Wernicke et al. 2004). Improved imaging during RT planning with MRI, dynamic contrast enhanced MRI or MRI-spectroscopy can enable us to identify the gross tumoral lesion (Futterer et al. 2006). As most recurrences occur within this lesion, overdosage of the lesion might improve outcome after RT (Cellini et al. 2002; De Meerleer et al. 2005). The use of MRI in prostate RT planning is currently still hampered by the limitations of CT-MRI co-registration software, especially for non-rigid co-registration (i.e. taking into account shape differences between CT and MRI).

References

Albertsen PC, Hanley JA, Fine J (2005) 20-year outcome following conservative management of clinically localized prostate cancer. JAMA 293:2095–2101

Arcangeli S, Strigari L, Soete G et al (2009) Clinical and dosimetric predictors of acute toxicity after a 4-week hypofractionated external beam radiotherapy regimen for prostate cancer: results from a multicentric prospective trial. Int J Radiat Oncol Biol Phys 73(1):39–45

Aubry JF, Beaulieu L, Girouard LM et al (2004) Measurements of intrafraction motion and interfraction and intrafraction rotation of prostate by three-dimensional analysis of daily portal imaging with radiopaque markers. Int J Radiat Oncol Biol Phys 60:30–39

Bel A, van Herk M, Lebesque J (1996) Target margins for random geometrical uncertainties in conformal radiotherapy. Med Phys 23:1537–1545

Bill-Axelson A, Holmberg L, Ruutu M et al (2005) Radical prostatectomy versus watchful waiting in early prostate cancer. N Engl J Med 352:1977–1984

Boersma LJ, van den Brink M, Bruce AM et al (1998) Estimation of the incidence of late bladder and rectum complications after high-dose (70–78 Gy) conformal for prostate cancer, using dose-volume histograms. Int J Radiat Oncol Biol Phys 41:83–92

Bolla M, Collette L, Blank L et al (2002) Long-term results with immediate androgen suppression and external irradiation in patients with locally advanced prostate cancer (an EORTC study): a phase III randomised trial. Lancet 360:103–108

Brenner DJ, Hall EJ (1999) Fractionation and protraction for radiotherapy of prostate carcinoma. Int J Radiat Oncol Biol Phys 43:1095–1101

Brenner DJ, Martinez AA, Edmundson GK et al (2002) Direct evidence that prostate tumours show high sensitivity to fractionation (low alpha/beta ratio), similar to late responding normal tissue. Int J Radiat Oncol Biol Phys 52:6–13

Cellini N, Morganti AG, Mattiucci GC et al (2002) Analysis of intraprostatic failures in patients treated with hormonal therapy and radiotherapy: implications for conformal therapy planning. Int J Radiat Oncol Biol Phys 53:595–599

Chappell R, Fowler J, Ritter M (2004) New data on the value of alpha/beta – evidence mounts that it is low. Int J Radiat Oncol Biol Phys 60:1002–1003

Court L, Rosen I, Mohan R et al (2003) Evaluation of mechanical precision and alignment uncertainties for an integrated CT/LINAC system. Med Phys 30:1198–1210

Cox JD, Stetz J, Pajak TF (1995) Toxicity criteria of the radiation therapy oncology group (RTOG) and the European organization for research and treatment of cancer (EORTC). Int J Radiat Oncol Biol Phys 31:1341–1346

D'Amico AV, Whittington R, Malkowicz SB et al (1999) Optimizing patient selection for dose escalation techniques using the prostate-specific antigen level, biopsy Gleason score, and clinical T-stage. Int J Radiat Oncol Biol Phys 45:1227–1233

D'Amico AV, Manola J, Loffredo M et al (2004) 6-month androgen suppression plus radiation therapy vs. radiation therapy alone for patients with clinically localized prostate cancer: a randomized controlled trial. JAMA 292:821–827

de Crevoisier R, Tucker SL, Dong L et al (2005) Increased risk of biochemical and local failure in patients with distended rectum on the planning CT for prostate cancer radiotherapy. Int J Radiat Oncol Biol Phys 62:965–973

De Meerleer G, Villeirs G, Bral S et al (2005) The magnetic resonance detected intraprostatic lesion in prostate cancer: planning and delivery of intensity-modulated radiotherapy. Radiother Oncol 75:325–333

Dearnaley DP, Hall E, Lawrence D et al (2005) Phase III pilot study of dose escalation using conformal radiotherapy in prostate cancer: PSA control and side effects. Br J Cancer 92:488–498

Engels B, Soete G, Verellen D et al (2009) Conformal arc radiotherapy for prostate cancer: increased biochemical failure in patients with distended rectum on the planning CT in spite of image guidance by implanted markers. Int J Radiat Oncol Biol Phys 74(2):388–391

Fiorino C, Sanguineti G, Cozzarini C et al (2003) Rectal dose-volume constraints in high-dose radiotherapy of localized prostate cancer. Int J Radiat Oncol Biol Phys 57:953–962

Fowler J, Chappell R, Ritter M et al (2001) Is alpha/beta for prostate tumours really low? Int J Radiat Oncol Biol Phys 50:1021–1031

Futterer JJ, Heijmink SW, Scheenen TW et al (2006) Prostate cancer localization with dynamic contrast-enhanced MR imaging and proton MR spectroscopic imaging. Radiology 241:449–458

Gibbs IC (2006) Frameless image-guided intracranial and extracranial radiosurgery using the Cyberknife robotic system. Cancer Radiothér 10:283–287

Hanks GE, Hanlon AL, Pinover WH et al (2000) Dose selection for prostate cancer patients based on dose comparison and dose response studies. Int J Radiat Oncol Biol Phys 46:823–832

Heemsbergen WD, Hoogeman MS, Witte MG et al (2007) Increased risk of biochemical and clinical failure for prostate patients with a large rectum at radiotherapy planning: results from the Dutch trial of 68 GY versus 78 Gy. Int J Radiat Oncol Biol Phys 67:1418–1424

Huang E, Dong L, Chandra A et al (2002) Intrafraction prostate motion during IMRT for prostate cancer. Int J Radiat Oncol Biol Phys 53:261–268

Hurkmans CW, Remeijer P, Lebesque JV et al (2001) Set-up verification using portal imaging; review of current clinical practice. Radiother Oncol 58:105–120

Jaffray DA, Siewerdsen JH, Wong JW et al (2002) Flat-panel cone-beam computed tomography for image-guided radiation therapy. Int J Radiat Oncol Biol Phys 53:1337–1349

Jemal A, Siegel R, Ward E et al (2006) Cancer statistics, 2006. CA Cancer J Clin 56:106–130

Kal HB, Van Gellekom MPR (2003) How low is the α/β ratio for prostate cancer? Int J Radiat Oncol Biol Phys 57: 1116–1121

Kattan MW, Eastham JA, Stapleton AM et al (1998) A preoperative nomogram for disease recurrence following radical prostatectomy for prostate cancer. J Natl Cancer Inst 90:766–771

Kattan MW, Zelefsky MJ, Kupelian PA et al (2000) Pretreatment nomogram for predicting the outcome of three-dimensional conformal radiotherapy in prostate cancer. J Clin Oncol 18:3352–3359

Kattan MW, Potters L, Blasko JC et al (2001) A preoperative nomogram for predicting freedom from recurrence after permanent prostate brachytherapy in prostate cancer. Urology 58:393–399

Kestin L, Goldstein N, Vicini F et al (2002) Treatment of prostate cancer with radiotherapy: should the entire seminal vesicles be included in the clinical target volume? Int J Radiat Oncol Biol Phys 54:686–697

King CR, Mayo CS (2000) Is the prostate α/β ratio of 1.5 from Brenner & Hall a modeling artifact? Int J Radiat Oncol Biol Phys 47:536–537

Kuban D, Pollack A, Huang E et al (2003) Hazards of dose escalation in prostate cancer radiotherapy. Int J Radiat Oncol Biol Phys 57:1260–1268

Kupelian PA, Potters L, Khuntia D et al (2004) Radical prostatectomy, external beam radiotherapy <72 Gy, external beam radiotherapy ≥ 72 Gy, permanent seed implantation or combined seeds/external beam radiotherapy for stage T1-T2 prostate cancer. Int J Radiat Oncol Biol Phys 58:25–33

Kupelian PA, Thakkar VV, Khuntia D et al (2005) Hypofractionated intensity-modulated radiotherapy (70 Gy at 2.5 Gy per fraction) for localized prostate cancer: long term outcomes. Int J Radiat Oncol Biol Phys 63:1463–1468

Kutcher GJ, Mageras GS, Leibel SA (1995) Control, correction, and modeling of setup errors and organ motion. Semin Radiat Oncol 5:134–145

Langen KM, Pouliot J, Anezinos C et al (2003) Evaluation of ultrasound-based prostate localization for image-guided radiotherapy. Int J Radiat Oncol Biol Phys 57:635–644

Lattanzi J, McNeeley S, Pinover W et al (1999) A comparison of daily CT localization to a daily ultrasound-based system in prostate cancer. Int J Radiat Oncol Biol Phys 43:719–725

Lauve AD, Siebers JV, Crimaldi AJ et al (2006) Dynamic compensation strategy to correct patient-positioning errors in conformal prostate radiotherapy. Med Phys 33:1879–1887

Linthout N, Verellen D, Tournel K et al (2007) Assessment of secondary patient motion induced by automated couch movement during on-line 6 dimensional repositioning in prostate cancer treatment. Radiother Oncol 83:68–74

Livsey JE, Cowan RA, Wylie JP et al (2003) Hypofractionated conformal radiotherapy in carcinoma of the prostate: five-year outcome analysis. Int J Radiat Oncol Biol Phys 57:1254–1259

Lloyd-Davies RW, Collins CD, Swan AV (1990) Carcinoma of the prostate treated by radical external beam radiotherapy using hypofractionation. Twenty-two years' experience (1962–1984). Urology 36:107–111

Lukka H, Hayter C, Julian JA et al (2005) Randomized trial comparing two fractionation schedules for patients with localized prostate cancer. J Clin Oncol 23:6132–6138

Lyons JA, Kupelian PA, Mohan DS et al (2000) Importance of high radiation doses (72 Gy or greater) in the treatment of stage T1-T3 adenocarcinoma of the prostate. Urology 55:85–90

Mackie TR, Kapatoes J, Ruchala K et al (2003) Image guidance for precise conformal radiotherapy. Int J Radiat Oncol Biol Phys 56:89–105

Mahadevan A, Kupelian P, Reddy C et al (2005) Comparison of two fractionation schedules for conformal radiation therapy for prostate cancer. Int J Radiat Oncol Biol Phys 63:S291

Mangar SA, Sydes MR, Tucker HL et al (2006) Evaluating the relationship between erectile dysfunction and dose received by the penile bulb: using data from a randomised controlled trial of conformal radiotherapy in prostate cancer (MRC RT01, ISRCTN47772397). Radiother Oncol 80:355–362

Merrick GS, Butler WM, Wallner KE et al (2005) Erectile function after prostate brachytherapy. Int J Radiat Oncol Biol Phys 62:437–447

Miller DC, Sanda MG, Dumn RL et al (2005) Long-term outcomes among localized prostate cancer survivors: health-related quality-of-life changes after radical prostatectomy, external radiation, and brachytherapy. J Clin Oncol 23:2772–2780

Partin AW, Kattan MW, Subong EN et al (1997) Combination of prostate-specific antigen, clinical stage, and Gleason score to predict pathological stage of localized prostate cancer. A multi-institutional update. JAMA 277:1445–1451

Peeters STH, Heemsbergen WD, Koper PCM et al (2006) Dose-response in radiotherapy for localized prostate cancer: results of the Dutch multicenter randomized phase III trial comparing 68 Gy of radiotherapy with 78 Gy. J Clin Oncol 24:1990–1996

Pilepich MV, Winter K, Lawton CA et al (2005) Androgen suppression adjuvant to definitive radiotherapy in prostate carcinoma – long-term results of phase III RTOG 85-31. Int J Radiat Oncol Biol Phys 61:1285–1290

Pollack A, Smith LG, von Eschenbach AC (2000) External beam radiotherapy dose response characteristics of 1127 men with prostate cancer treated in the PSA era. Int J Radiat Oncol Biol Phys 48:507–512

Pollack A, Zagars GK, Starkschall G et al (2002) Prostate cancer radiation dose response: results of the M. D. Anderson phase III randomized trial. Int J Radiat Oncol Biol Phys 53:1097–1105

Pollack A, Hanlon AL, Horwitz EM et al (2006) Dosimetry and preliminary acute toxicity in the first 100 men treated for prostate cancer on a randomized hypofractionation dose escalation trial. Int J Radiat Oncol Biol Phys 64:518–526

Potosky AL, Davis WW, Hoffman RM et al (2004) Five-year outcomes after prostatectomy or radiotherapy for prostate cancer: the prostate cancer outcomes study. J Natl Cancer Inst 96:1358–1367

Pouliot J, Morin O, Aubin M et al (2006) Megavoltage cone-beam CT: recent developments and clinical applications. Cancer Radiothér 10:258–268

Ritter MA, Chappell RJ, Tome WA et al (2005) A multi-institutional phase I/II trial of dose-per-fraction escalation for localized prostate cancer. Int J Radiat Oncol Biol Phys 63:S124

Roach M 3rd, DeSilvio M, Lawton C et al (2003) Phase III trial comparing whole-pelvic versus prostate-only radiotherapy versus adjuvant combined androgen suppression: radiation therapy oncology group 9413. J Clin Oncol 21:1904–1911

Roach M 3rd, Hanks G, Thames H Jr et al (2006) Defining biochemical failure following radiotherapy with or without hormonal therapy in men with clinically localized prostate cancer: recommendations of the RTOG-ASTRO Phoenix Consensus Conference. Int J Radiat Oncol Biol Phys 65:965–974

Shipley WU, Verhey LJ, Munzenrider JE et al (1995) Advanced prostate cancer - The results of a randomized comparative trial of high dose irradiation boosting with conformal protons compared with conventional dose irradiation using photons alone. Int J Radiat Oncol Biol Phys 32:3–12

Soete G, Van de Steene J, Verellen D et al (2002a) Initial clinical experience with infrared-reflecting skin markers in the positioning of patients treated by conformal radiotherapy for prostate cancer. Int J Radiat Oncol Biol Phys 52:694–698

Soete G, Verellen D, Michielsen D et al (2002b) Clinical use of stereoscopic X-ray positioning of patients treated with conformal radiotherapy for prostate cancer. Int J Radiat Oncol Biol Phys 54:948–952

Soete G, Arcangeli S, De Meerleer G et al (2006a) Phase II study of a four-week hypofractionated external beam radiotherapy regimen for prostate cancer: report on acute toxicity. Radiother Oncol 80:78–81

Soete G, Verellen D, Tournel K et al (2006b) Setup accuracy of stereoscopic X-ray positioning with automated correction for rotational errors in patients treated with conformal arc radiotherapy for prostate cancer. Radiother Oncol 80:371–373

Soete G, Verellen D, Michielsen D et al (2006c) Image-guided conformation arc therapy for prostate cancer: early side effects. Int J Radiat Oncol Biol Phys 66:S141–S144

Soete G, De Cock M, Verellen D et al (2007) X-ray assisted positioning of patients treated by conformal arc radiotherapy for prostate cancer: comparison of setup accuracy using implanted markers versus bony structures. Int J Radiat Oncol Biol Phys 67:823–827

Song WY, Schaly B, Bauman G et al (2006) Evaluation of image-guided radiation therapy (IGRT) technologies and their impact on the outcomes of hypofractionated prostate cancer treatments: a radiobiologic analysis. Int J Radiat Oncol Biol Phys 64:289–300

Talcott JA, Rieker P, Clark JA et al (1998) Patient-reported symptoms after primary therapy for early prostate cancer: results of a prospective cohort study. J Clin Oncol 16:275–283

Thames HD Jr, Withers HR, Peters LI et al (1982) Changes in early and late radiation responses with altered dose fractionation: implications for dose-survival relationships. Int J Radiat Oncol Biol Phys 8:219–226

Tsuji H, Yanagi T, Ishikawa H et al (2005) Hypofractionated radiotherapy with carbon ion beams for prostate cancer. Int J Radiat Oncol Biol Phys 63:1153–1160

van Herk M, Remeijer P, Rasch C et al (2000) The probability of correct target dosage: dose-population histograms for deriving treatment margins in radiotherapy. Int J Radiat Oncol Biol Phys 47:1121–1135

Verellen D, Linthout N, Soete G et al (2002) Considerations on treatment efficiency of different conformal radiation therapy techniques for prostate cancer. Radiother Oncol 63:27–36

Verellen D, Soete G, Linthout N et al (2003) Quality assurance of a system for improved target localization and patient setup that combines real-time infrared tracking and stereoscopic X-ray imaging. Radiother Oncol 67:129–141

van den Heuvel F, Powell T (2003) Independent verification of ultrasound based image-guided radiation treatment, using electronic portal imaging and implanted gold markers. Med Phys 30:2878–2887

Wallner KE, Merrick GS, Benson ML et al (2002) Penile bulb imaging. Int J Radiat Oncol Biol Phys 53:928–933

Wang JZ, Guerrero M, Li XA (2003) How low is the α/β ratio for prostate cancer? Int J Radiat Oncol Biol Phys 55:194–203

Wang L, Hricak H, Kattan MW et al (2006) Prediction of organ-confined prostate cancer: incremental value of MR imaging and MR spectroscopic imaging to staging nomograms. Radiology 238:597–603

Wernicke AG, Valicenti R, Dieva K et al (2004) Radiation dose delivered to the proximal penis as a predictor of the risk of erectile dysfunction after three-dimensional conformal radiotherapy for localized prostate cancer. Int J Radiat Oncol Biol Phys 60:1357–1363

Yeoh EE, Holloway RH, Fraser RJ et al (2006) Hypofractionated versus conventionally fractionated radiation therapy for prostate carcinoma: updated results of a phase III randomized trial. Int J Radiat Oncol Biol Phys 66:1072–1083

Zapatero A, Garcia-Vicente F, Modolell I et al (2004) Impact of mean rectal dose on late rectal bleeding after conformal radiotherapy for prostate cancer: dose-volume effect. Int J Radiat Oncol Biol Phys 59:1343–1351

Zelefsky MJ, Leibel SA, Gaudin PB et al (1998) Dose escalation with three-dimensional conformal radiation therapy affects the outcome in prostate cancer. Int J Radiat Oncol Biol Phys 41:491–500

Zietman AL, DeSilvio ML, Slater JD et al (2005) Comparison of conventional-dose vs high-dose conformal radiation therapy in clinically localized adenocarcinoma of the prostate: a randomized controlled trial. JAMA 294:1233–1239

Stereotactic Body Radiation Therapy (SBRT) for Tumors of the Liver

27

Percy Lee and Ronald W. Busuttil

27.1 Introduction

Surgical resection and liver transplantation are the standard of care for medically and technically operable hepatocellular carcinoma (HCC) as well as for oligometastatic disease from other primary cancers (i.e., colorectal, breast, lung, and other cancers) (Dawood et al. 2009). However, for patients who are not eligible for surgery, stereotactic body radiation therapy (SBRT) is emerging as an excellent alternative.

The liver is a common site for metastatic seeding from colorectal malignancies. This is because both the rectum and the colon drain through the portal vein (Dawood et al. 2009). For patients with metastatic disease confined to the liver, hepatic resection has been accepted as the standard of care for those who are able to undergo surgery (Rusthoven et al. 2009). There are data for long-term survivorship in well-selected patients using hepatic metastatectomy (Borasio et al. 2010). However, such patients are often not surgical candidates due to medical or technical reasons.

For HCC, surgical resection and liver transplantation are the most established treatment modalities associated with the best long-term outcomes (Lee et al. 2009). There are similar issues regarding medical and technical operability for HCC (Lee et al. 2009) compared to that for the treatment of oligometastatic disease to the liver. SBRT is emerging as a promising alternative for patients with unresectable primary HCC. For this disease, radiation dose escalation using standard fractionation was seen as possible and effective by a group in France (Mornex et al. 2005) who reported a phase II trial using conventionally fractionated external beam radiation therapy. They delivered a dose up to 66 Gy in 27 patients with HCC, 15 of who had received prior liver irradiation. Eighteen of the twenty-three evaluable patients had a complete response, and three patients achieved a partial response. One of the first groups of patients to receive SBRT for HCC was at the Karolinska Institute (Mornex et al. 2005) (nine patients with HCC, and two with other primary intrahepatic cancers). In these 11 patients, there were 20 tumors treated, with a dose ranging from 14 to 45 Gy in 1–3 fractions. Seventy percent of the patients had either a partial or complete response. Following this trend, the response to SBRT for primary HCC would likely be higher using higher total doses of radiation.

Recently, a group from Korea evaluated dose–volume parameters that were predictive of hepatic complications in patients with poor baseline liver function due to cirrhosis (Son et al. 2010). They concluded, in this patient population with primary HCC treated with SBRT, that keeping 800 mL of liver volume under 18 Gy was meaningful in reducing the risk of hepatic toxicity. Kavanagh et al. used a similar SBRT dosimetric constraint by requiring that 700 mL of the normal liver receive no more than a total of 15 Gy in a three-fraction regimen for liver SBRT. This critical volume-type restriction for the normal liver (Rusthoven et al. 2009) is comparable to liver surgeons requiring a certain predicted minimal volume of liver to remain in order to ensure that a patient has adequate and reasonable liver functional reserve after surgical resection.

From Indiana University, the results of a recent phase I feasibility study using SBRT for HCC have been reported (Cardenes et al. 2010). Patients with Child–Turcotte–Pugh's class A or B, who were not

P. Lee (✉) and R.W. Busuttil
Department of Radiation Oncology and Surgery,
David Geffen School of Medicine at UCLA, 200 UCLA
Medical Plaza, Suite B265, Los Angeles, CA 90095, USA
e-mail: percylee@mednet.ucla.edu

A.A.F. De Salles et al. (eds.), *Shaped Beam Radiosurgery*,
DOI: 10.1007/978-3-642-11151-8_27, © Springer-Verlag Berlin Heidelberg 2011

candidates for surgical resection, were eligible. Each patient enrolled and treated with SBRT on this study had one to three lesion(s), with the sum of all maximum individual tumor diameter less than or equal to 6 cm. Dose-limiting toxicity was defined as treatment-related Common Terminology Criteria for Adverse Events v3.0 grade 3 or higher toxicity. Seventeen patients with 25 lesions were treated on the protocol. SBRT dose was escalated from 36 Gy in 3 fractions (12 Gy per fraction) to 48 Gy in 3 fractions (16 Gy per fraction). Two patients with Child–Turcotte–Pugh's class B developed grade 3 hepatic toxicity at the 42 Gy in 3 fractions (16 Gy per fraction). Therefore, the protocol was amended for class B patients to receive a regimen of 5 fractions at 40 Gy (8 Gy per fraction). With a median follow-up of 2 years, the reported local control is 100%. Overall, the 1- and 2-year Kaplan–Meier estimates for overall survival are 75% and 60%, respectively. The researchers concluded that SBRT is a noninvasive, feasible, and well-tolerated therapy in adequately selected patients with HCC that are not eligible for surgery. Currently, a phase II trial is opened to accrual at this study center.

27.2 Oligometastatic Disease

Liver SBRT has also been used successfully for the treatment of oligometastatic disease to the liver from colorectal, lung, breast, and other primary cancers. At Heidelberg University, on a phase I/II dose escalation study where radiation dose was safely escalated from 14 to 26 Gy, 37 patients were treated with a single fraction SBRT for liver metastases (Herfarth et al. 2001). Median tumor volume was 10 mL, with a range from 1 to 132 mL. At 18 months, the actuarial tumor control rate for the entire cohort was 67%. In the USA, Schefter et al. recently reported a multicenter phase I/II dose escalation for liver SBRT for oligometastatic disease to the liver using a 3-fraction regimen (Rusthoven et al. 2009). Patients who had one to three discrete liver metastases, no prior radiation therapy to the liver, and no chemotherapy within the 2 weeks prior to SBRT were eligible. In addition, the sum of all maximum individual tumor diameters of the lesions treated was required to be less than 6 cm in aggregate. Radiation dose was escalated in a 3+3 design, with the first cohort receiving 36 Gy in 3 fractions. SBRT dose was safely escalated from a total dose of 36–60 Gy in 3 fractions. The total dose of 60 Gy in 3 fractions was predetermined at the onset of the protocol to be the maximum dose even if the maximum tolerated dose (MTD) was not reached. Dose-limiting toxicity was defined as any grade 3 liver, gastrointestinal, spinal cord toxicity, or any grade 4 toxicity related to SBRT. Therefore, since the MTD was not reached, the determined phase II total dose was 60 Gy, and the primary endpoint for the study was local control. At the time of the report, 63 tumors in 47 patients were treated. Median follow-up time was 16 months. There was local progression in only three lesions out of all the assessable lesions (assessable lesions were defined as lesions with at least 6 months of radiographic follow-up). The 1- and 2-year in-field local control rates were 95% and 92%, respectively. Among lesions with a maximal diameter of 3 cm or less, the 2-year local control rate was 100%. Median survival for the entire cohort was 20.5 months.

27.3 Technology and Workflow

Similar to SBRT for pancreatic tumors, at our institution, we utilize an advanced radiosurgical linear accelerator with image-guidance capabilities, Novalis TX™ (Brainlab AG, Feldkirchen, Germany; Varian Medical Systems, Palo Alto, CA) to deliver body radiosurgery for liver tumors. Essentially, most of the concepts relating to SBRT treatment planning for pancreas tumors apply to SBRT for liver tumors. Accurate and reproducible patient setup at the time of treatment simulation and treatment delivery is critical. At the time of treatment simulation, a concurrent PET-CT may be used to integrate biological treatment planning (i.e., for colorectal, lung, or breast metastases) in order to optimally target these liver tumor(s), and to assist in defining the gross tumor volume(s) (GTV). For HCC, a PET-CT simulation is of less utility due to the low FDG uptake for HCC in relationship to the uptake by the surrounding normal liver. With HCC, a specialized MRI of the abdomen with gadolinium or gadoxetate disodium is more useful to assist in defining the GTV. In addition, characterization of tumor and organ motion with a retrospectively correlated 4-dimensional CT scan at the time of CT simulation is important in order to assess the degree of tumor and organ motion for a particular patient. This study also helps to determine the best treatment strategy in order to optimize delivery of the radiation dose to the tumor while maximally sparing the normal tissue. The optimal way to accomplish the above is often utilizing either an intensity-modulated radiation therapy (IMRT) or volumetric modulated arc therapy (VMAT) treatment delivery strategy. The exact strategy is determined at the time of dosimetric plan optimization and using dose–volume histograms (DVHs) as a tool for plan evaluation.

At the time of SBRT delivery, various sophisticated image-guided radiation therapy (IGRT) options are employed to verify tumor and normal tissue location with respect to each other prior to and during treatment delivery. Novalis TX combines a conventional high-energy linear accelerator with a kV imager, cone beam CT, and the ability to delivery treatments with respiratory gating. Utilizing this type of multimodality IGRT customized to the individual patient, liver SBRT is delivered with extremely high accuracy and precision. These innovations allow us to eliminate uncertainties in tumor location, and we are able to use the Novalis TX to correct for real-time changes in tumor motion or patient motion using its 6-degree robotic treatment couch.

27.4 Conclusion

Surgical resection and liver transplantation are still the best options for patients with operable HCC or oligometastatic disease to the liver from other primary cancers. As far as a noninvasive approach, however, SBRT has been shown by recent publications to be a promising treatment for well-localized tumors in the liver. Up to three lesions may be treated in one sitting, delivering high doses of radiation in a few fractions with very little morbidity. Aggregate tumor diameter (sum of all maximum individual tumor diameters) of 6 cm or less appears to be a good way to select rationale target(s) for liver SBRT. In closing, an illustrative case study discussing the use of SBRT for a single metastatic lesion to the liver will be presented below.

27.5 Case Study

27.5.1 Patient

This is a 59-year-old woman, nonsmoker, with a distant history of bilateral breast cancer, who developed a right upper lobe stage I lung cancer 5 years prior to being seen in radiation oncology at our institution. She underwent an upper lobectomy of the right lung at that time for a 2-cm tumor, and pathology revealed an infiltrating adenocarcinoma, mixed with bronchoalveolar features, TTF1-positive, consistent with a lung primary. No adjuvant therapy was recommended. Routine image-based surveillance was performed for the next 4 years, and she was without evidence of disease. Six months prior to our consultation, a PET-CT scan was performed, which revealed a 6 × 5 × 5 cm intensely FDG-avid mass seen in the right medial lobe of the liver. A biopsy was performed, which revealed adenocarcinoma. Immunohistochemical staining was strongly positive for KI-67, TTF1, but not for keratin 20 or BRST-2. The tumor was also ER, PR, and Her-2/neu negative, consistent with an oligometastatic recurrence from her lung cancer. The patient then received 6 months of multi-agent chemotherapy (5 cycles). She was unable to complete a sixth cycle due to hematological toxicities. Two months prior to our consultation, a re-staging PET-CT scan was performed (after completion of her fifth cycle of chemotherapy). This revealed no evidence of further metastatic progression. However, the right liver mass now measured 7.5 × 6 × 5 cm, with a maximum SUV of 11.2. The patient was seen by an expert oncological liver surgeon at our institution, and the patient was deemed not a suitable candidate for liver resection. Therefore, she was referred to us for consideration for potential radiation therapy treatment.

27.5.2 Treatment

Stereotactic body radiation therapy for this oligometastatic lesion to the liver was recommended. The patient did not have further metastatic progression during her 6-months course of chemotherapy. However, radiographically, systemic therapy was not effective in order to control her liver-confined disease. A PET-CT, 4-dimensional CT simulation was performed for her liver SBRT. A dose of 60 Gy in 5 fractions (12 Gy per fraction) was delivered to the FDG-avid right liver tumor measuring 7.5 × 6 × 5 cm (superior–inferior, lateral, anterior–posterior dimension, respectively). More than 700 mL of normal liver received less than a total dose of 15 Gy (3 Gy per fraction) (Fig. 27.1). The patient experienced only grade 1 fatigue during treatment and did not experience nausea, abdominal pain, or diarrhea. She reports being able to resume her normal activity, including playing tennis, the day following her liver SBRT.

27.5.3 Results

One month following her liver SBRT, the patient was seen in follow-up, and was doing well clinically with a stable weight, and resolution of her mild fatigue. Two months post-SBRT, the patient received a repeat PET-CT scan in our clinic in order to assess for an early response to therapy (Fig. 27.1). This PET-CT scan revealed a near-complete metabolic response to her radiation therapy (Fig. 27.1). Six months post-SBRT, the repeat PET-CT scan revealed a complete metabolic response to therapy. To date, she continues to do well clinically and is without acute SBRT-related complications.

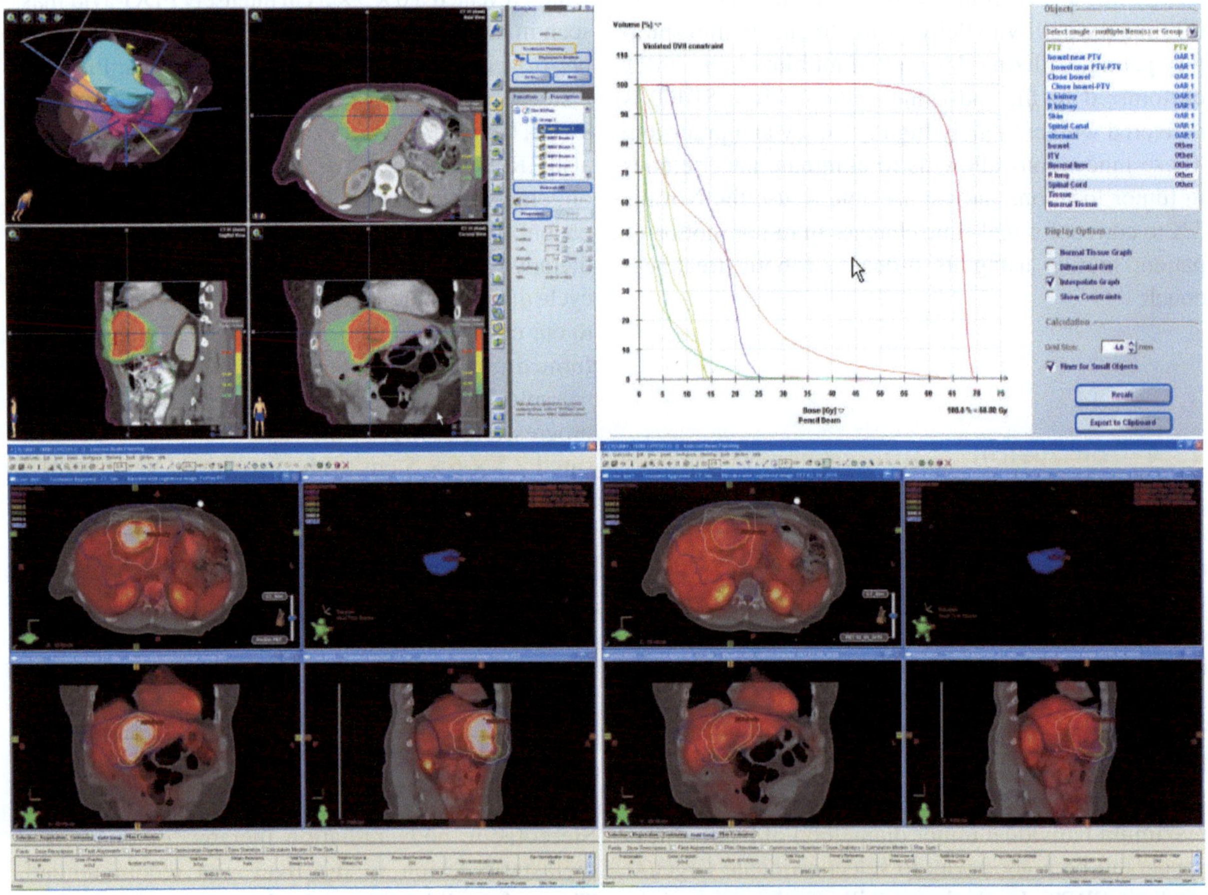

Fig. 27.1 Liver SBRT: 60 Gy delivered in 5 fractions. (*Top left*) SBRT treatment plan in dose color wash, showing total dose delivered. (*Top right*) Dose–volume histogram for the planning target volume (PTV), as well as the critical normal organs that require sparing. (*Bottom left*) Pretreatment planning PET-CT scan demonstrating the FDG-avid mass with overlay of the isodose lines. (*Bottom right*) Posttreatment PET-CT scan obtained 2 months post-SBRT demonstrating a near-complete metabolic response

References

Borasio P, Gisabella M, Billé A et al (2010) Role of surgical resection in colorectal lung metastases: analysis of 137 patients. Int J Colorectal Dis 26(2):183–190

Cardenes HR, Price TR, Perkins SM et al (2010) Phase I feasibility trial of stereotactic body radiation therapy for primary hepatocellular carcinoma. Clin Transl Oncol 12:218–225

Dawood O, Mahadevan A, Goodman KA (2009) Stereotactic body radiation therapy for liver metastases. Eur J Cancer 45:2947–2959

Herfarth KK, Debus J, Lohr F et al (2001) Stereotactic single-dose radiation therapy of liver tumors: results of a phase I/II trial. J Clin Oncol 19:164–170

Lee P, Kee S, Busuttil R (2009) Is downstaging prior to liver transplantation important in hepatocellular carcinoma? Am J Transplant 9:1703–1704

Mornex F, Girard N, Merle P et al (2005) Tolerance and efficacy of conformal radiotherapy for hepatocellular carcinoma in cirrhotic patients. Results of the French RTF1 phase II trial. Cancer Radiothér 9:470–476

Rusthoven KE, Kavanagh BD, Cardenes H et al (2009) Multi-institutional phase I/II trial of stereotactic body radiation therapy for liver metastases. J Clin Oncol 27:1572–1578

Son SH, Choi BO, Ryu MR et al (2010) Stereotactic body radiotherapy for patients with unresectable primary hepatocellular carcinoma: dose-volumetric parameters predicting the hepatic complication. Int J Radiat Oncol Biol Phys 78(4): 1073–1080

The Future of Radiosurgery and Radiotherapy

28

Antonio A.F. De Salles, Mark Sedrak, and Jean Jacques Lemaire

28.1 Introduction

Early diagnosis and disease prevention, thorough visualization and understanding of disease and societal affordability, are the focus of medicine in the years to come. The goals in treatments are precision, accuracy, non-invasive techniques, efficacy of treatment and no side effects. Radiosurgery's impact on the field of radiotherapy has imposed these goals over the last 60 years. The ingredients for the evolution of medicine hinges on our increasing ability to non-invasively see the intricacies of the human body, initially only bones, then soft-tissues, inside of organs, and now at the cellular and molecular level. Are we ready in the life science field for what society asks of us, to decrease suffering and enhance human life? There has been much progress in the last several decades in the technology and applicability of radiation and its uses in medicine. Since the first description of radiosurgery by Lars Leksell, the field has blossomed to include the treatment of tumors, vascular lesions, and various functional disorders (Leksell 1951). There is no doubt that the application of this technology has impacted the field of medicine and neurosurgery more than any other single modality. However, until now radiation has largely been used as an ablative technique, and its ability to modify cellular function at the genetic level continues in early stages of development.

Improvements in accuracy, targeting and comfort for each patient have tremendously advanced the field by improving patient outcome and satisfaction. Nevertheless, there are limitations to radiation treatments, and incorporation of nanotechnologies and adjuvant modalities such as Focused Ultrasound Surgery might play a key role.

28.2 Conformal Beam Shaping

We have seen remarkable advancements in beam conformity, dose analysis and delivery in the last several decades. Although metallic blocking helmets were initially used to direct radiation beams into the indicated region, the idea of focused beam radiation came many years later. The advantage of focused beam radiation is that each beam in isolation carries a low dose of radiation, but when many of these overlap in one focused region, the radiation in that region can be much higher carrying a therapeutic effect. The rigidity offered by the Leksell G or BRW Frames (Brown-Roberts-Wells) made stereotactic delivery of radiation readily feasible. Computer based systems have clearly added yet another element to identification and analysis of dose delivery prior to the treatment. Furthermore, many in the field have now seen the progression from frame-based systems to those that are frameless.

Certainly computerized and robotic processes brought the versatility of these systems and easily display computations for analysis by medical personnel, even before the treatment is performed. This exponentially expanding medical and technological age seems boundless in the years to come. In more recent years, frameless treatments came in use. This frameless technology has expedited patient care and improved

A.A.F. De Salles (✉), M. Sedrak, and J.J. Lemaire
Department of Neurosurgery and Radiation Oncology, David Geffen School of Medicine at UCLA, 10495 Le Conte Avenue, Suite 2120, Los Angeles, CA 90095, USA
e-mail: adesalles@mednet.ucla.edu

A.A.F. De Salles et al. (eds.), *Shaped Beam Radiosurgery*,
DOI: 10.1007/978-3-642-11151-8_28, © Springer-Verlag Berlin Heidelberg 2011

comfort, yet maintained critical accuracy needed for this technology (Agazaryan et al. 2008).

Advancements in multi-leaf collimation and intensity modulation have allowed further refining to conforming radiation. This rapidly adapting technology allows increased ability to tailor dosing to tumor shape and size. This improvement has reduced irradiation to unaffected tissue while allowing for increased doses to affected tissues (Kubo et al. 1999).

28.3 Targeting and Imaging Integration

Conformal beam radiation has clearly improved the physics of dose delivery to each treatment plan. Fundamental imaging techniques, CT or MRI, display tomographic images that are static in one point in time. It is from these images that information is extrapolated for treatments. Targeting is fundamentally more complicated than this because of motion, progression of disease, and inadequacy of target identification.

Integration of real-time imaging would correct for these real-life changes that occur during treatments. Respiration tracking and robotic motion compensation have been used to correct for gross movements during radiation delivery (Schweikard et al. 2000; Schweikard et al. 2004). This 4-D imaging, adding the element of time, has improved even further the delivery of radiation to the affected region. The most idealistic form of this would be integration of live MRI or CT during treatment.

Improvements in both anatomic detail and physiological and molecular information will be the next key steps to integrate into this technology and improve targeting. PET imaging is already routinely combined with CT and MRI for the treatment of many cancers (Grosu et al. 2003). However, we still see complete prostate irradiation, rather than direct targeting of only the prostate cancer, which is feasible from a beam shaping perspective.

Diffusion Tensor Imaging (DTI) is an MRI modality taking into account diffusion of water (Mori and Van Zijl 2002). DTI infers axon bundle orientation in white or grey matter. Much excitement has been seen using DTI for tumor analysis and surgical navigation (Lin et al. 2010). DTI may be integrated into radiosurgery planning and help improve treatments while lowering complications and side effects (Foroni et al. 2010). Functional MRI (fMRI) has been routinely combined with DTI imaging for neurosurgical practice in many tertiary centers. fMRI can help to identify areas of activation during certain tasks, such as speech and motor. This integration has yet to be exploited for radiosurgical planning (Fig. 28.1).

28.4 Nanotechnology

Nanotechnology also likely will have a major impact in the field of medicine this century. Potential uses for nanotechnology include manufacturing on a molecular level. This can be used for diagnostic and screening purposes, artificial receptors, DNA sequencing using nanopores, drug delivery, gene delivery, and tissue engineering (Emerich and Thanos 2003). It will likely have an impact on radiosurgery as well, both in terms of targeting and radiation efficacy.

Because nanotechnology can be used as a molecular marker for identification of tumors (Böckmann et al. 2001), this can make targeting of the tumor margins much more successful than currently available techniques. There is much excitement with the possibility of radio-sensitization of tumors or to radiation-guided delivery systems (Hoh et al. 2007; Stacy et al. 2004). These particles adhering to molecular changes on tumor cells can then be packaged with drug delivery systems when a certain threshold of radiation is delivered, for example. It may also serve to protect uninvolved tissue, or even for gene-guided therapies. This technology will add yet another powerful tool that will likely be used adjunctive to other modalities with seemingly endless possibilities.

28.5 Limitations of Photon and Proton Beam Radiation

Limitations to radiosurgery include tissue specific limitations. Indeed, optic apparatus, hypothalamic-pituitary axis, cochlea, brainstem, spinal cord, watershed regions of the brain, bowel, urinary pathway, major arteries in the lung and abdomen and biliary tract are just a few examples where dose limitations may alter the treatment strategy. In addition, there are

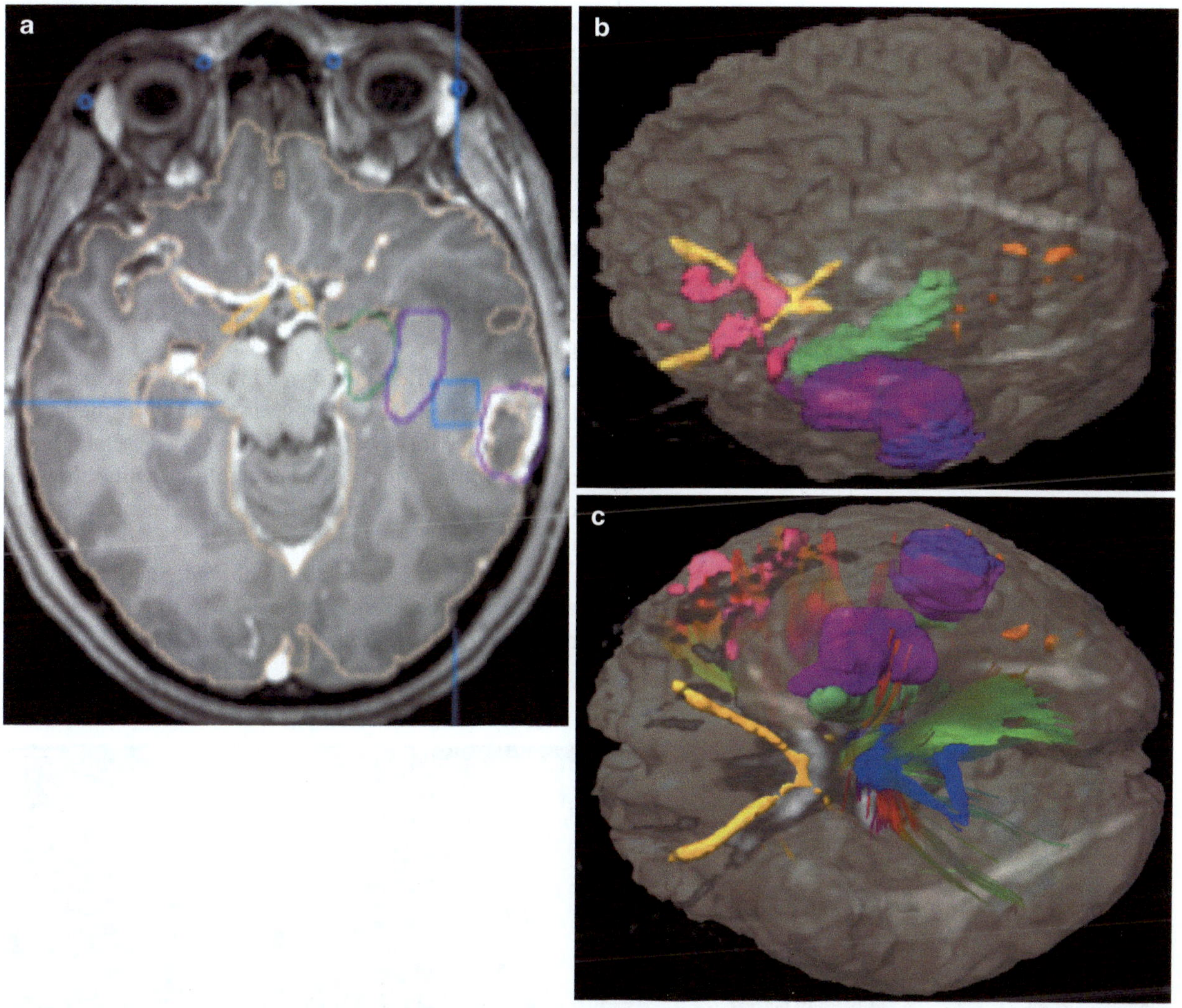

Fig. 28.1 Combination MR Imaging. (**a**) MRI with contrast demonstrated tumors outlined in purple. DTI imaging without anisotropy identified between tumor masses indicating possible tumor infiltrate or edema. Hippocampus outlined in green (**b**). Overall convexity appearance with superimposed fMRI. Orange indicated speech reception activation and pink with speech expression activation. (**c**) DTI demonstrating surrounding pathways

also limitations to re-dosing because of the risk of radiation toxicity and necrosis. Although fractionated therapies have improved dose delivery while preserving these tissues, there are still limitations and this approach has failed to cure substantial types of cancers.

Adjuvant forms of stereotactic treatments will play an important role in the future because of these inherent radiation limitations. Combination therapies using both photon beam and proton beam radiation in treatments may be one method of overcoming some of these limitations. Proton beam radiation takes advantage of Bragg peaks creating a sharp fall off of radiation beyond the lesion of interest. The technology carries much hope but has largely been limited by cost, allowing photon beam technologies to progress more rapidly. However, combination modalities is feasible and one can apply higher than standard doses of radiation safely (Bonnet et al. 2001; Park et al. 2006).

28.6 Focused Ultrasound Surgery

Focused Ultrasound Surgery (FUS) is an emerging field that does not use radiation and theoretically may be used adjunctively with radiosurgery (Jolesz and

Hynynen 2002). FUS is used in conjunction with magnetic resonance imaging (MRI) creating a powerful union to correctly localize tumors, optimally target acoustic energy, monitor deposition of energy in real time, and accurately control the thermal dose to the entire volume (Dong et al. 2004). It has already been in use for the treatment of various abdominal diseases and the application in neurological diseases is being tried (Hynynen et al. 2001; McDannold et al. 2010; Roberts 2005).

FUS already has theoretical applications for the treatment of brain tumors, stroke, and various functional disorders of the brain including epilepsy, pain and movement disorders to name a few. FUS can function in the form of both ablation and neuromodulation. Indeed, the growth of this technology is already occurring around the world and likely will impact in the indications of stereotactic radiation, either as a competitor for certain pathologies or as an adjuvant for others.

28.7 Conclusions

A combination of these modalities will likely paint the future. We are quite excited and optimistic about the times to come as these treatments represent a hope for the future. Numerous advancements in medicine have been guided by our understanding of anatomy, molecular biology, genetics and pharmacology. Radiation therapies have only augmented the field of medicine especially for its oncological applications. The convergence of many fields of science allow for advanced collaborative efforts to form a more definitive perspective on disease and improve treatments in medicine. A key for the future will be this continued collaboration across multiple fields, well exemplified with the work of physicists, radiation oncologists, and neurosurgeons in the field of radiosurgery.

Radiosurgery has no doubt affected surgeons and oncologist tremendously over the last several decades. The paradigm for treatment of some tumors

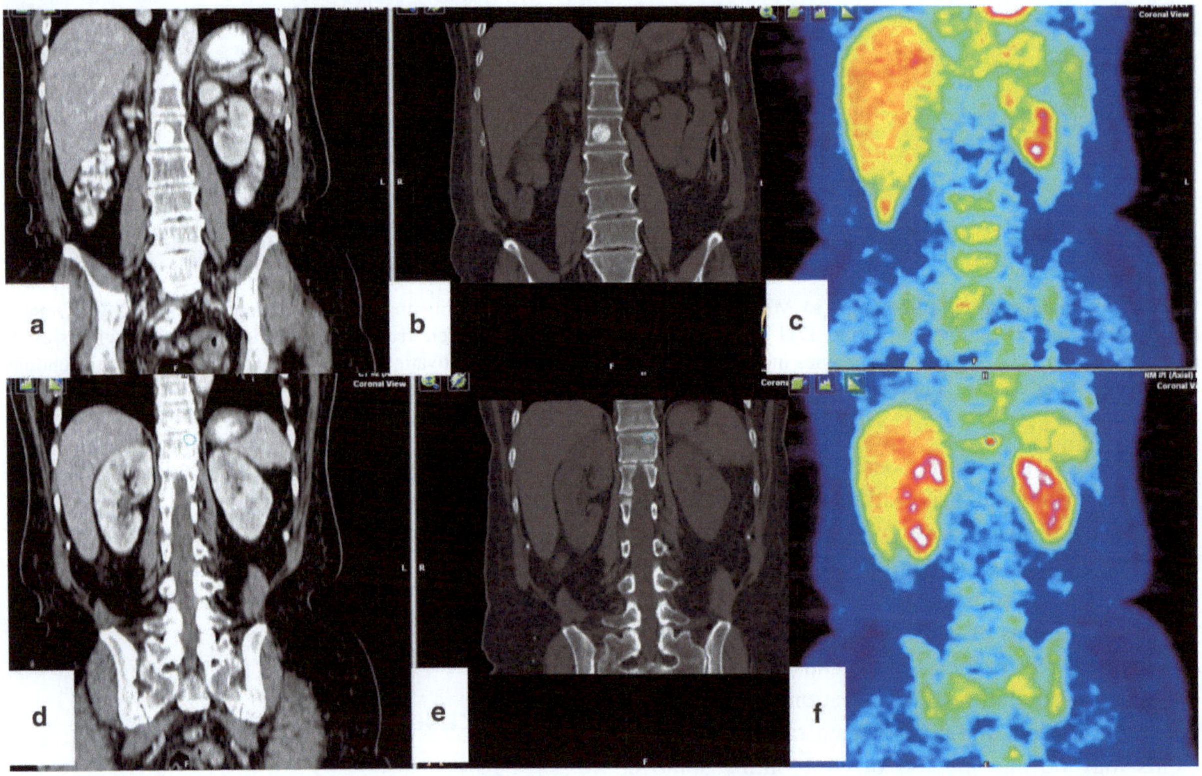

Fig. 28.2 Metastatic lesion of L2 treated with radiosurgery. Notice the lesion still seen on CT (**a**) and (**b**) but no longer seen on PET (**c**). Notice a new lesions previously not seen in the T12 vertebrae (**d**), but now seen with difficulty on CT (**e**) and well visualized on PET (**f**)

has changed from surgery followed by chemotherapy and radiation to chemotherapy and radiation followed by surgery. We have seen this in the treatment of sarcomas and colorectal cancer. Although some tumors are curable by surgery, some diseases are beyond surgical skill and surgery can even blur the margins of tumors and even seed other types of cancer. The paradigm may continue to switch, preparing tumors for surgery with irradiation. This may provide the toxic dose necessary to kill many tumor cells that are present on initial imaging, reducing the difficulty in identification after surgery. Many have even used radiation to "biopsy" tumors and deduce the likely pathologic diagnosis based on the responsiveness, an example is germinoma (Packer et al. 2000) (Fig. 28.2).

Indeed, we see the field of radiosurgery being used as front line for many cancers. Focused ultrasound surgery will likely be a competitor or partner in this fight. Nanotechnology will augment all these treatments and create a different age in medicine. Surgery will likely be reserved as an adjuvant therapy and used only when necessary for mass effect.

References

Agazaryan N, Tenn S, Desalles A, Selch M (2008) Image-guided radiosurgery for spinal tumors. Phys Med Biol 53:1715–1727

Böckmann B, Grill H, Giesing M (2001) Molecular characterization of minimal residual cancer cells in patients with solid tumors. Biomol Eng 17:95–111

Bonnet R, Bush D, Cheek G, Slater J, Panossian D, Franke C, Slater J (2001) Effects of proton and combined proton/photon beam radiation on pulmonary function in patients with resectable but medically inoperable non-small cell lung cancer. Chest 120:1803

Cohen M, Melnik K, Boiarski A, Ferrari M, Martin F (2003) Microfabrication of silicon-based nanoporous particulates for medical applications. Biomed Microdevices 5:253–259

Dong M, Wan BK, Zhang LX, Yong H (2004) Theoretical modeling study of the necrotic field during high-intensity focused ultrasound surgery. Med Sci Monit 10(2):MT19-23

Emerich D, Thanos C (2003) Nanotechnology and medicine. Expert Opin Biol Ther 3:655–663

Foroni R, Ricciardi G, Lupidi F, Sboarina A, De Simone A, Longhi M, Nicolato A, Pizzini F, Beltramello A, Gerosa M (2010) Diffusion-tensor imaging tractography of the corticospinal tract for evaluation of motor fiber tract radiation exposure in Gamma Knife® Radiosurgery treatment planning. Radiosurgery 7:128–138

Grosu A, Lachner R, Wiedenmann N, Stärk S, Thamm R, Kneschaurek P, Schwaiger M, Molls M, Weber W (2003) Validation of a method for automatic image fusion (BrainLAB System) of CT data and 11 C-methionine-PET data for stereotactic radiotherapy using a LINAC: first clinical experience. Int J Radiat Oncol Biol Phys 56:1450–1463

Hoh D, Liu C, Chen J, Pagnini P, Yu C, Wang M, Apuzzo M (2007) Chained lightning: Part III-emerging technology, novel therapeutic strategies, and new energy modalities for radiosurgery. Neurosurgery 61:1111

Hynynen K, Pomeroy O, Smith D, Huber P, McDannold N, Kettenbach J, Baum J, Singer S, Jolesz F (2001) MR imaging-guided focused ultrasound surgery of fibroadenomas in the breast: a feasibility study. Radiology 219:176

Jolesz F, Hynynen K (2002) Magnetic resonance image-guided focused ultrasound surgery. Cancer J 8:100–112

Kubo H, Wilder R, Pappas C (1999) Impact of collimator leaf width on stereotactic radiosurgery and 3D conformal radiotherapy treatment plans. Int J Radiat Oncol Biol Phys 44:937–945

Leksell L (1951) The stereotaxic method and radiosurgery of the brain. Acta Chir Scand 102:316

Lin YC, Wang CC, Wai YY, Wan YL, Ng SH, Chen YL, Liu HL, Wang JJ (2010) Significant temporal evolution of diffusion anisotropy for evaluating early response to radiosurgery in patients with vestibular schwannoma: findings from functional diffusion maps. Am J Neuroradiol 31(2):269–274

McDannold N, Clement GT, Black P, Jolesz F, Hynynen K (2010) Transcranial MRI-guided focused ultrasound surgery of brain tumors: initial findings in three patients. Neurosurgery 66(2):323–332

Mori S, Van Zijl P (2002) Fiber tracking: principles and strategies – a technical review. NMR Biomed 15:468–480

Packer R, Cohen B, Cooney K (2000) Intracranial germ cell tumors. Oncologist 5:312

Park L, DeLaney T, Liebsch N, Hornicek F, Goldberg S, Mankin H, Rosenberg A, Rosenthal D, Suit H (2006) Sacral chordomas: impact of high-dose proton/photon-beam radiation therapy combined with or without surgery for primary versus recurrent tumor. Int J Radiat Oncol Biol Phys 65: 1514–1521

Roberts W (2005) Focused ultrasound ablation of renal and prostate cancer: current technology and future directions. Urol Oncol 23:367–371, Elsevier

Schweikard A, Glosser G, Bodduluri M, Murphy M, Adler J (2000) Robotic motion compensation for respiratory movement during radiosurgery. Comput Aided Surg 5:263–277

Schweikard A, Shiomi H, Adler J (2004) Respiration tracking in radiosurgery. Med Phys 31:2738

Stacy D, Lu B, Hallahan D (2004) Radiation-guided drug delivery systems. Expert Rev Anticancer Ther 4:283–288

Index

A.A.F. De Salles et al. (eds.), *Shaped Beam Radiosurgery*,
DOI: 10.1007/978-3-642-11151-8, © Springer-Verlag Berlin Heidelberg 2011

MIX
Papier aus verantwortungsvollen Quellen
Paper from responsible sources
FSC® C105338
FSC
www.fsc.org

If you have any concerns about our products,
you can contact us on
ProductSafety@springernature.com

In case Publisher is established outside the EU,
the EU authorized representative is:
Springer Nature Customer Service Center GmbH
Europaplatz 3, 69115 Heidelberg, Germany

Printed by Libri Plureos GmbH
in Hamburg, Germany